Defining the Beginning and End of Life

Defining the Beginning and End of Life

Readings on Personal Identity and Bioethics

Edited by John P. Lizza

Professor, Department of Philosophy
Kutztown University of Pennsylvania
Kutztown, Pennsylvania

The Johns Hopkins University Press
Baltimore

In memory of Charles and Marie Lizza, whose love made me the person I am today

© 2009 The Johns Hopkins University Press
All rights reserved. Published 2009
Printed in the United States of America on acid-free paper
9 8 7 6 5 4 3 2 1

The Johns Hopkins University Press
2715 North Charles Street
Baltimore, Maryland 21218-4363
www.press.jhu.edu

ISBN 13: 978-0-8018-9336-0 (hardcover: alk. paper)
ISBN 10: 0-8018-9336-4 (hardcover: alk. paper)
ISBN 13: 978-0-8018-9337-7 (pbk.: alk. paper)
ISBN 10: 0-8018-9337-2 (pbk.: alk. paper)

Library of Congress Control Number: 2009920414

A catalog record for this book is available from the British Library.

Special discounts are available for bulk purchases of this book. For more information, please contact Special Sales at 410-516-6936 or specialsales@press.jhu.edu.

The Johns Hopkins University Press uses environmentally friendly book materials, including recycled text paper that is composed of at least 30 percent post-consumer waste, whenever possible. All of our book papers are acid-free, and our jackets and covers are printed on paper with recycled content.

Contents

Preface

The idea for this anthology was prompted by a telephone call from my cousin, Dr. Paul Manganiello, Director of Reproductive Endocrinology and Infertility at the Dartmouth-Hitchcock Medical Center, who was asked to testify before the State of New Hampshire's House Judiciary Committee in 2006. This legislative body was addressing a bill that would establish the definition of when human life begins. The legislature assumed that Manganiello, as a specialist in embryology, had some expertise in the matter of when a person's life begins or at least could provide them with a biological understanding of human embryology that would be helpful in their consideration of whether to accord the legal status of personhood to human embryos. My cousin was well aware that philosophers and theologians differ in their views on the nature of persons and the beginning and end of life. He had telephoned me with a request that I quickly provide him with a list of philosophical and theological references that he could use in his testimony to show this diversity of opinion.

As I scrambled to meet his request, I realized that there was no anthology that systematically represented various theoretical perspectives on persons and how those perspectives have figured in bioethical debates over the beginning and end of life. While there were anthologies that gave attention to the concept of personhood in the bioethical debate over abortion and stem cell research and other anthologies devoted to the theoretical treatment of personal identity, there was no anthology that did both and no anthology that specifically tracked how alternative views of the nature of persons have influenced the debate over the definition of death. Thus, I came to think that such an anthology might be useful, not only for government bodies considering issues of personhood, but also for undergraduate and graduate education. Indeed, the book should be useful to anyone interested in the definition and criteria of human life and death, including the general public, bioethicists, philosophers, health care professionals, attorneys engaged in medical or health-related issues, hospital ethics committees, and governmental committees or bodies who advise on policy and law concerning issues at the beginning and end of life. The book would be particularly appropriate for adoption in courses in bioethics, death and dying, metaphysics, persons, and ethics, at both the undergraduate and the graduate level, and in a variety of programs: bioethics, philosophy, religion, law, nursing, and medicine. In light of increased public awareness of these issues brought about by cases such as that of Terry Schiavo and *Roe v. Wade,* this anthology should be a timely addition to the literature and will help to meet important educational and societal needs. The bill that would have legally defined the beginning of life was defeated in the New Hampshire legislature.

Those familiar with this body of literature will notice that this volume does not include some of the important work that has addressed the issue of whether a human embryo, fetus, or individual in a permanent vegetative state deserves respect or has a right to life, independent of whether it is a person. The more narrow focus of this anthology is on theoretical and metaphysical considerations of persons and how those considerations affect the evaluation of practical cases. The anthology also does not represent to any great extent theoretical accounts of potentiality and their ethical relevance to the issue of when life begins and ends. While I believe that considerations of potentiality are highly relevant and complicate the bioethical discussion more at the beginning of life than at the end, there was simply not enough space in a single volume to do justice to the rich discussion of potentiality. I intend to compile a separate anthology that does exactly this.

I would like to thank the staff at The Hastings Center, especially Dan Callahan and Tom Murray, for their encouragement and suggestions in compiling this anthology. As an adjunct associate of The Hastings Center, I have benefited greatly from time at the center. I would also like to thank the Pennsylvania State

System of Higher Education for a summer research grant to work on this project. Aaron Mackler, Jason Eberl, and David Jones graciously agreed to contribute original articles for this collection, although they draw on some of their previously published work. I especially appreciated how quickly and professionally they were able to provide me with their contributions. I would also like to thank Laurel Delaney, secretary in the Department of Philosophy at Kutztown University, for her invaluable assistance in securing copyright permissions, organizing materials, and proofreading.

I am grateful to the authors or publishers for permission to reprint the following material from previously published works:

Chapter 1: Plato, Selections from *Phaedo*, trans. Benjamin Jowett, Project Gutenberg Etext prepared by Sue Asscher.

Chapter 2: René Descartes, *Meditations on First Philosophy,* 3rd edition, trans. Donald A. Cress, Hackett Publishing Company (1993): 17–24 and 49–58. Reprinted with permission of Hackett Publishing Company, Inc.

Chapter 3: Richard Swinburne, "Personal Identity: The Dualist Theory," in Sydney Shoemaker and Richard Swinburne, *Personal Identity*, Blackwell Publishing (1984): 22–34.

Chapter 4: St. Thomas Aquinas, Selections from *Summa Theologiae*, Section Ia, Question 29, Article 1 and Section Ia, Question 118, Article 2, trans. Fathers of the English Dominican Province, Benzinger Bros. edition (1947). Reprinted with the permission of Christian Classics Ethereal Library.

Chapter 5: Gilbert Meilaender, "*Terra es animata*: On Having a Life," *Hastings Center Report* 23:4 (1993): 25–32. Reprinted with the permission of Gilbert Meilaender and The Hastings Center Report.

Chapter 6: Eric T. Olson, "An Argument for Animalism," in Raymond Martin and John Barresi, eds., *Personal Identity*, Blackwell Publishing (2003): 318–334.

Chapter 7: John Locke, *An Essay Concerning Human Understanding*, Volume 1, Project Gutenburg Etext prepared by Steve Harris and David Widger.

Chapter 8: Derek Parfit, "The Unimportance of Identity," in Raymond Martin and John Barresi, eds., *Personal Identity*, Blackwell Publishing (2003): 292–317.

Chapter 9: P. F. Strawson, "Persons," in H. Feigel, M. Scriven, and G. Maxwell, eds., *Concepts, Theories and the Mind-Body Problem*, Minnesota

Studies in the Philosophy of Science, Vol. II, University of Minnesota Press (1957): 330–353.

Chapter 10: E. J. Lowe, "Real Selves: Persons as a Substantial Kind," in David Cockburn, ed., *Human Beings*, Cambridge University Press (1991): 87–107. Copyright 1991 by The Royal Institute of Philosophy. Reprinted with the permission of Cambridge University Press.

Chapter 11: Lynne Rudder Baker, "The Ontological Status of Persons," *Philosophy and Phenomenological Research* 65:2 (2002): 370–388. Copyright 2002 by International Phenomenological Society. Reprinted with the permission of Blackwell Publishing.

Chapter 12: G. H. Mead, *Mind, Self, and Society from the Standpoint of a Social Behaviorist*, University of Chicago Press (1934). Copyright 1934 by The University of Chicago.

Chapter 13: Clifford Geertz, "The Impact of the Concept of Culture on the Concept of Man," in John R. Platt, ed., *New Views on the Nature of Man*, University of Chicago Press (1965): 93–118.

Chapter 14: Rom Harré, *Personal Being*, Blackwell Publishing (1984): 209–216.

Chapter 15: Tom Kitwood, *Dementia Reconsidered: The Person Comes First*, Open University Press/McGraw-Hill Education (1997): 8–12, 14–19. Copyright 1997 by Tom Kitwood. Reprinted with the kind permission of Open University Press Publishing Company.

Chapter 16: Harry G. Frankfurt, "Freedom of the Will and the Concept of a Person," *Journal of Philosophy* 68:1 (1971): 5–20. Reprinted with the permission of Harry Frankfurt and Journal of Philosophy.

Chapter 18: Germain Grisez, "When Do People Begin?" *Proceedings of the American Catholic Philosophical Association* 63 (1989): 27–47. Reprinted with the permission of The Philosophy Documentation Center.

Chapter 20: Helga Kuhse and Peter Singer, "Individuals, Humans, and Persons: The Issue of Moral Status," in Peter Singer, Helga Kuhse, Stephen Buckle, Karen Dawson, and Pascal Kasimba, eds., *Embryo Experimentation*, Cambridge University Press (1990): 65–75. Reprinted with the permission of Cambridge University Press.

Chapter 21: Mary Anne Warren, "On the Moral and Legal Status of Abortion," *The Monist* 57:1 (1973): 43–61. Copyright 1973 *The Monist: An International Quarterly Journal of General Philosophical Inquiry*, Peru, Illinois 61354. Reprinted by permission.

Chapter 22: Nicola Poplawski and Grant Gillett, "Ethics and Embryos," *Journal of Medical Ethics* 17 (1991): 62–69. Reprinted with the permission of BMJ Publishing Group.

Chapter 23: Lynne Rudder Baker, "When Does a Person Begin?" *Social Philosophy and Policy* 22:2 (2005): 25–48. Copyright 2005 by Social Philosophy and Policy Foundation. Reprinted with the permission of Cambridge University Press.

Chapter 24: James L. Bernat, "The Biophilosophical Basis for Whole-Brain Death," *Social Philosophy and Policy* 19 (2002): 324–342. Copyright 2002 by Social Philosophy and Policy Foundation. Reprinted with the permission of Cambridge University Press.

Chapter 25: Fred Rosner, "The Definition of Death in Jewish Law," in Stuart J. Youngner, Robert M. Arnold, and Renie Schapiro, eds., *The Definition of Death*, Johns Hopkins University Press (1999): 210–221.

Chapter 27: William A. Wallace, "St. Thomas on the Beginning and Ending of Human Life," in A. Vari, ed., *Sanctus Thomas de Aquino Doctor Hodiernae Humanitatis, Studi Tomistici* 58 (1995): 394–407. Reprinted with the permission of Libreria Editrice Vaticana.

Chapter 28: Robert M. Veatch, "The Impending Collapse of the Whole-Brain Definition of Death," *The Hastings Center Report* 23:4 (1993): 18–24. Reprinted with the permission of Robert Veatch and The Hastings Center Report.

Chapter 29: Hans Jonas, "Against the Stream: Comments on the Definition and Redefinition of Death," in Hans Jonas, *Philosophical Essays: From Ancient Creed to Technological Man*, Prentice Hall (1974): 132–140. Copyright 1974 by Prentice-Hall, Inc. Reprinted with the permission of University of Chicago Press.

Chapter 30: Michael B. Green and Daniel Wikler, "Brain Death and Personal Identity," *Philosophy and Public Affairs* 9:2 (1980): 105–133. Copyright 1980 by Princeton University Press. Reprinted with the permission of Blackwell Publishing.

Chapter 32: President's Council on Bioethics, *Controversies in the Determination of Death: A White Paper*, www.bioethics.gov.

Authors

St. Thomas Aquinas (1225–1274), philosopher, theologian, doctor of the Church (Angelicus Doctor), Naples, Italy

Lynne Rudder Baker, Ph.D., Distinguished Professor, Department of Philosophy, University of Massachusetts Amherst, Amherst, Massachusetts

James L. Bernat, M.D., Dartmouth-Hitchcock Medical Center, Lebanon Neurology, Lebanon, New Hampshire

René Descartes (1596–1650), philosopher, mathematician, scientist, writer, Touraine, France

Jason T. Eberl, Ph.D., Associate Professor and Graduate Co-director, Department of Philosophy, Indiana University–Purdue University Indianapolis, Indianapolis, Indiana

Harry G. Frankfurt, Ph.D., Professor Emeritus, Department of Philosophy, Princeton University, Princeton, New Jersey

Clifford Geertz, Ph.D. (1926–2006), Professor Emeritus, School of Social Science, Institute for Advanced Study, Princeton, New Jersey

Grant Gillett, Ph.D., Senior Lecturer in Medical Ethics, Bioethics Research Centre, University of Otago, Dunedin, New Zealand

Michael B. Green, Ph.D., former Assistant Professor of Philosophy, University of Texas, Austin, Texas

Germain Grisez, Ph.D., Flynn Professor of Christian Ethics, Mount St. Mary's University, Emmitsburg, Maryland

Rom Harré, D.Litt., Professor Emeritus of Philosophy, Linacre College, University of Oxford, Oxford, United Kingdom; and Adjunct Professor of Philosophy, Georgetown University, Washington, D.C.

Hans Jonas, Ph.D. (1903–1993), Emeritus Alvin Johnson Professor of Philosophy, The New School for Social Research, New York, New York

David A. Jones, Ph.D., Senior Lecturer in Bioethics, St. Mary's College, University of Surrey Twickenham, London, United Kingdom

Tom Kitwood, Ph.D. (1937–1999), Senior Lecturer in Psychology, Bradford University, Bradford, United Kingdom

Helga Kuhse, Ph.D., Honorary Research Fellow, Monash University, Melbourne, Victoria, Australia

John P. Lizza, Ph.D., Professor, Department of Philosophy, Kutztown University of Pennsylvania, Kutztown, Pennsylvania

John Locke (1632–1704), philosopher, medical researcher, University of Oxford, Oxford, England

E. J. Lowe, D.Phil., Professor of Philosophy, University of Durham, Durham, United Kingdom

Aaron L. Mackler, Ph.D., Professor of Theology, Duquesne University, Pittsburgh, Pennsylvania

G. H. Mead, M.A. (1863–1931), Professor of Philosophy, University of Chicago, Chicago, Illinois

Gilbert Meilaender, Ph.D., Dusenberg Professor of Christian Ethics, Valparaiso University, Valparaiso, Indiana

Eric T. Olson, Ph.D., Lecturer in Philosophy and Churchill College Fellow, University of Cambridge, Cambridge, United Kingdom

Derek Parfit, M.A., Senior Research Fellow, All Souls College, University of Oxford, Oxford, United Kingdom; Fellow, British Academy; and Fellow, American Academy of Arts and Sciences

Plato (428?–347 BCE), Classical Greek philosopher and founder of the Academy in Athens, Athens, Greece

Nicola Poplawski, M.D., Clinical Geneticist and Senior Lecturer, Department of Pediatrics, University of Adelaide, Adelaide, New Zealand

Fred Rosner, M.D., Professor of Medicine, Mount Sinai School of Medicine, New York, New York; and Fellow, American Academy of Physicians

Peter Singer, M.A., B.Phil., Ira W. DeCamp Professor of Bioethics, Princeton University, Princeton, New Jersey; and Laureate Professor, Center for Applied Philosophy and Public Ethics, University of Melbourne, Melbourne, Victoria, Australia

P. F. Strawson, M.A. (1919–2006), Waynflete Professor of Metaphysical Philosophy, Magdalen College, University of Oxford, Oxford, United Kingdom

Richard Swinburne, B.Phil., Nolloth Professor Emeritus of the Philosophy of the Christian Religion, University of Oxford, Oxford, United Kingdom; Fellow Emeritus of Oriel College, Oxford, United Kingdom; and Fellow of the British Academy, United Kingdom

Robert M. Veatch, Ph.D., Professor of Medical Ethics, Kennedy Institute of Ethics, Georgetown University, Washington, D.C.

William A. Wallace, O.P., Ph.D., S.T.D., Professor Emeritus of Philosophy and History, Catholic University of America, Washington, D.C.; and Adjunct Professor of Philosophy, University of Maryland, College Park, Maryland

Mary Anne Warren, Ph.D., Professor Emeritus of Philosophy, San Francisco State University, San Francisco, California

Daniel Wikler, Ph.D., Mary B. Saltonstall Professor of Population Ethics and Professor of Ethics and Population Health, Harvard University, Cambridge, Massachusetts

Defining the Beginning and End of Life

Introduction

John P. Lizza

Advances in medical technology have posed significant challenges to how we fix the boundaries of the beginning and end of life. When does a person begin and cease to exist? Are human embryos,[1] artificially sustained whole-brain dead bodies, individuals in permanent vegetative state,[2] anencephalic individuals,[3] and individuals with advanced dementia living persons? In short, who should be counted among the living "we"?

Different answers to this fundamental question have figured prominently in the debate over abortion, the use of human embryos for research, and the definition and determination of death. Indeed, in many cases, alternative views of the nature of persons have determined one's position on these bioethical issues.[4] This work offers a selection of readings to explore the connection between some of the more theoretical perspectives on persons and practical cases in bioethics. Its aim is to encourage further reflection on how commitment to alternative theories of personhood and personal identity affect the evaluation of difficult cases at the beginning and end of life and how those cases may test and shape our theories. It is also offered in the hope of promoting greater understanding of why people differ on the bioethical issues.

This anthology is by no means comprehensive—that is a task that would take many volumes. Instead, perhaps more than anything, it reflects a kind of map of my own attempt to learn something about persons that may be helpful in addressing some of the difficult cases that have come with advances in medical technology. My investigation has been mainly in Western philosophy and religion. Accordingly, I have given more attention to the treatment of the concept of person in philosophy and religion and less to its treatment in anthropology, sociology, and psychology. The concept of person, however, is informed by all of these disciplines. If persons are naturally psychological, social, and cultural beings, then any account of their nature cannot be given independently of psychological, social, and cultural theories. I have therefore included several works in social psychology and cultural anthropology with the intent of at least showing the relevance of these disciplines to determining who and what "we" are.

Part I provides a selection of readings representing various views about the nature of persons that have been influential in the ontological and bioethical discussion. The first view is a dualist or "spiritualist" view that identifies the person with an immaterial spirit or soul. Dualists often appeal to the possibility that a person could acquire a completely new body or continue to exist with no body at all, as many religious accounts of life after death have maintained. If such possibilities are coherent, these theorists argue that we must be composed of bodily matter and some other kind of stuff (i.e., an immaterial soul) and that the continuation of this immaterial soul accounts for personal identity over time. The selections from Plato, Descartes, and Richard Swinburne represent this view.

The second "hylomorphic" view treats persons as "ensouled bodies" or "embodied souls." It is traditionally associated with Thomas Aquinas and finds modern expression in the selections from Gilbert Meilaender. In this view, a person is a human biological organism informed by a rational soul. Because the soul is what unifies and individuates living material organisms, the soul and the material body are inextricably linked. The soul (form) cannot exist separately from the matter; nor can the matter exist separately from the soul. Indeed, for Aquinas, personal resurrection after death requires flesh and bones. Personal identity over time thus consists in the continuation of an ensouled body.

The third view is a "species" or animalist view that identifies the person with the human body or organism. To be a person is to be a physical specimen of the human species. As with other organisms, the human specimen need not have any psychological traits to retain its organic integrity. Because our organisms existed and may continue to exist without psychological qualities or psychological continuity associated with them, our psychology is ultimately irrelevant to who and what we are. In this view, represented by Eric Olson, our identity consists in biological continuity.[5]

The fourth view is a "qualitative" or "functionalist" view that identifies the person with certain psychological abilities and qualities of awareness. It has its roots in the work of John Locke and David Hume and finds its contemporary expression most clearly in the work of Derek Parfit. It also has similarities with the Buddhist doctrine of *anattā* (no self).[6] These philosophers treat the person as a set of mental qualities, including consciousness and memories, rather than as a substantive entity or subject. Locke, for example, distinguishes the person from the human animal (organism). In his discussion of the hypothetical case of a prince and cobbler swapping bodies, Locke argues that personal identity travels with one's psychological states and memories.[7] Thus, if the body of the cobbler woke up one day with the psychological states and memories of the prince, and the body of the prince, with the psychological states and memories of the cobbler, Locke concludes that the prince and cobbler would have swapped bodies. For Locke, personal identity consists of the connectedness between psychological states evident in memories, regardless of whatever substance, material or immaterial, may underlie those psychological states over time.

Because the substantive matter underlying the psychological states is irrelevant to personal identity, Locke's view is a precursor to contemporary functionalist theories about the mind and personal identity. Functionalism as a philosophy of mind rejects the idea that the mind is a substantive entity, whether material (e.g., the brain) or immaterial (e.g., the soul). Instead, the mind is conceived as a function that can be described abstractly by a machine table of inputs, internal states, and outputs. While the function needs to be embodied in some medium (e.g., the neurophysiological processes of the brain), the function can be described independently of whatever underlies or instantiates the function. As K. T. Maslin explains, "The Lockean/Parfit proposal is analogous to treating you as a function or program run on the hardware of the brain, the material embodiment being strictly irrelevant to your identity and survival. You could go from body and brain to body and brain, just as information can be transferred intact to another disc if the original becomes damaged."[8]

The fifth view treats the person not as some qualitative or functional specification of some more basic kind of thing (e.g., a human organism), but as a primitive substance that has psychological and corporeal characteristics. This "substantive" view, reflected in selections from contemporary philosophers Peter Strawson and E. J. Lowe, differs from the "animalist" view in that it entails that the person must have the capacity or realistic potential for psychological functions. This cannot be said about some living members of the human species, such as anencephalics and individuals in permanent vegetative state. This view also differs from the dualist and hylomorphic views because it is not committed to the existence of an immaterial soul.

The sixth view treats persons as psychological beings constituted by bodies. Lynne Rudder Baker is the most prominent proponent of the "constitutive view" of the person.[9] In contrast to the "species" view, persons are not *identical* to the human organisms that constitute them. Instead, the relation between the person and human organism is one of constitution, similar to the relation between a work of art, such as a sculpture, and the matter that it is made of (e.g., a piece of marble). Persons and human organisms are therefore different kinds of things with different principles of individuation and identity. Baker holds that the capacity for subjectivity or a "first-person perspective" is essential to personhood. The constitutive view also allows for relational factors, such as recognition by others, to play a central role in their existence.

The seventh view is a "relational" view that treats persons as essentially social and cultural beings. The selections from G. H. Mead, Clifford Geertz, Rom Harré, and Tom Kitwood are illustrative of this approach. These theorists emphasize how relations to others embedded in diverse cultural contexts are part of what defines who we are. To attempt to define the person in ontological terms, independent of considerations of social relations and culture, would involve a distortion of our nature. Thus, whatever merit any of the previous six ontological views of the person might have, they will fall short if they fail to take into account the social and cultural dimension of persons.

The eighth and last view in Part I defines persons by the capacity for certain "higher order" or "self-conscious" psychological functions. For Harry Frankfurt, it is the capacity for having beliefs and desires about our beliefs and desires.[10] This capacity, in turn, provides the basis for freedom of the will. Persons are thus distinguished from other kinds of things by their particular kind of self-conscious psychology and freedom of will.

The first six views entail different ontological beliefs about the relation between mind and body. With the exception of the third view, which holds that psychology is irrelevant to the nature of persons, the seventh and eighth views are sometimes incorporated into the other theories as part of a more complete account of personhood.

The readings in Part II track how the debate over abortion and the moral status of embryos has turned on acceptance or rejection of one or more of these views about the nature of persons. Many opponents of abortion and research on embryos identify the person with an ensouled, human organism and link ensoulment with the beginning of human life. However, they differ on when a human organism begins to exist and consequently on when ensoulment takes place. As the readings by Aaron Mackler, Germain Grisez, and Jason Eberl illustrate, this disagreement is nowhere more evident than in the discussion that has taken place within the Judaeo-Christian tradition. Some (e.g., Grisez) fix the point of the beginning of a person's life at conception because, it is claimed, the zygote contains the human genotype and therewith the active potential for further development as a person. Although not represented in this anthology, others (e.g., Richard McCormick) fix the point at the formation of the primitive streak with implantation about fourteen days after fertilization.[11] They claim that there is no individual organism before then because up to that point there is just a group of individual totipotent cells and identical twinning is possible. Still others (e.g., Thomas Shannon, Allan Wolter, Joseph Donceel, and Hans-Martin Sass) fix the point even later.[12] Sass, for example, argues that because a biological prerequisite for rationality is necessary for personhood, the person exists no earlier than approximately eight weeks after fertilization, at which point subcortical and cortical structures begin to be more fully integrated. Finally, although most Jewish thinkers hold that the embryo has a significant moral status that generally prohibits abortion throughout gestation, all agree that it does not become a person until birth.

While proponents of the "species" or "animalist" view and the "ensouled body" view differ on the nature of a person, they are strange bedfellows when it comes to determining personhood because both look to biology for a determination of when human life begins. As noted above, the former is a materialist view that regards psychological characteristics, such as intellect and will, as irrelevant to the nature of a person. The latter, on the other hand, sees such characteristics as essential to the ensouled nature of persons. Theologically, characteristics like intellect and will are what make persons in God's image. For example, Eric Olson, perhaps the leading proponent of the animalist view, cites the biological analysis of Norman Ford, a Catholic, in support of his claim that a person begins to exist with the formation of the primitive streak.[13] Although Ford treats a person as an ensouled human being, his determination of when a person's life begins is informed by biological considerations. In contrast to Olson, Eberl tries to integrate Ford's biological analysis into a Thomistic metaphysics of personhood but ultimately rejects it as incompatible with a Thomistic account of active potentiality. However, in his article, "St. Thomas on the Beginning and Ending of Human Life," which appears as Chapter 27 in the third section of this anthology, William Wallace offers an alternative interpretation of Aquinas that is more compatible with Ford's and Olson's views.

Even though Catholic bioethicists such as McCormick and Ford hold that a human person does not begin to exist until the formation of the primitive streak, they disapprove of aborting and experimenting on pre-implanted embryos, as this would interrupt the generative process and interfere with the embryo's potential to develop into a person. Other theological beliefs, however, are invoked to explain why such an interruption in the generative process is wrong. For example, Ford states that it intentionally frustrates "the Creator's plan for the responsible transmission of human life as the fruit of an act of conjugal love."[14]

In contrast, bioethicists, such as Helga Kuhse and Peter Singer, agree that the early human embryo is not a person, but they see that as morally relevant to providing a justification for allowing abortion and experimentation on those embryos. Because in their view the possibility of fission, fusion, and the totipotency of the cells of the pre-implanted embryo provide grounds for denying the identity of the early embryo with any person that may later come into being, whatever interests, concerns, or moral status that the later person may have are not shared by the embryo. Thus, insofar as the nonidentity of the early embryo with any person is invoked to justify abortion and experimentation, the issue of identity plays a critical role in the debate.

In contrast to the "species" and "ensouled body" views, many who argue in favor of choice and research on embryos accept a qualitative or functionalist view of persons, linking personhood with certain capacities, such as consciousness, sentience, self-awareness, rationality, and agency. Because embryos, especially early in gestation, lack some or all of these qualities, they are not persons and therefore are not deserving of the same rights and protections accorded to persons. The seminal article by Mary Anne Warren is representative of this approach.

Nicola Poplawski and Grant Gillett appear to accept a substantive view of the person, as they treat the person as a being with a biological and psychological life history, a "longitudinal form" that, because it has value at some point in its history, has value throughout its history. Because these theorists maintain that the basis of the moral value of persons lies in "the human ability to interact with others in those situations where moral sense and morality are grounded," the relational nature of persons is also of central importance in their account.

In the final article in Part II, Lynne Rudder Baker applies the constitutive view of persons to the issue of the beginning of life. She argues that the constitutive view entails that human persons do not begin to exist until near birth, when the human organism begins to develop a rudimentary first-person perspective. She concludes with some reflections of the implications of this metaphysical view on the morality of abortion.

While not as evident as in the debate over the beginning of life, alternative views about the nature of persons can be traced in the contemporary debate over the definition and determination of death, that is, when a person no longer exists. Much of the contemporary debate has focused on the question of whether "brain death" or "total brain failure" is death. Part III begins with an article by James Bernat, which represents the "received" rationale for why "brain death" is death. Bernat accepts what he calls a "biological paradigm" of death, which holds that death is fundamentally a biological phenomenon. He defines death as "the permanent cessation of the critical systems of the organism as a whole" and accepts as a criterion of death "the permanent cessation of the clinical functions of the brain." He believes that when we artificially sustain whole-brain-dead human bodies, we are sustaining collections of human organs rather than the human organism as a whole. Bernat's article provides a useful framework for understanding the three main alternative criteria for determining death: irreversible loss of circulation and respiration, irreversible loss of all brain functions, including those of the brain stem, and irreversible loss of consciousness. The readings then track the discussion of how alternative views of personhood or humanity have been used to justify alternative views about the definition and criteria for death.

Paralleling the disagreement within religious traditions over when a person's life begins, there is disagreement in those traditions on when it ends. Fred Rosner points out that some Jews (e.g., Rabbi David Bleich) reject the whole-brain neurological criterion for death on grounds that the spirit has not left the body until respiration has ceased. Others in this tradition (e.g., Rabbis Moses Tendler and Moshe Feinstein) accept the neurological criterion on grounds that, if all brain functions have irreversibly ceased, then spontaneous respiration has also ceased—a kind of "physiological decapitation" has occurred.[15] According to Rosner, the consciouness-related criterion for death (what is sometimes referred to as "cerebral death") is generally not accepted in Judaism, because "unconsciousness does not remove the humanhood or personhood from a patient."

Among Christians, there is also disagreement. David Jones holds that the divine spirit of a person, what endows a human body with the potential for intellect and will, is not dependent on the brain. He therefore rejects the current whole-brain criterion for death. As D. Alan Shewmon, who holds a similar view, puts it, "as long as the human body is alive (from the biological perspective of somatic integrative unity) then the person is alive."[16] The loss of all brain functions is insufficient to conclude with any moral certainty that the soul has departed from the body.[17] In this view, death is defined as the separation of the soul from the body. It is interesting to note that some Japanese view the spirit as diffused throughout the body and not located in any particular organ, such as the brain.[18] In their view, the spirit is present in the artificially sustained, whole-brain-dead body and therefore the person is still alive.

Many other Christians, who also have an "ensouled body" view of the person, accept the current whole-brain neurological criterion for death. Although not represented in this anthology, Paul Ramsay, for example, believes that when we artificially sustain whole-brain-dead human bodies, we are sustaining collections of human organs rather than the person (i.e., the human organism as a whole).[19] If all brain functions are lost, including the integrative functions of the brainstem, then the person has died. Death is understood as the irreversible loss of organic integration. Ramsay holds that even though individuals in permanent vegetative state and those with anencephaly may permanently lack consciousness, they are still living persons. Death has not occurred, because these individuals retain brainstem functions and thus the human organism (i.e., the person) has not lost its organic integration.

Finally, William Wallace and Robert Veatch argue in favor of acceptance of a consciousness-related or "higher-brain" formulation of death. Wallace suggests that just as Aquinas held a view of delayed hominization, he also accepted the possibility of early dehominization. Wallace believes that this view is most consistent with a consciousness-related formulation of death. Veatch invokes the Judeo-Christian understanding of the human being as a substantial union of mind and body. He argues that if the capacity for consciousness is irreversibly destroyed, as can be said about individuals in permanent vegetative state, then the essential union of mind and body is destroyed and therefore death has occurred. Veatch's article, like the following article by Hans Jonas, is noteworthy, because it contains a strong argument for why defining death is not a strictly biological matter.

Disagreement over the criteria and definition of death is also found in the secular tradition. For example, Hans Jonas accepts a species view of the person that identifies the person with the human organism. Consequently, he holds that because the whole-brain-dead organism may retain its organic integration (entropy has not set in), the person (human organism) has not died. Jonas also opines that the issue of how to treat individuals who have lost all brain functions is an axiological matter and cannot be settled simply by appeal to clinical fact. Others who accept a species-related concept of death challenge the neurological criterion by pointing to cases of post-mortem pregnancy[20] and the extraordinary case of a whole-brain-dead body sustained for over twenty years.[21] They argue that a person may continue to exist, despite the loss of all brain functions. Such persons retain their organic integration, albeit through artificial life support. Accordingly, these theorists accept only the traditional criterion of irreversible cessation of respiration and circulation for a determination of death.

In contrast to those who accept a "species" or "ensouled body" concept of person, bioethicists who identify the person with a set of psychological functions define a person's life and death in terms of the beginning, continuation, and cessation of certain psychological functions. Thus, Green and Wikler argue in favor of a consciousness-related or "higher-brain" formulation of death that would consider individuals who have lost all brain function, as well as individuals in permanent vegetative state, as dead. Because individuals in permanent vegetative state are no longer psychologically continuous with their former selves, those former selves have ceased to exist (i.e., they have died).

Some prominent critics of this higher-brain formulation of death and proponents of the whole-brain formulation of death, such as James Bernat, Charles Culver, and Bernard Gert, accept the functionalist or qualitative view of the person that Green and Wikler invoke, but reject the implication that individuals who have irreversibly lost consciousness and every other mental function have "died." Bernat, Culver, and Gert distinguish the person from the human organism and hold that individuals in permanent vegetative state are not persons. However, they object to characterizing individuals in permanent vegetative state as "dead" on grounds that this would be an incorrect use of the term *dead*. They define "death" as "the permanent cessation of functioning of the organism as a whole" and claim that "death" is a strictly biological concept, applicable to human organisms but not to persons. Thus, they criticize the consciousness-related, neurological formulation of death as involving a metaphorical use of "death," "applying it to an organism which has ceased to be a person but has not died."[22] In their view, "death" cannot be applied literally to persons, because death is a biological concept appropriate to biological organisms, not to roles, functions, abilities, or qualities of awareness. Just as a human organism may cease to be a banker or basketball player without dying, Bernat, Culver, and Gert hold that a human organism can cease to be a person without dying.[23]

The "substantive" concept of person treats the person neither as some qualitative or functional specification of some more basic kind of thing (e.g., a human organism) nor as identical to a human organism. Instead, in this view, a person is a primitive substance that necessarily has psychological and corporeal characteristics. P. F. Strawson's definition of a person as an individual to which we can apply both predicates that ascribe psychological characteristics (P-predicates) and predicates that ascribe corporeal characteristics (M-predicates) is an example of the use of "person" in this substantive sense.[24] In Strawson's view, it is neither a category mistake nor a metaphor to predicate death to persons. This view of the person is reflected in common expressions such as "people die every day." Also, as noted earlier, it differs from the "species meaning" in that it entails that the person must have the capacity or realistic potential for psychological functions. This cannot be said about a corpse or about some living members of the biological species *Homo sapiens* (e.g., anencephalic individuals and individuals in permanent vegetative state).

In the context of the debate over the definition of death, Tristam Engelhardt,[25] Karen Gervais,[26] Jeff McMahan,[27] and I[28] have invoked this substantive view of the person and have distinguished the death of the person from that of the human organism. Because persons must have the capacity or realistic potential for consciousness and other mental functions, the irreversible loss of that capacity or potential would mean the ceasing to exist or death of the person. Persons whose brains have been destroyed to the point where they have lost the potential for consciousness and every other mental function are therefore dead. Technology may sustain human or humanoid bodies that have irreversibly lost the potential for consciousness, but this should not obscure the reality that the person, understood as a substantive being, has died. My contribution, which also offers a broader challenge to the "biological paradigm" of death, is representative of this view.

Recently, the President's Council on Bioethics (2008) considered the issue of whether individuals who satisfy the currently accepted neurological criterion for death, what the council now calls "total brain failure," are really dead. A large part of the council's white paper, *Controversies in the Determination of Death* (2008), is devoted to addressing the challenges raised by cases in which individuals with total brain failure have been artificially sustained for weeks, months, and, in the one case reported by Shewmon, over twenty years. In contrast to the view of James Bernat and the influential 1981 President's Commission for the Study of Ethical Problems in Medicine and Biomedical and Behavioral Research, the President's council accepts that artificially sustained individuals with total brain failure may retain internal organic integration and cannot be understood simply as collections of organic parts. Nonetheless, the council maintains that these individuals are correctly classified as dead. It offers a novel rationale in support of its view. The council holds that what distinguishes an organism's being alive from being dead is its ability to engage in commerce with the surrounding world to secure its sustenance. Because individuals with total brain failure lack the spontaneous drive and "felt need" to breathe or interact with the world in other life-sustaining ways, they are no longer alive. Whether this alternative rationale for the neurological criterion for determining death will hold up· under critical scrutiny remains to be seen. Chapter 4 of the council's white paper is the final selection in this anthology.

Because the concept of person is pivotal in these discussions of the beginning and end of life, an assessment of which concept of person makes the most sense is unavoidable. Failure to address the issue would leave us with parties in the debate essentially talking past each other by proposing definitions of life and death for different kinds of things. Disagreement over whether a human embryo, artificially sustained whole-brain-dead body, anencephalic, or individual in permanent vegetative state is a person may lead to irreconcilable disagreement over the morality of abortion, the definition of death, and the treatment of these individuals. Indeed, when the discussion of personhood in the debate over abortion was perhaps at its height, Ruth Macklin concluded that we had reached an impasse on differences over the concept of personhood and that continued focus on personhood would be of little help in making progress or reaching any kind of consensus on abortion.[29] Although Macklin provides a perceptive account of certain aspects of the disagreement over concepts of personhood and the role that the concept has played in bioethics, I think that her conclusions were premature.

While I agree with Macklin that there will probably always be disagreement over the concept of person, I am generally skeptical about calling disagreement at any point "fundamental" or incapable of making progress toward consensus on.[30] Further analysis often reveals how our beliefs are tied to other beliefs, and critical reflection on those other beliefs may lead to revision in the beliefs that we thought were different in a "fundamental" or foundational sense. We sometimes find that what we initially consider to be a "fundamental disagreement" turns out to be not so fundamental or even a disagreement after all. Indeed, because the concept of personhood is so central to our moral, metaphysical, and cultural systems of thought, it has a depth to it that we have only begun to explore. Because our concept of personhood is tied to other descriptive and prescriptive beliefs, we need to examine exactly what those beliefs are and whether they are consistent with how we wish to use the term *person*.

Daniel Callahan has pointed out that persons cannot be understood or defined by a single character or essential nature.[31] Callahan cites Ernest Becker, who observes, "In the human sciences man must be seen at all times in the total social-cultural-historical context, precisely because it is this that forms his 'self' or nature."[32] This social-cultural-historical depth to the concept of person has been insufficiently explored, especially in the context of advances in life-sustaining technology that affect our understanding of when a person lives and dies.

In addition, instead of examining how the social-cultural-historical context informs our notions of persons and personal identity, contemporary philosophers addressing issues of personhood and personal identity have spent much more time considering conceptual puzzles about personal identity that ignore the social-cultural-historical context in which persons appear. While some theorists, such as G. H. Mead, Jean-Paul Sartre, Ludwig Wittgenstein, Clifford Geertz, Rom Harré, Ken Gergen, and many feminist scholars (e.g., Diana Meyers and Virginia Held) have emphasized the relational and cultural nature of persons, most contemporary debate over criteria for personhood and personal identity in the philosophical literature has assumed that the criteria must be something internal to the person (e.g., internally related, psychological or bodily states).[33] Much less attention has been paid to how moral considerations, external factors, such as an individual's relation to others, and cultural factors, may determine the nature and identity of persons. Examination of such factors may lead to a greater consensus or an acceptance of pluralism concerning the nature of persons and what it means for them to die. In fact, one of the main reasons for accepting the view that persons are "constituted by" human organisms may be that it allows relational factors to play an essential role in the identity and individuation of persons.[34]

There is a legitimate concern, of course, that if relational or cultural factors are allowed to determine in part the nature of persons and who counts as a person, certain individuals will be excluded for no good reason. Haven't slaves, for example, been treated as nonpersons because others were in a position of power and the attitudes of the powerful carried the day? There are, however, resources within our moral and political theories to respond to this concern. For example, as Jean-Paul Sartre demonstrates, racist and sexist beliefs are often grounded in factually mistaken beliefs about the nature of the individuals who are the focus of the racist and sexist attitudes (e.g., that women are intellectually inferior to men or that Jews are the cause of all social ills).[35] Also, these beliefs can often be traced to self-interested motivations to exercise power over others—motivations that are subject to strong critique from our moral and political systems of thought.

Personhood is a dynamic concept that is subject to change in light of new knowledge and possibilities. If our nature is not fixed and we can create, at least in part, who we are, personhood and personal identity should be approached more as open-ended projects, rather than realities that are determined by factors independent of the choices that we make.[36] Thus, although examining our tradition is important for evaluating the new phenomena created by advances in medical technology, especially when it poses challenges to our basic concepts of life, death, and who we are, it is insufficient. We need to also ask what it is that we want to become.

As Christopher Gill points out, David Wiggins has suggested that our theory of personhood tries to hold together in a single focus three aspects of persons:

1. an object of biological, anatomical, and neurophysiological inquiry;
2. a subject of consciousness; and
3. a locus of all sorts of moral attributes and the source or conceptual origin of all value.[37]

Callahan, Geertz, Harré, and others suggest a fourth aspect to this triadic nature:

4. an essentially relational nature as a social and cultural being

Wiggins's approach is helpful because it suggests that, when faced with problematic cases that challenge the range of our concept of person (e.g., the whole-brain dead, individuals in permanent vegetative state, or human embryos), we need to examine to what extent these beings are like ourselves in the four senses that inform our concept of person. We also need to examine how these features are interconnected. Too often, theorists will focus on one of these aspects and ignore the others. This is particularly evident in the philosophical discussion about personal identity over the last fifty years. As noted above, the thought experiments that challenge our concept of persons and personal identity and that have dominated contemporary philosophical discussion of personal identity tend to sunder persons from the cultural and moral context in which they appear. If Wiggins and these other theorists are right, we should not expect to have an account of the nature of a person independent of our values and culture.

People will likely continue to differ on whether certain individuals are dead or alive, because they will continue to differ on their views of the nature of persons. However, this should not lead to acceptance of a naïve relativism about persons or the idea that ontology, values, and cultural practices cannot or should not be changed. The new cases dished up by advances in medical technology should force us to reflect on our beliefs and practices and, in some cases, to revise them. Thus, on reflection, some beliefs and practices may be determined to be inconsistent with other things we believe about persons and how they should be treated. The beliefs and practices may also be based on mistaken beliefs about other matters. For example, a view that treats persons as essentially having a conscious, subjective nature is inconsistent with treating human organisms that have irreversibly lost the capacity for subjectivity as living persons.

This anthology aims to promote a greater understanding of the diversity of opinion concerning the nature of persons and why people differ about the practical cases. Again, this is not to encourage acceptance of a moral or cultural relativism in which the beliefs of others are seen as simply the products of different tastes and culture that we have no hope of understanding and that we must simply accept without criticism. Instead, it is to encourage greater understanding of the fact that, as Isaiah Berlin puts it, "there are many different ends that men may seek and still be fully rational, fully men, capable of understanding each other and sympathizing and deriving light from each other."[38] Such understanding, as Berlin explains, is critical if we are to hold in check the dangers that come when one individual, group, or civilization seeks to promotes its view of the good as a final solution.

Whether human embryos, anencephalics, individuals in permanent vegetative state, and the artificially sustained whole-brain dead are persons may not be readily answered by some discovery about the nature of persons. Because *person* is not a univocal term and there is no universally agreed-upon theory about the nature of persons, it may only be possible to criticize alternative views about persons by showing how those views conflict with the rules of usage of the terms within a given theory of personhood or how they conflict with other accepted ethical or metaphysical beliefs. In other words, the question may be answered by how consistent our application of the term is with other important values and ontological commitments and the implications that our view has for respecting those commitments and realizing those values.[39] Indeed, the adequacy of any concept of person may depend on how successfully it manages to hold in a "single focus" our nature as biological, psychological, moral, and cultural beings.

NOTES

1. A critical ontological issue is whether the zygote can be identified with the implanted embryo and the fetus at later stages of development. Without begging this issue, I use the term *embryo* to refer to the zygote and what exists at all developmental stages from fertilization to birth. Whether what exists at any of these stages can be individuated as a "person" is, of course, another critical issue.

2. I use the term *permanent vegetative state* to refer to extreme cases of persistent vegetative state (PVS) in which the diagnosis of the irreversible loss of consciousness and other cognitive functions can be determined with a high degree of probability. The Multi-Society Task Force on PVS states that "a permanent vegetative state . . . means an irreversible state, which like all clinical diagnoses in medicine, is based on probabilities, not absolutes. A patient in a persistent vegetative state becomes permanently vegetative when the diagnosis of irreversibility can be established with a high degree of clinical certainty—that is when the chance that the patient will regain consciousness is exceedingly small" (Multi-Society Task Force on PVS, "Medical aspects of the persistent vegetative state: Parts 1 and 2," *New England Journal of Medicine* 330 (1994): 1501).

J.-M. Guérit identifies such cases pathophysiologically by their absence of all primary components of cortical evoked potentials (EPs): "We know that, for metabolic reasons, the sensitivity to anoxia of the primary sensory cortices is intermediate between that of association cortex and brain stem [F. Plum and J. Posner, *The Diagnosis of Stupor and Coma*, 3rd ed., Philadelphia: F. A. Davis Co., 1980: 87–151]. This implies that brain anoxia sufficient to destroy the primary cortex should be sufficient to destroy all association cortex, irrespective of brain stem status. This irreversible situation is incompatible with any consciousness. . . . Significantly, this situation can be reliably identified at the patient's bedside with multimodality or, more specifically, somatosensory EPs, which show the absence of any cortical components (what we labeled as post-anoxic Grade 4 in our EP classification [J.-M. Guerit, M. de Tourtcharinoff, L. Soveges, and P. Mahieu, "The prognostic value of three-modality evoked potentials (TMEPs) in anoxia and traumatic coma," *Neurophysiologic Clinique* 23 (1993): 209–226]. One major advantage of this approach is that Grade 4 somatosensory EPs constitute a pattern clearly distinct from all others, eliminating any 'slippery slope'" (J.-M. Guérit, "The concept of brain death," in C. Machado and D. A. Shewmon, eds., *Brain Death and Disorders of Consciousness*. New York: Kluwer, 2004, 20).

Despite Guérit's confidence, however, there is debate in neurology over whether we can know that individuals in PVS lack consciousness, temporarily or irreversibly. See A. Howsepian, "Philosophical reflections on coma," *Review of Metaphysics* 47 (1994): 735–755, and "The 1994 Multi-Society Task Force consensus statement on the persistent vegetative state: A critical analysis," *Issues in Law and Medicine* 12 (1996): 3–29; C. Borthwick, "The permanent vegetative state: Ethical crux, medical fiction?", *Issues in Law and Medicine* 12 (1996): 167–185; D. A. Shewmon, "The ABC of PVS," in C. Machado and D. A. Shewmon, eds., *Brain Death and Disorders of Consciousness* (New York: Kluwer, 2004); and S. Laureys et al., "Brain function in the vegetative state," in C. Machado and D. A. Shewmon, eds., *Brain Death and Disorders of Consciousness* (New York: Kluwer, 2004).

3. Anencephaly is defined as "a severe and uniformly fatal abnormality resulting in the congenital absence of skull, scalp, and forebrain. Although some telencephalic tissue may be present, by the time of birth, there is no functional cortex but only a hemorrhagic mass of neurons and glia" (S. Shinnar and J. Arras, "Ethical issues in the use of anencephalic

infants as organ donors," *Neurologic Clinics* 7 (1989): 730). Guérit ("The Concept of Brain Death," 19–20) expresses the widely accepted view in neurology that anencephaly constitutes a "pathophysiological process known to be incompatible with consciousness, irrespective of whether the brain stem is functioning or not." However, there is some debate over whether the plasticity of the brain may enable some infants lacking cortical structures to have experiences that would normally be mediated by them in adults. See, for example, D. A. Shewmon, "Anencephaly: Selected medical aspects," *Hastings Center Report* 18:5 (1988): 11–18. Indeed, Shewmon, in "The ABC of PVS," reports three remarkable cases in which children without cortical structures exhibited conscious behavior.

Shewmon, in "Anencephaly," estimates that approximately 1,125 anencephalic infants are born each year in the United States. About one-half are stillborn. Of the other half, most studies report that 90 to 100 percent die in the first week. Survival beyond a few weeks, however, has been reported in some cases. See Shinnar and Arras, "Ethical issues"; P. A. Baird and A. D. Sadovnik, "Survival in infants with anencephaly," *Clinical Pediatrics* 23 (1984): 268–271; J. M. Elwood and J. H. Elwood, *Epidemiology of Anencephalics and Spina Bifida* (Oxford: Oxford University Press, 1980); and J. L. Peabody and J. R. Emery, "Experience with anencephalic infants as prospective organ donors," *New England Journal of Medicine* 321 (1989): 344–350.

4. Settling the issue of personhood does not solve all the ethical problems. For example, as Judith Jarvis Thomson has pointed out, even if the embryo is a person with a right to life, its right to life may not entail a right to whatever means are necessary for it to survive. (See Judith Jarvis Thomson, "A defense of abortion," *Philosophy and Public Affairs* 1:1 (1971): 47–66.) Also, even if the embryo is not a person, it may still deserve moral consideration and protection.

5. For a related view, emphasizing how personal identity may consist in bodily continuity, see Bernard Williams, "The self and the future," *The Philosophical Review* 79:2 (1970): 161–180.

6. See, for example, Richard Taylor, "The anattā doctrine and personal identity," *Philosophy East and West* 19:4 (1969): 359–366.

7. John Locke, *An Essay Concerning Human Understanding*, 2nd edition, Book II, Chapter 27, Paragraph 15 ([1694] 1975).

8. K. T. Maslin, *An Introduction to the Philosophy of Mind* (Malden, MA: Blackwell, 2001), 275.

9. I have also argued in favor of this view. See John P. Lizza, *Metaphysical and Cultural Aspects of Persons*, Ph.D. diss., Columbia University (Ann Arbor: University Microfilms International, 1991), and Chapter 5 of John P. Lizza, *Persons, Humanity, and the Definition of Death* (Baltimore: Johns Hopkins University Press, 2006).

10. Another influential approach that emphasizes a higher-order function as definitive of persons appears in the work of Peter French. French defines persons as intentional agents (i.e., beings whose behavior can be given an intentional description). See Peter French, "Kinds and persons," *Philosophy and Phenomenological Research* 44:2 (1983): 241–254. In this view, ontological considerations, such as the relation between the mind and body that are central to other views about the nature of persons, are essentially irrelevant. Corporations, for example, are treated as persons, because their action can be understood in intentional terms and they can be held morally and legally responsible. Concern about whether they have an organic or spiritual nature is entirely misplaced.

11. Richard McCormick, "Who or what is the pre-embryo?" *Kennedy Institute of Ethics Journal* 1:1 (1991): 1–15.

12. Cf. Thomas A. Shannon and Allan B. Wolter, "Reflections on the moral status of the pre-embryo," *Theological Studies* 51 (1990): 603–626; Bernard Haring, *Medical Ethics* (Fides: Notre Dame, 1973); Joseph Donceel, "Immediate animation and delayed hominization," *Theological Studies* 31 (1970): 76–105; Hans-Martin Sass, "Brain life and brain death: A proposal for a normative agreement," *Journal of Medicine and Philosophy* 14 (1989): 45–59.

13. Norman Ford, *When Did I Begin? Conception of the Human Individual in History, Philosophy, and Science* (Cambridge: Cambridge University Press, 1988).

14. Norman Ford, "When did I begin?—A reply to Nicholas Tonti-Filippini," *Linacre Quarterly* 57:4 (1990): 65.

15. The characterization of the loss of all brain function as "physiological decapitation" was used by Rabbi Tendler in his testimony before the President's Commission for the Study of Ethical Problems in Medicine and Biomedical and Behavioral Research. See the Commission's 1981 report, *Defining Death* (Washington, DC: U.S. Government Printing Office, 1981), 11.

16. D. Alan Shewmon, "Recovery from 'brain death': A neurologist's apologia," *Linacre Quarterly* 64:1 (1997): 74.

17. Cf. Josef Seifert, "Is 'brain death' actually death?", *Monist* 76: 175–202.

18. Margaret Lock, *Twice Dead* (Berkeley: University of California Press, 2002), 227–228.

19. Chapter 2 of Paul Ramsay, *The Patient as Person* (New Haven: Yale University Press, 1970).

20. See, for example, D. R. Field, E. A. Gates, R. K. Creasy, K. R. Jonsen, and R. K. Laros, "Maternal brain death during pregnancy," *Journal of the American Medical Association* 260 (1988): 816–822; and A. Anstötz, "Should a brain-dead pregnant woman carry her child to full term? The case of the 'Erlanger baby'," *Bioethics* 7 (1993): 340–350.

21. D. Alan Shewmon, "'Brainstem death,' 'brain death,' and death: A critical reevaluation of the purported evidence," *Issues in Law and Medicine* 14 (1998): 125–146.

22. Charles M. Culver and Bernard Gert, *Philosophy and Medicine: Conceptual and Ethical Issues in Medicine and Psychiatry* (New York: Oxford University Press, 1982), 182–183.

23. In their most recent writing, Bernard Gert and Charles Culver have amended the earlier definition of death that they had proposed with James Bernat. Gert and Culver (joined by K. Danner Clouser) now define death as "the permanent cessation of all observable natural functioning of the organism as a whole, and the permanent absence of consciousness in the organism as a whole, or in any part of that organism." Bernard Gert, Charles M. Culver, and K. Danner Clouser, *Bioethics: A Systematic Approach* (New York: Oxford University Press, 2006), 290. These authors believe that it is now necessary to postulate this special definition of death for human beings and other higher-order organisms, because of the importance that consciousness plays in the life of these types of organisms. For a critique of how this amendment is inconsistent with the "biological paradigm" of death and leads to acceptance of a consciousness-related formulation of death, see John Lizza, "On the Definition of Death," Chapter 31 in this volume.

24. P. F. Strawson, *Individuals* (London: Methuen, 1959), 87–116. See also P. F. Strawson, "Persons," in H. Feigl, M. Scriven, and G. Maxwell, eds., *Concepts, Theories and the Mind-Body Problem*, Minnesota Studies in the Philosophy of Science, vol. 2 (Minneapolis: University of Minnesota Press, 1958), reprinted in D. M. Rosenthal, ed., *The Nature of Mind* (New York: Oxford University Press, 1991) and Chapter 9 in this volume.

25. H. T. Engelhardt, "Defining death: A philosophical problem for medicine and law," *American Review of Respiratory Diseases* 112 (1975): 587–590.

26. Karen Granstrand Gervais, *Redefining Death* (New Haven: Yale University Press, 1986).

27. Jeff McMahan, "The metaphysics of brain death," *Bioethics* 9 (1995): 91–126. See also Jeff McMahan, *The Ethics of Killing* (Oxford: Oxford University Press, 2002), 423–455.

28. John P. Lizza, "Defining death for persons and human organisms," *Theoretical Medicine and Bioethics* 20 (1999): 439–453; "The conceptual basis for brain death revisited: Loss of organic integration or loss of consciousness?", in C. Machado and D. Alan Shewmon, eds., *Brain Death and Disorders of Consciousness* (New York: Kluwer, 2004); and *Persons, Humanity, and the Definition of Death* (Baltimore: Johns Hopkins University Press, 2006).

29. Ruth Macklin, "Personhood in the bioethics literature," *Milbank Memorial Fund Quarterly* 6 (1983): 35–57.

30. Macklin does not explicitly say that the disagreement over personhood is "fundamental." However, her conclusion that no further progress can be made through further investigation of the alternative concepts of personhood appears to imply as much. Otherwise, what reason would there be for such a claim?

31. Daniel Callahan, "The 'beginning' of human life," in M. F. Goodman, ed., *What Is a Person?* (Clifton, NJ: Humana Press, 1988), 29–55.

32. Ibid., 47.

33. G. H. Mead, "The genesis of self and social control," *International Journal of Ethics* 35 (1925): 251–273, and *Mind, Self, and Society from the Standpoint of a Social Behaviorist* (Chicago: University of Chicago Press, 1934); Jean-Paul Sartre, *Being and Nothingness*, trans. H. E. Barnes (New York: Gramercy Books, [1942] 1994), *No Exit*, trans. S. Gilbert (New York: Vantage, [1945] 1995), and *L'existentialisme est un humanisme*, Repr. (Paris: Les Editions Nagel, [1946] 1970); Ludwig Wittgenstein, *Philosophical Investigations*, trans. G. E. M. Anscombe (Oxford: Blackwell, 1953); Clifford Geertz, "The transition to humanity," in S. Tax, ed., *Horizons of Anthropology* (Chicago: Aldine, 1964), and "The impact of the concept of culture on the concept of man," in Clifford Geertz, *The Interpretation of Cultures* (New York: Basic Books, 1973), 33–54; Rom Harré, *Personal Being: A Theory for Individual Psychology* (Cambridge: Harvard University Press, 1984), and "The 'self' as a theoretical concept," in M. Krauz, ed., *Relativism: Interpretation and Confrontation* (Notre Dame, IN: University of Notre Dame Press, 1989); K. J. Gergen, *The Saturated Self: Dilemmas of Identity in Contemporary Life* (New York: Basic Books, 1991), and "The social construction of self-knowledge," in D. Kolak and R. Martin, eds., *Self and Identity* (New York: Macmillan, 1991); Diana T. Meyers, *Self, Society, and Personal Choice* (New York: Columbia University Press, 1989); and Virginia Held, *Feminist Morality* (Chicago: University of Chicago Press, 1993).

34. See Chapter 2 of Lynne Rudder Baker, *Persons and Bodies* (Cambridge: Cambridge University Press, 2000), and Chapter 5 of John P. Lizza, *Persons, Humanity, and the Definition of Death* (Baltimore: Johns Hopkins University Press, 2006).

35. Jean-Paul Sartre, *Anti-Semite and Jew*, trans. George J. Becker (New York: Schocken Books, 1948).

36. The idea that our nature is not fixed and that we are responsible for the kind of being that we are is a theme that runs through existentialist philosophy. For example, Jean-Paul Sartre writes, "Man is nothing else but what he makes of himself. Such is the first principle of existentialism. . . . But what do we mean by this, if not that man has a

greater dignity than a stone or table? For we mean that man first exists, that is, that man first of all is the being who hurls himself towards a future and who is conscious of imagining himself as being in the future. Man is at the start a plan which is aware of itself, rather than a piece of garbage, or a cauliflower; nothing exists prior to this plan." Jean-Paul Sartre, *Existentialism and Human Emotions*, trans. Bernard Frechtman (New York: The Philosophical Library, 1957), 15–16.

37. Christopher Gill, "The human being as an ethical norm," in C. Gill, ed., *The Person and the Human Mind* (Oxford: Oxford University Press, 1990), 156. Gill's reference is to David Wiggins, "The person as object of science, subject of experience, and as the locus of value," in A. Peacocke and G. Gillett, eds., *Persons and Personality: A Contemporary Inquiry* (Oxford: Oxford University Press, 1987).

38. Isaiah Berlin, *The Crooked Timber of Humanity* (New York: Vintage Books, 1992), 11. I thank Eric Parens for his suggestion of how this anthology may support Berlin's point.

39. I thank Daniel Callahan for help in formulating the point in this way.

Part I / Theories of Persons

PERSONS AS IMMATERIAL SOULS
OR MINDS

CHAPTER ONE

Selections from the *Phaedo*

Plato

Translated by Benjamin Jowett

Socrates: Do we believe that there is such a thing as death?

To be sure, replied Simmias.

Is it not the separation of soul and body? And to be dead is the completion of this; when the soul exists in herself, and is released from the body and the body is released from the soul, what is this but death?

Just so, he replied.

There is another question, which will probably throw light on our present inquiry if you and I can agree about it:—Ought the philosopher to care about the pleasures—if they are to be called pleasures—of eating and drinking?

Certainly not, answered Simmias.

And what about the pleasures of love—should he care for them?

By no means.

And will he think much of the other ways of indulging the body, for example, the acquisition of costly raiment, or sandals, or other adornments of the body? Instead of caring about them, does he not rather despise anything more than nature needs? What do you say?

I should say that the true philosopher would despise them.

Would you not say that he is entirely concerned with the soul and not with the body? He would like, as far as he can, to get away from the body and to turn to the soul.

Quite true.

In matters of this sort philosophers, above all other men, may be observed in every sort of way to dissever the soul from the communion of the body.

Very true.

Whereas, Simmias, the rest of the world are of opinion that to him who has no sense of pleasure and no part in bodily pleasure, life is not worth having; and that he who is indifferent about them is as good as dead.

That is also true.

What again shall we say of the actual acquirement of knowledge?—is the body, if invited to share in the enquiry, a hinderer or a helper? I mean to say, have sight and hearing any truth in them? Are they not, as the poets are always telling us, inaccurate witnesses? and yet, if even they are inaccurate and indistinct, what is to be said of the other senses?—for you will allow that they are the best of them?

Certainly, he replied.

Then when does the soul attain truth?—for in attempting to consider anything in company with the body she is obviously deceived.

True.

Then must not true existence be revealed to her in thought, if at all?

Yes.

And thought is best when the mind is gathered into herself and none of these things trouble her—neither sounds nor sights nor pain nor any pleasure,—when she takes leave of the body, and has as little as possible to do with it, when she has no bodily sense or desire, but is aspiring after true being?

Certainly.

And in this the philosopher dishonours the body; his soul runs away from his body and desires to be alone and by herself?

That is true.

Well, but there is another thing, Simmias: Is there or is there not an absolute justice?

Assuredly there is.

And an absolute beauty and absolute good?

Of course.

But did you ever behold any of them with your eyes?

Certainly not.

Or did you ever reach them with any other bodily sense?—and I speak not of these alone, but of absolute greatness, and health, and strength, and of the essence or true nature of everything. Has the reality of them ever been perceived by you through the bodily organs? or rather, is not the nearest approach to the knowledge of their several natures made by him who so orders his intellectual vision as to have the most exact conception of the essence of each thing which he considers?

Certainly.

And he attains to the purest knowledge of them who goes to each with the mind alone, not introducing or intruding in the act of thought sight or any other sense together with reason, but with the very light of the mind in her own clearness searches into the very truth of each; he who has got rid, as far as he can, of eyes and ears and, so to speak, of the whole body, these being in his opinion distracting elements which when they infect the soul hinder her from acquiring truth and knowledge—who, if not he, is likely to attain the knowledge of true being?

What you say has a wonderful truth in it, Socrates, replied Simmias.

And when real philosophers consider all these things, will they not be led to make a reflection which they will express in words something like the following? "Have we not found," they will say, "a path of thought which seems to bring us and our argument to the conclusion, that while we are in the body, and while the soul is infected with the evils of the body, our desire will not be satisfied? and our desire is of the truth. For the body is a source of endless trouble to us by reason of the mere requirement of food; and is liable also to diseases which overtake and impede us in the search after true being: it fills us full of loves, and lusts, and fears, and fancies of all kinds, and endless foolery, and in fact, as men say, takes away from us the power of thinking at all. Whence come wars, and fightings, and factions? whence but from the body and the lusts of the body? wars are occasioned by the love of money, and money has to be acquired for the sake and in the service of the body; and by reason of all these impediments we have no time to give to philosophy; and, last and worst of all, even if we are at leisure and betake ourselves to some speculation, the body is always breaking in upon us, causing turmoil and confusion in our enquiries, and so amazing us that we are prevented from seeing the truth. It has been proved to us by experience that if we would have pure knowledge of anything we must be quit of the body—the soul in herself must behold things in themselves: and then we shall attain the wisdom which we desire, and of which we say that we are lovers, not while we live, but after death; for if while in company with the body, the soul cannot have pure knowledge, one of two things follows—either knowledge is not to be attained at all, or, if at all, after death. For then, and not till then, the soul will be parted from the body and exist in herself alone. In this present life, I reckon that we make the nearest approach to knowledge when we have the least possible intercourse or communion with the body, and are not surfeited with the bodily nature, but keep ourselves pure until the hour when God himself is pleased to release us. And thus having got rid of the foolishness of the body we shall be pure and hold converse with the pure, and know of ourselves the clear light everywhere, which is no other than the light of truth." For the impure are not permitted to approach the pure. These are the sort of words, Simmias, which the true lovers of knowledge cannot help saying to one another, and thinking. You would agree; would you not?

Undoubtedly, Socrates.

But, O my friend, if this is true, there is great reason to hope that, going whither I go, when I have come to the end of my journey, I shall attain that which has been the pursuit of my life. And therefore I go on my way rejoicing, and not I only, but every other man who believes that his mind has been made ready and that he is in a manner purified.

Certainly, replied Simmias.

And what is purification but the separation of the soul from the body, as I was saying before; the habit of the soul gathering and collecting herself into herself from all sides out of the body; the dwelling in her own place alone, as in another life, so also in this, as far as she can;—the release of the soul from the chains of the body?

Very true, he said.

And this separation and release of the soul from the body is termed death?

To be sure, he said.

And the true philosophers, and they only, are ever seeking to release the soul. Is not the separation and release of the soul from the body their especial study?

That is true.

And, as I was saying at first, there would be a ridiculous contradiction in men studying to live as nearly as they can in a state of death, and yet repining when it comes upon them.

Clearly.

And the true philosophers, Simmias, are always occupied in the practice of dying, wherefore also to them least of all men is death terrible. Look at the matter thus:—if they have been in every way the enemies of the body, and are wanting to be alone with the soul, when this desire of theirs is granted, how inconsistent would they be if they trembled and repined, instead of rejoicing at their departure to that place where, when they arrive, they hope to gain that which in life they desired—and this was wisdom— and at the same time to be rid of the company of their enemy. Many a man has been willing to go to the world below animated by the hope of seeing there an earthly love, or wife, or son, and conversing with them. And will he who is a true lover of wisdom, and is strongly persuaded in like manner that only in the world below he can worthily enjoy her, still repine at death? Will he not depart with joy? Surely he will, O my friend, if he be a true philosopher. For he will have a firm conviction that there and there only, he can find wisdom in her purity. And if this be true, he would be very absurd, as I was saying, if he were afraid of death.

. . .

The lovers of knowledge are conscious that the soul was simply fastened and glued to the body—until philosophy received her, she could only view real existence through the bars of a prison, not in and through herself; she was wallowing in the mire of every sort of ignorance; and by reason of lust had become the principal accomplice in her own captivity. This was her original state; and then, as I was saying, and as the lovers of knowledge are well aware, philosophy, seeing how terrible was her confinement, of which she was to herself the cause, received and gently comforted her and sought to release her, pointing out that the eye and the ear and the other senses are full of deception, and persuading her to retire from them, and abstain from all but the necessary use of them, and be gathered up and collected into herself, bidding her trust in herself and her own pure apprehension of pure existence, and to mistrust whatever comes to her through other channels and is subject to variation; for such things are visible and tangible, but what she sees in her own nature is intelligible and invisible. And the soul of the true philosopher thinks that she ought not to resist this deliverance, and therefore abstains from pleasures and desires and pains and fears, as far as she is able; reflecting that when a man has great joys or sorrows or fears or desires, he suffers from them, not merely the sort of evil which might be anticipated—as for example, the loss of his health or property which he has sacrificed to his lusts—but an evil greater far, which is the greatest and worst of all evils, and one of which he never thinks.

What is it, Socrates? said Cebes.

The evil is that when the feeling of pleasure or pain is most intense, every soul of man imagines the objects of this intense feeling to be then plainest and truest: but this is not so, they are really the things of sight.

Very true.

And is not this the state in which the soul is most enthralled by the body?

How so?

Why, because each pleasure and pain is a sort of nail which nails and rivets the soul to the body, until she becomes like the body, and believes that to be true which the body affirms to be true; and from agreeing with the body and having the same delights she is obliged to have the same habits and haunts, and is not likely ever to be pure at her departure to the world below, but is always infected by the body; and so she sinks into another body and there germinates and grows, and has therefore no part in the communion of the divine and pure and simple.

Most true, Socrates, answered Cebes.

And this, Cebes, is the reason why the true lovers of knowledge are temperate and brave; and not for the reason which the world gives.

Certainly not.

Certainly not! The soul of a philosopher will reason in quite another way; she will not ask philosophy to release her in order that when released she may deliver herself up again to the thraldom of pleasures and pains, doing a work only to be undone again, weaving instead of unweaving her Penelope's web. But she will calm passion, and follow reason, and dwell in the contemplation of her, beholding the true and divine (which is not matter of opinion), and thence deriving nourishment. Thus she seeks to live while she lives, and after death she hopes to go to her own kindred and to that which is like her, and to be freed from human ills. Never fear, Simmias and Cebes, that a soul which has been thus nurtured and has had these pursuits, will at her departure from the body be scattered and blown away by the winds and be nowhere and nothing.

CHAPTER TWO

Selections from *Meditations on First Philosophy*

René Descartes

Meditation Two: Concerning the Nature of the Human Mind: That It Is Better Known Than the Body

Yesterday's meditation has thrown me into such doubts that I can no longer ignore them, yet I fail to see how they are to be resolved. It is as if I had suddenly fallen into a deep whirlpool; I am so tossed about that I can neither touch bottom with my foot, nor swim up to the top. Nevertheless I will work my way up and will once again attempt the same path I entered upon yesterday. I will accomplish this by putting aside everything that admits of the least doubt, as if I had discovered it to be completely false. I will stay on this course until I know something certain, or, if nothing else, until I at least know for certain that nothing is certain. Archimedes sought but one firm and immovable point in order to move the entire earth from one place to another. Just so, great things are also to be hoped for if I succeed in finding just one thing, however slight, that is certain and unshaken.

Therefore I suppose that everything I see is false. I believe that none of what my deceitful memory represents ever existed. I have no senses whatever. Body, shape, extension, movement, and place are all chimeras. What then will be true? Perhaps just the single fact that nothing is certain.

But how do I know there is not something else, over and above all those things that I have just reviewed, concerning which there is not even the slightest occasion for doubt? Is there not some God, or by whatever name I might call him, who instills these very thoughts in me? But why would I think that, since I myself could perhaps be the author of these thoughts? Am I not then at least something? But I have already denied that I have any senses and any body. Still I hesitate; for what follows from this? Am I so tied to a body and to the senses that I cannot exist without them? But I have persuaded myself that there is absolutely nothing in the world: no sky, no earth, no minds, no bodies. Is it then the case that I too do not exist? But doubtless I did exist, if I persuaded myself of something. But there is some deceiver or other who is supremely powerful and supremely sly and who is always deliberately deceiving me. Then too there is no doubt that I exist, if he is deceiving me. And let him do his best at deception, he will never bring it about that I am nothing so long as I shall think that I am something. Thus, after everything has been most carefully weighed, it must finally be established that this pronouncement "I am, I exist" is necessarily true every time I utter it or conceive it in my mind.

But I do not yet understand sufficiently what I am—I, who now necessarily exist. And so from this point on, I must be careful lest I unwittingly mistake something else for myself, and thus err in that very item of knowledge that I claim to be the most certain and evident of all. Thus, I will meditate once more on what I once believed myself to be, prior to embarking upon these thoughts. For this reason, then, I will set aside whatever can be weakened even to the slightest degree by the arguments brought forward, so that eventually all that remains is precisely nothing but what is certain and unshaken.

What then did I use to think I was? A man, of course. But what is a man? Might I not say a "rational animal"? No, because then I would have to inquire what "animal" and "rational" mean. And thus from one question I would slide into many more difficult ones. Nor do I now have enough free time that I want to waste it on subtleties of this sort. Instead, permit me to focus here on what came spontaneously and naturally into my thinking whenever I pondered what I was. Now it occurred to me first that I had a face, hands, arms, and this entire mechanism of bodily members: the very same as are discerned in a corpse, and which I referred to by the name "body." It next occurred to me that I took in food, that I walked about, and that I sensed and thought various things; these actions I used to attribute to the soul. But as to what this soul might be, I either did not think about it or else I imagined it a rarified I-know-not-what, like a wind, or a fire, or ether, which had been infused into my coarser parts. But as to the body I was not in any doubt. On the contrary, I was under the impression that I knew its nature distinctly. Were I perhaps tempted to describe this nature such as I conceived it in my mind, I would have described it thus: by "body," I understand all that is capable of being bounded by some shape, of being enclosed in a place, and of filling up a space in such a way as to exclude any other body from it; of being perceived by touch, sight, hearing, taste, or smell; of being moved in several ways, not, of course, by itself, but by whatever else impinges upon it. For it was my view that the power of self-motion, and likewise of sensing or of thinking, in no way belonged to the nature of the body. Indeed I used rather to marvel that such faculties were to be found in certain bodies.

But now what am I, when I suppose that there is some supremely powerful and, if I may be permitted to say so, malicious deceiver who deliberately tries to fool me in any way he can? Can I not affirm that I possess at least a small measure of all those things which I have already said belong to the nature of the body? I focus my attention on them, I think about them, I review them again, but nothing comes to mind. I am tired of repeating this to no purpose. But what about those things I ascribed to the soul? What about being nourished or moving about? Since I now do not have a body, these are surely nothing but fictions. What about sensing? Surely this too does not take place without a body; and I seemed to have sensed in my dreams many things that I later realized I did not sense. What about thinking? Here I make my discovery: thought exists; it alone cannot be separated from me. I am; I exist—this is certain. But for how long? For as long as I am thinking; for perhaps it could also come to pass that if I were to cease all thinking I would then utterly cease to exist. At this time I admit nothing that is not necessarily true. I am therefore precisely nothing but a thinking thing; that is, a mind, or intellect, or understanding, or reason—words of whose meanings I was previously ignorant. Yet I am a true thing and am truly existing; but what kind of thing? I have said it already: a thinking thing.

What else am I? I will set my imagination in motion. I am not that concatenation of members we call the human body. Neither am I even some subtle air infused into these members, nor a wind, nor a fire, nor a vapor, nor a breath, nor anything I devise for myself. For I have supposed these things to be nothing. The assumption still stands; yet nevertheless I am something. But is it perhaps the case that these very things which I take to be nothing, because they are unknown to me, nevertheless are in fact no different from that "me" that I know?

This I do not know, and I will not quarrel about it now. I can make a judgment only about things that are known to me. I know that I exist; I ask now who is this "I" whom I know? Most certainly, in the strict sense the knowledge of this "I" does not depend upon things of whose existence I do not yet have knowledge. Therefore it is not dependent upon any of those things that I simulate in my imagination. But this word "simulate" warns me of my error. For I would indeed be simulating were I to "imagine" that I was something, because imagining is merely the contemplating of the shape or image of a corporeal thing. But I now know with certainty that I am and also that all these images—and, generally, everything belonging to the nature of the body—could turn out to be nothing but dreams. Once I have realized this, I would seem to be speaking no less foolishly were I to say: "I will use my imagination in order to recognize more distinctly who I am," than were I to say: "Now I surely am awake, and I see something true; but since I do not yet see it clearly enough, I will deliberately fall asleep so that my dreams might represent it to me more truly and more clearly." Thus I realize that none of what I can grasp by means of the imagination pertains to this knowledge that I have of myself. Moreover, I realize that I must be most diligent about withdrawing my mind from these things so that it can perceive its nature as distinctly as possible.

But what then am I? A thing that thinks. What is that? A thing that doubts, understands, affirms, denies, wills, refuses, and that also imagines and senses.

Indeed it is no small matter if all of these things belong to me. But why should they not belong to me? Is it not the very same "I" who now doubts almost everything, who nevertheless understands something, who affirms that this one thing is true, who denies other things, who desires to know more, who wishes not to be deceived, who imagines many things even against my will, who also notices many things which appear to come from the senses? What is there in all of this that is not every bit as true as the fact that I exist—even if I am always asleep or even if my creator makes every effort to mislead me? Which of these things is distinct from my thought? Which of them can be said to be separate from myself? For it is so obvious that it is I who doubt, I who understand, and I who will, that there is nothing by which it could be explained more clearly. But indeed it is also the same "I" who imagines; for although perhaps, as I supposed before, absolutely nothing that I imagined is true, still the very power of imagining really does exist, and constitutes a part of my thought. Finally, it is this same "I" who senses or who is cognizant of bodily things as if through the senses. For example, I now see a light, I hear a noise, I feel heat. These things are false, since I am asleep. Yet I certainly do seem to see, hear, and feel warmth. This cannot be false. Properly speaking, this is what in me is called "sensing." But this, precisely so taken, is nothing other than thinking.

From these considerations I am beginning to know a little better what I am. But it still seems (and I cannot resist believing) that corporeal things—whose images are formed by thought, and which the senses themselves examine—are much more distinctly known than this mysterious "I" which does not fall within the imagination. And yet it would be strange indeed were I to grasp the very things I consider to be doubtful, unknown, and foreign to me more distinctly than what is true, what is known—than, in short, myself. But I see what is happening: my mind loves to wander and does not yet permit itself to be restricted within the confines of truth. So be it then; let us just this once allow it completely free rein, so that, a little while later, when the time has come to pull in the reins, the mind may more readily permit itself to be controlled. . . .

Meditation Six: Concerning the Existence of Material Things, and the Real Distinction between Mind and Body

. . . But now, having begun to have a better knowledge of myself and the author of my origin, I am of the opinion that I must not rashly admit everything that I seem to derive from the senses; but neither, for that matter, should I call everything into doubt.

First, I know that all the things that I clearly and distinctly understand can be made by God such as I understand them. For this reason, my ability clearly and distinctly to understand one thing without another suffices to make me certain that the one thing is different from the other, since they can be separated from each other, at least by God. The question as to the sort of power that might effect such a separation is not relevant to their being thought to be different. For this reason, from the fact that I know that I exist, and that at the same time I judge that obviously nothing else belongs to my nature or essence except that I am a thinking thing, I rightly conclude that my essence consists entirely in my being a thinking thing. And although perhaps (or rather, as I shall soon say, assuredly) I have a body that is very closely joined to me, nevertheless, because on the one hand I have a clear and distinct idea of myself, insofar as I am merely a thinking thing and not an extended thing, and because on the other hand I have a distinct idea of a body, insofar as it is merely an extended thing and not a thinking thing, it is certain that I am really distinct from my body, and can exist without it.

Moreover, I find in myself faculties for certain special modes of thinking, namely the faculties of imagining and sensing. I can clearly and distinctly understand myself in my entirety without these faculties, but not vice versa: I cannot understand them clearly and distinctly without me, that is, without a substance endowed with understanding in which they inhere, for they include an act of understanding in their formal concept. Thus I perceive them to be distinguished from me as modes from a thing. I also acknowledge that there are certain other faculties, such as those of moving from one place to another, of taking on various shapes, and so on, that, like sensing or imagining, cannot be understood apart from some substance in which they inhere, and hence without which they cannot exist. But it is clear that these faculties, if in fact they exist, must be in a corporeal or extended substance, not in a substance endowed with understanding. For some extension is contained in a clear and distinct concept of them, though certainly not any understanding. Now there clearly is in me a passive faculty of sensing, that is, a faculty for receiving and knowing the ideas of sensible things; but I could not use it unless there also existed, either in me or in something else, a certain active faculty of producing or bringing about these ideas. But this faculty surely cannot be in me, since it clearly presupposes no act of understanding, and these ideas are produced without my cooperation and often even against my will. Therefore the only alternative is that it is in some substance different from me, containing either formally or eminently all the reality that exists objectively in the ideas produced by that faculty, as I have just noted above. Hence this substance is either a body, that is, a corporeal nature, which contains formally all that is contained objectively in the ideas, or else it is God, or some other creature more noble than a body, which contains eminently all that is contained objectively in the ideas. But since God is not a deceiver, it is patently obvious that he does not send me these ideas either immediately by himself, or even through the mediation of some creature that contains the objective reality of these ideas not formally but only eminently. For since God has given me no faculty whatsoever for making this determination, but instead has given me a great inclination to believe that these ideas issue from corporeal things, I fail to see how God could be understood not to be a deceiver, if these ideas were to issue from a source other than corporeal things. And consequently corporeal things exist. Nevertheless, perhaps not all bodies exist exactly as I grasp them by sense, since this sensory grasp is in many cases very obscure and confused. But at least they do contain everything I clearly and distinctly understand—that is, everything, considered in a general sense, that is encompassed in the object of pure mathematics.

As far as the remaining matters are concerned, which are either merely particular (for example, that the sun is of such and such a size or shape, and so on) or less clearly understood (for example, light, sound, pain, and the like), even though these matters are very doubtful and uncertain, nevertheless the fact that God is no deceiver (and thus no falsity can be found in my opinions, unless there is also in me a faculty given me by God for the purpose of rectifying this falsity) offers me a definite hope of reaching the truth even in these matters. And surely there is no doubt that all that I am taught by nature has some truth to it; for by "nature," taken generally, I understand nothing other than God himself or the ordered network of created things which was instituted by God. By my own particular nature I understand nothing other than the combination of all the things bestowed upon me by God.

There is nothing that this nature teaches me more explicitly than that I have a body that is ill-disposed when I feel pain, that needs food and drink when I suffer hunger or thirst, and the like. Therefore, I should not doubt that there is some truth in this.

By means of these sensations of pain, hunger, thirst and so on, nature also teaches not merely that I am present to my body in the way a sailor is present in a ship, but that I am most tightly joined and, so to speak, commingled with it, so much so that I and the body constitute one single thing. For if this were not the case, then I, who am only a thinking thing, would not sense pain when the body is injured; rather, I would perceive the wound by means of the pure intellect, just as a sailor perceives by sight whether anything in his ship is broken. And when the body is in need of food or drink, I should understand this explicitly, instead of having confused sensations of hunger and thirst. For clearly these sensations of thirst, hunger, pain, and so on are nothing but certain confused modes of thinking arising from the union and, as it were, the commingling of the mind with the body.

Moreover, I am also taught by nature that various other bodies exist around my body, some of which are to be pursued, while others are to be avoided. And to be sure, from the fact that I sense a wide variety of colors, sounds, odors, tastes, levels of heat, and grades of roughness, and the like, I rightly conclude that in the bodies from which these different perceptions of the senses proceed there are differences corresponding to the different perceptions—though perhaps the latter do not resemble the former. And from the fact that some of these perceptions are pleasant while others are unpleasant, it is plainly certain that my body, or rather my whole self, insofar as I am comprised of a body and a mind, can be affected by various beneficial and harmful bodies in the vicinity.

Granted, there are many other things that I seem to have been taught by nature; nevertheless it was not really nature that taught them to me but a certain habit of making reckless judgments. And thus it could easily happen that these judgments are false: for example, that any space where there is absolutely nothing happening to move my senses is empty; or that there is something in a hot body that bears an exact likeness to the idea of heat that is in me; or that in a white or green body there is the same whiteness or greenness that I sense; or that in a bitter or sweet body there is the same taste, and so on; or that stars and towers and any other distant bodies have the same size and shape that they present to my senses, and other things of this sort. But to ensure that my perceptions in this matter are sufficiently distinct, I ought to define more precisely what exactly I mean when I say that I am "taught something by nature." For I am taking "nature" here more narrowly than the combination of everything bestowed on me by God. For this combination embraces many things that belong exclusively to my mind, such as my perceiving that what has been done cannot be undone, and everything else that is known by the light of nature. That is not what I am talking about here. There are also many things that belong exclusively to the body, such as that it tends to move downward, and so on. I am not dealing with these either, but only with what God has bestowed on me insofar as I am comprised of mind and body. Accordingly, it is this nature that teaches me to avoid things that produce a sensation of pain and to pursue things that produce a sensation of pleasure, and the like. But it does not appear that nature teaches us to conclude anything, besides these things, from these sense perceptions unless the intellect has first conducted its own inquiry regarding things external to us. For it seems to belong exclusively to the mind, and not to the composite of mind and body, to know the truth in these matters. Thus, although a star affects my eye no more than does the flame from a small torch, still there is no real or positive tendency in my eye toward believing that the star is no larger than the flame. Yet, ever since my youth, I have made this judgment without any reason for doing so. And although I feel heat as I draw closer to the fire, and I also feel pain upon drawing too close to it, there is not a single argument that persuades me that there is something in the fire similar to that heat, any more than to that pain. On the contrary, I am convinced only that there is something in the fire that, regardless of what it finally turns out to be, causes in us those sensations of heat or pain. And although there may be nothing in a given space that moves the senses, it does not therefore follow that there is no body in it. But I see that in these and many other instances I have been in the habit of subverting the order of nature. For admittedly I use the perceptions of the senses (which are properly given by nature only for signifying to the mind what things are useful or harmful to the composite of which it is a part, and to that extent they are clear and distinct enough) as reliable rules for immediately discerning what is the essence of bodies located outside us. Yet they signify nothing about that except quite obscurely and confusedly.

I have already examined in sufficient detail how it could happen that my judgments are false, despite the goodness of God. But a new difficulty now arises regarding those very things that nature shows me are either to be sought out or avoided, as well as the internal sensations where I seem to have detected errors, as for example, when someone is deluded by a food's pleasant taste to eat the poison hidden inside it. In this case, however, he is driven by nature only toward desiring the thing in which the pleasurable taste is found, but not toward the poison, of which he obviously is unaware. I can only conclude that this nature is not omniscient. This is not remarkable, since man is a limited thing, and thus only what is of limited perfection befits him.

But we not infrequently err even in those things to which nature impels us. Take, for example, the case of those who are ill and who desire food or drink that will soon afterwards be injurious to them. Perhaps it could be said here that they erred because their nature was corrupt. However, this does not remove our difficulty, for a sick man is no less a creature of God than a healthy one, and thus it seems no less inconsistent that the sick man got a deception-prone nature from God. And a clock made of wheels and counter-weights follows all the laws of nature no less closely when it has been badly constructed and does not tell time accurately than it does when it completely satisfies the wish of its maker. Likewise, I might regard a man's body as a kind of mechanism that is outfitted with and composed of bones, nerves, muscles, veins, blood and skin in such a way that, even if no mind existed in it, the man's body would still exhibit all the same motions that are in it now except for those motions that proceed either from a command of the will or, consequently, from the mind. I easily recognize that it would be natural for this body, were it, say, suffering from dropsy and experiencing dryness in the throat (which typically produces a thirst sensation in the mind), and also so disposed by its nerves and other parts to take something to drink, the result of which would be to exacerbate the illness. This is as natural as for a body without any such illness to be moved by the same dryness in the throat to take something to drink that is useful to it. And given the intended purpose of the clock, I could say that it deviates from its nature when it fails to tell the right time. And similarly, considering the mechanism of the human body in terms of its being equipped for the motions that typically occur in it, I may think that it too is deviating from its nature, if its throat were dry when having something to drink is not beneficial to its conservation. Nevertheless, I am well aware that this last use of "nature" differs greatly from the other. For this latter "nature" is merely a designation dependent on my thought, since it compares a man in poor health and a poorly constructed clock with the ideas of a healthy man and of a well-made clock, a designation extrinsic to the things to which it is applied. But by "nature" taken in the former sense, I understand something that is really in things, and thus is not without some truth.

When we say, then, in the case of the body suffering from dropsy, that its "nature" is corrupt, given the fact that it has a parched throat and yet does not need something to drink, "nature" obviously is merely an extrinsic designation. Nevertheless, in the case of the composite, that is, of a mind joined to such a body, it is not a pure designation, but a true error of nature that this body should be thirsty when having something to drink would be harmful to it. It therefore remains to inquire here how the goodness of God does not prevent "nature," thus considered, from being deceptive.

Now my first observation here is that there is a great difference between a mind and a body in that a body, by its very nature, is always divisible. On the other hand, the mind is utterly indivisible. For when I consider the mind, that is, myself insofar as I am only a thinking thing, I cannot distinguish any parts within me; rather, I understand myself to be manifestly one complete thing. Although the entire mind seems to be united to the entire body, nevertheless, were a foot or an arm or any other bodily part to be amputated, I know that nothing has been taken away from the mind on that account. Nor can the faculties of willing, sensing, understanding, and so on be called "parts" of the mind, since it is one and the same mind that wills, senses, and understands. On the other hand, there is no corporeal or extended thing I can think of that I may not in my thought easily divide into parts; and in this way I understand that it is divisible. This consideration alone would suffice to teach me that the mind is wholly diverse from the body, had I not yet known it well enough in any other way.

My second observation is that my mind is not immediately affected by all the parts of the body, but only by the brain, or perhaps even by just one small part of the brain, namely, by that part where the "common" sense is said to reside. Whenever this part of the brain is disposed in the same manner, it presents the same thing to the mind, even if the other parts of the body are able meanwhile to be related in diverse ways. Countless experiments show this, none of which need be reviewed here.

My next observation is that the nature of the body is such that whenever any of its parts can be moved by another part some distance away, it can also be moved in the same manner by any of the parts that lie between them, even if this more distant part is doing nothing. For example, in the cord ABCD, if the final part D is pulled, the first part A would be moved in exactly the same manner as it could be, if one of the intermediate parts B or C were pulled, while the end part D remained immobile. Likewise, when I feel a pain in my foot, physics teaches me that this sensation took place by means of nerves distributed throughout the foot, like stretched cords extending from the foot all the way to the brain. When these nerves are pulled in the foot, they also pull on the inner parts of the brain to which they extend, and produce a certain motion in them. This motion has been constituted by nature so as to affect the mind with a sensation of pain, as if it occurred in the foot. But because these nerves need to pass through the shin, thigh, loins, back, and neck to get from the foot to the brain, it can happen that even if it is not the part in the foot but merely one of the intermediate parts that is being struck, the very same movement will occur in the brain that would occur were the foot badly injured. The inevitable result will be that the mind feels the same pain. The same opinion should hold for any other sensation.

My final observation is that, since any given motion occurring in that part of the brain immediately affecting the mind produces but one sensation in it, I can think of no better arrangement than that it produces the one sensation that, of all the ones it is able to produce, is most especially and most often conducive to the maintenance of a healthy man. Moreover, experience shows that all the sensations bestowed on us by nature are like this. Hence there is absolutely nothing to be found in them that does not bear witness to God's power and goodness. Thus, for example, when the nerves in the foot are agitated in a violent and unusual manner, this motion of theirs extends through the marrow of the spine to the inner reaches of the brain, where it gives the mind the sign to sense something, namely, the pain as if it is occurring in the foot. This provokes the mind to do its utmost to move away from the cause of the pain, since it is seen as harmful to the foot. But the nature of man could have been so constituted by God that this same motion in the brain might have indicated something else to the mind: for example, either the motion itself as it occurs in the brain, or in the foot, or in some place in between, or something else entirely different. But nothing else would have served so well the maintenance of the body. Similarly, when we need something to drink, a certain dryness arises in the throat that moves the nerves in the throat, and, by means of them, the inner parts of the brain. And this motion affects the mind with a sensation of thirst, because in this entire affair nothing is more useful for us to know than that we need something to drink in order to maintain our health; the same holds in the other cases.

From these considerations it is utterly apparent that, notwithstanding the immense goodness of God, the nature of man, insofar as it is composed of mind and body, cannot help being sometimes mistaken. For if some cause, not in the foot but in some other part through which the nerves extend from the foot to the brain, or perhaps even in the brain itself, were to produce the same motion that would normally be produced by a badly injured foot, the pain will be felt as if it were in the foot, and the senses will naturally be deceived. For since an identical motion in the brain can only bring about an identical sensation in the mind, and it is more frequently the case that this motion is wont to arise on account of a cause that harms the foot than on account of some other thing existing elsewhere, it is reasonable that the motion should always show pain to the mind as something belonging to the foot rather than to some other part. And if dryness in the throat does not arise, as is normal, because taking something to drink contributes to bodily health, but from a contrary cause, as happens in the case of someone with dropsy, then it is far better that it should deceive on that occasion than that it should always be deceptive when the body is in good health. The same holds for the other cases. . . .

CHAPTER THREE

Selections from "Personal Identity: The Dualist Theory"

Richard Swinburne

The brain transplant considerations of the first section leading to the simple view of personal identity showed that significant continuity of brain and memory was not enough to ensure personal identity. They did not show that continuity of brain or memory were totally dispensable; that P_2 at time t_2 could be the same person as P_1 at an earlier time t_1, even though P_2 had none of the brain matter (or other bodily matter) of P_1 and had no apparent memory of P_1's actions and experiences. A number of more extravagant thought-experiments do, however, show that there is no contradiction in this latter supposition.

There seems no contradiction in the supposition that a person might acquire a totally new body (including a completely new brain)—as many religious accounts of life after death claim that men do. To say that this body, sitting at the desk in my room is my body is to say two things. First it is to say that I can move parts of this body (arms, legs, etc.), just like that, without having to do any other intentional action and that I can make a difference to other physical objects only by moving parts of this body. By holding the door handle and turning my hand, I open the door. By bending my leg and stretching it I kick the ball and make it move into the goal. But I do not turn my hand or bend my leg by doing some other intentional action; I just do these things.[1] Secondly, it is to say that my knowledge of states of the world outside this body is derived from their effects on this body—I learn about the positions of physical objects by seeing them, and seeing them involves light rays reflected by them impinging on my eyes and setting up nervous impulses in my optic nerve. My body is the vehicle of my agency in the world and my knowledge of the world. But then is it not coherent to suppose that I might suddenly find that my present body no longer served this function, that I could no longer acquire information through these eyes or move these limbs, but might discover that another body served the same function? I might find myself moving other limbs and acquiring information through other eyes. Then I would have a totally new body. If that body, like my last body, was an occupant of the Earth, then we would have a case of reincarnation, as Eastern religions have understood that. If that body was an occupant of some distant planet, or an environment which did not belong to the same space[2] as our world, then we would have a case of resurrection as on the whole Western religions (Christianity, Judaism and Islam) have understood that.

This suggestion of a man acquiring a new body (with brain) may be more plausible, to someone who has difficulty in grasping it, by supposing the event to occur gradually. Suppose that one morning a man wakes up to find himself unable to control the right side of his body, including his right arm and leg. When he tries to move the right-side parts of his body, he finds that the corresponding left-side parts of his body move; and when he tries to move the left-side parts, the corresponding right-side parts of his wife's body move. His knowledge of the world comes to depend on stimuli to his left side and to his wife's right side (e.g., light rays stimulating his left eye and his wife's right eye). The bodies fuse to some extent physiologically as with Siamese twins, while the man's wife loses control of her right side. The focus of the man's control of and knowledge of the world is shifting. One may suppose the process completed as the man's control is shifted to the wife's body, while the wife loses control of it.

Equally coherent, I suggest, is the supposition that a person might become disembodied. A person has a body if there is one particular chunk of matter through which he has to operate on and learn about the world. But suppose that he finds himself able to operate on and learn about the world within some small finite region, without having to use one particular chunk of matter for this purpose. He might find himself with knowledge of the position of objects in a room (perhaps by having visual sensations, perhaps not), and able to move such objects just like that, in the ways in which we know about the positions of our limbs and can move them. But the room would not be, as it were, the person's body; for we may suppose that simply by choosing to do so he can gradually shift the focus of his knowledge and control, e.g., to the next room. The person would be in no way limited to operating and learning through one particular chunk of matter. Hence we may term him disembodied. The supposition that a person might become disembodied also seems coherent.

I have been arguing so far that it is coherent to suppose that a person could continue to exist with an entirely new body or with no body at all. . . . Could a person continue to exist without any apparent memory of his previous doings? Quite clearly, we do allow not merely the logical possibility, but the frequent actuality of amnesia—a person forgetting all or certain stretches of his past life. Despite Locke, many a person does forget much of what he has done. But, of course, we normally only suppose this to happen in cases where there is the normal bodily and brain continuity. Our grounds for supposing that a person forgets what he has done are that the evidence of bodily and brain continuity suggests that he was the previous person who did certain things, which he now cannot remember having done. And in the absence of both of the main kinds of evidence for personal identity, we would not be justified in supposing that personal identity held. . . . For that reason I cannot describe a case where we would have good reason to suppose that P_2 was identical with P_1, even though there was neither brain continuity nor memory continuity between them. However, only given verificationist dogma, is there any reason to suppose that the only things which are true are those of whose truth we can have evidence, and . . . that there is no good reason for believing verificationism to be true. We can make sense of states of affairs being true, of which we can have no evidence that they are true. And among them surely is the supposition that the person who acquires another body loses not merely control of the old one, but memories of what he did with its aid. Again, many religions have taken seriously stories of persons passing through the waters of Lethe (a river whose waters made a person forget all his previous life) and then acquiring a new body. Others who have heard these stories may not have believed them true; but they have usually claimed to understand them, and (unless influenced by philosophical dogma) have not suspected them of involving contradiction.

Those who hope to survive their death, despite the destruction of their body, will not necessarily be disturbed if they come to believe that they will then have no memory of their past life on Earth; they may just want to survive and have no interest in continuing to recall life on Earth. Again, apparently, there seems to be no contradiction involved in their belief. It seems to be a coherent belief (whether or not true or justified). Admittedly, there may be stories or beliefs which involve a hidden contradiction when initially they do not seem to do so. But the fact that there seems (and to so many people) to be no contradiction hidden in these stories is good reason for supposing that there is no contradiction hidden in them—until a contradiction is revealed. If this were not a good reason for believing there to be no contradiction, we would have no good reason for believing any sentence at all to be free of hidden contradiction.

Not merely is it not logically necessary that a person have a body made of certain matter, or have certain apparent memories, if he is to be the person which he is; it is not even necessitated by laws of nature.[3] For let us assume that natural laws dictated the course of evolution and the emergence of consciousness. In 4000 million BC the Earth was a cooling globe of inanimate atoms. Natural laws then, we assume, dictated how this globe would evolve, and so which arrangements of matter will be the bodies of conscious men, and just how apparent memories of conscious men depend on their brain states. My point now is that what natural laws in no way determine is which animate body is yours and which is mine. Just the same arrangement of matter and just the same laws could have given to me the body (and so the apparent memories) which are now yours, and to you the body (and so the apparent memories) which are now mine. It needs either God or chance to allocate bodies to persons; the most that natural laws determine is that bodies of a certain construction are the bodies of some person or other, who in consequence of this construction have certain apparent memories. Since the body which is presently yours (together with the associated apparent memories) could have been mine (logic and even natural laws allow), that shows that none of the matter of which my body is presently made (nor the apparent memories) is essential to my being the person I am. That must be determined by something else.

The view that personal identity is something ultimate, unanalyzable in terms of such observable and experienceable phenomena as bodily continuity and continuity of memory, was put forward in the eighteenth century by Butler, and, slightly less explicitly, by Reid. In recent years R. M. Chisholm (1969) has put forward a similar view.

I could just leave my positive theory at that—that personal identity is unanalyzable. But it will, I hope, be useful to express it in another way, to bring out more clearly what it involves and to connect it with another whole tradition of philosophical thought.

In section I, I set out Aristotle's account of the identity of substances: that a substance at one time is the same substance as a substance at an earlier time if and only if the later substance has the same form as, and continuity of matter. . . . with, the earlier substance. On this view a person is the same person as an earlier person if he has the same form as the earlier person (i.e., both are persons) and has continuity of matter with him (i.e., has the same body).

Certainly, to be the same person as an earlier person, a later person has to have the same form—i.e., has to be a person. If my arguments for the logical possibility of there being disembodied persons are correct, then the essential characteristics of a person constitute a narrower set than those which Aristotle would have included. My arguments suggest that all that a person needs to be a person are certain mental capacities—for having conscious experiences (e.g., thoughts or sensations) and performing intentional actions. Thought-experiments of the kind described earlier allow that a person might lose his body, but they describe his continuing to have conscious experiences and his performing or being able to perform intentional actions, i.e., to do actions which he means to do, bring about effects for some purpose.

Yet if my arguments are correct, showing that two persons can be the same, even if there is no continuity between their bodily matter, we must say that in the form stated the Aristotelian account of identity applies only to inanimate objects and plants and has no application to personal identity.[4] We are then faced with a choice either of saying that the criteria of personal identity are different from those for other substances, or of trying to give a more general account than Aristotle's of the identity of substances which would cover both persons and other substances. It is possible to widen the Aristotelian account so that we can do the latter. We have only to say that two substances are the same if and only if they have the same form and there is continuity of the stuff of which they are made, and allow that there may be kinds of stuff other than matter. I will call this account of substance identity the wider Aristotelian account. We may say that there is a stuff of another kind, immaterial stuff, and that persons are made of both normal bodily matter and of this immaterial stuff but that it is the continuity of the latter which provides that continuity of stuff which is necessary for the identity of the person over time.

This is in essence the way of expressing the simple theory which is adopted by those who say that a person living on Earth consists of two parts—a material part, the body; and an immaterial part, the soul. The soul is the essential part of a person, and it is its continuing which constitutes the continuing of the person. While on Earth, the soul is linked to a body (by the body being the vehicle of the person's knowledge of and action upon the physical world). But, it is logically possible, the soul can be separated from the body and exist in a disembodied state (in the way described earlier) or linked to a new body. This way of expressing things has been used in many religious traditions down the centuries, for it is a very natural way of expressing what is involved in being a person once you allow that a person can survive the death of his body. Classical philosophical statements of it are to be found in Plato and, above all, in Descartes. I shall call this view classical dualism.

I wrote that "in essence" classical dualism is the view that there is more stuff to the person than bodily matter, and that it is the continuing of this stuff which is necessary for the continuing of the person, because a writer such as Descartes did not distinguish between the immaterial stuff, let us call it soul-stuff, and that stuff being organized (with or without a body) as one soul. Descartes and other classical dualists however did not make this distinction, because they assumed (implicitly) that it was not logically possible that persons divide—i.e., that an earlier person could be in part the same person as each of two later persons. Hence they implicitly assumed that soul-stuff comes in essentially indivisible units. That is indeed what one has to say about soul-stuff, if one makes the supposition . . . , that it is not logically possible that persons divide. There is nothing odd about supposing that soul-stuff comes in essentially indivisible units. Of any chunk of matter, however small, it is always logically, if not physically, possible that it be divided into two. Yet it is because matter is extended, that one can always make sense of it being divided. For a chunk of matter necessarily takes up a finite volume of space. A finite volume of space necessarily is composed of two half-volumes. So it always makes sense to suppose that part of the chunk which occupies the left half-volume of space to be separated from that part of the chunk which occupies the right half-volume. But that kind of consideration has no application to immaterial stuff. There is no reason why there should not be a kind of immaterial stuff which necessarily is indivisible; and if the supposition is correct, the soul-stuff will have that property.

So then—once we modify the Aristotelian understanding of the criteria for the identity of substances, the simple view of personal identity finds a natural expression in classical dualism. The arguments which Descartes gave in support of his account of persons are among the arguments which I have given in favour of the simple theory and since they take for granted the wider Aristotelian framework, they yield classical dualism as a consequence. Thus Descartes argues:

> Just because I know certainly that I exist, and that meanwhile I do not remark that any other thing necessarily pertains to my nature or essence, excepting that I am

a thinking thing, I rightly conclude that my essence consists solely in the fact that
I am a thinking thing. And although possibly . . . I possess a body with which I am
very intimately conjoined, yet because, on the one side, I have a clear and distinct
idea of myself inasmuch as I am only a thinking and unextended thing, and as, on
the other, I possess a distinct idea of body, inasmuch as it is only an extended and
unthinking thing, it is certain that this I [that is to say, my soul by which I am what
I am], is entirely and absolutely distinct from my body, and can exist without it.[5]

Descartes is here saying that he can describe a thought-experiment in which
he continues to exist, although his body does not. I have also described such a
thought-experiment and have argued, as Descartes in effect does, that it follows
that his body is not logically necessary for his existence, that it is not an essential
part of himself. Descartes can go on "thinking" (i.e., being conscious) and so
existing without it. Now if we take the wider Aristotelian framework for granted
that the continuing of a substance involves the continuing of some of the stuff
of which it is made, and since the continuing existence of Descartes does not
involve the continuing of bodily matter, it follows that there must now be as
part of Descartes some other stuff, which he calls his soul, which forms the
essential part of Descartes.

Given that for any present person who is currently conscious, there is no
logical impossibility, whatever else may be true now of that person, that that
person continue to exist without his body, it follows that that person must now
actually have a part other than a bodily part which can continue, and which we
may call his soul—and so that his possession of it is entailed by his being a
conscious thing. For there is not even a logical possibility that if I now consist
of nothing but matter and the matter is destroyed, that I should nevertheless
continue to exist. From the mere logical possibility of my continued existence
there follows the actual fact that there is now more to me than my body; and
that more is the essential part of myself. A person's being conscious is thus to
be analyzed as an immaterial core of himself, his soul being conscious.[6]

So Descartes argues, and his argument seems to me correct—given the wider
Aristotelian framework. If we are prepared to say that substances can be the
same, even though none of the stuff (in a wide sense) of which they are made is
the same, the conclusion does not follow. The wider Aristotelian framework
provides a partial definition of "stuff" rather than a factual truth.

To say that a person has an immaterial soul is not to say that if you examine
him closely enough under an acute enough microscope you will find some very
rarefied constituent which has eluded the power of ordinary microscopes. It is

just a way of expressing the point within a traditional framework of thought that persons can—it is logically possible—continue, when their bodies do not. It does, however, seem a very natural way of expressing the point—especially once we allow that persons can become disembodied. Unless we adopt a wider Aristotelian framework, we shall have to say that there can be substances which are not made of anything, and which are the same substances as other substances which are made of matter.

It does not follow from all this that a person's body is no part of him. Given that what we are trying to do is to elucidate the nature of those entities which we normally call "persons," we must say that arms and legs and all other parts of the living body are parts of the person. My arms and legs are parts of me. The crucial point that Descartes was making is that the body is only, contingently and possibly temporarily, part of the person; it is not an essential part. However, Descartes does seem in a muddle about this. In the passage from the *Meditations* just cited, as elsewhere in his works,[7] he claims sometimes (wrongly) that my body is no part of me, and at other times (correctly) that my body is not an essential part of me.

The other arguments which I have given for the "simple theory," e.g., that two embodied persons can be the same despite there being no bodily continuity between them, can also, like the argument of Descartes just discussed, if we assume the wider Aristotelian framework, be cast into the form of arguments for classical dualism.

As we have seen, classical dualism is the way of expressing the simple view of personal identity within what I called the wider Aristotelian framework. However, this framework is a wider one than Aristotle himself would have been happy with, allowing a kind of stuff other than Aristotle would have countenanced. There has been in the history of thought a different and very influential way of modifying Aristotle, to take account of the kind of point made by the simple view. This way was due to St. Thomas Aquinas (see, e.g., *Summa contra Gentiles*). Aquinas accepted Aristotle's general doctrine that substances are made of matter, organized by a form; the desk is the desk which it is because of the matter of which it is made and the shape which is imposed upon it. The form was normally a system of properties, universals which had no existence except in the particular substances in which they were instantiated. However, Aquinas claimed that for man the form of the body, which he called the soul, was separable from the body and capable of independent existence. The soul of man, unlike the souls of animals or plants, was in Aquinas's terminology, an "intellectual substance."

However, if we are going to modify Aristotle to make his views compatible with the simple theory of personal identity, this seems definitely the less satisfactory way of doing so. Properties seem by their very nature to be universals and so it is hard to give any sense to their existing except when conjoined to some stuff. Above all, it is hard to give sense to their being individual—a universal can be instantiated in many different substances. What makes the substances differ is the different stuff of which they are composed. The form of man can be instantiated in many different men. But Aquinas wants a form which is a particular, and so could only be combined with one body. All of this seems to involve a greater distortion of Aristotle's system than does classical dualism. Aquinas's system does have some advantages over classical dualism—for example, it enables him to bring out the naturalness of a person being embodied and the temporary and transitory character of any disembodiment—but the disadvantages of taking Aristotle's approach and then distorting it to this unrecognizable extent are in my view very great. Hence my preference for what I have called classical dualism. I shall in future express the simple view in the form of classical dualism, in order to locate this view within the philosophical tradition which seems naturally to express it.

There is, however, one argument often put forward by classical dualists—their argument from the indivisibility of the soul to its natural immortality—from which I must dissociate myself. Before looking at this argument, it is necessary to face the problem of what it means to say that the soul continues to exist. Clearly the soul continues to exist if a person exercises his capacities for experience and action, by having experiences and performing actions. But can the soul continue to exist when the person does not exercise those capacities? Presumably it can. For we say that an unconscious person (who is neither having experiences or acting) is still a person. We say this on the grounds that natural processes (i.e., processes according with the laws of nature) will, or at any rate may, lead to his exercising his capacities again—e.g., through the end of normal sleep or through some medical or surgical intervention. Hence a person, and so his soul, if we talk thus, certainly exists while natural processes may lead to his exercising those capacities again. But what when the person is not exercising his capacities, and no natural processes (whether those operative in our present material universe or those operative in some new world to which the person has moved) will lead to his exercising his capacities? We could say that the person and so his soul still exists on the grounds that there is the logical possibility of his coming to life again. To my mind, the more natural alternative is to say that when ordinary natural processes cannot lead to his exercising his capacities again, a person and so his soul has ceased to exist; but there remains the logical possibility that he may come into existence again (perhaps through God causing him to exist again). One argument against taking the latter alternative is the argument that no substance can have two beginnings of existence. If a person really ceases to exist, then there is not even the logical possibility of his coming into existence again. It would follow that the mere logical possibility of the person coming into existence again has the consequence that a person once existent, is always existent (even when he has no capacity for experience and action). But this principle— that no substance can have two beginnings of existence—is one which I see no good reason for adopting; and if we do not adopt it, then we must say that souls cease to exist when there is no natural possibility of their exercising their capacities. But that does not prevent souls which have ceased to exist coming into existence again. This way of talking does give substantial content to claims that souls do or do not exist, when they are not exercising their capacities.

Now classical dualists assumed (in my view, on balance, correctly) that souls cannot be divided. But they often argued from this, that souls were indestructible,[8] and hence immortal, or at any rate naturally immortal (i.e., immortal as a result of the operation of natural processes, and so immortal barring an act of God to stop those processes operating). That does not follow. Material bodies may lose essential properties without being divided—an oak tree may die and become fossilized without losing its shape. It does not follow from a soul's being indivisible that it cannot lose its capacity for experience and action—and so cease to be a soul. Although there is (I have been arguing) no logical necessity that a soul be linked to a body, it may be physically necessary that a soul be linked to one body if it is to have its essential properties (of capacity for experience and action) and so continue to exist. . . .

NOTES

1. Following A. C. Danto (1965), philosophers call those intentional actions which we just do, not by doing some other intentional action, basic actions, and those which we do by doing some other intentional action, mediated actions. An intentional action is one which an agent does, meaning to do. No doubt certain events have to happen in our nerves and muscles if we are to move our arms and legs, but we do not move our arms and legs by intentionally making these events occur.

2. Two objects belong to the same space if they are at some distance from each other, if you can get from one to the other by going along a path in space which joins them. For a fuller account of the meaning of the claim that an object occupies a different space from our space, see Swinburne 1981, chs 1 and 2.

3. I owe this argument to Knox 1969.

4. I do not discuss the difficult issue of whether the Aristotelian account applies to animals other than man, e.g., whether continuity of matter and form is necessary and sufficient for the identity of a dog at a later time with a dog at an earlier time.

5. Descartes, *Meditations*, p. 190. The clause in square brackets occurs only in the French translation, approved by Descartes.

6. It may be useful, in case anyone suspects the argument of this paragraph of committing some modal fallacy, to set it out in a more formal logical shape. I use the usual logical symbols—'.' means 'and', '~' means 'not', '◇' means 'it is logically possible'. I then introduce the following definitions:

p='I am a conscious person, and I exist in 1984'
q=my body is destroyed at the end of 1984
r=I have a soul in 1984
s=I exist in 1985
x ranges over all consistent propositions compatible with (p. q) and describing 1984
    states of affairs
("(*x*)" is to be read in the normal way as "for all states *x* . . .")

The argument may now be set out as follows:

p	Premise (1)
(*x*) ◇ (p.q.x.s)	Premise (2)
~ ◇ (p.q.~r.s)	Premise (3)

∴ ~r is not within the range of x.

But since ~r describes a state of affairs in 1984, it is not compatible with (p.q). But q can hardly make a difference to whether or not r. So p is incompatible with ~r.

∴ r

The argument is designed to show that r follows from p; and so, more generally, that every conscious person has a soul. Premise (3) is justified by the wider Aristotelian principle that if I am to continue, some of the stuff out of which I am made has to continue. As I argued in the text, that stuff must be non-bodily stuff. The soul is defined as that non-bodily part whose continuing is essential for my continuing.

Premise (2) relies on the intuition that whatever else might be the case in 1984, compatible with (p.q), my stream of consciousness could continue thereafter.

If you deny (2) and say that r is a state of affairs not entailed by (p.q), but which has to hold if it is to be possible that s, you run into this difficulty. There may be two people in 1984, Oliver who has a soul, and Fagin, who does not. Both are embodied and conscious, and to all appearances indistinguishable. God (who can do all things logically possible, compatible with how the world is up to now), having forgotten to give Fagin a soul, has, as he annihilates Fagin's body at the end of 1984, no power to continue his stream of thought. Whereas he has the power to continue Oliver's stream of thought. This seems absurd.

7. For examples and commentary, see pp. 63–6 of Smart 1977.

8. Thus Berkeley: 'We have shown that the soul is indivisible, incorporeal, unextended, and it is consequently incorruptible' (*Principles*, § 141).

REFERENCES

Aquinas, St. Thomas. *Summa contra Gentiles*, II, 56, 57, 68, 70, 79, 80, 81. Translated under the title *On the Truth of the Catholic Faith,* Book II, translated by James F. Anderson. New York, 1956.
Aristotle. *De Anima*, Books II and III, translated with an introduction and notes by D. W. Hamlyn. Oxford, 1968.
Aristotle. *Metaphysics*, Book 7.
Berkeley, George. *Principles of Human Knowledge.*
Butler, Joseph. "Of Personal Identity," in J. H. Bernard (ed.), *The Works of Bishop Butler*, Volume II. London, 1900. Also reprinted in Perry 1975.
Chisholm, R. M. 1969. "The Loose and Popular and the Strict and Philosophical Senses of Identity," in N. S. Care and R. H. Grimm (eds.), *Perception and Personal Identity*. Cleveland, Ohio.
Danto, A. C. 1965. "Basic Actions," *American Philosophical Quarterly*, 2, pp. 141–8.
Descartes, René. *Meditations on the First Philosophy*, in *The Philosophical Works of Descartes*, Volume I, translated by E. S. Haldane and G. R. T. Ross. Cambridge, 1911.
Knox, John, Jr. 1969. "Can the Self Survive the Death of Its Mind?" *Religious Studies*, 5, pp. 85–97.
Locke, John. *An Essay Concerning Human Understanding*, ed. P. H. Nidditch, Book II, Chapter XXVII. Oxford, 1975. Reprinted in Perry 1975.
Perry, John (ed.). 1975. *Personal Identity*. Berkeley, Los Angeles, and London.
Plato. *Phaedo.*
Plato. *Timaeus.*
Reid, Thomas. *Essays on the Intellectual Powers of Man*, Essay III, chapters 4 and 6. Reprinted in Perry 1975.
Smart, Brian. 1977. "How Can Persons Be Ascribed M-Predicates?" *Mind*, 86, pp. 49–66.
Swinburne, Richard. 1981. *Space and Time*, second edition. London.

PERSONS AS ENSOULED BODIES

CHAPTER FOUR

Selections from *Summa Theologiae*

St. Thomas Aquinas

Section Ia, Question 29, Article 1:
The Definition of "Person"

Objection 1: It would seem that the definition of person given by Boethius (De Duab. Nat.) is insufficient—that is, "a person is an individual substance of a rational nature." For nothing singular can be subject to definition. But "person" signifies something singular. Therefore person is improperly defined.

Objection 2: Further, substance as placed above in the definition of person, is either first substance, or second substance. If it is the former, the word "individual" is superfluous, because first substance is individual substance; if it stands for second substance, the word "individual" is false, for there is contradiction of terms; since second substances are the "genera" or "species." Therefore this definition is incorrect.

Objection 3: Further, an intentional term must not be included in the definition of a thing. For to define a man as "a species of animal" would not be a correct definition; since man is the name of a thing, and "species" is a name of an intention. Therefore, since person is the name of a thing (for it signifies a substance of a rational nature), the word "individual" which is an intentional name comes improperly into the definition.

Objection 4: Further, "Nature is the principle of motion and rest, in those things in which it is essentially, and not accidentally," as Aristotle says (Phys. ii). But person exists in things immovable, as in God, and in the angels. Therefore the word "nature" ought not to enter into the definition of person, but the word should rather be "essence."

Objection 5: Further, the separated soul is an individual substance of the rational nature; but it is not a person. Therefore person is not properly defined as above.

I answer that, Although the universal and particular exist in every genus, nevertheless, in a certain special way, the individual belongs to the genus of substance. For substance is individualized by itself; whereas the accidents are individualized by the subject, which is the substance; since this particular whiteness is called "this," because it exists in this particular subject. And so it is reasonable that the individuals of the genus substance should have a special name of their own; for they are called "hypostases," or first substances.

Further still, in a more special and perfect way, the particular and the individual are found in the rational substances which have dominion over their own actions; and which are not only made to act, like others; but which can act of themselves; for actions belong to singulars. Therefore also the individuals of the rational nature have a special name even among other substances; and this name is "person."

Thus the term "individual substance" is placed in the definition of person, as signifying the singular in the genus of substance; and the term "rational nature" is added, as signifying the singular in rational substances.

Reply to Objection 1: Although this or that singular may not be definable, yet what belongs to the general idea of singularity can be defined; and so the Philosopher (De Praedic., cap. De substantia) gives a definition of first substance; and in this way Boethius defines person.

Reply to Objection 2: In the opinion of some, the term "substance" in the definition of person stands for first substance, which is the hypostasis; nor is the term "individual" superfluously added, forasmuch as by the name of hypostasis or first substance the idea of universality and of part is excluded. For we do not say that man in general is an hypostasis, nor that the hand is since it is only a part. But where "individual" is added, the idea of assumptibility is excluded from person; for the human nature in Christ is not a person, since it is assumed by a greater—that is, by the Word of God. It is, however, better to say that substance is here taken in a general sense, as divided into first and second, and when "individual" is added, it is restricted to first substance.

Reply to Objection 3: Substantial differences being unknown to us, or at least unnamed by us, it is sometimes necessary to use accidental differences in the place of substantial; as, for example, we may say that fire is a simple, hot, and dry body: for proper accidents are the effects of substantial forms, and make them known. Likewise, terms expressive of intention can be used in defining realities if used to signify things which are unnamed. And so the term "individual" is placed in the definition of person to signify the mode of subsistence which belongs to particular substances.

Reply to Objection 4: According to the Philosopher (Metaph. v, 5), the word "nature" was first used to signify the generation of living things, which is called nativity. And because this kind of generation comes from an intrinsic principle, this term is extended to signify the intrinsic principle of any kind of movement. In this sense he defines "nature" (Phys. ii, 3). And since this kind of principle is either formal or material, both matter and form are commonly called nature. And as the essence of anything is completed by the form; so the essence of anything, signified by the definition, is commonly called nature. And here nature is taken in that sense. Hence Boethius says (De Duab. Nat.) that, "nature is the specific difference giving its form to each thing," for the specific difference completes the definition, and is derived from the special form of a thing. So in the definition of "person," which means the singular in a determined "genus," it is more correct to use the term "nature" than "essence," because the latter is taken from being, which is most common.

Reply to Objection 5: The soul is a part of the human species; and so, although it may exist in a separate state, yet since it ever retains its nature of unibility, it cannot be called an individual substance, which is the hypostasis or first substance, as neither can the hand nor any other part of man; thus neither the definition nor the name of person belongs to it.

Section Ia, Question 118, Article 2: Whether the Intellectual Soul is Produced from the Semen?

Objection 1: It would seem that the intellectual soul is produced from the semen. For it is written (Gn. 46:26): "All the souls that came out of [Jacob's] thigh, sixty-six." But nothing is produced from the thigh of a man, except from the semen. Therefore the intellectual soul is produced from the semen.

Objection 2: Further, as shown above (Q[76], A[3]), the intellectual, sensitive, and nutritive souls are, in substance, one soul in man. But the sensitive soul in man is generated from the semen, as in other animals; wherefore the Philosopher says (De Gener. Animal. ii, 3) that the animal and the man are not made at the same time, but first of all the animal is made having a sensitive soul. Therefore also the intellectual soul is produced from the semen.

Objection 3: Further, it is one and the same agent whose action is directed to the matter and to the form: else from the matter and the form there would not result something simply one. But the intellectual soul is the form of the human body, which is produced by the power of the semen. Therefore the intellectual soul also is produced by the power of the semen.

Objection 4: Further, man begets his like in species. But the human species is constituted by the rational soul. Therefore the rational soul is from the begetter.

Objection 5: Further, it cannot be said that God concurs in sin. But if the rational soul be created by God, sometimes God concurs in the sin of adultery, since sometimes offspring is begotten of illicit intercourse. Therefore the rational soul is not created by God.

On the contrary, It is written in De Eccl. Dogmat. xiv that "the rational soul is not engendered by coition."

I answer that, It is impossible for an active power existing in matter to extend its action to the production of an immaterial effect. Now it is manifest that the intellectual principle in man transcends matter; for it has an operation in which the body takes no part whatever. It is therefore impossible for the seminal power to produce the intellectual principle.

Again, the seminal power acts by virtue of the soul of the begetter according as the soul of the begetter is the act of the body, making use of the body in its operation. Now the body has nothing whatever to do in the operation of the intellect. Therefore the power of the intellectual principle, as intellectual, cannot reach the semen. Hence the Philosopher says (De Gener. Animal. ii, 3): "It follows that the intellect alone comes from without."

Again, since the intellectual soul has an operation independent of the body, it is subsistent, as proved above (Q[75], A[2]): therefore to be and to be made are proper to it. Moreover, since it is an immaterial substance it cannot be caused through generation, but only through creation by God. Therefore to hold that the intellectual soul is caused by the begetter, is nothing else than to hold the soul to be non-subsistent and consequently to perish with the body. It is therefore heretical to say that the intellectual soul is transmitted with the semen.

Reply to Objection 1: In the passage quoted, the part is put instead of the whole, the soul for the whole man, by the figure of synecdoche.

Reply to Objection 2: Some say that the vital functions observed in the embryo are not from its soul, but from the soul of the mother; or from the formative power of the semen. Both of these explanations are false; for vital functions such as feeling, nourishment, and growth cannot be from an extrinsic principle. Consequently it must be said that the soul is in the embryo; the nutritive soul from the beginning, then the sensitive, lastly the intellectual soul.

Therefore some say that in addition to the vegetative soul which existed first, another, namely the sensitive, soul supervenes; and in addition to this, again another, namely the intellectual soul. Thus there would be in man three souls of which one would be in potentiality to another. This has been disproved above (Q[76], A[3]).

Therefore others say that the same soul which was at first merely vegetative, afterwards through the action of the seminal power, becomes a sensitive soul; and finally this same soul becomes intellectual, not indeed through the active seminal power, but by the power of a higher agent, namely God enlightening (the soul) from without. For this reason the Philosopher says that the intellect comes from without. But this will not hold. First, because no substantial form is susceptible of more or less; but addition of greater perfection constitutes another species, just as the addition of unity constitutes another species of number. Now it is not possible for the same identical form to belong to different species. Secondly, because it would follow that the generation of an animal would be a continuous movement, proceeding gradually from the imperfect to the perfect, as happens in alteration. Thirdly, because it would follow that the generation of a man or an animal is not generation simply, because the subject thereof would be a being in act. For if the vegetative soul is from the beginning in the matter of offspring, and is subsequently gradually brought to perfection; this will imply addition of further perfection without corruption of the preceding perfection. And this is contrary to the nature of generation properly so called. Fourthly, because either that which is caused by the action of God is something subsistent: and thus it must needs be essentially distinct from the pre-existing form, which was non-subsistent; and we shall then come back to the opinion of those who held the existence of several souls in the body—or else it is not subsistent, but a perfection of the pre-existing soul: and from this it follows of necessity that the intellectual soul perishes with the body, which cannot be admitted.

There is again another explanation, according to those who held that all men have but one intellect in common: but this has been disproved above (Q[76], A[2]).

We must therefore say that since the generation of one thing is the corruption of another, it follows of necessity that both in men and in other animals, when a more perfect form supervenes the previous form is corrupted: yet so that the supervening form contains the perfection of the previous form, and something in addition. It is in this way that through many generations and corruptions we arrive at the ultimate substantial form, both in man and other animals. This indeed is apparent to the senses in animals generated from putrefaction. We conclude therefore that the intellectual soul is created by God at the end of human generation, and this soul is at the same time sensitive and nutritive, the pre-existing forms being corrupted.

Reply to Objection 3: This argument holds in the case of diverse agents not ordered to one another. But where there are many agents ordered to one another, nothing hinders the power of the higher agent from reaching to the ultimate form; while the powers of the inferior agents extend only to some disposition of matter: thus in the generation of an animal, the seminal power disposes the matter, but the power of the soul gives the form. Now it is manifest from what has been said above (Q[105], A[5]; Q[110], A[1]) that the whole of corporeal nature acts as the instrument of a spiritual power, especially of God. Therefore nothing hinders the formation of the body from being due to a corporeal power, while the intellectual soul is from God alone.

Reply to Objection 4: Man begets his like, forasmuch as by his seminal power the matter is disposed for the reception of a certain species of form.

Reply to Objection 5: In the action of the adulterer, what is of nature is good; in this God concurs. But what there is of inordinate lust is evil; in this God does not concur.

CHAPTER FIVE

Terra es animata

On Having a Life

Gilbert Meilaender

For the past quarter century bioethics has been a booming business in this country. In part that may be because humanists found here a field in which they could compete with scientists for grant money. In larger part, it is surely because medical advance has forced certain problems upon our attention. But, at least in part, it must also be because some of the concerns of bioethics impinge upon everyday life—upon the lives of most people, and at some of the crucial moments of life, in particular birth and death. Bioethics could not have boomed as it has were it not a reflection of some of our central concerns.

I will examine some of the issues that have emerged in bioethical discussions of death, dying, and care for the dying as a way of thinking about what it means to have a life. In particular, I will focus on a concept that has risen to great prominence in our thinking: the concept of a person. Two competing visions of the person—and the relation of person to body—have unfolded as bioethics has developed, and in my view, the wrong one has begun to triumph. We have tried to handle our substantive disagreements on this question by turning to procedural solutions—in particular, advance directives—trusting that they presume no answer to the disputed question. We are, however, beginning to see how problematic such a procedural solution is, how flawed and even contradictory much thinking about advance directives has been. What we need, I will suggest, is to recapture the connection between our person and the natural trajectory of bodily life.

That will be the course of my argument. But, as a way of framing the issues, I begin in what is likely to seem a strange place: with the thought of some of the early Christian Fathers about heaven and the resurrection of the dead. They were attempting to relate the body's history to their concept of the person's optimal development. In so doing, they provide a different and illuminating angle from which to see our present concerns.

Patristic Images of the Resurrection of the Body

In his *City of God* Saint Augustine describes the human being as *terra animata,* "animated earth."[1] Such a description, contrary in many ways to trends in bioethics over the last several decades, ought to give pause to anyone inclined to characterize Augustine's thought simply in terms of a Neoplatonic dualism that ignores the personal significance of the body. It may, in fact, be our own constant talk of "personhood" that betrays a more powerful tendency toward dualism of body and self.

This same Augustine, however, found himself puzzled at the thought of the resurrected body. What sort of body will one who dies in childhood have in the resurrection? "As for little children," Augustine wrote, "I can only say that they will not rise again with the tiny bodies they had when they died. By a marvelous and instantaneous act of God they will gain that maturity they would have attained by the slow lapse of time" (22.14). This is, in fact, a question to which a number of the Church Fathers devoted thought.[2]

Origen, for example, understood that throughout life our material bodies are constantly changing. How, then, can the body be raised? He appealed (in good Platonic fashion) to the *eidos,* the unchanging form of the body. Despite the body's material transformations, its *eidos* remains the same as we grow from infancy, through childhood and adulthood, to old age. (For Origen this *eidos* is not the soul; it is the bodily form united with the soul in this life and again in the resurrection. J. N. D. Kelly comments that Origen was charged with having held that resurrected bodies would be spherical; he may have held such a view, in keeping with the Platonic theory that a sphere is the perfect shape.)

From here it is not a long step to suppose that since the *eidos* of each resurrected body will be perfect, it will in every instance be identical in qualities and characteristics. Thus, Gregory of Nyssa, though differing from Origen in some respects, held that in the resurrection our bodies will be freed from all the consequences of sin—including not only death and infirmity, but also deformity and difference of age. This is a view not unlike Augustine's. Bodies may have a (natural) history, but the bodily form is unchanging. That form is the human being at his or her optimal stage of development, the person as he or she is truly meant to be. (I write "he or she" not simply to conform to current canons but because Augustine, for example, took trouble to note that the sexual distinction—but not the lust which, in our experience, accompanies it—would remain in the resurrection. All defects would be removed from the resurrected body, but "a woman's sex is not a defect" [*CD* 22.17]. And although intercourse and childbirth will be no more in the resurrection, "the female organs . . . will be part of a new beauty." This is perhaps what C. S. Lewis had in mind when he wrote of the resurrection: "What is no longer needed for biological purposes may be expected to survive for splendour."[3]

Against Origen's notion that the resurrected body would be a purely spiritual *eidos*, Methodius of Olympus held that the body itself—not just its form—would be restored in the resurrection. He based his claim less on a developed philosophical argument than on the resurrection of Jesus, who was raised in the same body that had been crucified (complete, we may recall, with the nail prints in his hands).

Such issues continued to occupy the attention of theologians for centuries to come. For Saint Thomas, the form of the body is the rational soul, and the body reunited with that soul in the resurrection need not reassume all the matter that had ever been its own during temporal life. Rather, as Thomas suggests in the *Summa contra gentiles*, the resurrected man "need assume from that matter only what suffices to complete the quantity due."[4] The "quantity due" is whatever is "consistent with the form and species of humanity." This means that if one had died at an early age "before nature could bring him to the quantity due," or if one had suffered mutilation, "the divine power will supply this from another source" (4.81.12). Saint Thomas is emphatic—against what may have been Origen's view—that our risen bodies will not be purely spiritual. Like Christ's they will have flesh and bones, but in these bodies there will not be "any corruption, any deformity, any deficiency" (4.86.4). Nor, it appears, will there be differences of age; for all will rise "in the age of Christ, which is that of youth [young adulthood], by reason of the perfection of nature which is found in that age alone. For the age of boyhood has not yet achieved the perfection of nature through increase; and by decrease old age has already withdrawn from that perfection" (4.88.5).

Modern Images of the Resurrection

At least to my knowledge, this sort of speculation becomes much rarer after the Reformation—perhaps because Protestants were less inclined to go beyond biblical warrants, even when an intriguing and potentially significant question beckoned. In the fifteenth and last of his charity sermons, Jonathan Edwards does say of heaven: "There shall be none appearing with any defects either natural or moral."[5] And more recently Austin Farrer has approached these questions by asking how it is possible for us to "relate to the mercy of God beings who never enjoy a glimmer of reason."[6] If there never was a speaking and loving person, Farrer asks, where is the creature for God to immortalize? He is less troubled by those who have lost the speaking and loving personhood that once was theirs; God can immortalize them, though Farrer does not tell us whether they are immortalized free of defects or even age differences. But what of those in whom reason never developed? "The baby smiled before it died. Will God bestow immortality on a smile?" Farrer contemplates, without being satisfied by, the possibility that "every human birth, however imperfect, is the germ of a personality, and that God will give it an eternal future"—a speculation not entirely unlike that of some of the early Fathers. And he realizes that there may be some who, though retarded, are not completely without reason—though he never asks, then, what sort of eternal future might be theirs.

If we can overcome both our Enlightened bemusement at such speculation and our Protestant refusal to learn from questions that admit of no answer, if instead we enter into the spirit of such questioning, we may find ourselves rather puzzled. Could such a monochromatic heaven really be heavenly? All of us thirty-five-years old, well endowed with (identical?) reasoning capacities? If each of the saints is to see God and to praise the vision of God that is uniquely his or hers, and if the joy of heaven is not only to see God but to be enriched by each other's vision, then why should we not look through the eyes of persons who are very different indeed? Is not the praise of a five-year-old different from that of a thirty-five-year-old, and, again, from that of a seventy-five-year-old? Why should not these distinct and different visions be part of the vast friendship that is heaven? Perhaps it is easier to understand the tendency to eliminate any defects from heaven, but even there, when they closely touch personal identity, we may find ourselves rather puzzled. Edwards was, for example, confident that there would be neither moral nor *natural* defect in heaven. Yet he was willing to grant that friends will know each other there. But if the stump that should have been my leg has shaped the person who I am, the person who has been your friend for forty years, it is hard to know exactly what our heavenly reunion is to be like when the stump is replaced by a perfectly formed leg. "Will God bestow immortality on a smile?" As likely, I should think, as that the mother of that child will meet one upon whom God has, in Augustine's words, bestowed in "a marvelous and instantaneous act . . . that maturity they would have attained by the slow lapse of time." We might set against Farrer's view the comment of his fellow Anglican David Smith, who writes that "at the very least it would be hard for Anglicans to hold that a being who might be baptized was lacking in human dignity."[7]

Perhaps I begin to wax too enthusiastic in my own speculations, but the point is worth pondering. To live the risen life with God is, presumably, to be what we are meant to be. It is the fulfillment and completion of one's personal history. To try to think from that vantage point, therefore, is to imagine human life in its full dignity. And to try, however clumsy the speculation, to adopt this vantage point for a moment is to think about what it means to have a life. The questions I have been considering invite us to think about our person, our individual self. Does it have a kind of timeless form? A moment in life to which all prior development leads and from which all future development is decline? A moment, then, in which we are uniquely ourselves? Or is our person simply our personal history, whether long or short, a history inseparable from the growth, development, and decline of our body?

There is some reason to think—or so I shall suggest in what follows—that much contemporary thought in ethics has a great deal in common with Origen. In an age supposedly dominated by modes of thought more natural and historical than metaphysical, we have allowed ourselves to think of personhood in terms quite divorced from our biological nature or the history of our embodied self. In the words of Holmes Rolston, our "humanistic disdain for the organic sector" is "less rational, more anthropocentric, not really *bio*-ethical at all," when compared to a view that takes nature and history into our understanding of the person.[8] Or, put in a more literary vein, the view I will try to explicate is that expressed by Ozy Froats in Robertson Davies's novel, *The Rebel Angels*. Froats, a scientist, is discussing his theories about body types with Simon Darcourt, priest and scholar. Froats believes there is little one can do to alter one's body type, a dismaying verdict for Darcourt, who had hoped by diet and exercise to alter his tendency toward a round, fat body. Froats says of such hopes:

> To some extent. Not without more trouble than it would probably be worth. That's what's wrong with all these diets and body-building courses and so forth. You can

go against your type, and probably achieve a good deal as long as you keep at it. . . . You can keep in good shape for what you are, but radical change is impossible. Health isn't making everybody into a Greek ideal; it's living out the destiny of the body.[9]

Terra es animata.

Ozy Froats's notion of having a life is not, however, the vision that seems to be triumphing in bioethics. And, to the degree that developments in bioethics both reflect and shape larger currents of thought in our society, those developments merit our attention.

Contra Ozy Froats

The language of personhood has been central to much of the last quarter century's developments in bioethics. It was there at the outset when, in 1972, in the second volume of the *Hastings Center Report,* Joseph Fletcher published his "Indicators of Humanhood: A Tentative Profile of Man." The language had not yet solidified, since Fletcher could still use "human" and "person" interchangeably. But the heart of his view was precisely that which would, in years to come, distinguish clearly between the class of human beings and the (narrower) class of persons.

Among the important indicators (by 1974 Fletcher would declare it fundamental[10]) was "neo-cortical function." Apart from cortical functioning, "the *person* is non-existent." Having a life requires such function, for "to be dead 'humanly' speaking is to be ex-cerebral, no matter how long the body remains alive." And, in fact, being a person has more to do with being in control than with being embodied. Among the indicators Fletcher discusses are self-awareness, self-control (lacking which, one has a life "about on a par with a paramecium"), and control of existence ("to the degree that a man lacks control he is not responsible, and to be irresponsible is to be subpersonal"). Human beings are neither essentially sexual nor parental, but the technological impulse *is* central to their being. ("A baby made artificially, by deliberate and careful contrivance, would be more *human* than one resulting from sexual roulette.")

Even if, in the briskness with which he can set forth his claims, Fletcher makes an easy target, he was not without considerable influence—and it may be that he discerned and articulated where bioethics was heading well before the more fainthearted were prepared to develop the full consequences of their views. Certainly the understanding of personhood that he represents is very different from Augustine's "animated earth" or Ozy Froats's sense that one must live out the destiny of the body. Views of that sort have generally been labeled "vitalism," and their inadequacy assumed.

This is especially evident in our attitude toward death and toward those who are dying. To confront our own mortality or that of those we love is to be compelled to think about our embodiment and about what it means to have a life.[11] How we face death, and how we care for the dying, are not just isolated problems about which decisions must be made. These are also occasions in which we come to terms with who we are, recognizing that we may soon be no more. The approach of death may seem to mock our pretensions to autonomy; at the least, we are invited to wonder whether wisdom really consists in one last effort to assert our autonomy by taking control of the timing of our death. Contemplation of mortality reminds us that our identity has been secured through bodily ties—in nature, with those from whom we are descended; in history, with those whose lives have intertwined with ours. We are forced to ask whether the loss of these ties must necessarily mean the end of the person we are. Such issues, fundamental in most people's lives, have been involved in arguments about how properly to care for the dying, as we can see if we attempt to bring to the surface two contrasting views within bioethics about what it means to have a life.

Having a Life: View 1

For some time the distinction between "ordinary" and "extraordinary" care dominated bioethical discussions of care for the dying. It provided categories by which to think about end-of-life decisions. When this language began to be widely used—and, indeed, it did filter quite often into ordinary, everyday conversation—its chief purpose was a simple one. The perception, in many ways accurate, was that patients needed moral language capable of asserting their independence over against the medical establishment. They needed to be able to have ways of justifying treatment refusals, ways of resisting overly zealous—even if genuinely concerned—medical caregivers. A widespread sense that patients found themselves confronting a runaway medical establishment lay behind arguments that "extraordinary" or "heroic" care could rightly be refused and that no one had a moral obligation to accept such care. Over against a runaway and powerful medical establishment, this language sought to restore a sense of limits and an acceptance of life's natural trajectory. The language proved inadequate, however, meaning too many different things to different people. But it was not simply inadequate; it was also a language that did not, taken by itself, lend stature to the increasingly prominent concept of personhood. And that concept has been used to broaden significantly the meaning of "useless" or "futile" treatment, by divorcing the person from the life of the body.

In recent years we have seen a spate of articles seeking to define futility in medical care. Care that is futile or useless has in the past been considered "extraordinary" and could be refused or withheld. But what do we mean by futility? Years ago, when I was younger and more carefree, I used to enjoy going out at night in the midst of a hard snowstorm to shovel my driveway. In a sense, this was far from futile, since its psychological benefits were, I thought, considerable. But if the aim was a driveway clear of snow, it was close to futile. Well before I had finished, if the snow was coming hard, the driveway would again be covered. Sometimes I'd do it again before coming in, though aware that those inside were laughing at me. But if the goal was a driveway clear of snow, it just could not be accomplished, no matter how hard I worked while the snow was falling. "In Greek mythology, the daughters of Danaus were condemned in Hades to draw water in leaky sieves. . . . A futile action is one that cannot achieve the goals of the action, no matter how often repeated."[12]

This sense of futility we all understand, even if we realize that it may be difficult to apply with precision in some circumstances. Thus, for example, the comatose person (unlike the person in a persistent vegetative state) is reasonably described as "terminally ill." Because the cough, gag, and swallowing reflexes of the comatose patient are impaired, he or she is highly susceptible to respiratory infections and has a life span usually "limited to weeks or months."[13] Because these reflexes are not similarly impaired in the PVS patient, he or she may live years if nourished and cared for. It makes sense, therefore, to describe most medical care for the comatose person as futile, and we understand readily, I think, the language of futility in that context. It is not as obvious, however, that the same language is appropriate in referring to the PVS patient.

Recent discussions make clear that, in light of such problems, "futility" has gradually come to mean something else—and something quite different. If the sense of futility described above is termed "quantitative" (referring to the improbability that treatment could preserve life for long), a rather different sense of futility is now termed "qualitative." Thus, some have argued, treatment that preserves "continued biologic life without conscious autonomy" is qualitatively futile.[14] It is effective in keeping the earth that is the body animated—effective, but, so the argument goes, not beneficial because what is central to being a person cannot be restored.

How ambivalent we remain on these questions becomes evident, however, when we contrast that view with a recent article, "New Directions in Nursing Home Ethics."[15] The authors argue that the standard view of autonomy that has governed so much of our thinking about acute care in the hospital context is not applicable to the nursing home patient. There we need a new notion of "autonomy within community." This may not be the best language to make their point, however, since the authors want to do more than just envision the person within his community of care. They are also concerned to see his medical condition, his chronic needs, his dependence, as internal to the person. Thus, they seek a

> notion of moral personhood that is not abstracted from the individual's social context or state or physical and mental capacity. . . . For now the caring constitutes the fabric of the person's life . . . and the reality of the moral situation is that the person must embrace dependency rather than resisting it as a temporary, external threat.

The aim here is no longer to fend off the threat external to his person and return the patient to an autonomous condition; instead, the aim is to rethink autonomy, to take into it a loss of self-mastery, to accept dependence in order "to give richer meaning to the lives of individuals who can no longer be self-reliant." Perhaps we might even say that the aim is to help the chronically ill person live out the destiny of the body.

How can it be, in essentially the same time and place where this argument is put forward, that we should be moving rapidly away from such an understanding of the person in so many discussions of "futile" medical care? When Dr. Timothy Quill assisted his patient Diane to commit suicide, he did it, he said, to help her "maintain . . . control on her own terms until death." The hands are the hands of Dr. Quill, but the voice is that of Joseph Fletcher, an increasingly powerful voice in our society.

Having a Life: View 2

Around the time that Fletcher was publishing his indicators of humanhood, one of the other great figures in the early years of the bioethics movement, also a theologian, was writing that the human being is "a sacredness in the natural biological order. He is a person who within the ambience of the flesh claims our care. He is an embodied soul or an ensouled body."[16] In those words of Paul Ramsey the vision of the human being as *terra animata* was forcefully articulated. As "embodied souls" we long for a fulfillment never fully given in human history, for the union with God that is qualitatively different from this life—which longing can never, therefore, be satisfied by a greater quantity of this life. But as "ensouled bodies" our lives also have a shape, a trajectory, that is the body's. Our identity is marked, first, by the bodily union of our parents, a relationship that then gradually takes on a history. We are a "someone who"—a someone who has a history—and though we may long for that qualitatively different fulfillment, we never fully transcend the body's history in this life. To come to know who we are, therefore, one must enter that history.

It is a history that may be cut short at any time by accident or illness, but in its natural pattern it moves through youth and adulthood toward old age and, finally, decline and death. That is the body's destiny. As Hans Jonas has suggested, we exist as living bodies, as organisms, not simply by perduring but by a constant encounter with the possibility of death.[17] We constantly give up the component parts of our self to renew them, and our continued life always carries within itself the possibility that these exchanges may fail us. Eventually we are worn down, unable any longer to manage the necessary exchanges. The fire goes out, and we are no longer "animated" earth.

To point to some moment in this history as the moment in which we are most truly ourselves, the vantage point from which the rest of our life is to be judged—not just another of the many moments in which we are persons, but a moment at which, presumably, we have personhood—is to suppose that we can somehow extricate ourselves from the body's natural history, can see ourselves whole. It is even, perhaps, to suppose that in such a moment we are rather like God, no longer having our personal presence in the body.

It is not too much to say that two quite different visions of the person—Fletcher's and Ramsey's—have been at war with each other during the three decades or so that bioethics has been a burgeoning movement. But it is equally clear that one view has begun to predominate within the bioethics world and perhaps within our culture more generally. Among the peculiarities of our historicist and purportedly antiessentialist age is the rise to prominence of an ahistorical and essentialist concept of the person. On this view, it is not the natural history of the embodied self but the presence or absence of certain capacities that makes the person. Indeed, we tend to think and speak not of being a person but of having personhood, which becomes a quality added to being. The view gaining ascendancy does not think of dependence or illness as something to be taken into the fabric of the person and lived out as part of one's personal history. It pictures the real person—like Origen's spherical *eidos*—as separate from that history, free to accept or reject it as part of one's person and life. Moreover, to be without the capacity to make such a decision is to fall short of personhood.

This view is not required by any of the standard approaches to bioethical reasoning or any of the basic principles (such as autonomy, beneficence, and justice) so commonly in use. What we do with such principles depends on the background beliefs we bring to them. Those beliefs determine how wide will be the circle of our beneficence and whether our notion of autonomy will be able to embrace dependence. The problems we face lie less with the principles than with ourselves. We have lost touch with the natural history of bodily life—a strange upshot for *bio*ethics, as Holmes Rolston noted. How wrong we would be to suppose that ours is a materialistic age, when everything we hold central to our person is separated from the animated earth that is the body.

Embodied Souls sans Competence

It might be, however, that I have overlooked something important. If in some cases we judge care futile when the capacity for independence is gone, and if in other cases of chronic illness we take the need for continual care into the very meaning of personal life, perhaps—one might suggest—the difference lies in what different people want, how they choose to live. One patient chooses to live on; another sees no point in doing so. Hence, the key is autonomous choice, which remains at the heart of personhood. All we need do is get people to state their wishes—enact advance directives—while they are able. Then, if the day comes when others must make decisions for them, we will not have to delve into disputed background beliefs about the meaning of personhood. We will have a procedure in place to deal with such circumstances.

In the wider sweep of history, living wills are a very recent innovation, but the debate about their usefulness or wisdom coincides with the quarter century in which bioethics has grown as a movement.[18] And when we are told that, within a month after the Supreme Court's *Cruzan* decision, 100,000 people sought information about living wills from the Society for the Right to Die, we can understand that this is not an issue for specialized academic disciplines alone. The term "living will" was coined in 1969, and the nation's first living will law (in California) was passed in 1976—prompted, it seems, by the Karen Quinlan case. By now most states have enacted laws giving legal standing to living wills, and in 1991 the federal Patient Self-Determination Act went into effect, requiring hospitals to advise patients upon admission of their right to enact an advanced directive. In a relatively short period of time, therefore, the idea of living wills (and other forms of advance directives, such as the health care power of attorney) seems to have scored an impressive triumph. If we have no substantive agreement on what it means to be a person or have a life, the living will offers a process whereby we can deal with substantive disagreement. Each of us autonomously decides when our life would be so lacking in personal dignity as to be no longer worth preserving, and we pretend that such a process masks no substantive vision of what personhood means.

But it does, of course. Such a procedural approach brings with it a certain vision of the person: to be a person is to be, or have the capacity to be, an autonomous chooser, to take control over one's personal history, determining its bounds and limits. This substantive view turns out to have a life of its own and—we are beginning to see—can lead in several quite different directions. For a time, perhaps, all choices of once autonomous patients are honored. You choose to die when your ability to live independently and with "dignity" wanes; I choose to live on even when my rational capacities are gone. Each of us is treated as we have stipulated in advance. But then a day comes—and, indeed, is upon us—when the vision of the person hidden in this process comes to the fore.

The Paradox of Autonomy

If the person is essentially an autonomous chooser, then we will not forever be allowed to choose to live on when our personhood (so defined) has been lost. Living wills had, for the most part, been understood as a means by which we could ensure that we were not given care we would no longer have wanted, care that preserved a life regarded as subpersonal and no longer worth having. But in principle, after all, the process could be used to other ends. One could execute a living will directing that everything possible be done to keep oneself alive, even when one's "personal" capacities had been irretrievably lost. What then?

In a case somewhat like this, Helga Wanglie's caregivers answered that question by seeking a court order to stop the respirator and feeding tube that were sustaining her life. Mrs. Wanglie was an eighty-seven-year-old woman who, because of a respiratory attack, lost oxygen to her brain. She did not recover and remained in a persistent vegetative state. Although the costs of her care were covered by the family's insurance policy, the hospital still sought permission to remove life support. In some relatively minor ways, her case does not fit perfectly the hypothetical situation I considered above, for she had no living will. What she had, though, was a husband who was her guardian and who refused to consent to the withdrawal of treatment, believing she would not have wanted him to do so. Also, the medical caregivers went to court challenging her husband's suitability as guardian, rather than directly seeking court approval to terminate treatment.[19] But as Alexander Morgan Capron notes, when the caregivers first announced their intention to go to court, they stated that "they did not 'want to give medical care they described as futile.'"

Thus, in the Wanglie case, at least in the minds of the caregivers, personhood defined in terms of the right autonomously to determine one's future gave way to personhood defined in terms of the present possession of certain capacities.[20] For those who lack such rational capacities, further care is understood as futile—whatever they might previously have stipulated while competent. Similarly, when Schneiderman and his colleagues develop their "qualitative" understanding of futility, they make clear its impact on cases like this one. "The patient has no right to be sustained in a state in which he or she has no purpose other than mere vegetative survival; the physician has no obligation to offer this option or services to achieve it.'[21] Ironies abound here. At the heart of the bioethics movement has been an assertion of personal autonomy for patients, which was, of course, ordinarily understood as ensuring their ability to be rid of unwanted treatment. But having built autonomy into the center of our understanding of personhood, having indeed (after *Roe v. Wade*) claimed that such autonomy flows from our right of privacy and may be asserted on our behalf even by others when we are unable to assert our wishes, having used patient autonomy as a hammer to bludgeon into submission paternalistic physicians, we suddenly rediscover the responsibility of physicians to consider what is really best for the patient, to make judgments about when care is futile. We suddenly do an about face. Against past autonomous patient choice for continued treatment even after "personhood" has been lost, we now assert medical responsibility not to provide present care that is "futile."

Helga Wanglie's caregivers and those who would assert a "qualitative" notion of personhood are both right and wrong—though not in the ways they suppose. They are right in that there is no reason to think that my physicians should forever be bound by what I stipulate (when I am forty-five and in good health) about my future care. That is, they are right in thinking that autonomy alone is far too thin an account of the person and that physicians must concern themselves with patients' best interests, not just their requests or directives. But they are wrong in supposing that care for me becomes futile simply because I have irretrievably lost the higher human capacities for reasoning and self-awareness. They are also confused; for the vision of the person guiding them where they are right is incompatible with the vision of the person at work where they are wrong. In supposing that care for me becomes futile when I have lost my powers of reason (even though I may not be terminally ill), they express a vision of the person that divorces personhood from organic bodily life. They decline to take into their understanding of the person defect, dependence, or disability. But in judging that caregivers need not be bound forever by directions I have stipulated in advance, when my condition was quite different from what it has now become, they accept the need to live out the body's history, and they decline to give privileged status to the person's existence at one earlier moment in time.

Rethinking the *Eidos*

If we could develop an increased sense of irony about the course the bioethics movement has taken, we might be well positioned to think about the important questions for everyday life with which it here deals. The ironies are a clue to our confusions. Is it not striking that just at the moment when the idea of living wills seems to have triumphed, when federal law has required hospitals to make certain we know of our right to execute an advance directive, bioethicists should begin to wonder whether living wills are not themselves problematic? Having gotten what we thought we wanted—a law undergirded by a certain vision of the person—we begin to discern problems.

Thus, for example, John A. Robertson has had "Second Thoughts on Living Wills."[22] There are, he notes, spheres of life in which we do not hold a person to an understanding he or she had previously stated. We do not, for example, hold surrogate mothers to contracts. Yet, we are reluctant to recognize that when Meilaender becomes incompetent—severely demented, let us say—his interests may well shift. We prefer to suppose that his person was complete and perfect at some earlier point in his development—when, say, at age forty-five he executed a living will. We hesitate to consider that what the forty-five-year-old Meilaender thought should be done to and for a demented Meilaender may not be in the latter's best interest. His life circumstances have changed drastically; he has become more simply and completely organism and less neocortex. If we would care for him, we must take that into account. And if we do not take it into our reckoning, if we blindly follow whatever directions the forty-five-year-old Meilaender gave, it is not clear that we can really claim to have the best interests of *this* patient—the Meilaender now before us—at the center of our concern.

Something like that is Robertson's argument, and it makes good sense. For it essentially denies that we should think of the person as a perfect *eidos* captured at a moment in time, and, less directly, it invites us to think of the person as a someone who has a history, as animated earth. But that is not really Robertson's intent. He sees that the living will has become essentially "a device that functions to avoid assessing incompetent patient interests," but his real aim is to encourage us to take up "the difficult task of determining which incompetent states of existence are worth protecting." This can only land him back in the muddle from which he is trying to escape. He is back to thinking of personhood as something added to existence—and well on his way, therefore, to the conception of personhood that gave rise to an emphasis on autonomy, which in turn suggested the living will as a useful way to exercise our autonomy, which—or so he thinks—is a path strewn with "conceptual frailties." He wants us not to live out the destiny of the body but to escape it.

Life as "Someone Who"

To have a life is to be *terra animata,* a living body whose natural history has a trajectory. It is to be a someone who has a history, not a someone with certain capacities or characteristics. In our history this understanding of the person was most fully developed when Christians had to make sense of the claim that in Jesus of Nazareth both divine and human natures were joined in one person.[23] Christians did not wish to say that there were really two persons (two sets of personal characteristics) in Christ; hence, they could not formulate his personal identity in terms of capacities or characteristics. They could speak of his person only as an individual with a history, a "someone who." The personal is not just an example of the universal form; rather, the general characteristics exist in and through the individual person. And we can come to know such persons only by entering into their history, by personal engagement and commitment to them, not by measuring them against an ideal of health or personhood.

Perhaps such an understanding of the person is also available to us through reflection upon our life as embodied beings. "Embodiment is a curse only for those who believe they deserve to be gods."[24] If Origen's account of the resurrected body seems to have lost much of what we mean by embodiment, he had at least this excuse: he genuinely believed that God intended to make humankind divine. That bioethics—and our culture more generally—is in danger of losing the body in search of the person is harder to understand, unless in our own way we believe that we deserve to be gods.

James Rachels, arguing that ethics must and can get along quite well without God, has recently distinguished between biological and biographical life, arguing that only the second of these is of any value to us.[25] Biological life has instrumental value, since apart from it there is no possibility of realizing biographical life, but biological life without the possibility of self-consciousness and self-control can be of no value to us. In such a state we no longer have any interest in living, and we cannot be harmed if our life is not preserved.

Perhaps, though, such arguments do not take seriously enough the *terra* of which we are made. What Rachels never explains, for example, is why one's period of decline is not part of one's personal history, one's biography. As John Kleinig suggests, "Karen Ann Quinlan's biography did not end in 1975, when she became permanently comatose. It continued for another ten years. That was part of the tragedy of her life."[26] From zygote to irreversible coma, each life is a single personal history. We may, Kleinig notes, distinguish different points in this story, from potentiality to zenith to residuality. But the zenith is not the person. "Human beings are continuants, organisms with a history that extends beyond their immediate present, usually forward and backward. What has come to be seen as 'personhood,' a selected segment of that organismic trajectory, is connected to its earlier and later phases by a complex of factors—physical, social, psychological—that constitutes part of a single history."

Indeed, it is not at all strange to suggest that even the unaware living body has "interests." For the living body takes in nourishment and uses it; the living body struggles against infection and injury. And if we remember "the somatic dimensions of personality, as expressed for instance in face and hands,"[27] we may recognize in the living body the place—the only place—through which the person is present with us. This does not mean that the person is "merely" body; indeed, in such contexts the word "merely" is always a dangerous word. As bodies we are located in time, space, and history; yet, we also transcend that location to some degree. Indeed, from the Christian perspective with which I began, it is right to say that, precisely because we are made for God, we indefinitely transcend our historical location. But it is as embodied creatures that we do so, and our person cannot be divorced from the body and its natural trajectory. This is not vitalism; it is "the wisdom of the body"[28]. It is the wisdom to see that every human life is a story and has a narrative quality—a plot to be lived out. That story begins before we are conscious of it, and, for many of us, continues after we have lost consciousness of it. Yet, each narrative is the story of "someone who"—someone who, as a living body, has a history.

Caught as we are within the midst of our own life stories, and unable as we are to grasp anyone else's story as a single whole, we have to admit that only God can see us as the persons we are—can catch the self and hold it still. What exactly we will be like when we are with God is, therefore, always beyond our capacity to say. But it will be the completion of the someone who we were and are, and we should not, therefore, settle for any more truncated vision of the person even here and now.

NOTES

1. St. Augustine, *De civitate Dei,* trans. Henry Bettenson (New York: Penguin Books, 1972), 20.20. Future citations will be given by book and chapter number within parentheses in the body of the text.

2. For much of what follows about the early Fathers I draw upon J. N. D. Kelly, *Early Christian Doctrines* (New York: Harper & Row, 1960), pp. 464–79. I am indebted to Robert Wilken for drawing my attention to Kelly's discussion.

3. C. S. Lewis, *Miracles* (New York: Macmillan, 1947), p. 166.

4. Saint Thomas Aquinas, *Summa contra gentiles,* trans. Charles J. O'Neil (Notre Dame: University of Notre Dame Press, 1975), 4.81.12. Future citations will be given by book, chapter, and paragraph number within parentheses in the body of the text.

5. Jonathan Edwards, *Works,* vol. 8, *Ethical Writings,* ed. Paul Ramsey (New Haven: Yale University Press, 1989), p. 371.

6. Austin Farrer, *Love Almighty and Ills Unlimited* (Garden City, N.Y.: Doubleday & Company, 1961), p. 166. For his discussion more generally, see the Appendix, "Imperfect Lives," pp. 166–68.

7. David H. Smith, *Health and Medicine in the Anglican Tradition* (New York: Crossroad, 1986), p. 10.

8. Holmes Rolston III, "The Irreversibly Comatose: Respect for the Subhuman in Human Life," *Journal of Medicine and Philosophy* 7 (1982): 337–54.

9. Robertson Davies, *The Rebel Angels* (New York: Penguin Books, 1983), pp. 249ff.

10. Joseph Fletcher, "Four Indicators of Humanhood: The Enquiry Matures," *Hastings Center Report* 4, no. 6 (1974): 4–7.

11. I have discussed this from another angle in chapter 8 of *Faith and Faithfulness* (Notre Dame: University of Notre Dame Press, 1991).

12. Lawrence J. Schneiderman, Nancy S. Jecker, and Albert R. Jonsen, "Medical Futility: Its Meaning and Ethical Implications," *Annals of Internal Medicine* 112 (June 1990): 949–54.

13. Ronald E. Cranford, "The Persistent Vegetative State: The Medical Reality (Getting the Facts Straight)," *Hastings Center Report* 18, no. 1 (1988): 27–32.

14. Schneiderman et al., "Medical Futility," p. 952.

15. Bart Collopy, Philip Boyle, and Bruce Jennings, "New Directions in Nursing Home Ethics," special supplement, *Hastings Center Report* 21, no. 2 (1991): 1–16.

16. Paul Ramsey, *The Patient as Person* (New Haven: Yale University Press, 1970), p. xiii.

17. Hans Jonas, "The Burden and Blessing of Mortality," *Hastings Center Report* 22, no. 1 (1992): 34–40.

18. For the historical information that follows I rely upon George J. Annas, "The Health Care Proxy and the Living Will," *NEJM* 324 (25 April 1991): 1210–13.

19. Alexander Morgan Capron, "In Re Helga Wanglie," *Hastings Center Report* 21, no. 5 (1991): 26–28.

20. My distinction here bears some similarities to James Childress's distinction between autonomy as an end state and autonomy as a side constraint. Cf. his *Who Should Decide? Paternalism in Health Care* (New York: Oxford University Press, 1982), p. 64.

21. Schneiderman et al., "Medical Futility," p. 952.

22. John A. Robertson, "Second Thoughts on Living Wills." *Hastings Center Report* 21, no. 6 (1991): 6–9.

23. I have discussed this point more fully (and acknowledged my indebtedness for it to Oliver O'Donovan) in *Faith and Faithfulness*, pp. 45–47.

24. Leon R. Kass, *Toward a More Natural Science* (New York: Free Press, 1985), p. 293.

25. James Rachels, *Created from Animals: The Moral Implications of Darwinism* (New York: Oxford University Press, 1990), pp. 198ff.

26. John Kleinig, *Valuing Life* (Princeton: Princeton University Press, 1991), p. 201.

27. Rolston, "Irreversibly Comatose," p. 352.

28. Rolston, "Irreversibly Comatose," p. 338. [Editor's Note: Rolston attributes the phrase "the wisdom of the body" to W. B. Cannon, *The Wisdom of the Body* (New York: W.W. Norton, 1932, 1963).]

PERSONS AS HUMAN ORGANISMS

An Argument for Animalism

Eric T. Olson

It is a truism that you and I are human beings. It is also a truism that a human being is a kind of animal: roughly a member of the primate species *Homo sapiens*. It would seem to follow that we are animals. Yet that claim is deeply controversial. Plato, Augustine, Descartes, Spinoza, Leibniz, Locke, Berkeley, Hume, Kant, and Hegel all denied it. With the notable exception of Aristotle and his followers, it is hard to find a major figure in the history of Western philosophy who thought that we are animals. The view is no more popular in non-Western traditions. And probably nine out of ten philosophers writing about personal identity today either deny outright that we are animals or say things that are clearly incompatible with it.

This is surprising. Isn't it obvious that we are animals? I will try to show that it isn't obvious, and that Plato and the others have their reasons for thinking otherwise. Before doing that I will explain how I understand the claim that we are animals. My main purpose, though, is to make a case for this unpopular view. I won't rely on the brief argument I began with. My strategy is to ask what it would mean if we weren't animals. Denying that we are animals is harder than you might think.

1. What Animalism Says

When I say that we are animals, I mean that each of us is numerically identical with an animal. There is a certain human organism, and that organism is you. You and it are one and the same. This view has been called "animalism" (not a very nice name, but I haven't got a better one). Simple though it may appear, this is easily misunderstood. Many claims that sound like animalism are in fact different.

First, some say that we are animals and yet reject animalism.[1] How is that possible? How can you be an animal, and yet not be one? The idea is that there is a sense of the verb *to be* in which something can "be" an animal without being identical with any animal. Each of us "is" an animal in the sense of "being constituted by" one. That means roughly that you are in the same place and made of the same matter as an animal. But you and that animal could come apart (more on this later). And since a thing can't come apart from itself, you and the animal are not identical.

I wish people wouldn't say things like this. If you are not identical with a certain animal, that animal is something other than you. And I doubt whether there is any interesting sense in which you can *be* something other than yourself. Even if there is, expressing a view on which no one is identical with an animal by saying that we *are* animals is badly misleading. It discourages us from asking important questions: what we *are* identical with, if not animals, for instance. Put plainly and honestly, these philosophers are saying that each of us is a non-animal that relates in some intimate way to an animal. They put it by saying that we *are* animals because that sounds more plausible. This is salesman's hype, and we shouldn't be fooled. In any case, the "constitutionalists" do not say that we are animals in the straightforward sense in which I mean it. They are not animalists.

The existence of the "constitution view" shows that animalism is not the same as *materialism*. Materialism is the view that we are material things; and we might be material things but not animals. Animalism implies materialism (animals are material things), but not vice versa. It may seem perverse for a materialist to reject animalism. If we are material things of any sort, surely we are animals? Perverse or not, though, the view that we are material non-organisms is widely held.

Animalism says that *we* are animals. That is compatible with the existence of non-animal people (or persons, if you prefer). It is often said that to be a person is to have certain mental qualities: to be rational, intelligent, and self-conscious, say. Perhaps a person must also be morally responsible, and have free will. If something like that is right, then gods or angels might be people but not animals.

Nor does our being animals imply that all animals, or even all human animals, are people. Human beings in a persistent vegetative state are biologically alive, but their mental capacities are permanently destroyed. They are certainly human animals. But we might not want to call them people. The same goes for human embryos.

So the view that we are animals does not imply that to be a person is nothing other than to be an animal of a certain sort—that being an animal is part of what it is to be a person. Inconveniently enough, this view has also been called animalism. It isn't the animalism that I want to defend. In fact it looks rather implausible. I don't know whether there could be inorganic people, as for instance traditional theism asserts. But mere reflection on what it is to be a person doesn't seem to rule it out. Of course, if people are animals by definition, it follows that we are animals, since we are obviously people. But the reverse entailment doesn't hold: we might be animals even if something could be a person without being an animal.

If I don't say that all people are animals, which people do I mean? Is animalism the mere tautology that all animal people are animals? No. I say that you and I and the other people who walk the earth are animals. If you like, all *human* people are animals, where a human person is roughly someone who relates to a human animal in the way that you and I do, whatever way that is. (Even idealists can agree that we are in some sense human, and not, say, feline or angelic.) Many philosophers deny that *any* people are animals. So there is nothing trivial about this claim.

"Animalism" is sometimes stated as the view that we are *essentially or most fundamentally* animals. We are essentially animals if we couldn't possibly exist without being animals. It is less clear what it is for us to be most fundamentally animals, but this is usually taken to imply at least that our identity conditions derive from our being animals, rather than from our being, say, people or philosophers or material objects—even though we *are* people and philosophers and material objects.

Whether our being animals implies that we are essentially or most fundamentally animals depends on whether human animals are essentially or most fundamentally animals. If the animal that you are is essentially an animal, then so are you. If it is only contingently an animal, then you are only contingently an animal. Likewise, you are most fundamentally an animal if and only if the animal that you are is most fundamentally an animal. The claim that each of us is identical with an animal is neutral on these questions. Most philosophers think that every animal is essentially and most fundamentally an animal, and I am inclined to agree. But you could be an animalist in my sense without accepting this.

Is animalism the view that we are identical with our bodies? That depends on what it is for something to be someone's body. If a person's body is by definition a sort of animal, then I suppose being an animal amounts to being one's body. It is often said, though, that someone could have a partly or wholly inorganic body. One's body might include plastic or metal limbs. Someone might even have an entirely robotic body. I take it that no animal could be partly or wholly inorganic. If you cut off an animal's limb and replace it with an inorganic prosthesis, the animal just gets smaller and has something inorganic attached to it. So perhaps after having some or all of your parts replaced by inorganic gadgets of the right sort you would be identical with your body, but would not be an animal. Animalism may imply that you are your body, but you could be your body without being an animal. Some philosophers even say that being an animal rules out being identical with one's body. If you replaced enough of an animal's parts with new ones, they say, it would end up with a different body from the one it began with.

Whether these claims about bodies are true depends on what it is for something to be someone's body. What does it *mean* to say that your body is an animal, or that someone might have a robotic body? I have never seen a good answer to this question (see van Inwagen 1980 and Olson 1997: 144–49). So I will talk about people and animals, and leave bodies out of it.

Finally, does animalism say that we are *merely* animals? That we are nothing more than biological organisms? This is a delicate point. The issue is whether being "more than just" or "not merely" an animal is compatible with being an animal—that is, with being identical with an animal.

If someone complains that the committee is more than just the chairman, she means that it is not the chairman: it has other members too. If we are more than just animals in something like this sense, then we are not animals. We have parts that are not parts of any animal: immaterial souls, perhaps.

On the other hand, we say that Descartes was more than just a philosopher: he was also a mathematician, a Frenchman, a Roman Catholic, and many other things. That is of course compatible with his being a philosopher. We can certainly be more than "mere" animals in this sense, and yet still be animals. An animal can have properties other than being an animal, and which don't follow from its being an animal. Our being animals does not rule out our being mathematicians, Frenchmen, or Roman Catholics—or our being people, socialists, mountaineers, and many other things. At least there is no evident reason why it should. Animalism does not imply that we have a fixed, "animal" nature, or that we have only biological or naturalistic properties, or that we are no different, in any important way, from other animals. There may be a vast psychological and moral gulf between human animals and organisms of other species. We may be very special animals. But special animals are still animals.

2. Alternatives

One reason why it may seem obvious that we are animals is that it is unclear what else we could be. If we're not animals, what are we? What are the alternatives to animalism? This is a question that philosophers ought to ask more often. Many views about personal identity clearly rule out our being animals, but leave it a mystery what sort of things we might be instead. Locke's account is a notorious example. His detailed account of personal identity doesn't even tell us whether we are material or immaterial.

Well, there is the traditional idea that we are simple immaterial substances, or, alternatively, compound things made up of an immaterial substance and a biological organism.

There is the view, mentioned earlier, that we are material objects constituted by human animals. You and a certain animal are physically indistinguishable. Nonetheless you and it are two different things.

Some say that we are temporal parts of animals. Animals and other persisting objects exist at different times by having different temporal parts or "stages" located at those times. You are made up of those stages of a human animal (or, in science fiction, of several animals) that are "psychologically interconnected" (Lewis 1976). Since your animal's embryonic stages have no mental properties at all, they aren't psychologically connected with anything, and so they aren't parts of you. Hence, you began later than the animal did.

Hume famously proposed that each of us is "a bundle or collection of different perceptions, which succeed each other with an inconceivable rapidity, and are in a perpetual flux and movement" (1888: 252). Strictly speaking you are not made of bones and sinews, or of atoms, or of matter. You are literally composed of thoughts. Whether Hume actually believed this is uncertain; but some do (e.g., Quinton 1962).

Every teacher of philosophy has heard it said that we are something like computer programs. You are a certain complex of information "realized" in your brain. (How else could you survive Star-Trek teletransportation?) That would mean that you are not a concrete object at all. You are a universal. There could literally be more than one of you, just as there is more than one concrete instance of the web browser *Netscape 6.2.*

There is even the paradoxical view that we don't really exist at all. There are many thoughts and experiences, but no beings that *have* those thoughts or experiences. The existence of human people is an illusion—though of course no one is deluded about it. Philosophers who have denied or at least doubted their own existence include Parmenides, Spinoza, Hume, Hegel (as I read them, anyway), Russell (1985: 50), and Unger (1979). We also find the view in Indian Buddhism.

There are other views about what we might be, but I take these to be animalism's main rivals. One of these claims, or another one that I haven't mentioned, must be true. There must be *some* sort of thing that we are. If there is anything sitting in your chair and reading these words, it must have some basic properties or other.

For those who enjoy metaphysics, these are all fascinating proposals. Whatever their merits, though, they certainly are strange. No one but a philosopher could have thought of them. And it would take quite a bit of philosophy to get anyone to believe one of them. Compared with these claims, the idea that we are animals looks downright sensible. That makes its enduring unpopularity all the more surprising.

3. Why Animalism Is Unpopular

Why is animalism so unpopular? Historically, the main reason (though by no means the only one) is hostility to materialism. Philosophers have always found it hard to believe that a material object, no matter how physically complex, could produce thought or experience. And an animal is a material object (I assume that vitalism is false). Since it is plain enough that *we* can think, it is easy to conclude that we couldn't be animals.

But why do modern-day materialists reject animalism, or at least say things that rule it out? The main reason, I believe, is that when they think about personal identity they don't ask what sort of things we are. They don't ask whether we are animals, or what we might be if we aren't animals, or how we relate to the human animals that are so intimately connected with us. Or at least they don't ask that first. No one who *began* by asking what we are would hit on the idea that we must be computer programs or bundles of thoughts or non-animals made of the same matter as animals.

The traditional problem of personal identity is not what we are, but what it takes for us to persist. It asks what is necessary, and what is sufficient, for a person existing at one time to be identical with something present at another time: what sorts of adventures we could survive, and what would inevitably bring our existence to an end. Many philosophers seem to think that an answer to this question would tell us all there is to know about the metaphysics of personal identity. This is not so. Claims about what it takes for us to persist do not by themselves tell us what other fundamental properties we have: whether we are material or immaterial, simple or composite, abstract or concrete, and so on. At any rate, the single-minded focus on our identity over time has tended to put other metaphysical questions about ourselves out of philosophers' minds.

What is more, the most popular solution to this traditional problem rules out our being animals. It is that we persist by virtue of some sort of psychological continuity. You are, necessarily, that future being that in some sense inherits its mental features—personality, beliefs, memories, values, and so on—from you. And you are that past being whose mental features you have inherited. Philosophers disagree about what sort of inheritance this has to be: whether those mental features must be continuously physically realized, for instance. But most accept the general idea. The persistence of a human animal, on the other hand, does not consist in mental continuity.

The fact that each human animal starts out as an unthinking embryo and may end up as an unthinking vegetable shows that no sort of mental continuity is necessary for a human animal to persist. No human animal is mentally continuous with an embryo or a vegetable.

To see that no sort of mental continuity is sufficient for a human animal to persist, imagine that your cerebrum is put into another head. The being who gets that organ, and he alone, will be mentally continuous with you on any account of what mental continuity is. So if mental continuity of any sort suffices for you to persist, you would go along with your transplanted cerebrum. You wouldn't stay behind with an empty head.

What would happen to the human animal associated with you? Would *it* go along with its cerebrum? Would the surgeons pare that animal down to a small chunk of yellowish-pink tissue, move it across the room, and then supply it with a new head, trunk, and other parts? Surely not. A detached cerebrum is no more an organism than a detached liver is an organism. The empty-headed thing left behind, by contrast, *is* an animal. It may even remain alive, if the surgeons are careful to leave the lower brain intact. The empty-headed being into which your cerebrum is implanted is also an animal. It looks for all the world like there are two human animals in the story. One of them loses its cerebrum and gets an empty head. The other has its empty head filled with that organ. No animal moves from one head to another. The surgeons merely move an organ from one animal to another. If this is right, then no sort of psychological continuity suffices for the identity of a human animal over time. One human animal could be mentally continuous with another one (supposing that they can have mental properties at all).

If we tell the story in the right way, it is easy enough to get most people, or at any rate most Western-educated philosophy students, to say that *you* would go along with your transplanted cerebrum. After all, the one who got that organ would act like you and think she was you. Why deny that she would be the person she thinks she is? But "your" animal—the one you would be if you were any animal—would stay behind. That means that you and that animal could go your separate ways. And a thing and itself can never go their separate ways.

It follows that you are not that animal, or indeed any other animal. Not only are you not essentially an animal. You are not an animal at all, even contingently. Nothing that is even contingently an animal would move to a different head if its cerebrum were transplanted. The human animals in the story stay where they are and merely lose or gain organs.[2]

So the thought that leads many contemporary philosophers to reject animalism—or that would lead them to reject it if they accepted the consequences of what they believe—is something like this: You would go along with your transplanted cerebrum; but no human animal would go along with its transplanted cerebrum. More generally, some sort of mental continuity suffices for us to persist, yet no sort of mental continuity suffices for an animal to persist. It follows that we are not animals. If we were animals, we should have the identity conditions of animals. Those conditions have nothing to do with psychological facts. Psychology would be irrelevant to our identity over time. That goes against 300 years of thinking about personal identity.

This also shows that animalism is a substantive metaphysical thesis with important consequences. There is nothing harmless about it.

4. The Thinking-Animal Argument

I turn now to my case for animalism. It seems evident that there *is* a human animal intimately related to you. It is the one located where you are, the one we point to when we point to you, the one sitting in your chair. It seems equally evident that human animals can think. They can act. They can be aware of themselves and the world. Those with mature nervous systems in good working order can, anyway. So there is a thinking, acting human animal sitting where you are now. But you think and act. *You* are the thinking being sitting in your chair.

It follows from these apparently trite observations that you are an animal. In a nutshell, the argument is this: (1) There is a human animal sitting in your chair. (2) The human animal sitting in your chair is thinking. (If you like, every human animal sitting there is thinking.) (3) You are the thinking being sitting in your chair. The one and only thinking being sitting in your chair is none other than you. Hence, you are that animal. That animal is you. And there is nothing special about you: we are all animals. If anyone suspects a trick, here is the argument's logical form:

1. $(\exists x)$ (x is a human animal & x is sitting in your chair)
2. (x) ((x is a human animal & x is sitting in your chair) $\supset$ x is thinking)
3. (x) ((x is thinking & x is sitting in your chair) $\supset$ x=you)
4. $(\exists x)$ (x is a human animal & x=you)

The reader can verify that it is formally valid. (Compare: A man entered the bank vault. The man who entered the vault—any man who did—stole the money. Snodgrass, and no one else, entered the vault and stole the money. Doesn't it follow that Snodgrass is a man?)

Let us be clear about what the "thinking-animal" argument purports to show. Its conclusion is that we are human animals. That is, one of the things true of you is that you are (identical with) an animal. That of course leaves many metaphysical questions about ourselves unanswered. It doesn't by itself tell us whether we are essentially or most fundamentally animals, for instance, or what our identity conditions are. That depends on the metaphysical nature of human animals: on whether human animals are essentially animals, and what their identity conditions are. These are further questions. I argued in the previous section that no sort of mental continuity is either necessary or sufficient for a human animal to persist. If that is right, then our being animals has important and highly contentious metaphysical implications. But it might be disputed, even by those who agree that we are animals. The claim that we are animals is not the end of the story about personal identity. It is only the beginning. Still, it is important to begin in the right place.

The thinking-animal argument is deceptively simple. I suspect that its very simplicity has prevented many philosophers from seeing its point. But there is nothing sophistical about it. It has no obvious and devastating flaw that we teach our students. It deserves to be better known.[3]

In any case, the argument has three premisses, and so there are three ways of resisting it. One could deny that there is any human animal sitting in your chair. One could deny that any such animal thinks. Or one could deny that you are the thinking being sitting there. Anyone who denies that we are animals is committed to accepting one of these claims. They are not very plausible. But let us consider them.

5. Alternative One: There Are No Human Animals

Why suppose that there is no human animal sitting in your chair? Presumably because there are no human animals anywhere. If there are any human animals at all, there is one sitting there. (I assume that you aren't a Martian foundling.) And if there are no human animals, it is hard to see how there could be any organisms of other sorts. So denying the argument's first premise amounts to denying that there are, strictly speaking, any organisms. There appear to be, of course. But that is at best a well-founded illusion.

There are venerable philosophical views that rule out the existence of organisms. Idealism, for instance, denies that there are any material objects at all (so I should describe it, anyway). And there is the view that nothing can have different parts at different times (Chisholm 1976: 86–113, 145–58). Whenever something appears to lose or gain a part, the truth of the matter is that one object, made of the first set of parts, ceases to exist (or becomes scattered) and is instantly replaced by a numerically different object made of the second set of parts. Organisms, if there were such things, would constantly assimilate new particles and expel others. If nothing can survive a change of any of its parts, organisms are metaphysically impossible. What we think of as an organism is in reality only a succession of different "masses of matter" that each take on organic form for a brief moment—until a single particle is gained or lost—and then pass that form on to a numerically different mass.

But few opponents of animalism deny the existence of animals. They have good reason not to, quite apart from the fact that this is more or less incredible. Anything that would rule out the existence of animals would also rule out most of the things we might be if we are not animals. If there are no animals, there are no beings constituted by animals, and no temporal parts of animals. And whatever rules out animals may tell against Humean bundles of perceptions as well. If there are no animals, it is not easy to see what we *could* be.

6. Alternative Two: Human Animals Can't Think

The second alternative is that there is an animal sitting in your chair, but it isn't thinking. (Let any occurrence of a prepositional attitude, such as the belief that it's raining or the hope that it won't, count as "thinking.") *You* think, but the animal doesn't. The reason for this can only be that the animal can't think. If it were able to think, it would be thinking now. And if *that* animal can't think—despite its healthy, mature human brain, lengthy education, surrounding community of thinkers, and appropriate evolutionary history—then no human animal can. And if no human animal can think, no animal of any sort could. (We can't very well say that dogs can think but human animals can't.) Finally, if no animal could ever think—not even a normal adult human animal—it is hard to see how any organism could have any mental property whatever. So if your animal isn't thinking, that is apparently because it is impossible for any organism to have mental properties.

The claim, then, is that animals, including human animals, are no more intelligent or sentient than trees. We could of course say that they are "intelligent" in the sense of being the bodies of intelligent people who are not themselves animals. And we could call organisms like dogs "sentient" in the sense of being the bodies of sentient non-animals that stand to those animals as you and I stand to human animals. But that is loose talk. The strict and sober truth would be that only non-organisms could ever think.

This is rather hard to believe. Anyone who denies that animals can think (or that they can think in the way that we think) needs to explain why they can't. What stops a typical human animal from using its brain to think? Isn't that what that organ is *for*?

Traditionally, those who deny that animals can think deny that any material object could do so. That seems natural enough: if *any* material thing could think, it would be an animal. Thinking things must be immaterial, and so must we. Of course, simply denying that any material thing could think does nothing to explain why it couldn't. But again, few contemporary opponents of animalism believe that we are immaterial.

Someone might argue like this: "The human animal sitting in your chair is just your body. It is absurd to suppose that your body reads or thinks about philosophy. The thinking thing there—you—must therefore be something other than the animal. But that doesn't mean that you are immaterial. You might be a material thing other than your body."

It may be false to say that your body is reading. There is certainly *something* wrong with that statement. What is less clear is whether it is wrong because the phrase "your body" denotes something that you in some sense have—a certain human organism—that is unable to read. Compare the word "body" with a closely related one: *mind*. It is just as absurd to say that Alice's mind weighs 120 pounds, or indeed any other amount, as it is to say that Alice's body is reading. (If that seems less than obvious, consider the claim that Alice's mind is sunburned.) Must we conclude that Alice has something—a clever thing, for Alice has a clever mind—that weighs nothing? Does this show that thinking beings have no mass? Surely not. I think we should be equally wary of drawing metaphysical conclusions from the fact that the phrase "Alice's body" cannot always be substituted for the name "Alice." In any case, the "body" argument does nothing to explain why a human animal should be unable to think.

Anyone who claims that some material objects can think but animals cannot has his work cut out for him. Shoemaker (1984: 92–97; 1999) has argued that animals cannot think because they have the wrong identity conditions. Mental properties have characteristic causal roles, and these, he argues, imply that psychological continuity must suffice for the bearers of those properties to persist. Since this is not true of any organism, no organism could have mental properties. But material things with the right identity conditions *can* think, and organisms can "constitute" such things. I have discussed this argument in another place (Olson 2002b). It is a long story, though, and I won't try to repeat it here.

7. Alternative Three: You Are Not Alone

Suppose, then, that there is a human animal sitting in your chair. And suppose that it thinks. Is there any way to resist the conclusion that you are that thinking animal? We can hardly say that the animal thinks but you don't. (If anything thinks, you do.) Nor can we deny that you exist, when there is a rational animal thinking your thoughts. How, then, could you fail to be that thinking animal? Only if you are not the only thinker there. If you are not *the* thinking thing sitting there, you must be one of at least two such thinkers. You exist. You think. There is also a thinking human animal there. Presumably it has the same psychological qualities as you have. But it isn't you. There are two thinking beings wherever we thought there was just one. There are two philosophers, you and an animal, sitting there and reading this. You are never truly alone: wherever you go, a watchful human animal goes with you.

This is not an attractive picture. Its adherents may try to comfort us by proposing linguistic hypotheses. Whenever two beings are as intimately related as you and your animal are, they will say, we "count them as one" for ordinary purposes (Lewis 1976). When I write on the copyright form that I am the sole author of this essay, I don't mean that every author of this essay is numerically identical with me. I mean only that every author of this essay bears some relation to me that does not imply identity: that every such author is co-located with me, perhaps. My wife is not a bigamist, even though she is, I suppose, married both to me and to the animal. At any rate it would be seriously misleading to describe our relationship as a *ménage à quatre*.

This is supposed to show that the current proposal needn't contradict anything that we say or believe when engaged in the ordinary business of life. Unless we are doing metaphysics, we don't distinguish strict numerical identity from the intimate relation that each of us bears to a certain human animal. Ordinary people have no opinion about how many numerically different thinking beings there are. Why should they? What matters in real life is not how many thinkers there are strictly speaking, but how many *non-overlapping* thinkers.

Perhaps so. Still, it hardly makes the current proposal easy to believe. Is it not strange to suppose that there are two numerically different thinkers wherever we thought there was just one?

In any event, the troubles go beyond mere overcrowding. If there really are two beings, a person and an animal, now thinking your thoughts and performing your actions, you ought to wonder which one you are. You may think you're the person (the one that isn't an animal). But doesn't the animal think that *it* is a person? It has all the same reasons for thinking so as you have. Yet it is mistaken. If you *were* the animal and not the person, you'd still think you were the person. For all you know, *you*'re the one making the mistake. Even if you are a person and not an animal, you could never have any reason to believe that you are.[4]

For that matter, if your animal can think, that ought to make *it* a person. It has the same mental features as you have. (Otherwise we should expect an explanation for the difference, just as we should if the animal can't think at all.)

It is, in Locke's words, "a thinking intelligent being, that has reason and reflection, and can consider itself as itself, the same thinking thing, in different times and places" (1975: 335). It satisfies every ordinary definition of "person." But it would be mad to suppose that the animal sitting in your chair is a *person* numerically different from you—that each human person shares her location and her thoughts with *another* person. If nothing else, this would contradict the claim that people—all people—have psychological identity conditions, thus sweeping away the main reason for denying that we are animals in the first place.

On the other hand, if rational human animals are not people, familiar accounts of what it is to be a person are all far too permissive. Having the psychological and moral features that you and I have would not be enough to make something a person. There could be rational, intelligent, self-conscious *non*-people. In fact there would be at least one such rational non-person for every genuine person. That would deprive personhood of any psychological or moral significance.

8. Hard Choices

That concludes my argument for animalism. We could put the same point in another way. There are about six billion human animals walking the earth. Those animals are just like ourselves. They sit in our chairs and sleep in our beds. They work, and talk, and take holidays. Some of them do philosophy. They have just the mental and physical attributes that we take ourselves to have. So it seems, anyway. This makes it hard to deny that *we* are those animals. The apparent existence of rational human animals is an inconvenient fact for the opponents of animalism. We might call it the *problem of the thinking animal.*

But what of the case against animalism? It seems that you would go along with your cerebrum if that organ were transplanted. More generally, some sort of mental continuity appears to suffice for us to persist.[5] And that is not true of any animal. Generations of philosophers have found this argument compelling. How can they have gone so badly wrong?

One reason, as I have said, is that they haven't asked the right questions. They have thought about what it takes for us to persist through time, but not about what we are.

Here is another. If someone is mentally just like you, that is strong evidence for his being you. All the more so if there is continuously physically realized mental continuity between him and you. In fact it is conclusive evidence, given that brain transplants belong to science fiction. Moreover, most of us find mental continuity more interesting and important than brute physical continuity. When we hear a story, we don't much care which person at the end of the tale is the same animal as a given person at the beginning. We care about who is psychologically continuous with that person. If mental and animal continuity often came apart, we might think differently. But they don't.

These facts can easily lead us to suppose that the one who remembers your life in the transplant story is you. Easier still if we don't know how problematic that claim is—if we don't realize that it would rule out our being animals. To those who haven't reflected on the problem of the thinking animal—and that includes most philosophers—it can seem dead obvious that we persist by virtue of mental continuity. But if we are animals, this is a mistake, though an understandable one.

Of course, opponents of animalism can play this game too. They can attempt to explain why it is natural to suppose that there are human animals, or that human animals can think, or that you are the thinking thing sitting in your chair, in a way that does not imply that those claims are true. (That is the point of the linguistic hypotheses I mentioned earlier.) What to do? Well, I invite you to compare the thinking-animal argument with the transplant argument. Which is more likely? That there are no animals? That no animal could ever think? That you are one of at least two intelligent beings sitting in your chair? Or that you would not, after all, go along with your transplanted cerebrum?

9. What It Would Mean If We Were Animals

What would it mean if we were animals? The literature on personal identity gives the impression that this is a highly counter-intuitive, "tough-minded" idea, radically at odds with our deepest convictions. It is certainly at odds with most of that literature. But I doubt whether it conflicts with anything that we all firmly believe.

If animalism conflicts with any popular beliefs, they will be beliefs about the conditions of our identity over time. As we have seen, the way we react (or imagine ourselves reacting) to certain fantastic stories suggests that we take ourselves to persist by virtue of mental continuity. Our beliefs about *actual* cases, though, suggest no such thing. In every actual case, the number of people we think there are is just the number of human animals. Every actual case in which we take someone to survive or perish is a case where a human animal survives or perishes.

If anything, the way we regard actual cases suggests a conviction that our identity does not consist in mental continuity, or at any rate that mental continuity is unnecessary for us to persist. When someone lapses into a persistent vegetative state, his friends and relatives may conclude that his life no longer has any value. They may even conclude that he has ceased to exist *as a person*. But they don't ordinarily suppose that their loved one no longer exists at all, and that the living organism on the hospital bed is something numerically different from him—even when they come to believe that there is no mental continuity between the vegetable and the person. *That* would be a tough-minded view.

And most of us believe that we were once fetuses. When we see an ultrasound picture of a twelve-week-old fetus, it is easy to believe we are seeing something that will, if all goes well, be born, learn to talk, go to school, and eventually become an adult human person. Yet none of us is in any way mentally continuous with a twelve-week-old fetus.

Animalism may conflict with religious beliefs: in reincarnation or resurrection, for instance (though whether there is any real conflict is less obvious than it may seem: see van Inwagen 1978). But few accounts of personal identity are any more compatible with those beliefs. If resurrection and reincarnation rule out our being animals, they probably rule out our being anything except immaterial substances, or perhaps computer programs. On this score animalism is no worse off than its main rivals.

And don't we have a strong conviction that we are animals? We all think that we are human beings. And until the philosophers got hold of us, we took human beings to be animals. We *seem* to be animals. It is the opponents of animalism who insist that this appearance is deceptive: that the animal you see in the mirror is not really you. That we are animals ought to be the default position. If anything is hard to believe, it's the alternatives.[6]

NOTES

1. E.g., Shoemaker 1984: 113f. For what it's worth, my opinion of "constitutionalism" can be found in Olson 2001.

2. For more on this crucial point see Olson 1997: 114–19.

3. The argument is not entirely new. As I see it, it only makes explicit what is implicit in Carter 1989, Ayers 1990: 283f, Snowdon 1990, and Olson 1997: 100–109.

4. Some say that revisionary linguistics can solve this problem, too (Noonan 1998). The idea is roughly this. First, not just any rational, self-conscious being is a person, but only those that have psychological identity conditions. Human animals, despite their

mental properties, are not people because they lack psychological identity conditions. Second, the word "I" and other personal pronouns refer only to people. Thus, when the animal associated with you says "I," it doesn't refer to itself. Rather, it refers to you, the person associated with it. When it says, "I am a person," it does not say falsely that *it* is a person, but truly that *you* are. So the animal is not mistaken about which thing it is, and neither are you. You can infer that you are a person from the linguistic facts that you are whatever you refer to when you say "I," and that "I" refers only to people. I discuss this ingenious proposal in Olson 2002a.

5. In fact this is not so. Let the surgeons transplant each of your cerebral hemispheres into a different head. Both offshoots will be mentally continuous with you. But they can't both *be* you, for the simple reason that one thing (you) cannot be identical with two things. We cannot say in general that anyone who is mentally continuous with you must be you. Exceptions are possible. So it ought to come as no great surprise if the original cerebrum transplant is another exception.

6. I thank Trenton Merricks and Gonzalo Rodriguez-Pereyra for comments on an earlier version of this paper.

REFERENCES

Ayers, M. 1990. *Locke*, vol. 2. London: Routledge.
Carter, W. R. 1989. How to change your mind. *Canadian Journal of Philosophy* 19: 1–14.
Chisholm, R. 1976. *Person and Object*. La Salle, IL: Open Court.
Hume, D. 1888. *Treatise of Human Nature* (1739), ed. L. A. Selby-Bigge. Oxford: Clarendon Press. Partly repr. in Perry 1975: 159–78.
Lewis, D. 1976. Survival and identity. In A. Rorty, ed., *The Identities of Persons,* Berkeley: University of California Press, pp. 17–40. Repr. in his *Philosophical Papers*, vol. 1, New York: Oxford University Press, 1983, pp. 55–77.
Locke, J. 1975. *An Essay Concerning Human Understanding*, 2nd edn (1694), ed. P. Nidditch. Oxford: Clarendon Press. Partly repr. in Perry 1975: 33–52.
Noonan, Harold. 1998. Animalism versus Lockeanism: a current controversy. *Philosophical Quarterly* 48: 302–18.
Olson, E. 1997. *The Human Animal: Personal Identity without Psychology.* New York: Oxford University Press.
———. 2001. Material coincidence and the indiscernibility problem. *Philosophical Quarterly* 51: 337–55.
———. 2002a. Thinking animals and the reference of "I." *Philosophical Topics* 30.
———. 2002b. What does functionalism tell us about personal identity? *Noûs* 36.
Perry, J., ed. 1975. *Personal Identity.* Berkeley: University of California Press.
Quintan, A. 1962. The soul. *Journal of Philosophy* 59: 393–403. Repr. in Perry 1975: 53–72.
Russell, B. 1985. *The Philosophy of Logical Atomism* (1918). La Salle, IL: Open Court.
Shoemaker, S. 1984. Personal identity: a materialist's account. In S. Shoemaker and R. Swinburne, *Personal Identity*, Oxford: Blackwell, pp. 67–132.
———. 1999. Self, body, and coincidence. *Proceedings of the Aristotelian Society*, supp. vol. 73: 287–306.
Snowdon, Paul. 1990. Persons, animals, and ourselves. In C. Gill, ed., *The Person and the Human Mind*, Oxford: Clarendon Press, pp. 83–107.

Unger, P. 1979. I do not exist. In G. F. MacDonald, ed., *Perception and Identity,* London: Macmillan, pp. 235–51. Repr. in M. Rea, ed., *Material Constitution,* Lanham, MD: Rowman and Littlefield, 1997, pp. 175–90.

van Inwagen, P. 1978. The possibility of resurrection. *International Journal for the Philosophy of Religion* 9: 114–21. Repr. in his *The Possibility of Resurrection and Other Essays in Christian Apologetics,* Boulder, CO: Westview, 1997, pp. 45–51.

———. 1980. Philosophers and the words "human body." In van Inwagen, ed., *Time and Cause,* Dordrecht: Reidel, pp. 283–99.

PERSONS AS PSYCHOLOGICAL QUALITIES
OR FUNCTIONS

CHAPTER SEVEN

Selection from *An Essay Concerning Human Understanding*

John Locke

Chapter XXVII. of Identity and Diversity.

1. Wherein Identity consists.

ANOTHER occasion the mind often takes of comparing, is the very being of things, when, considering ANYTHING AS EXISTING AT ANY DETERMINED TIME AND PLACE, we compare it with ITSELF EXISTING AT ANOTHER TIME, and thereon form the ideas of IDENTITY and DIVERSITY. When we see anything to be in any place in any instant of time, we are sure (be it what it will) that it is that very thing, and not another which at that same time exists in another place, how like and undistinguishable soever it may be in all other respects: and in this consists IDENTITY, when the ideas it is attributed to vary not at all from what they were that moment wherein we consider their former existence, and to which we compare the present. For we never finding, nor conceiving it possible, that two things of the same kind should exist in the same place at the same time, we rightly conclude, that, whatever exists anywhere at any time, excludes all of the same kind, and is there itself alone. When therefore we demand whether anything be the SAME or no, it refers always to something that existed such a time in such a place, which it was certain, at that instant, was the same with itself, and no other. From whence it follows, that one thing cannot have two beginnings of existence, nor two things one beginning; it being impossible for two things of the same kind to be or exist in the same instant, in the very same place; or one and the same thing in different places. That, therefore, that had one beginning, is the same thing; and that which had a different beginning in time and place from that, is not the same, but diverse. That which has made the difficulty about this relation has been the little care and attention used in having precise notions of the things to which it is attributed.

2. Identity of Substances.

We have the ideas but of three sorts of substances: 1. GOD. 2. FINITE INTELLIGENCES. 3. BODIES.

First, GOD is without beginning, eternal, unalterable, and everywhere, and therefore concerning his identity there can be no doubt.

Secondly, FINITE SPIRITS having had each its determinated time and place of beginning to exist, the relation to that time and place will always determine to each of them its identity, as long as it exists.

Thirdly, The same will hold of every PARTICLE OF MATTER, to which no addition or subtraction of matter being made, it is the same. For, though these three sorts of substances, as we term them, do not exclude one another out of the same place, yet we cannot conceive but that they must necessarily each of them exclude any of the same kind out of the same place: or else the notions and names of identity and diversity would be in vain, and there could be no such distinctions of substances, or anything else one from another. For example: could two bodies be in the same place at the same time; then those two parcels of matter must be one and the same, take them great or little; nay, all bodies must be one and the same. For, by the same reason that two particles of matter may be in one place, all bodies may be in one place: which, when it can be supposed, takes away the distinction of identity and diversity of one and more, and renders it ridiculous. But it being a contradiction that two or more should be one, identity and diversity are relations and ways of comparing well founded, and of use to the understanding.

3. Identity of modes and relations.

All other things being but modes or relations ultimately terminated in substances, the identity and diversity of each particular existence of them too will be by the same way determined: only as to things whose existence is in succession, such as are the actions of finite beings, v.g. MOTION and THOUGHT, both which consist in a continued train of succession, concerning THEIR diversity there can be no question: because each perishing the moment it begins, they cannot exist in different times, or in different places, as permanent beings can at different times exist in distant places; and therefore no motion or thought, considered as at different times, can be the same, each part thereof having a different beginning of existence.

4. Principium Individuationis.

From what has been said, it is easy to discover what is so much inquired after, the PRINCIPIUM INDIVIDUATIONIS; and that, it is plain, is existence itself; which determines a being of any sort to a particular time and place, incommunicable to two beings of the same kind. This, though it seems easier to conceive in simple substances or modes; yet, when reflected on, is not more difficult in compound ones, if care be taken to what it is applied: v.g. let us suppose an atom, i.e. a continued body under one immutable superficies, existing in a determined time and place; it is evident, that, considered in any instant of its existence, it is in that instant the same with itself. For, being at that instant what it is, and nothing else, it is the same, and so must continue as long as its existence is continued; for so long it will be the same, and no other. In like manner, if two or more atoms be joined together into the same mass, every one of those atoms will be the same, by the foregoing rule: and whilst they exist united together, the mass, consisting of the same atoms, must be the same mass, or the same body, let the parts be ever so differently jumbled. But if one of these atoms be taken away, or one new one added, it is no longer the same mass or the same body. In the state of living creatures, their identity depends not on a mass of the same particles, but on something else. For in them the variation of great parcels of matter alters not the identity: an oak growing from a plant to a great tree, and then lopped, is still the same oak; and a colt grown up to a horse, sometimes fat, sometimes lean, is all the while the same horse: though, in both these cases, there may be a manifest change of the parts; so that truly they are not either of them the same masses of matter, though they be truly one of them the same oak, and the other the same horse. The reason whereof is, that, in these two cases—a MASS OF MATTER and a LIVING BODY—identity is not applied to the same thing.

5. Identity of Vegetables.

We must therefore consider wherein an oak differs from a mass of matter, and that seems to me to be in this, that the one is only the cohesion of particles of matter any how united, the other such a disposition of them as constitutes the parts of an oak; and such an organization of those parts as is fit to receive and distribute nourishment, so as to continue and frame the wood, bark, and leaves, etc., of an oak, in which consists the vegetable life. That being then one plant which has such an organization of parts in one coherent body, partaking of one common life, it continues to be the same plant as long as it partakes of the same life, though that life be communicated to new particles of matter vitally united to the living plant, in a like continued organization conformable to that sort of plants. For this organization, being at any one instant in any one collection of matter, is in that particular concrete distinguished from all other, and IS that individual life, which existing constantly from that moment both forwards and backwards, in the same continuity of insensibly succeeding parts united to the living body of the plant, it has that identity which makes the same plant, and all the parts of it, parts of the same plant, during all the time that they exist united in that continued organization, which is fit to convey that common life to all the parts so united.

6. Identity of Animals.

The case is not so much different in BRUTES but that any one may hence see what makes an animal and continues it the same. Something we have like this in machines, and may serve to illustrate it. For example, what is a watch? It is plain it is nothing but a fit organization or construction of parts to a certain end, which, when a sufficient force is added to it, it is capable to attain. If we would suppose this machine one continued body, all whose organized parts were repaired, increased, or diminished by a constant addition or separation of insensible parts, with one common life, we should have something very much like the body of an animal; with this difference, That, in an animal the fitness of the organization, and the motion wherein life consists, begin together, the motion coming from within; but in machines the force coming sensibly from without, is often away when the organ is in order, and well fitted to receive it.

7. The Identity of Man.

This also shows wherein the identity of the same MAN consists; viz. in nothing but a participation of the same continued life, by constantly fleeting particles of matter, in succession vitally united to the same organized body. He that shall place the identity of man in anything else, but, like that of other animals, in one fitly organized body, taken in any one instant, and from thence continued, under one organization of life, in several successively fleeting particles of matter united to it, will find it hard to make an embryo, one of years, mad and sober, the SAME man, by any supposition, that will not make it possible for Seth, Ismael, Socrates, Pilate, St. Austin, and Caesar Borgia, to be the same man. For if the identity of SOUL ALONE makes the same MAN; and there be nothing in the nature of matter why the same individual spirit may not be united to different bodies, it will be possible that those men, living in distant ages, and of different tempers, may have been the same man: which way of speaking must be from a very strange use of the word man, applied to an idea out of which body and shape are excluded. And that way of speaking would agree yet worse with the notions of those philosophers who allow of transmigration, and are of opinion that the souls of men may, for their miscarriages, be detruded into the bodies of beasts, as fit habitations, with organs suited to the satisfaction of their brutal inclinations. But yet I think nobody, could he be sure that the SOUL of Heliogabalus were in one of his hogs, would yet say that hog were a MAN or Heliogabalus.

8. Idea of Identity suited to the Idea it is applied to.

It is not therefore unity of substance that comprehends all sorts of identity, or will determine it in every case; but to conceive and judge of it aright, we must consider what idea the word it is applied to stands for: it being one thing to be the same SUBSTANCE, another the same MAN, and a third the same PERSON, if PERSON, MAN, and SUBSTANCE, are three names standing for three different ideas;—for such as is the idea belonging to that name, such must be the identity; which, if it had been a little more carefully attended to, would possibly have prevented a great deal of that confusion which often occurs about this matter, with no small seeming difficulties, especially concerning PERSONAL identity, which therefore we shall in the next place a little consider.

9. Same man.

An animal is a living organized body; and consequently the same animal, as we have observed, is the same continued LIFE communicated to different particles of matter, as they happen successively to be united to that organized living body. And whatever is talked of other definitions, ingenious observation puts it past doubt, that the idea in our minds, of which the sound man in our mouths is the sign, is nothing else but of an animal of such a certain form. Since I think I may be confident, that, whoever should see a creature of his own shape or make, though it had no more reason all its life than a cat or a parrot, would call him still a MAN; or whoever should hear a cat or a parrot discourse, reason, and philosophize, would call or think it nothing but a CAT or a PARROT; and say, the one was a dull irrational man, and the other a very intelligent rational parrot.

10. Same man.

For I presume it is not the idea of a thinking or rational being alone that makes the IDEA OF A MAN in most people's sense: but of a body, so and so shaped, joined to it; and if that be the idea of a man, the same successive body not shifted all at once, must, as well as the same immaterial spirit, go to the making of the same man.

11. Personal Identity.

This being premised, to find wherein personal identity consists, we must consider what PERSON stands for;—which, I think, is a thinking intelligent being, that has reason and reflection, and can consider itself as itself, the same thinking thing, in different times and places; which it does only by that consciousness which is inseparable from thinking, and, as it seems to me, essential to it: it being impossible for any one to perceive without PERCEIVING that he does perceive. When we see, hear, smell, taste, feel, meditate, or will anything, we know that we do so. Thus it is always as to our present sensations and perceptions: and by this every one is to himself that which he calls SELF:—it not being considered, in this case, whether the same self be continued in the same or divers substances. For, since consciousness always accompanies thinking, and it is that which makes every one to be what he calls self, and thereby distinguishes himself from all other thinking things, in this alone consists personal identity, i.e. the sameness of a rational being: and as far as this consciousness can be extended backwards to any past action or thought, so far reaches the identity of that person; it is the same self now it was then; and it is by the same self with this present one that now reflects on it, that that action was done.

12. Consciousness makes personal Identity.

But it is further inquired, whether it be the same identical substance. This few would think they had reason to doubt of, if these perceptions, with their consciousness, always remained present in the mind, whereby the same thinking thing would be always consciously present, and, as would be thought, evidently the same to itself. But that which seems to make the difficulty is this, that this consciousness being interrupted always by forgetfulness, there being no moment of our lives wherein we have the whole train of all our past actions before our eyes in one view, but even the best memories losing the sight of one part whilst they are viewing another; and we sometimes, and that the greatest part of our lives, not reflecting on our past selves, being intent on our present thoughts, and in sound sleep having no thoughts at all, or at least none with that consciousness which remarks our waking thoughts,—I say, in all these cases, our consciousness being interrupted, and we losing the sight of our past selves, doubts are raised whether we are the same thinking thing, i.e. the same SUBSTANCE or no. Which, however reasonable or unreasonable, concerns not PERSONAL identity at all. The question being what makes the same person; and not whether it be the same identical substance, which always thinks in the same person, which, in this case, matters not at all: different substances, by the same consciousness (where they do partake in it) being united into one person, as well as different bodies by the same life are united into one animal, whose identity is preserved in that change of substances by the unity of one continued life. For, it being the same consciousness that makes a man be himself to himself, personal identity depends on that only, whether it be annexed solely to one individual substance, or can be continued in a succession of several substances. For as far as any intelligent being CAN repeat the idea of any past action with the same consciousness it had of it at first, and with the same consciousness it has of any present action; so far it is the same personal self. For it is by the consciousness it has of its present thoughts and actions, that it is SELF TO ITSELF now, and so will be the same self, as far as the same consciousness can extend to actions past or to come; and would be by distance of time, or change of substance, no more two persons, than a man be two men by wearing other clothes to-day than he did yesterday, with a long or a short sleep between: the same consciousness uniting those distant actions into the same person, whatever substances contributed to their production.

13. Personal Identity in Change of Substance.

That this is so, we have some kind of evidence in our very bodies, all whose particles, whilst vitally united to this same thinking conscious self, so that WE FEEL when they are touched, and are affected by, and conscious of good or harm that happens to them, are a part of ourselves; i.e. of our thinking conscious self. Thus, the limbs of his body are to every one a part of himself; he sympathizes and is concerned for them. Cut off a hand, and thereby separate it from that consciousness he had of its heat, cold, and other affections, and it is then no longer a part of that which is himself, any more than the remotest part of matter. Thus, we see the SUBSTANCE whereof personal self consisted at one time may be varied at another, without the change of personal identity; there being no question about the same person, though the limbs which but now were a part of it, be cut off.

14. Personality in Change of Substance.

But the question is, Whether if the same substance which thinks be changed, it can be the same person; or, remaining the same, it can be different persons?

And to this I answer: First, This can be no question at all to those who place thought in a purely material animal constitution, void of an immaterial substance. For, whether their supposition be true or no, it is plain they conceive personal identity preserved in something else than identity of substance; as animal identity is preserved in identity of life, and not of substance. And therefore those who place thinking in an immaterial substance only, before they can come to deal with these men, must show why personal identity cannot be preserved in the change of immaterial substances, or variety of particular immaterial substances, as well as animal identity is preserved in the change of material substances, or variety of particular bodies: unless they will say, it is one immaterial spirit that makes the same life in brutes, as it is one immaterial spirit that makes the same person in men; which the Cartesians at least will not admit, for fear of making brutes thinking things too.

15. Whether in Change of thinking Substances there can be one Person.

But next, as to the first part of the question, Whether, if the same thinking substance (supposing immaterial substances only to think) be changed, it can be the same person? I answer, that cannot be resolved but by those who know what kind of substances they are that do think; and whether the consciousness of past actions can be transferred from one thinking substance to another. I grant were the same consciousness the same individual action it could not: but it being a present representation of a past action, why it may not be possible, that that may be represented to the mind to have been which really never was, will remain to be shown. And therefore how far the consciousness of past actions is annexed to any individual agent, so that another cannot possibly have it, will be hard for us to determine, till we know what kind of action it is that cannot be done without a reflex act of perception accompanying it, and how performed by thinking substances, who cannot think without being conscious of it. But that which we call the same consciousness, not being the same individual act, why one intellectual substance may not have represented to it, as done by itself, what IT never did, and was perhaps done by some other agent—why, I say, such a representation may not possibly be without reality of matter of fact, as well as several representations in dreams are, which yet whilst dreaming we take for true—will be difficult to conclude from the nature of things. And that it never is so, will by us, till we have clearer views of the nature of thinking substances, be best resolved into the goodness of God; who, as far as the happiness or misery of any of his sensible creatures is concerned in it, will not, by a fatal error of theirs, transfer from one to another that consciousness which draws reward or punishment with it. How far this may be an argument against those who would place thinking in a system of fleeting animal spirits, I leave to be considered. But yet, to return to the question before us, it must be allowed, that, if the same consciousness (which, as has been shown, is quite a different thing from the same numerical figure or motion in body) can be transferred from one thinking substance to another, it will be possible that two thinking substances may make but one person. For the same consciousness being preserved, whether in the same or different substances, the personal identity is preserved.

16. Whether, the same immaterial Substance remaining, there can be two Persons.

As to the second part of the question, Whether the same immaterial substance remaining, there may be two distinct persons; which question seems to me to be built on this,—Whether the same immaterial being, being conscious of the action of its past duration, may be wholly stripped of all the consciousness of its past existence, and lose it beyond the power of ever retrieving it again: and so as it were beginning a new account from a new period, have a consciousness that CANNOT reach beyond this new state. All those who hold pre-existence are evidently of this mind; since they allow the soul to have no remaining consciousness of what it did in that pre-existent state, either wholly separate from body, or informing any other body; and if they should not, it is plain experience would be against them. So that personal identity, reaching no further than consciousness reaches, a pre-existent spirit not having continued so many ages in a state of silence, must needs make different persons. Suppose a Christian Platonist or a Pythagorean should, upon God's having ended all his works of creation the seventh day, think his soul hath existed ever since; and should imagine it has revolved in several human bodies; as I once met with one, who was persuaded his had been the SOUL of Socrates (how reasonably I will not dispute; this I know, that in the post he filled, which was no inconsiderable one, he passed for a very rational man, and the press has shown that he wanted not parts or learning;)—would any one say, that he, being not conscious of any of Socrates's actions or thoughts, could be the same PERSON with Socrates? Let any one reflect upon himself, and conclude that he has in himself an immaterial spirit, which is that which thinks in him, and, in the constant change of his body keeps him the same: and is that which he calls HIMSELF: let him also suppose it to be the same soul that was in Nestor or Thersites, at the siege of Troy, (for souls being, as far as we know anything of them, in their nature indifferent to any parcel of matter, the supposition has no apparent absurdity in it,) which it may have been, as well as it is now the soul of any other man: but he now having no consciousness of any of the actions either of Nestor or Thersites, does or can he conceive himself the same person with either of them? Can he be concerned in either of their actions? attribute them to himself, or think them his own more than the actions of any other men that ever existed? So that this consciousness, not reaching to any of the actions of either of those men, he is no more one SELF with either of them than of the soul of immaterial spirit that now informs him had been created, and began to exist, when it began to inform his present body; though it were never so true, that the same SPIRIT that informed Nestor's or Thersites' body were numerically the same that now informs his. For this would no more make him the same person with Nestor, than if some of the particles of matter that were once a part of Nestor were now a part of this man the same immaterial substance, without the same consciousness, no more making the same person, by being united to any body, than the same particle of matter, without consciousness, united to any body, makes the same person. But let him once find himself conscious of any of the actions of Nestor, he then finds himself the same person with Nestor.

17. The body, as well as the soul, goes to the making of a Man.

And thus may we be able, without any difficulty, to conceive the same person at the resurrection, though in a body not exactly in make or parts the same which he had here,—the same consciousness going along with the soul that inhabits it. But yet the soul alone, in the change of bodies, would scarce to any one but to him that makes the soul the man, be enough to make the same man. For should the soul of a prince, carrying with it the consciousness of the prince's past life, enter and inform the body of a cobbler, as soon as deserted by his own soul, every one sees he would be the same PERSON with the prince, accountable only for the prince's actions: but who would say it was the same MAN? The body too goes to the making the man, and would, I guess, to everybody determine the man in this case, wherein the soul, with all its princely thoughts about it, would not make another man: but he would be the same cobbler to every one besides himself. I know that, in the ordinary way of speaking, the same person, and the same man, stand for one and the same thing. And indeed every one will always have a liberty to speak as he pleases, and to apply what articulate sounds to what ideas he thinks fit, and change them as often as he pleases. But yet, when we will inquire what makes the same SPIRIT, MAN, or PERSON, we must fix the ideas of spirit, man, or person in our minds; and having resolved with ourselves what we mean by them, it will not be hard to determine, in either of them, or the like, when it is the same, and when not.

18. *Consciousness alone unites actions into the same Person.*

But though the same immaterial substance or soul does not alone, wherever it be, and in whatsoever state, make the same MAN; yet it is plain, consciousness, as far as ever it can be extended—should it be to ages past—unites existences and actions very remote in time into the same PERSON, as well as it does the existences and actions of the immediately preceding moment: so that whatever has the consciousness of present and past actions, is the same person to whom they both belong. Had I the same consciousness that I saw the ark and Noah's flood, as that I saw an overflowing of the Thames last winter, or as that I write now, I could no more doubt that I who write this now, that saw the Thames overflowed last winter, and that viewed the flood at the general deluge, was the same SELF,—place that self in what SUBSTANCE you please—than that I who write this am the same MYSELF now whilst I write (whether I consist of all the same substance material or immaterial, or no) that I was yesterday. For as to this point of being the same self, it matters not whether this present self be made up of the same or other substances—I being as much concerned, and as justly accountable for any action that was done a thousand years since, appropriated to me now by this self-consciousness, as I am for what I did the last moment.

19. *Self depends on Consciousness, not on Substance.*

SELF is that conscious thinking thing,—whatever substance made up of, (whether spiritual or material, simple or compounded, it matters not)—which is sensible or conscious of pleasure and pain, capable of happiness or misery, and so is concerned for itself, as far as that consciousness extends. Thus every one finds that, whilst comprehended under that consciousness, the little finger is as much a part of himself as what is most so. Upon separation of this little finger, should this consciousness go along with the little finger, and leave the rest of the body, it is evident the little finger would be the person, the same person; and self then would have nothing to do with the rest of the body. As in this case it is the consciousness that goes along with the substance, when one part is separate from another, which makes the same person, and constitutes this inseparable self: so it is in reference to substances remote in time. That with which the consciousness of this present thinking thing CAN join itself, makes the same person, and is one self with it, and with nothing else; and so attributes to itself, and owns all the actions of that thing, as its own, as far as that consciousness reaches, and no further; as every one who reflects will perceive.

20. Persons, not Substances, the Objects of Reward and Punishment.

In this personal identity is founded all the right and justice of reward and punishment; happiness and misery being that for which every one is concerned for HIMSELF, and not mattering what becomes of any SUBSTANCE, not joined to, or affected with that consciousness. For, as it is evident in the instance I gave but now, if the consciousness went along with the little finger when it was cut off, that would be the same self which was concerned for the whole body yesterday, as making part of itself, whose actions then it cannot but admit as its own now. Though, if the same body should still live, and immediately from the separation of the little finger have its own peculiar consciousness, whereof the little finger knew nothing, it would not at all be concerned for it, as a part of itself, or could own any of its actions, or have any of them imputed to him.

21. Which shows wherein Personal identity consists.

This may show us wherein personal identity consists: not in the identity of substance, but, as I have said, in the identity of consciousness, wherein if Socrates and the present mayor of Queenborough agree, they are the same person: if the same Socrates waking and sleeping do not partake of the same consciousness, Socrates waking and sleeping is not the same person. And to punish Socrates waking for what sleeping Socrates thought, and waking Socrates was never conscious of, would be no more of right, than to punish one twin for what his brother-twin did, whereof he knew nothing, because their outsides were so like, that they could not be distinguished; for such twins have been seen.

22. *Absolute oblivion separates what is thus forgotten from the person, but not from the man.*

But yet possibly it will still be objected,—Suppose I wholly lose the memory of some parts of my life, beyond a possibility of retrieving them, so that perhaps I shall never be conscious of them again; yet am I not the same person that did those actions, had those thoughts that I once was conscious of, though I have now forgot them? To which I answer, that we must here take notice what the word "I" is applied to; which, in this case, is the MAN only. And the same man being presumed to be the same person, I is easily here supposed to stand also for the same person. But if it be possible for the same man to have distinct incommunicable consciousness at different times, it is past doubt the same man would at different times make different persons; which, we see, is the sense of mankind in the solemnest declaration of their opinions, human laws not punishing the mad man for the sober man's actions, nor the sober man for what the mad man did,—thereby making them two persons: which is somewhat explained by our way of speaking in English when we say such an one is "not himself," or is "beside himself"; in which phrases it is insinuated, as if those who now, or at least first used them, thought that self was changed; the selfsame person was no longer in that man.

23. *Difference between Identity of Man and of Person.*

But yet it is hard to conceive that Socrates, the same individual man, should be two persons. To help us a little in this, we must consider what is meant by Socrates, or the same individual MAN.

First, it must be either the same individual, immaterial, thinking substance; in short, the same numerical soul, and nothing else.

Secondly, or the same animal, without any regard to an immaterial soul.

Thirdly, or the same immaterial spirit united to the same animal.

Now, take which of these suppositions you please, it is impossible to make personal identity to consist in anything but consciousness; or reach any further than that does.

For, by the first of them, it must be allowed possible that a man born of different women, and in distant times, may be the same man. A way of speaking which, whoever admits, must allow it possible for the same man to be two distinct persons, as any two that have lived in different ages without the knowledge of one another's thoughts.

By the second and third, Socrates, in this life and after it, cannot be the same man any way, but by the same consciousness; and so making human identity to

consist in the same thing wherein we place personal identity, there will be difficulty to allow the same man to be the same person. But then they who place
human identity in consciousness only, and not in something else, must consider how they will make the infant Socrates the same man with Socrates after
the resurrection. But whatsoever to some men makes a man, and consequently
the same individual man, wherein perhaps few are agreed, personal identity can
by us be placed in nothing but consciousness, (which is that alone which makes
what we call SELF,) without involving us in great absurdities.

24. *Drunk and Sober Man.*

But is not a man drunk and sober the same person? why else is he punished for
the fact he commits when drunk, though he be never afterwards conscious of
it? Just as much the same person as a man that walks, and does other things in
his sleep, is the same person, and is answerable for any mischief he shall do in
it. Human laws punish both, with a justice suitable to THEIR way of knowledge;—
because, in these cases, they cannot distinguish certainly what is real, what
counterfeit: and so the ignorance in drunkenness or sleep is not admitted as a
plea. But in the Great Day, wherein the secrets of all hearts shall be laid open, it
may be reasonable to think, no one shall be made to answer for what he knows
nothing of; but shall receive his doom, his conscience accusing or excusing
him.

25. *Consciousness alone unites remote existences into one Person.*

Nothing but consciousness can unite remote existences into the same person:
the identity of substance will not do it; for whatever substance there is, however
framed, without consciousness there is no person: and a carcass may be a person, as well as any sort of substance be so, without consciousness.

Could we suppose two distinct incommunicable consciousnesses acting the
same body, the one constantly by day, the other by night; and, on the other side,
the same consciousness, acting by intervals, two distinct bodies: I ask, in the
first case, whether the day and the night—man would not be two as distinct
persons as Socrates and Plato? And whether, in the second case, there would not
be one person in two distinct bodies, as much as one man is the same in two
distinct clothings? Nor is it at all material to say, that this same, and this distinct
consciousness, in the cases above mentioned, is owing to the same and distinct
immaterial substances, bringing it with them to those bodies; which, whether
true or no, alters not the case: since it is evident the personal identity would
equally be determined by the consciousness, whether that consciousness were

annexed to some individual immaterial substance or no. For, granting that the thinking substance in man must be necessarily supposed immaterial, it is evident that immaterial thinking thing may sometimes part with its past consciousness, and be restored to it again: as appears in the forgetfulness men often have of their past actions; and the mind many times recovers the memory of a past consciousness, which it had lost for twenty years together. Make these intervals of memory and forgetfulness to take their turns regularly by day and night, and you have two persons with the same immaterial spirit, as much as in the former instance two persons with the same body. So that self is not determined by identity or diversity of substance, which it cannot be sure of, but only by identity of consciousness.

26. Not the substance with which the consciousness may be united.

Indeed it may conceive the substance whereof it is now made up to have existed formerly, united in the same conscious being: but, consciousness removed, that substance is no more itself, or makes no more a part of it, than any other substance; as is evident in the instance we have already given of a limb cut off, of whose heat, or cold, or other affections, having no longer any consciousness, it is no more of a man's self than any other matter of the universe. In like manner it will be in reference to any immaterial substance, which is void of that consciousness whereby I am myself to myself: so that I cannot upon recollection join with that present consciousness whereby I am now myself, it is, in that part of its existence, no more MYSELF than any other immaterial being. For, whatsoever any substance has thought or done, which I cannot recollect, and by my consciousness make my own thought and action, it will no more belong to me, whether a part of me thought or did it, than if it had been thought or done by any other immaterial being anywhere existing.

27. Consciousness unites substances, material or spiritual, with the same personality.

I agree, the more probable opinion is, that this consciousness is annexed to, and the affection of, one individual immaterial substance.

But let men, according to their diverse hypotheses, resolve of that as they please. This every intelligent being, sensible of happiness or misery, must grant—that there is something that is HIMSELF, that he is concerned for, and would have happy; that this self has existed in a continued duration more than one instant, and therefore it is possible may exist, as it has done, months and years to come, without any certain bounds to be set to its duration; and may be the same self, by the same consciousness continued on for the future. And thus, by this consciousness he finds himself to be the same self which did such and such an action some years since, by which he comes to be happy or miserable now. In all which account of self, the same numerical SUBSTANCE is not considered a making the same self; but the same continued CONSCIOUSNESS, in which several substances may have been united, and again separated from it, which, whilst they continued in a vital union with that wherein this consciousness then resided, made a part of that same self. Thus any part of our bodies, vitally united to that which is conscious in us, makes a part of ourselves: but upon separation from the vital union by which that consciousness is communicated, that which a moment since was part of ourselves, is now no more so than a part of another man's self is a part of me: and it is not impossible but in a little time may become a real part of another person. And so we have the same numerical substance become a part of two different persons; and the same person preserved under the change of various substances. Could we suppose any spirit wholly stripped of all its memory of consciousness of past actions, as we find our minds always are of a great part of ours, and sometimes of them all; the union or separation of such a spiritual substance would make no variation of personal identity, any more than that of any particle of matter does. Any substance vitally united to the present thinking being is a part of that very same self which now is; anything united to it by a consciousness of former actions, makes also a part of the same self, which is the same both then and now.

28. *Person a forensic Term.*

PERSON, as I take it, is the name for this self. Wherever a man finds what he calls himself, there, I think, another may say is the same person. It is a forensic term, appropriating actions and their merit; and so belongs only to intelligent agents, capable of a law, and happiness, and misery. This personality extends itself beyond present existence to what is past, only by consciousness,—whereby it becomes concerned and accountable; owns and imputes to itself past actions, just upon the same ground and for the same reason as it does the present. All which is founded in a concern for happiness, the unavoidable concomitant of consciousness; that which is conscious of pleasure and pain, desiring that that self that is conscious should be happy. And therefore whatever past actions it cannot reconcile or APPROPRIATE to that present self by consciousness, it can be no more concerned in than if they had never been done: and to receive pleasure or pain, i.e. reward or punishment, on the account of any such action, is all one as to be made happy or miserable in its first being, without any demerit at all. For, supposing a MAN punished now for what he had done in another life, whereof he could be made to have no consciousness at all, what difference is there between that punishment and being CREATED miserable? And therefore, conformable to this, the apostle tells us, that, at the great day, when every one shall "receive according to his doings, the secrets of all hearts shall be laid open." The sentence shall be justified by the consciousness all persons shall have, that THEY THEMSELVES, in what bodies soever they appear, or what substances soever that consciousness adheres to, are the SAME that committed those actions, and deserve that punishment for them.

29. Suppositions that look strange are pardonable in our ignorance.

I am apt enough to think I have, in treating of this subject, made some suppositions that will look strange to some readers, and possibly they are so in themselves. But yet, I think they are such as are pardonable, in this ignorance we are in of the nature of that thinking thing that is in us, and which we look on as OURSELVES. Did we know what it was; or how it was tied to a certain system of fleeting animal spirits; or whether it could or could not perform its operations of thinking and memory out of a body organized as ours is; and whether it has pleased God that no one such spirit shall ever be united to any but one such body, upon the right constitution of whose organs its memory should depend; we might see the absurdity of some of those suppositions I have made. But taking, as we ordinarily now do (in the dark concerning these matters,) the soul of a man for an immaterial substance, independent from matter, and indifferent alike to it all; there can, from the nature of things, be no absurdity at all to suppose that the same SOUL may at different times be united to different BODIES, and with them make up for that time one MAN: as well as we suppose a part of a sheep's body yesterday should be a part of a man's body to-morrow, and in that union make a vital part of Meliboeus himself, as well as it did of his ram.

30. The Difficulty from ill Use of Names.

To conclude: Whatever substance begins to exist, it must, during its existence, necessarily be the same: whatever compositions of substances begin to exist, during the union of those substances, the concrete must be the same: whatsoever mode begins to exist, during its existence it is the same: and so if the composition be of distinct substances and different modes, the same rule holds. Whereby it will appear, that the difficulty or obscurity that has been about this matter rather rises from the names ill-used, than from any obscurity in things themselves. For whatever makes the specific idea to which the name is applied, if that idea be steadily kept to, the distinction of anything into the same and divers will easily be conceived, and there can arise no doubt about it.

31. Continuance of that which we have made to be our complex idea of man makes the same man.

For, supposing a rational spirit be the idea of a MAN, it is easy to know what is the same man, viz. the same spirit—whether separate or in a body—will be the SAME MAN. Supposing a rational spirit vitally united to a body of a certain conformation of parts to make a man; whilst that rational spirit, with that vital conformation of parts, though continued in a fleeting successive body, remains, it will be the SAME MAN. But if to any one the idea of a man be but the vital union of parts in a certain shape; as long as that vital union and shape remain in a concrete, no otherwise the same but by a continued succession of fleeting particles, it will be the SAME MAN. For, whatever be the composition whereof the complex idea is made, whenever existence makes it one particular thing under any denomination, THE SAME EXISTENCE CONTINUED preserves it the SAME individual under the same denomination.

The Unimportance of Identity

Derek Parfit

We can start with some science fiction. Here on Earth, I enter the Teletransporter. When I press some button, a machine destroys my body, while recording the exact states of all my cells. The information is sent by radio to Mars, where another machine makes, out of organic materials, a perfect copy of my body. The person who wakes up on Mars seems to remember living my life up to the moment when I pressed the button, and he is in every other way just like me.

Of those who have thought about such cases, some believe that it would be I who would wake up on Mars. They regard Teletransportation as merely the fastest way of travelling. Others believe that, if I chose to be Teletransported, I would be making a terrible mistake. On their view, the person who wakes up would be a mere Replica of me.

{ I }

That is a disagreement about personal identity. To understand such disagreements, we must distinguish two kinds of sameness. Two white billiard balls may be qualitatively identical, or exactly similar. But they are not numerically identical, or one and the same ball. If I paint one of these balls red, it will cease to be qualitatively identical with itself as it was; but it will still be one and the same ball. Consider next a claim like, "Since her accident, she is no longer the same person." That involves both senses of identity. It means that *she*, one and the same person, is *not* now the same person. That is not a contradiction. The claim is only that this person's character has changed. This numerically identical person is now qualitatively different.

When psychologists discuss identity, they are typically concerned with the kind of person someone is, or wants to be. That is the question involved, for example, in an identity crisis. But, when philosophers discuss identity, it is numerical identity they mean. And, in our concern about our own futures, that is what we have in mind. I may believe that, after my marriage, I shall be a different person. But that does not make marriage death. However much I change, I shall still be alive if there will be someone living who will be me. Similarly, if I was Teletransported, my Replica on Mars would be qualitatively identical to me; but, on the sceptic's view, he wouldn't *be* me. *I* shall have ceased to exist. And that, we naturally assume, is what matters.

Questions about our numerical identity all take the following form. We have two ways of referring to a person, and we ask whether these are ways of referring to the same person. Thus we might ask whether Boris Nikolayevich is Yeltsin. In the most important questions of this kind, our two ways of referring to a person pick out a person at different times. Thus we might ask whether the person to whom we are speaking now is the same as the person to whom we spoke on the telephone yesterday. These are questions about identity over time.

To answer such questions, we must know the *criterion* of personal identity: the relation between a person at one time, and a person at another time, which makes these one and the same person.

Different criteria have been advanced. On one view, what makes me the same, throughout my life, is my having the same body. This criterion requires uninterrupted bodily continuity. There is no such continuity between my body on Earth and the body of my Replica on Mars; so, on this view, my Replica would not be me. Other writers appeal to psychological continuity. Thus Locke claimed that, if I was conscious of a past life in some other body, I would be the person who lived that life. On some versions of this view, my Replica would be me.

Supporters of these different views often appeal to cases where they conflict. Most of these cases are, like Teletransportation, purely imaginary. Some philosophers object that, since our concept of a person rests on a scaffolding of facts, we should not expect this concept to apply in imagined cases where we think those facts away. I agree. But I believe that, for a different reason, it is worth considering such cases. We can use them to discover, not what the truth is, but what we believe. We might have found that, when we consider science fiction cases, we simply shrug our shoulders. But that is not so. Many of us find that we have certain beliefs about what kind of fact personal identity is.

These beliefs are best revealed when we think about such cases from a first-person point of view. So, when I imagine something's happening to me, you should imagine its happening to you. Suppose that I live in some future century, in which technology is far advanced, and I am about to undergo some operation. Perhaps my brain and body will be remodelled, or partially replaced. There will be a resulting person, who will wake up tomorrow. I ask, "Will that person be me? Or am I about to die? Is this the end?" I may not know how to answer this question. But it is natural to assume that there must *be* an answer. The resulting person, it may seem, must be either me, or someone else. And the answer must be all-or-nothing. That person cannot be *partly* me. If that person is in pain tomorrow, this pain cannot be partly mine. So, we may assume, either I shall feel that pain, or I won't.

If this is how we think about such cases, we assume that our identity must be *determinate*. We assume that, in every imaginable case, questions about our identity must have answers, which must be either, and quite simply, Yes or No.

Let us now ask: "Can this be true?" There is one view on which it might be. On this view, there are immaterial substances: souls, or Cartesian Egos. These entities have the special properties once ascribed to atoms: they are indivisible, and their continued existence is, in its nature, all-or-nothing. And such an Ego is what each of us really is.

Unlike several writers, I believe that such a view might have been true. But we have no good evidence for thinking that it is, and some evidence for thinking that it isn't; so I shall assume here that no such view is true.

If we do not believe that there are Cartesian Egos, or other such entities, we should accept the kind of view which I have elsewhere called *Reductionist*. On this view

(1) A person's existence just consists in the existence of a body, and the occurrence of a series of thoughts, experiences, and other mental and physical events.

Some Reductionists claim

(2) Persons just *are* bodies.

This view may seem not to be Reductionist, since it does not reduce persons to something else. But that is only because it is hyper-Reductionist: it reduces persons to bodies in so strong a way that it doesn't even distinguish between them. We can call it *Identifying* Reductionism.

Such a view seems to me too simple. I believe that we should combine (1) with

(3) A person is an entity that has a body, and has thoughts and other experiences.

On this view, though a person is distinct from that person's body, and from any series of thoughts and experiences, the person's existence just *consists* in them. So we can call this view *Constitutive* Reductionism.

It may help to have other examples of this kind of view. If we melt down a bronze statue, we destroy this statue, but we do not destroy this lump of bronze. So, though the statue just consists in the lump of bronze, these cannot be one and the same thing. Similarly, the existence of a nation just consists in the existence of a group of people, on some territory, living together in certain ways. But the nation is not the same as that group of people, or that territory.

Consider next *Eliminative* Reductionism. Such a view is sometimes a response to arguments against the Identifying view. Suppose we start by claiming that a nation just is a group of people on some territory. We are then persuaded that this cannot be so: that the concept of a nation is the concept of an entity that is distinct from its people and its territory. We may conclude that, in that case, there are really no such things as nations. There are only groups of people, living together in certain ways.

In the case of persons, some Buddhist texts take an Eliminative view. According to these texts

(4) There really aren't such things as persons: there are only brains and bodies, and thoughts and other experiences.

For example:

Buddha has spoken thus: "O brethren, actions do exist, and also their consequences, but the person that acts does not. . . . There exists no Individual, it is only a conventional name given to a set of elements."

Or:

The mental and the material are really here,
But here there is no person to be found.

For it is void and merely fashioned like a doll,

Just suffering piled up like grass and sticks.

Eliminative Reductionism is sometimes justified. Thus we are right to claim that there were really no witches, only persecuted women. But Reductionism about some kind of entity is not often well expressed with the claim that there are no such entities. We should admit that there are nations, and that we, who are persons, exist.

Rather than claiming that there are no entities of some kind, Reductionists should distinguish kinds of entity, or ways of existing. When the existence of an X just consists in the existence of a Y, or Ys, though the X is *distinct* from the Y or Ys, it is not an *independent* or *separately existing* entity. Statues do not exist separately from the matter of which they are made. Nor do nations exist separately from their citizens and their territory. Similarly, I believe,

(5) Though persons are distinct from their bodies, and from any series of mental events, they are not independent or separately existing entities.

Cartesian Egos, if they existed, would not only be distinct from human bodies, but would also be independent entities. Such Egos are claimed to be like physical objects, except that they are wholly mental. If there were such entities, it would make sense to suppose that they might cease to be causally related to some body, yet continue to exist. But, on a Reductionist view, persons are not in that sense independent from their bodies. (That is not to claim that our thoughts and other experiences are merely changes in the states of our brains. Reductionists, while not believing in purely mental substances, may be dualists.)

We can now return to personal identity over time, or what constitutes the continued existence of the same person. One question here is this. What explains the unity of a person's mental life? What makes thoughts and experiences, had at different times, the thoughts and experiences of a single person? According to some Non-Reductionists, this question cannot be answered in other terms. We must simply claim that these different thoughts and experiences are all had by the same person. This fact does not consist in any other facts, but is a bare or ultimate truth.

If each of us was a Cartesian Ego, that might be so. Since such an Ego would be an independent substance, it could be an irreducible fact that different experiences are all changes in the states of the same persisting Ego. But that could not be true of persons, I believe, if, while distinct from their bodies, they are not separately existing entities. A person, so conceived, is not the kind of entity about which there could be such irreducible truths. When experiences at different times are all had by the same person, this fact must consist in certain other facts.

If we do not believe in Cartesian Egos, we should claim

(6) Personal identity over time just consists in physical and/or psychological continuity.

That claim could be filled out in different ways. On one version of this view, what makes different experiences the experiences of a single person is their being either changes in the states of, or at least directly causally related to, the same embodied brain. That must be the view of those who believe that persons just are bodies. And we might hold that view even if, as I think we should, we distinguish persons from their bodies. But we might appeal, either in addition or instead, to various psychological relations between different mental states and events, such as the relations involved in memory, or in the persistence of intentions, desires, and other psychological features. That is what I mean by psychological continuity.

On Constitutive Reductionism, the fact of personal identity is distinct from these facts about physical and psychological continuity. But, since it just consists in them, it is not an independent or separately obtaining fact. It is not a further difference in what happens.

To illustrate that distinction, consider a simpler case. Suppose that I already know that several trees are growing together on some hill. I then learn that, because that is true, there is a copse on this hill. That would not be new factual information. I would have merely learnt that such a group of trees can be called a "copse." My only new information is about our language. That those trees can be called a copse is not, except trivially, a fact about the trees.

Something similar is true in the more complicated case of nations. In order to know the facts about the history of a nation, it is enough to know what large numbers of people did and said. Facts about nations cannot be barely true: they must consist in facts about people. And, once we know these other facts, any remaining questions about nations are not further questions about what really happened.

I believe that, in the same way, facts about people cannot be barely true. Their truth must consist in the truth of facts about bodies, and about various interrelated mental and physical events. If we knew these other facts, we would have all the empirical input that we need. If we understood the concept of a person, and had no false beliefs about what persons are, we would then know, or would be able to work out, the truth of any further claims about the existence or identity of persons. That is because such claims would not tell us more about reality.

That is the barest sketch of a Reductionist view. These remarks may become clearer if we return to the so-called "problem cases" of personal identity. In such a case, we imagine knowing that, between me now and some person in the future, there will be certain kinds of degrees of physical and/or psychological continuity or connectedness. But, though we know these facts, we cannot answer the question whether that future person would be me.

Since we may disagree on which the problem cases are, we need more than one example. Consider first the range of cases that I have elsewhere called the *Physical Spectrum*. In each of these cases, some proportion of my body would be replaced, in a single operation, with exact duplicates of the existing cells. In the case at the near end of this range, no cells would be replaced. In the case at the far end, my whole body would be destroyed and replicated. That is the case with which I began: Teletransportation.

Suppose we believe that in that case, where my whole body would be replaced, the resulting person would not be me, but a mere Replica. If no cells were replaced, the resulting person would be me. But what of the cases in between, where the percentage of the cells replaced would be, say, 30, or 50, or 70 percent? Would the resulting person here be me? When we consider some of these cases, we will not know whether to answer Yes or No.

Suppose next that we believe that, even in Teletransportation, my Replica would be me. We should then consider a different version of that case, in which the Scanner would get its information without destroying my body, and my Replica would be made while I was still alive. In this version of the case, we may agree that my Replica would not be me. That may shake our view that, in the original version of the case, he *would* be me.

If we still keep that view, we should turn to what I have called the *Combined Spectrum*. In this second range of cases, there would be all the different degrees of both physical and psychological connectedness. The new cells would not be exactly similar. The greater the proportion of my body that would be replaced, the less like me would the resulting person be. In the case at the far end of this range, my whole body would be destroyed, and they would make a Replica of some quite different person, such as Greta Garbo. Garbo's Replica would clearly *not* be me. In the case at the near end, with no replacement, the resulting person would be me. On any view, there must be cases in between where we could not answer our question.

For simplicity, I shall consider only the Physical Spectrum, and I shall assume that, in some of the cases in this range, we cannot answer the question whether the resulting person would be me. My remarks could be transferred, with some adjustment, to the Combined Spectrum.

As I have said, it is natural to assume that, even if *we* cannot answer this question, there must always *be* an answer, which must be either Yes or No. It is natural to believe that, if the resulting person will be in pain, either I shall feel that pain, or I won't. But this range of cases challenges that belief. In the case at the near end, the resulting person would be me. In the case at the far end, he would be someone else. How could it be true that, in all the cases in between, he must be either me, or someone else? For that to be true, there must be, somewhere in this range, a sharp borderline. There must be some critical set of cells such that, if only those cells were replaced, it would be me who would wake up, but that in the very next case, with only just a few more cells replaced, it would be, not me, but a new person. That is hard to believe.

Here is another fact, which makes it even harder to believe. Even if there were such a borderline, no one could ever discover where it is. I might say, "Try replacing half of my brain and body, and I shall tell you what happens." But we know in advance that, in every case, since the resulting person would be exactly like me, he would be inclined to believe that he was me. And this could not show that he *was* me, since any mere Replica of me would think that too.

Even if such cases actually occurred, we would learn nothing more about them. So it does not matter that these cases are imaginary. We should try to decide now whether, in this range of cases, personal identity could be determinate. Could it be true that, in every case, the resulting person either would or would not be me?

If we do not believe that there are Cartesian Egos, or other such entities, we seem forced to answer No. It is not true that our identity must be determinate. We can always ask, 'Would that future person be me?' But, in some of these cases,

(7) This question would have no answer. It would be neither true nor false that this person would be me.

And

(8) This question would be *empty*. Even without an answer, we could know the full truth about what happened.

If our questions were about such entities as nations or machines, most of us would accept such claims. But, when applied to ourselves, they can be hard to believe. How could it be neither true nor false that I shall still exist tomorrow? And, without an answer to our question, how could I know the full truth about my future?

Reductionism gives the explanation. We naturally assume that, in these cases, there are different possibilities. The resulting person, we assume, might be me, or he might be someone else, who is merely like me. If the resulting person will be in pain, either I shall feel that pain, or I won't. If these really were different possibilities, it would be compelling that one of them must be the possibility that would in fact obtain. How could reality fail to choose between them? But, on a Reductionist view,

> (9) Our question is not about different possibilities. There is only a single possibility, or course of events. Our question is merely about different possible descriptions of this course of events.

That is how our question has no answer. We have not yet decided which description to apply. And, that is why, even without answering this question, we could know the full truth about what would happen.

Suppose that, after considering such examples, we cease to believe that our identity must be determinate. That may seem to make little difference. It may seem to be a change of view only about some imaginary cases, that will never actually occur. But that may not be so. We may be led to revise our beliefs about the nature of personal identity; and that would be a change of view about our own lives.

In nearly all actual cases, questions about personal identity have answers, so claim (7) does not apply. If we don't know these answers, there is something that we don't know. But claim (8) still applies. Even without answering these questions, we could know the full truth about what happens. We would know that truth if we knew the facts about both physical and psychological continuity. If, implausibly, we still didn't know the answer to a question about identity, our ignorance would only be about our language. And that is because claim (9) still applies. When we know the other facts, there are never different possibilities at the level of what happens. In all cases, the only remaining possibilities are at the linguistic level. Perhaps it would be correct to say that some future person would be me. Perhaps it would be correct to say that he would not be me. Or perhaps neither would be correct. I conclude that in *all* cases, if we know the other facts, we should regard questions about our identity as merely questions about language.

That conclusion can be misunderstood. First, when we ask such questions, that is usually because we *don't* know the other facts. Thus, when we ask if we are about to die, that is seldom a conceptual question. We ask that question because we don't know what will happen to our bodies, and whether, in particular, our brains will continue to support consciousness. Our question becomes conceptual only when we already know about such other facts.

Note next that, in certain cases, the relevant facts go beyond the details of the case we are considering. Whether some concept applies may depend on facts about other cases, or on a choice between scientific theories. Suppose we see something strange happening to an unknown animal. We might ask whether this process preserves the animal's identity, or whether the result is a new animal (because what we are seeing is some kind of reproduction). Even if we knew the details of this process, that question would not be merely conceptual. The answer would depend on whether this process is part of the natural development of this kind of animal. And that may be something we have yet to discover.

If we identify persons with human beings, whom we regard as a natural kind, the same would be true in some imaginable cases involving persons. But these are not the kind of case that I have been discussing. My cases all involve artificial intervention. No facts about natural development could be relevant here. Thus, in my Physical Spectrum, if we knew which of my cells would be replaced by duplicates, all of the relevant empirical facts would be in. In such cases any remaining questions would be conceptual.

Since that is so, it would be clearer to ask these questions in a different way. Consider the case in which I replace some of the components of my audio system, but keep the others. I ask, "Do I still have one and the same system?" That may seem a factual question. But, since I already know what happened, that is not really so. It would be clearer to ask, "Given that I have replaced those components, would it be correct to call this the same system?"

The same applies to personal identity. Suppose that I know the facts about what will happen to my body, and about any psychological connections that there will be between me now and some person tomorrow. I may ask, "Will that person be me?" But that is a misleading way to put my question. It suggests that I don't know what's going to happen. When I know these other facts, I should ask, "Would it be correct to call that person me?" That would remind me that, if there's anything that I don't know, that is merely a fact about our language.

I believe that we can go further. Such questions are, in the belittling sense, merely verbal. Some conceptual questions are well worth discussing. But questions about personal identity, in my kind of case, are like questions that we would all think trivial. It is quite uninteresting whether, with half its components replaced, I still have the same audio system. In the same way, we should regard it as quite uninteresting whether, if half of my body were simultaneously replaced, I would still exist. As questions about reality, these are entirely empty. Nor, as conceptual questions, do they need answers.

We might need, for legal purposes, to *give* such questions answers. Thus we might decide that an audio system should be called the same if its new components cost less than half its original price. And we might decide to say that I would continue to exist as long as less than half my body were replaced. But these are not answers to conceptual questions; they are mere decisions.

(Similar remarks apply if we are Identifying Reductionists, who believe that persons just are bodies. There are cases where it is a merely verbal question whether we still have one and the same human body. That is clearly true in the cases in the middle of the Physical Spectrum.)

It may help to contrast these questions with one that is not merely verbal. Suppose we are studying some creature which is very unlike ourselves, such as an insect, or some extraterrestrial being. We know all the facts about this creature's behavior, and its neurophysiology. The creature wriggles vigorously, in what seems to be a response to some injury. We ask, "Is it conscious, and in great pain? Or is it merely like an insentient machine?" Some Behaviourist might say, "That is a merely verbal question. These aren't different possibilities, either of which might be true. They are merely different descriptions of the very same state of affairs." That I find incredible. These descriptions give us, I believe, two quite different possibilities. It could not be an empty or a merely verbal question whether some creature was unconscious or in great pain.

It is natural to think the same about our own identity. If I know that some proportion of my cells will be replaced, how can it be a merely verbal question whether I am about to die, or shall wake up again tomorrow? It is because that is hard to believe that Reductionism is worth discussing. If we become Reductionists, that may change some of our deepest assumptions about ourselves.

These assumptions, as I have said, cover actual cases, and our own lives. But they are best revealed when we consider the imaginary problem cases. It is worth explaining further why that is so.

In ordinary cases, questions about our identity have answers. In such cases, there is a fact about personal identity, and Reductionism is one view about what kind of fact this is. On this view, personal identity just consists in physical and/ or psychological continuity. We may find it hard to decide whether we accept this view, since it may be far from clear when one fact just consists in another. We may even doubt whether Reductionists and their critics really disagree.

In the problem cases, things are different. When we cannot answer questions about personal identity, it is easier to decide whether we accept a Reductionist view. We should ask: Do we find such cases puzzling? Or do we accept the Reductionist claim that, even without answering these questions, if we knew the facts about the continuities, we would know what happened?

Most of us do find such cases puzzling. We believe that, even if we knew those other facts, if we could not answer questions about our identity, there would be something that we didn't know. That suggests that, on our view, personal identity does *not* just consist in one or both of the continuities, but is a separately obtaining fact, or a further difference in what happens. The Reductionist account must then leave something out. So there is a real disagreement, and one that applies to all cases.

Many of us do not merely find such cases puzzling. We are inclined to believe that, in all such cases, questions about our identity must have answers, which must be either Yes or No. For that to be true, personal identity must be a separately obtaining fact of a peculiarly simple kind. It must involve some special entity, such as a Cartesian Ego, whose existence must be all-or-nothing.

When I say that we have these assumptions, I am *not* claiming that we believe in Cartesian Egos. Some of us do. But many of us, I suspect, have inconsistent beliefs. If we are asked whether we believe that there are Cartesian Egos, we may answer No. And we may accept that, as Reductionists claim, the existence of a person just involves the existence of a body, and the occurrence of a series of interrelated mental and physical events. But, as our reactions to the problem cases show, we don't fully accept that view. Or, if we do, we also seem to hold a different view.

Such a conflict of beliefs is quite common. At a reflective or intellectual level, we may be convinced that some view is true; but at another level, one that engages more directly with our emotions, we may continue to think and feel as if some different view were true. One example of this kind would be a hope, or fear, that we know to be groundless. Many of us, I suspect, have such inconsistent beliefs about the metaphysical questions that concern us most, such as free will, time's passage, consciousness, and the self.

{ II }

I turn now from the nature of personal identity to its importance. Personal identity is widely thought to have great rational and moral significance. Thus it is the fact of identity which is thought to give us our reason for concern about our own future. And several moral principles, such as those of desert or distributive justice, presuppose claims about identity. The separateness of persons, or the non-identity of different people, has been called "the basic fact for morals."

I can comment here on only one of these questions: what matters in our survival. I mean by that, not what makes our survival good, but what makes our survival matter, whether it will be good or bad. What is it, in our survival, that gives us a reason for special anticipatory or prudential concern?

We can explain that question with an extreme imaginary case. Suppose that, while I care about my whole future, I am especially concerned about what will happen to me on future Tuesdays. Rather than suffer mild pain on a future Tuesday, I would choose severe pain on any other future day. That pattern of concern would be irrational. The fact that a pain will be on a Tuesday is no reason to care about it more. What about the fact that a pain will be *mine*? Is *this* a reason to care about it more?

Many people would answer Yes. On their view, what gives us a reason to care about our future is, precisely, that it will be our future. Personal identity is what matters in survival.

I reject this view. Most of what matters, I believe, are two other relations: the psychological continuity and connectedness that, in ordinary cases, hold between the different parts of a person's life. These relations only roughly coincide with personal identity, since, unlike identity, they are in part matters of degree. Nor, I believe, do they matter as much as identity is thought to do.

There are different ways to challenge the importance of identity.

One argument can be summarized like this:

(1) Personal identity just consists in certain other facts.

(2) If one fact just consists in certain others, it can only be these other facts which have rational or moral importance. We should ask whether, in themselves, these other facts matter.

Therefore

(3) Personal identity cannot be rationally or morally important. What matters can only be one or more of the other facts in which personal identity consists.

Mark Johnston rejects this argument.[1] He calls it an *Argument from Below,* since it claims that, if one fact justs consists in certain others, it can only be these other lower level facts which matter. Johnston replies with what he calls an *Argument from Above.* On his view, even if the lower-level facts do not in themselves matter, the higher-level fact may matter. If it does, the lower-level facts will have a derived significance. They will matter, not in themselves, but because they constitute the higher-level fact.

To illustrate this disagreement, we can start with a different case. Suppose we ask what we want to happen if, through brain damage, we become irreversibly unconscious. If we were in this state, we would still be alive. But this fact should be understood in a Reductionist way. It may not be the same as the fact that our hearts would still be beating, and our other organs would still be functioning. But it would not be an independent or separately obtaining fact. Our being still alive, though irreversibly unconscious, would just consist in these other facts.

On my Argument from Below, we should ask whether those other facts in themselves matter. If we were irreversibly unconscious, would it be either good for us, or good for others, that our hearts and other organs would still be functioning? If we answer No, we should conclude that it would not matter that we were still alive.

If Johnston were right, we could reject this argument. And we could appeal to an Argument from Above. We might say:

> It may not be in itself good that our hearts and other organs would still be functioning. But it is good to be alive. Since that is so, it is rational to hope that, even if we could never regain consciousness, our hearts would go on beating for as long as possible. That would be good because it would constitute our staying alive.

I believe that, of these arguments, mine is more plausible.

Consider next the moral question that such cases raise. Some people ask, in their living wills, that if brain damage makes them irreversibly unconscious, their hearts should be stopped. I believe that we should do what these people ask. But many take a different view. They could appeal to an Argument from Above. They might say:

> Even if such people can never regain consciousness, while their hearts are still beating, they can be truly called alive. Since that is so, stopping their hearts would be an act of killing. And, except in self-defence, it is always wrong to kill.

On this view, we should leave these people's hearts to go on beating, for months or even years.

As an answer to the moral question, this seems to me misguided. (It is a separate question what the law should be.) But, for many people, the word "kill" has such force that it seems significant whether it applies.

Turn now to a different subject. Suppose that, after trying to decide when people have free will, we become convinced by either of two compatibilist views. On one view, we call choices "unfree" if they are caused in certain ways, and we call them "free" if they are caused in certain other ways. On the other view, we call choices "unfree" if we know how they were caused, and we call them "free" if we have not yet discovered this.

Suppose next that, when we consider these two grounds for drawing this distinction, we believe that neither, in itself, has the kind of significance that could support making or denying claims about guilt, or desert. There seems to us no such significance in the difference between these kinds of causal determination; and we believe that it cannot matter whether a decision's causes have already been discovered. (Note that, in comparing the Arguments from Above and Below, we need not actually accept these claims. We are asking whether, *if* we accepted the relevant premises, we ought to be persuaded by these arguments.)

On my Argument from Below, if the fact that a choice is free just consists in one of those other facts, and we believe that those other facts cannot in themselves be morally important, we should conclude that it cannot be important whether some person's choice was free. Either choices that are unfree can deserve to be punished, or choices that are free cannot. On a Johnstonian Argument from Above, even if those other facts are not in themselves important—even if, in themselves, they are trivial—they can have a derived importance if and because they constitute the fact that some person's choice was free. As before, the Argument from Below seems to me more plausible.

We can now consider the underlying question on which this disagreement turns.

As I have claimed, if one fact just consists in certain others, the first fact is not an independent or separately obtaining fact. And, in the cases with which we are concerned, it is also, in relation to these other facts, merely a conceptual fact. Thus, if someone is irreversibly unconscious, but his heart is still beating, it is a conceptual fact that this person is still alive. When I call this fact conceptual, I don't mean that it is a fact about our concepts. That this person is alive is a fact about this person. But, if we have already claimed that this person's heart is still beating, when we claim that he is still alive, we do not give further information about reality. We only give further information about our use of the words "person" and "alive."

When we turn to ask what matters, the central question is this. Suppose we agree that it does not matter, in itself, that such a person's heart is still beating. Could we claim that, in another way, this fact does matter, because it makes it correct to say that this person is still alive? If we answer Yes, we are treating language as more important than reality. We are claiming that, even if some fact does not in itself matter, it may matter if and because it allows a certain word to be applied.

This, I believe, is irrational. On my view, what matters are the facts about the world, given which some concept applies. If the facts about the world have no rational or moral significance, and the fact that the concept applies is not a further difference in what happens, this conceptual fact cannot be significant.

Johnston brings a second charge against my argument. If physicalism were true, he claims, all facts would just consist in facts about fundamental particles. Considered in themselves, these facts about particles would have no rational or moral importance. If we apply an Argument from Below, we must conclude that nothing has any importance. He remarks: "this is not a proof of nihilism. It is a *reductio ad absurdum.*"

Given what I have suggested here, this charge can, I think, be answered. There may perhaps be a sense in which, if physicalism were true, all facts would just consist in facts about fundamental particles. But that is not the kind of reduction which I had in mind. When I claim that personal identity just consists in certain other facts, I have in mind a closer and partly conceptual relation. Claims about personal identity may not mean the same as claims about physical and/or psychological continuity. But, if we knew the facts about these continuities, and understood the concept of a person, we would thereby know, or would be able to work out, the facts about persons. Hence my claim that, if we know the other facts, questions about personal identity should be taken to be questions, not about reality, but only about our language. These claims do not apply to facts about fundamental particles. It is not true for example that, if we knew how the particles moved in some person's body, and understood our concepts, we would thereby know, or be able to work out, all of the relevant facts about this person. To understand the world around us, we need more than physics and a knowledge of our own language.

My argument does not claim that, whenever there are facts at different levels, it is always the lowest-level facts which matter. That is clearly false. We are discussing cases where, relative to the facts at some lower level, the higher-level fact is, in the sense that I have sketched, merely conceptual. My claim is that such conceptual facts cannot be rationally or morally important. What matters is reality, not how it is described. So this view might be called *realism about importance.*

If we are Reductionists about persons, and Realists about importance, we should conclude that personal identity is not what matters. Can we accept that conclusion?

Most of us believe that we should care about our future because it will be *our* future. I believe that what matters is not identity but certain other relations. To help us to decide between these views, we should consider cases where identity and those relations do not coincide.

Which these cases are depends on which criterion of identity we accept. I shall start with the simplest form of the Physical Criterion, according to which a person continues to exist if and only if that person's body continues to exist. That must be the view of those who believe that persons just are bodies. And it is the view of several of the people who identify persons with human beings. Let's call this the *Bodily Criterion.*

Suppose that, because of damage to my spine, I have become partly paralyzed. I have a brother, who is dying of a brain disease. With the aid of new techniques, when my brother's brain ceases to function, my head could be grafted onto the rest of my brother's body. Since we are identical twins, my brain would then control a body that is just like mine, except that it would not be paralyzed.

Should I accept this operation? Of those who assume that identity is what matters, three groups would answer No. Some accept the Bodily Criterion. These people believe that, if this operation were performed, I would die. The person with my head tomorrow would be my brother, who would mistakenly think that he was me. Other people are uncertain what would happen. They believe that it would be risky to accept this operation, since the resulting person might not be me. Others give a different reason why I should reject this operation: that it would be indeterminate whether that person would be me. On all these views, it matters who that person would be.

On my view, that question is unimportant. If this operation were performed, the person with my head tomorrow would not only believe that he was me, seem to remember living my life, and be in every other way psychologically like me. These facts would also have their normal cause, the continued existence of my brain. And this person's body would be just like mine. For all these reasons, his life would be just like the life that I would have lived, if my paralysis had been cured. I believe that, given these facts, I should accept this operation. It is irrelevant whether this person would be me.

That may seem all important. After all, if he would not be me, I shall have ceased to exist. But, if that person would not be me, this fact would just consist in another fact. It would just consist in the fact that my body will have been replaced below the neck. When considered on its own, is that second fact important? Can it matter in itself that the blood that will keep my brain alive will circulate, not through my own heart and lungs, but through my brother's heart and lungs? Can it matter in itself that my brain will control, not the rest of my body, but the rest of another body that is exactly similar?

If we believe that these facts would amount to my non-existence, it may be hard to focus on the question whether, in themselves, these facts matter. To make that easier, we should imagine that we accept a different view. Suppose we are convinced that the person with my head tomorrow *would* be me. Would we then believe that it would matter greatly that my head would have been grafted onto this other body? We would not. We would regard my receiving a new torso, and new limbs, as like any lesser transplant, such as receiving a new heart, or new kidneys. As this shows, if it would matter greatly that what will be replaced is not just a few such organs, but my whole body below the neck, that could only be because, if that happened, the resulting person would *not* be me.

According to my argument, we should now conclude that neither of these facts could matter greatly. Since it would not be in itself important that my head would be grafted onto this body, and that would be all there was to the fact that the resulting person would not be me, it would not be in itself important that this person would not be me. Perhaps it would not be irrational to regret these facts a little. But, I believe, they would be heavily outweighed by the fact that, unlike me, the resulting person would not be paralyzed.

When it is applied to our own existence, my argument is hard to accept. But, as before, the fundamental question is the relative importance of language and reality.

On my view, what matters is what is going to happen. If I knew that my head could be grafted onto the rest of a body that is just like mine, and that the resulting person would be just like me, I would know enough to decide whether to accept this operation. I need not ask whether the resulting person could be correctly called me. That is not a further difference in what is going to happen.

That may seem a false distinction. What matters, we might say, is whether the resulting person would *be* me. But that person would be me if and only if he could be correctly called me. So, in asking what he could be called, we are not merely asking a conceptual question. We *are* asking about reality.

This objection fails to distinguish two kinds of case. Suppose that I ask my doctor whether, while I receive some treatment, I shall be in pain. That is a factual question. I am asking what will happen. Since pain can be called "pain," I *could* ask my question in a different way. I could say, "While I am being treated, will it be correct to describe me as in pain?" But that would be misleading. It would suggest that I am asking how we use the word "pain."

In a different case, I might ask that conceptual question. Suppose I know that, while I am crossing the Channel, I shall be feeling sea-sick, as I always do. I might wonder whether that sensation could be correctly called "pain." Here too, I could ask my question in a different way. I could say, "While I am crossing the Channel, shall I be in pain?" But that would be misleading, since it would suggest that I am asking what will happen.

In the medical case, I don't know what conscious state I shall be in. There are different possibilities. In the Channel crossing case, there aren't different possibilities. I already know what state I shall be in. I am merely asking whether that state could be redescribed in a certain way.

It matters whether, while receiving the medical treatment, I shall be in pain. And it matters whether, while crossing the Channel, I shall be sea-sick. But it does not matter whether, in feeling sea-sick, I can be said to be in pain.

Return now to our main example. Suppose I know that my head will be successfully grafted onto my brother's headless body. I ask whether the resulting person will be me. Is this like the medical case, or the case of crossing the Channel? Am I asking what will happen, or whether what I know will happen could be described in a certain way?

On my view, I should take myself to be asking the second. I already know what is going to happen. There will be someone with my head and my brother's body. It is a merely verbal question whether that person will be me. And that is why, even if he won't be me, that doesn't matter.

It may now be objected: "By choosing this example, you are cheating. Of course you should accept this operation. But that is because the resulting person *would* be you. We should reject the Bodily Criterion. So this case cannot show that identity is not what matters."

Since there are people who accept this criterion, I am not cheating. It is worth trying to show these people that identity is not what matters. But I accept part of this objection. I agree that we should reject the Bodily Criterion.

Of those who appeal to this criterion, some believe that persons just are bodies. But, if we hold this kind of view, it would be better to identify a person with that person's brain, or nervous system. Consider next those who believe that persons are animals of a certain kind, viz. human beings. We could take this view, but reject the Bodily Criterion. We could claim that animals continue to exist if there continue to exist, and to function, the most important parts of their bodies. And we could claim that, at least in the case of human beings, the brain is so important that its survival counts as the survival of this human being. On both these views, in my imagined case, the person with my head tomorrow would be me. And that is what, on reflection, most of us would believe.

My own view is similar. I would state this view, not as a claim about reality, but as a conceptual claim. On my view, it would not be incorrect to call this person me; and this would be the best description of this case.

If we agree that this person would be me, I would still argue that this fact is not what matters. What is important is not identity, but one or more of the other facts in which identity consists. But I concede that, when identity coincides with these other facts, it is harder to decide whether we accept that argument's conclusion. So, if we reject the Bodily Criterion, we must consider other cases.

Suppose that we accept the Brain-Based version of the Psychological Criterion. On this view, if there will be one future person who is psychologically continuous with me, because he will have enough of my brain, that person will be me. But psychological continuity without its normal cause, the continued existence of enough of my brain, does not suffice for identity. My Replica would not be me.

Remember next that an object can continue to exist even if all its components are gradually replaced. Suppose that, every time some wooden ship comes into port, a few of its planks are replaced. Before long, the same ship may be entirely composed of different planks.

Assume, once again, that I need surgery. All of my brain cells have a defect which, in time, would be fatal. Surgeons could replace all these cells, inserting new cells that are exact replicas, except that they have no defect.

The surgeons could proceed in either of two ways. In *Case One*, there would be a hundred operations. In each operation, the surgeons would remove a hundredth part of my brain, and insert replicas of those parts. In *Case Two*, the surgeons would first remove all the existing parts of my brain and then insert all of their replicas.

There is a real difference here. In Case One, my brain would continue to exist, like a ship with all of its planks gradually replaced. In Case Two, my brain would cease to exist, and my body would be given a new brain.

This difference, though, is much smaller than that between ordinary survival and teletransportation. In both cases, there will later be a person whose brain will be just like my present brain, but without the defects, and who will therefore be psychologically continuous with me. And, in *both* cases, this person's brain will be made of the very same new cells, each of which is a replica of one of my existing cells. The difference between the cases is merely the way in which these new cells are inserted. In Case One, the surgeons alternate between removing and inserting. In Case Two, they do all the removing before all the inserting.

On the Brain-Based Criterion, this is the difference between life and death. In Case One, the resulting person would be me. In Case Two he would *not* be me, so I would cease to exist.

Can this difference matter? Reapply the Argument from Below. This difference consists in the fact that, rather than alternating between removals and insertions, the surgeon does all the removing before all the inserting. Considered on its own, can this matter? I believe not. We would not think it mattered if it did not constitute the fact that the resulting person would not be me. But if this fact does not in itself matter, and that is all there is to the fact that in Case Two I would cease to exist, I should conclude that my ceasing to exist does not matter.

Suppose next that you regard these as problem cases, ones where you do not know what would happen to me. Return to the simpler Physical Spectrum. In each of the cases in this range, some proportion of my cells will be replaced with exact duplicates. With some proportions—20 per cent, say, or 50, or 70—most of us would be uncertain whether the resulting person would be me. (As before, if we do not believe that here, my remarks could be transferred, with adjustments, to the Combined Spectrum.)

On my view, in all of the cases in this range, it is a merely conceptual question whether the resulting person would be me. Even without answering this question, I can know just what is going to happen. If there is anything that I don't know, that is merely a fact about how we could describe what is going to happen. And that conceptual question is not even, I believe, interesting. It is merely verbal, like the question whether, if I replaced some of its parts, I would still have the same audio system.

When we imagine these cases from a first-person point of view, it may still be hard to believe that this is merely a verbal question. If I don't know whether, tomorrow, I shall still exist, it may be hard to believe that I know what is going to happen. But what is it that I don't know? If there are different possibilities, at the level of what happens, what is the difference between them? In what would that difference consist? If I had a soul, or Cartesian Ego, there might be different possibilities. Perhaps, even if *n* percent of my cells were replaced, my soul would keep its intimate relation with my brain. Or perhaps another soul would take over. But, we have assumed, there are no such entities. What else could the difference be? When the resulting person wakes up tomorrow, what could make it either true, or false, that he is me?

It may be said that, in asking what will happen, I am asking what I can expect. Can I expect to wake up again? If that person will be in pain, can I expect to feel that pain? But this does not help. These are just other ways of asking whether that person will or will not be me. In appealing to what I can expect, we do not explain what would make these different possibilities.

We may believe that this difference needs no explanation. It may seem enough to say: Perhaps that person will be me, and perhaps he won't. Perhaps I shall exist tomorrow, and perhaps I shan't. It may seem that these must be different possibilities.

That, however, is an illusion. If I shall still exist tomorrow, that fact must consist in certain others. For there to be two possibilities, so that it might be either true or false that I shall exist tomorrow, there must be some other difference between these possibilities. There would be such a difference, for example, if, between now and tomorrow, my brain and body might either remain unharmed, or be blown to pieces. But, in our imagined case, there is no such other difference. I already know that there will be someone whose brain and body will consist partly of these cells, and partly of new cells, and that this person will be psychologically like me. There aren't, at the level of what happens, different possible outcomes. There is no further essence of me, or property of me-ness, which either might or might not be there.

If we turn to the conceptual level, there *are* different possibilities. Perhaps that future person could be correctly called me. Perhaps he could be correctly called someone else. Or perhaps neither would be correct. That, however, is the only way in which it could be either true, or false, that this person would be me.

The illusion may persist. Even when I know the other facts, I may want reality to go in one of two ways. I may want it to be true that I shall still exist tomorrow. But all that could be true is that we use language in one of two ways. Can it be rational to care about that?

{ III }

I am now assuming that we accept the Brain-Based Psychological Criterion. We believe that, if there will be one future person who will have enough of my brain to be psychologically continuous with me, that person would be me. On this view, there is another way to argue that identity is not what matters.

We can first note that, just as I could survive with less than my whole body, I could survive with less than my whole brain. People have survived, and with little psychological change, even when, through a stroke or injury, they have lost the use of half their brain.

Let us next suppose that the two halves of my brain could each fully support ordinary psychological functioning. That may in fact be true of certain people. If it is not, we can suppose that, through some technological advance, it has been made true of me. Since our aim is to test our beliefs about what matters, there is no harm in making such assumptions.

We can now compare two more possible operations. In the first, after half my brain is destroyed, the other half would be successfully transplanted into the empty skull of a body that is just like mine. Given our assumptions, we should conclude that, here too, I would survive. Since I would survive if my brain were transplanted, and I would survive with only half my brain, it would be unreasonable to deny that I would survive if that remaining half were transplanted. So, in this *Single Case*, the resulting person would be me.

Consider next the *Double Case*, or *My Division*. Both halves of my brain would be successfully transplanted, into different bodies that are just like mine. Two people would wake up, each of whom has half my brain, and is, both physically and psychologically, just like me.

Since these would be two different people, it cannot be true that each of them is me. That would be a contradiction. If each of them was me, each would be one and the same person: me. So they could not be two different people.

Could it be true that only one of them is me? That is not a contradiction. But, since I have the same relation to each of these people, there is nothing that could make me one of them rather than the other. It cannot be true, of either of these people, that he is the one who could be correctly called me.

How should I regard these two operations? Would they preserve what matters in survival? In the Single Case, the one resulting person would be me. The relation between me now and that future person is just an instance of the relation between me now and myself tomorrow. So that relation would contain what matters. In the Double Case, my relation to that person would be just the same.

So this relation must still contain what matters. Nothing is missing. But that person cannot here be claimed to be me. So identity cannot be what matters.

We may object that, if that person isn't me, something *is* missing. *I'm* missing. That may seem to make all the difference. How can everything still be there if *I'm* not there?

Everything is still there. The fact that I'm not there is not a real absence. The relation between me now and that future person is in itself the same. As in the Single Case, he has half my brain, and he is just like me. The difference is only that, in this Double Case, I also have the same relation to the other resulting person. Why am I not there? The explanation is only this. When this relation holds between me now and a single person in the future, we can be called one and the same person. When this relation holds between me now and *two* future people, I cannot be called one and the same as each of these people. But that is not a difference in the nature or the content of this relation. In the Single Case, where half my brain will be successfully transplanted, my prospect is survival. That prospect contains what matters. In the Double Case, where both halves will be successfully transplanted, nothing would be lost.

It can be hard to believe that identity is not what matters. But that is easier to accept when we see why, in this example, it is true. It may help to consider this analogy. Imagine a community of persons who are like us, but with two exceptions. First, because of facts about their reproductive system, each couple has only two children, who are always twins. Second, because of special features of their psychology, it is of great importance for the development of each child that it should not, through the death of its sibling, become an only child. Such children suffer psychological damage. It is thus believed, in this community, that it matters greatly that each child should have a twin.

Now suppose that, because of some biological change, some of the children in this community start to be born as triplets. Should their parents think this a disaster, because these children don't have twins? Clearly not. These children don't have twins only because they each have *two* siblings. Since each child has two siblings, the trio must be called, not twins, but triplets. But none of them will suffer damage as an only child. These people should revise their view. What matters isn't having a twin: it is having at least one sibling.

In the same way, we should revise our view about identity over time. What matters isn't that there will be someone alive who will be me. It is rather that there will be at least one living person who will be psychologically continuous with me as I am now, and/or who has enough of my brain. When there will be only one such person, he can be described as me. When there will be two such people, we cannot claim that each will be me. But that is as trivial as the fact that, if I had two identical siblings, they could not be called my twins.[2]

{ IV }

If, as I have argued, personal identity is not what matters, we must ask what does matter. There are several possible answers. And, depending on our answer, there are several further implications. Thus there are several moral questions which I have no time even to mention. I shall end with another remark about our concern for our own future.

That concern is of several kinds. We may want to survive partly so that our hopes and ambitions will be achieved. We may also care about our future in the kind of way in which we care about the well-being of certain other people, such as our relatives or friends. But most of us have, in addition, a distinctive kind of egoistic concern. If I know that my child will be in pain, I may care about his pain more than I would about my own future pain. But I cannot fearfully anticipate my child's pain. And if I knew that my Replica would take up my life where I leave off, I would not look forward to that life.

This kind of concern may, I believe, be weakened, and be seen to have no ground, if we come to accept a Reductionist view. In our thoughts about our own identity, we are prone to illusions. That is why the so-called "problem cases" seem to raise problems: why we find it hard to believe that, when we know the other facts, it is an empty or a merely verbal question whether we shall still exist. Even after we accept a Reductionist view, we may continue, at some level, to think and feel as if that view were not true. Our own continued existence may still seem an independent fact, of a peculiarly deep and simple kind. And that belief may underlie our anticipatory concern about our own future.

There are, I suspect, several causes of that illusory belief. I have discussed one cause here: our conceptual scheme. Though we need concepts to think about reality, we sometimes confuse the two. We mistake conceptual facts for facts about reality. And, in the case of certain concepts, those that are most loaded with emotional or moral significance, we can be led seriously astray. Of these loaded concepts, that of our own identity is, perhaps, the most misleading.

Even the use of the word "I" can lead us astray. Consider the fact that, in a few years, I shall be dead. This fact can seem depressing. But the reality is only this. After a certain time, none of the thoughts and experiences that occur will be directly causally related to this brain, or be connected in certain ways to these present experiences. That is all this fact involves. And, in that redescription, my death seems to disappear.[3]

NOTES

1. In his "Human Concerns without Superlative Selves," in Jonathan Dancy, *Reading Parfit* (Oxford: Blackwell, 1997), pp. 149–79.

2. In many contexts, we need to distinguish two senses of "what matters in survival." What matters in the *prudential* sense is what gives us reason for special concern about our future. What matters in the *desirability* sense is what makes our survival good. But, in the examples I have been discussing, these two coincide. On my view, even if we won't survive, we could have what matters *in* survival. If there will be at least one living person who will both be psychologically continuous with me, and have enough of my brain, my relation to that person contains what matters in the prudential sense. So it also preserves what matters in the desirability sense. It is irrelevant whether that person will be me.

3. Some of this essay draws from Part Three of my *Reasons and Persons* (Oxford University Press, 1984).

PERSONS AS PSYCHOLOGICAL SUBSTANCES

CHAPTER NINE

Persons

P. F. Strawson

{ I }

In the *Tractatus* (5.631–5.641), Wittgenstein writes of the I which occurs in philosophy, of the philosophical idea of the subject of experiences. He says first: "The thinking, presenting subject—there is no such thing." Then, a little later: "*In an important sense* there is no subject." This is followed by: "The subject does not belong to the world, but is a limit of the world." And a little later comes the following paragraph: "There is [therefore] really a sense in which in philosophy we can talk non-psychologically of the I. The I occurs in philosophy through the fact that the 'world is my world.' The philosophical I is not the man, not the human body, or the human soul of which psychology treats, but the metaphysical subject, the limit—not a part of the world." These remarks are impressive, but also puzzling and obscure. Reading them, one might think: Well, let's settle for the human body and the human soul of which psychology treats, and which is a part of the world, and let the metaphysical subject go. But again we might think: No, when I talk of myself, I do after all talk of that which has all of my experiences, I do talk of the subject of my experiences—and yet also of something that is part of the world in that it, but not the world, comes to an end when I die. The limit of my world is not—and is not so thought of by me—the limit of the world. It may be difficult to explain the idea of something which is both a subject of experiences and a part of the world. But it is an idea we have: it should be an idea we can explain.

Let us think of some of the ways in which we ordinarily talk of ourselves, of some of the things which we ordinarily ascribe to ourselves. They are of many kinds. We ascribe to ourselves *actions and intentions* (I am doing, did, shall do this); *sensations* (I am warm, in pain); *thoughts and feelings* (I think, wonder, want this, am angry, disappointed, contented); *perceptions and memories* (I see this, hear the other, remember that). We ascribe to ourselves, in two senses, position: *location* (I am on the sofa) and *attitude* (I am lying down). And of course we ascribe to ourselves not only temporary conditions, states, and situations, like most of these, but also enduring characteristics, including such physical characteristics as height, coloring, shape, and weight. That is to say, among the things we ascribe to ourselves are things of a kind that we also ascribe to material bodies to which we would not dream of ascribing others of the things that we ascribe to ourselves. Now there seems nothing needing explanation in the fact that the particular height, coloring, and physical position which we ascribe to ourselves, should be ascribed to *something or other;* for that which one calls one's body is, at least, a body, a material thing. It can be picked out from others, identified by ordinary physical criteria and described in ordinary physical terms. But it can seem, and has seemed, to need explanation that one's states of consciousness, one's thoughts and sensations, are ascribed *to the very same thing* as that to which these physical characteristics, this physical situation, is ascribed. Why are one's states of consciousness ascribed to the very same thing as certain corporeal characteristics, a certain physical situation, etc.? And once this question is raised, another question follows it, viz.: Why are one's states of consciousness ascribed to (said to be of, or to belong to) anything at all? It is not to be supposed that the answers to these questions will be independent of one another.

It might indeed be thought that an answer to both of them could be found in the unique role which each person's body plays in his experience, particularly his perceptual experience. All philosophers who have concerned themselves with these questions have referred to the uniqueness of this role. (Descartes was well enough aware of its uniqueness: "I am *not* lodged in my body like a pilot in a vessel.") In what does this uniqueness consist? Well, of course, in a great many facts. We may summarize some of these facts by saying that for each person there is one body which occupies a certain *causal* position in relation to that person's perceptual experience, a causal position which is in various ways unique in relation to each of the various kinds of perceptual experience he has; and—as a further consequence—that this body is also unique for him as an *object* of the various kinds of perceptual experience which he has. This complex uniqueness of the single body appears, moreover, to be a contingent matter, or rather a cluster of contingent matters; we can, or it seems that we can, imagine many peculiar combinations of dependence and independence of aspects of our perceptual experience on the physical states or situation of more than one body.

Now I must say, straightaway, that this cluster of apparently contingent facts about the unique role which each person's body plays in his experience does not seem to me to provide, *by itself,* an answer to our questions. Of course these facts explain *something.* They provide a very good reason why a subject of experience should have a very *special regard* for just one body, why he should think of it as unique and perhaps more important than any other. They explain—if I may be permitted to put it so—why I feel *peculiarly attached* to what in fact I call my own body; they even might be said to explain why, granted that I am going to speak of one body as *mine,* I should speak of this body (the body that I do speak of as mine) as mine. But they do not explain why I should have the concept of *myself* at all, why I should ascribe my thoughts and experiences to *anything.* Moreover, even if we were satisfied with some other explanation of why one's states of consciousness (thoughts and feelings and perceptions) were ascribed to *some-thing,* and satisfied that the facts in question sufficed to explain why the "possession" of a particular body should be ascribed to the *same* thing (i.e., to explain why a particular body should be spoken of as standing in some special relation, called "being possessed by" to that thing), yet the facts in question still do not explain why we should, as we do, ascribe certain corporeal characteristics not simply to the body standing in this special relation to the thing to which we ascribe thoughts, feelings, etc., but to the thing itself to which we ascribe those thoughts and feelings. (For we say "I am bald" as well as "I am cold," "I am lying on the hearthrug" as well as "I see a spider on the ceiling.") Briefly, the facts in question explain why a subject of experience should pick out one body from others, give it, perhaps, an honored name and ascribe to it whatever characteristics it has; but they do not explain why the experiences should be ascribed to any subject at all; and they do not explain why, if the experiences are to be ascribed to something, they *and* the corporeal characteristics which might be truly ascribed to the favored body, should be ascribed to the same thing. So the facts in question do not explain the use that we make of the word "I," or how any word has the use that word has. They do not explain the concept we have of a person.

{ II }

A possible reaction at this point *is* to say that the concept we have is wrong or confused, or, if we make it a rule not to say that the concepts we have are confused, that the usage we have, whereby we ascribe, or seem to ascribe, such different kinds of predicate to one and the same thing, is confusing, that it conceals the true nature of the concepts involved, or something of this sort. This reaction can be found in two very important types of view about these matters. The first type of view is Cartesian, the view of Descartes and of others who think like him. Over the attribution of the second type of view I am more hesitant; but there is some evidence that it was held, at one period, by Wittgenstein and possibly also by Schlick. On both of these views, one of the questions we are considering, namely "Why do we ascribe our states of consciousness to the very same thing as certain corporeal characteristics, etc.?" is a question which does not arise; for on both views it is only a linguistic illusion that both kinds of predicate are properly ascribed to one and the same thing, that there is a common owner, or subject, of both types of predicate. And on the second of these views, the other question we are considering, namely "Why do we ascribe our states of consciousness to anything at all?" is also a question which does not arise; for on this view, it is only a linguistic illusion that one ascribes one's states of consciousness at all, that there is any proper subject of these apparent ascriptions, that states of consciousness belong to, or are states of, anything.

That Descartes held the first of these views is well enough known. When we speak of a person, we are really referring to one or both of two distinct substances (two substances of different types), each of which has its own appropriate type of states and properties; and none of the properties or states of either can be a property or state of the other. States of consciousness belong to one of these substances, and not to the other. I shall say no more about the Cartesian view at the moment—what I have to say about it will emerge later on—except to note again that while it escapes one of our questions, it does not escape, but indeed invites, the other: "Why are one's states of consciousness *ascribed* at all, to *any* subject?"

The second of these views I shall call the "no-ownership" or "no-subject" doctrine of the self. Whether or not anyone has explicitly held this view, it is worth reconstructing, or constructing, in outline.[1] For the errors into which it falls are instructive. The "no-ownership" theorist may be presumed to start his explanations with facts of the sort which illustrate the unique causal position of a certain material body in a person's experience. The theorist maintains that the uniqueness of this body is sufficient to give rise to the idea that one's experiences can be ascribed to some particular individual thing, can be said to be possessed by, or owned by, that thing. This idea, he thinks, though infelicitously and misleadingly expressed in terms of ownership, would have some validity, would make some sort of sense, so long as we thought of this individual thing, the possessor of the experiences, as the body itself. So long as we thought in this way, then to ascribe a particular state of consciousness to this body, this individual thing, would at least be to say something contingent, something that might be, or might have been, false. It might have been a misascription; for the experience in question might be, or might have been, causally dependent on the state of some other body; in the present admissible, though infelicitous, sense of "belong," it might have belonged to some other individual thing. But now, the theorist suggests, one becomes confused: one slides from this admissible, though infelicitous, sense in which one's experiences may be said to belong to, or be possessed by, some particular thing, to a wholly inadmissible and empty sense of these expressions; and in this new and inadmissible sense, the particular thing which is supposed to possess the experiences is not thought of as a body, but as something else, say an ego.

Suppose we call the first type of possession, which is really a certain kind of causal dependence, "having$_1$," and the second type of possession, "having$_2$"; and call the individual of the first type "B" and the supposed individual of the second type "E." Then the difference is that while it is genuinely a contingent matter that *all my experiences are had$_1$ by B,* it appears as a necessary truth that *all my experiences are had$_2$ by E.* But the belief in E and in having$_2$ is an illusion. Only those things whose ownership is logically transferable can be owned at all. So experiences are not owned by anything except in the dubious sense of being causally dependent on the state of a particular body. This is at least a genuine relationship to a thing, in that they might have stood in it to another thing. Since the whole function of E was to own experiences in a logically nontransferable sense of "own," and since experiences are not owned by anything in this sense, for there is no such sense of "own," E must be eliminated from the picture altogether. It only came in because of a confusion.

I think it must be clear that this account of the matter, though it contains *some* of the facts, is not coherent. It is not coherent, in that one who holds it is forced to make use of that sense of possession of which he denies the existence, in presenting his case for the denial. When he tries to state the contingent fact, which he thinks gives rise to the illusion of the "ego," he has to state it in some such form as "All *my* experiences are had₁ by (uniquely dependent on the state of) body B." For any attempt to eliminate the "my," or some other expression with a similar possessive force, would yield something that was not a contingent fact at all. The proposition that *all* experiences are causally dependent on the state of a single body B, for example, is just false. The theorist means to speak of all the experiences *had by a certain person* being contingently so dependent. And the theorist cannot consistently argue that "all the experiences of person P" means the *same thing* as "all experiences contingently dependent on a certain body B"; for then his proposition would not be contingent, as his theory requires, but analytic. He must mean to be speaking of some class of experiences of the members of which it is in fact contingently true that they are all dependent on body B. And the defining characteristic of this class is in fact that they are "*my* experiences" or "the experiences of some person," where the sense of "possession" is the one he calls into question.

This internal incoherence is a serious matter when it is a question of denying what prima facie is the case: that is, that one does genuinely ascribe one's states of consciousness to something, viz., oneself, and that this kind of ascription is precisely such as the theorist finds unsatisfactory, i.e., is such that it does not seem to make sense to suggest, for example, that the identical pain which was in fact one's own might have been another's. We do not have to seek far in order to understand the place of this logically non-transferable kind of ownership in our general scheme of thought. For if we think of the requirements of identifying reference, in speech, to *particular* states of consciousness, or private experiences, we see that such particulars cannot be thus identifyingly referred to except as the states or experiences *of* some identified person. States, or experiences, one might say, owe their identity as particulars to the identity of the person whose states or experiences they are. And from this it follows immediately that if they can be identified as particular states or experiences at all, they must be possessed or ascribable in just that way which the no-ownership theorist ridicules, i.e., in such a way that it is logically impossible that a particular state or experience in fact possessed by someone should have been possessed by anyone else. The requirements of identity rule out logical transferability of ownership. So the theorist could maintain his position only by denying that we could ever refer to particular states or experiences at all. And *this* position is ridiculous.

We may notice, even now, a possible connection between the no-ownership doctrine and the Cartesian position. The latter is, straightforwardly enough, a

dualism of two subjects (two types of subject). The former could, a little paradoxically, be called a dualism too: a dualism of one subject (the body) and one
non-subject. We might surmise that the second dualism, paradoxically so called,
arises out of the first dualism, nonparadoxically so called; in other words, that
if we try to think of that to which one's states of consciousness are ascribed
as something utterly different from that to which certain corporeal characteristics are ascribed, then indeed it becomes difficult to see why states of consciousness should be ascribed, thought of as belonging to, anything at all. And when
we think of this possibility, we may also think of another: viz., that both the
Cartesian and the no-ownership theorist are profoundly wrong in holding, as
each must, that there are two uses of "I" in one of which it denotes something
which it does not denote in the other.

{ III }

The no-ownership theorist fails to take account of all the facts. He takes account
of some of them. He implies, correctly, that the unique position or role of a
single body in one's experience is not a sufficient explanation of the fact that
one's experiences, or states of consciousness, are ascribed to something which
has them, with that peculiar non-transferable kind of possession which is here
in question. It may be a necessary part of the explanation, but it is not, by itself,
a sufficient explanation. The theorist, as we have seen, goes on to suggest that
it is perhaps a sufficient explanation of something else: viz., of our confusedly
and mistakenly *thinking* that states of consciousness are to be ascribed to something in this special way. And this suggestion, as we have seen, is incoherent:
for it involves the denial that someone's states of consciousness are anyone's. We
avoid the incoherence of this denial, while agreeing that the special role of a
single body in someone's experience does not suffice to explain why that experience should be ascribed to anybody. The fact that there is this special role does
not, by itself, give a sufficient reason why what we think of as a subject of experience should have any use for the conception of himself as such a subject.

   When I say that the no-ownership theorist's account fails through not reckoning with all the facts, I have in mind a very simple but, in this question, a very
central, thought: viz., that it is a necessary condition of one's ascribing states of
consciousness, experiences, to oneself, in the way one does, that one should also
ascribe them (or be prepared to ascribe them) to others who are not oneself.[2]
This means not less than it says. It means, for example, that the ascribing phrases
should be used in just the same sense when the subject is another, as when the

subject is oneself. Of course the thought that this is so gives no trouble to the non-philosopher: the thought, for example, that "in pain" means the same whether one says "I am in pain" or "He is in pain." The dictionaries do not give two sets of meanings for every expression which describes a state of consciousness: a first-person meaning, and a second- and third-person meaning. But to the philosopher this thought has given trouble; indeed it has. How could the sense be the same when the method of verification was so different in the two cases—or, rather, when there was a method of verification in the one case (the case of others) and not, properly speaking, in the other case (the case of oneself)? Or, again, how can it be right to talk of *ascribing* in the case of oneself? For surely there can be a question of ascribing only if there is or could be a question of identifying that to which the ascription is made? And though there may be a question of identifying the one who is in pain when that one is another, how can there be such a question when that one is oneself? But this last query answers itself as soon as we remember that we speak primarily to others, for the information of others. In one sense, indeed, there is no question of my having to *tell who it is* who is in pain, when I am. In another sense I may have to *tell who it is*, i.e., to let others know who it is.

What I have just said explains, perhaps, how one may properly be said to ascribe states of consciousness to oneself, given that one ascribes them to others. But how is it that one can ascribe them to others? Well, one thing is certain: that *if* the things one ascribes states of consciousness to, in ascribing them to others, are thought of as a set of Cartesian egos to which *only* private experiences can, in correct logical grammar, be ascribed, *then* this question is unanswerable and this problem insoluble. If, in identifying the things to which states of consciousness are to be ascribed, private experiences are to be all one has to go on, then, just for the very same reason as that for which there is, from one's own point of view, no question of telling that a private experience is one's own, there is also no question of telling that a private experience is another's. All private experiences, all states of consciousness, will be mine, i.e., no one's. To put it briefly: one can ascribe states of consciousness to oneself only if one can ascribe them to others; one can ascribe them to others only if one can identify other subjects of experience; and one cannot identify others if one can identify them *only* as subjects of experience, possessors of states of consciousness.

It might be objected that this way with Cartesianism is too short. After all, there is no difficulty about distinguishing bodies from one another, no difficulty about identifying bodies. And does not this give us an indirect way of identifying subjects of experience, while preserving the Cartesian mode? Can we not identify such a subject as, for example, "the subject that stands to that body in the same special relation as I stand to this one"; or, in other words, "the subject of those experiences which stand in the same unique causal relation to body N as my experiences stand to body M"? But this suggestion is useless. It requires me to have noted that *my* experiences stand in a special relation to body M, when it is just the right to speak of *my* experiences at all that is in question. (It requires me to have noted that my experiences stand in a special relation to body M; but it requires me to have noted this as a condition of being able to identify other subjects of experience, i.e., as a condition of having the idea of myself as a subject of experience, i.e., as a condition of thinking of any experience as *mine*.) So long as we persist in talking, in the mode of this explanation, of experiences on the one hand, and bodies on the other, the most I may be allowed to have noted is that experiences, *all* experiences, stand in a special relation to body M, that body M is unique in just this way, that this is what makes body M unique among bodies. (This "most" is, perhaps, too much—because of the presence of the word "experiences.") The proffered explanation runs: "Another subject of experience is distinguished and identified as the subject of those experiences which stand in the same unique causal relationship to body N as *my* experiences stand to body M." And the objection is: "But what is the word 'my' doing in this explanation? (It could not get on without it.)"

What we have to acknowledge, in order to begin to free ourselves from these difficulties, is the *primitiveness* of the concept of a person. What I mean by the concept of a person is the concept of a type of entity such that *both* predicates ascribing states of consciousness and predicates ascribing corporeal characteristics, a physical situation, etc. are equally applicable to a single individual of that single type. And what I mean by saying that this concept is primitive can be put in a number of ways. One way is to return to those two questions I asked earlier: viz., (1) why are states of consciousness ascribed to anything at all? and (2) why are they ascribed to the very same thing as certain corporeal characteristics, a certain physical situation, etc.? I remarked at the beginning that it was not to be supposed that the answers to these questions were independent of each other. And now I shall say that they are connected in this way: that a necessary condition of states of consciousness being ascribed at all is that they should be ascribed to the very *same things* as certain corporeal characteristics, a certain physical situation, etc. That is to say, states of consciousness could not be ascribed at all, *unless* they were ascribed to persons, in the sense I have claimed for this word. We are tempted to think of a person as a sort of compound of two kinds of subject—a subject of experiences (a pure consciousness, an ego), on the one hand, and a subject of corporeal attributes on the other.

Many questions arise when we think in this way. But, in particular, when we ask ourselves how we come to frame, to get a use for, the concept of this compound of two subjects, the picture—if we are honest and careful—is apt to change from the picture of two subjects to the picture of one subject and one non-subject. For it becomes impossible to see how we could come by the idea of different, distinguishable, identifiable subjects of experiences—different consciousnesses—*if this idea is thought of as logically primitive,* as a logical ingredient in the compound idea of a person, the latter being composed of two subjects. For there could never be any question of assigning an experience, as such, to any subject other than oneself; and therefore never any question of assigning it to oneself either, never any question of ascribing it to a subject at all. So the concept of the pure individual consciousness—the pure ego—is a concept that cannot exist; or, at least, cannot exist as a primary concept in terms of which the concept of a person can be explained or analyzed. It can only exist, if at all, as a secondary, non-primitive concept, which itself is to be explained, analyzed, in terms of the concept of a person. It was the entity corresponding to this illusory primary concept of the pure consciousness, the ego-substance, for which Hume was seeking, or ironically pretending to seek, when he looked into himself, and complained that he could never discover himself without a perception and could never discover anything but the perception. More seriously—and this time there was no irony, but a confusion, a Nemesis of confusion for Hume—it was this entity of which Hume vainly sought for the principle of unity, confessing himself perplexed and defeated; sought vainly because there is no principle of unity where there is no principle of differentiation. It was this, too, to which Kant, more perspicacious here than Hume, accorded a purely formal ("analytic") unity: the unity of the "I think" that accompanies all my perceptions and therefore might just as well accompany none. And finally it is this, perhaps, of which Wittgenstein spoke when he said of the subject, first, that there is no such thing, and, second, that it is not a part of the world, but its limit.

So, then, the word "I" never refers to this, the pure subject. But this does not mean, as the no-ownership theorist must think and as Wittgenstein, at least at one period, seemed to think, that "I" in some cases does not refer at all. It refers, because I am a person among others. And the predicates which would, *per impossible,* belong to the pure subject if it could be referred to, belong properly to the person to which "I" does refer.

The concept of a person is logically prior to that of an individual conscious-ness. The concept of a person is not to be analyzed as that of an animated body or of an embodied anima. This is not to say that the concept of a pure individual consciousness might not have a logically secondary existence, if one thinks, or finds, it desirable. We speak of a dead person—a body—and in the same second-ary way we might at least think of a disembodied person, retaining the logical benefit of individuality from having been a person.[3]

{ IV }

It is important to realize the full extent of the acknowledgment one is making in acknowledging the logical primitiveness of the concept of a person. Let me rehearse briefly the stages of the argument. There would be no question of as-cribing one's own states of consciousness, or experiences, to anything, unless one also ascribed states of consciousness, or experiences, to other individual entities of the same logical type as that thing to which one ascribes one's own states of consciousness. The condition of reckoning oneself as a subject of such predicates is that one should also reckon others as subjects of such predicates. The condition, in turn, of this being possible, is that one should be able to dis-tinguish from one another (pick out, identify) different subjects of such predi-cates, i.e., different individuals of the type concerned. And the condition, in turn, of this being possible is that the individuals concerned, including oneself, should be of a certain unique type: of a type, namely, such that to each indi-vidual of that type there must be ascribed, or ascribable, both states of con-sciousness and corporeal characteristics. But this characterization of the type is still very opaque and does not at all clearly bring out what is involved. To bring this out, I must make a rough division, into two, of the kinds of predicates prop-erly applied to individuals of this type. The first kind of predicate consists of those which are also properly applied to material bodies to which we would not dream of applying predicates ascribing states of consciousness. I will call this first kind M-predicates: and they include things like "weighs 10 stone," "is in the drawing room," and so on. The second kind consists of all the other predicates we apply to persons. These I shall call P-predicates. And P-predicates, of course, will be very various. They will include things like "is smiling," "is go-ing for a walk," as well as things like "is in pain," "is thinking hard," "believes in God," and so on.

So far I have said that the concept of a person is to be understood as the con-cept of a type of entity such that *both* predicates ascribing states of consciousness and predicates ascribing corporeal characteristics, a physical situation, etc. are equally applicable to an individual entity of that type. And all I have said about the meaning of saying that this concept is primitive is that it is not to be analyzed in a certain way or ways. We are not, for example, to think of it as a secondary kind of entity in relation to two primary kinds, viz., a particular consciousness and a particular human body. I implied also that the Cartesian error is just a special case of a more general error, present in a different form in theories of the no-ownership type, of thinking of the designations, or apparent designations, of persons as not denoting precisely the same thing, or entity, for all kinds of predicate ascribed to the entity designated. That is, if we are to avoid the general form of this error we must not think of "I" or "Smith" as suffering from type-ambiguity. (If we want to locate type-ambiguity somewhere, we would do better to locate it in certain predicates like "is in the drawing room," "was hit by a stone," etc., and say they mean one thing when applied to material objects and another when applied to persons.)

This is all I have so far said or implied about the meaning of saying that the concept of a person is primitive. What has to be brought out further is what the implications of saying this are as regards the logical character of those predicates in which we ascribe states of consciousness. And for this purpose we may well consider P-predicates in general. For though not all P-predicates are what we should call "predicates ascribing states of consciousness" (for example, "going for a walk" is not), they may be said to have this in common, that they imply the possession of consciousness on the part of that to which they are ascribed.

What then are the consequences of this view as regards the character of P-predicates? I think they are these. Clearly there is no sense in talking of identifiable individuals of a special type, a type, namely, such that they possess both M-predicates and P-predicates, unless there is in principle some way of telling, with regard to any individual of that type, and any P-predicate, whether that individual possesses that P-predicate. And, in the case of at least some P-predicates, the ways of telling must constitute in some sense logically adequate kinds of criteria for the ascription of the P-predicate. For suppose in no case did these ways of telling constitute logically adequate kinds of criteria. Then we should have to think of the relation between the ways of telling and what the P-predicate ascribes (or a part of what it ascribes) always in the following way: we should have to think of the ways of telling as signs of the presence, in the individual concerned, of this different thing (the state of consciousness). But then we could only know that the way of telling was a sign of the presence of the different thing ascribed by the P-predicate, by the observation of correlations between the two. But this observation we could each make only in one case, namely, our own. And now we are back in the position of the defender of Cartesianism, who thought our way with it was too short. For what, now, does "our own case" mean? There is no sense in the idea of ascribing states of consciousness to oneself, or at all, unless the ascriber already knows how to ascribe at least some states of consciousness to others. So he cannot (or cannot generally) argue "from his own case" to conclusions about how to do this; for unless he already knows how to do this, he has no conception of *his own case,* or any *case* (i.e., any subject of experiences). Instead, he just has evidence that pain, etc. may be expected when a certain body is affected in certain ways and not when others are.

The conclusion here is, of course, not new. What I have said is that one ascribes P-predicates to others on the strength of observation of their behavior; and that the behavior criteria one goes on are not just signs of the presence of what is meant by the P-predicate, but are criteria of a logically adequate kind for the ascription of the P-predicate. On behalf of this conclusion, however, I am claiming that it follows from a consideration of the conditions necessary for any ascription of states of consciousness to anything. The point is not that we must accept this conclusion in order to avoid skepticism, but that we must accept it in order to explain the existence of the conceptual scheme in terms of which the skeptical problem is stated. But once the conclusion is accepted, the skeptical problem does not arise. (And so with the generality of skeptical problems: their statement involves the pretended acceptance of a conceptual scheme and at the same time the silent repudiation of one of the conditions of its existence. This is why they are, in the terms in which they are stated, insoluble.) But this is only half the picture about P-predicates.

Now let us turn to the other half. For of course it is true, at least of some important classes of P-predicates, that when one ascribes them to oneself, one does not do so on the strength of observation of those behavior criteria on the strength of which one ascribes them to others. This is not true of all P-predicates. It is not, in general, true of those which carry assessments of character and capability: these, when self-ascribed, are in general ascribed on the same kind of basis as that on which they are ascribed to others. And of those P-predicates of which it is true that one does not generally ascribe them to oneself on the basis of the criteria on the strength of which one ascribes them to others, there are many of which it is also true that their ascription is liable to correction by the self-ascriber on this basis. But there remain many cases in which one has an entirely adequate basis for ascribing a P-predicate to oneself, and yet in which this basis is quite distinct from those on which one ascribes the predicate to another. (Thus one says, reporting a present state of mind or feeling: "I feel tired, am depressed, am in pain.") How can this fact be reconciled with the doctrine that the criteria on the strength of which one ascribes P-predicates to others are criteria of a logically adequate kind for this ascription?

The apparent difficulty of bringing about this reconciliation may tempt us in many directions. It may tempt us, for example, to deny that these self-ascriptions are really ascriptions at all; to *assimilate* first-person ascriptions of states of consciousness to those other forms of behavior which constitute criteria on the basis of which one person ascribes P-predicates to another. This device seems to avoid the difficulty; it is not, in all cases, entirely inappropriate. But it obscures the facts, and is needless. It is merely a sophisticated form of failure to recognize the special character of P-predicates (or at least of a crucial class of P-predicates). For just as there is not (in general) one primary process of learning, or teaching oneself, an inner private meaning for predicates of this class, then another process of learning to apply such predicates to others on the strength of a correlation, noted in one's own case, with certain forms of behavior, so—and equally— there is not (in general) one primary process of learning to apply such predicates to others on the strength of behavior criteria, and then another process of acquiring the secondary technique of exhibiting a new form of behavior, viz., first-person P-utterances. Both these pictures are refusals to acknowledge the unique logical character of the predicates concerned.

Suppose we write "Px" as the general form of propositional function of such a predicate. Then according to the first picture, the expression which primarily replaces "x" in this form is "I," the first-person singular pronoun; its uses with other replacements are secondary, derivative, and shaky. According to the second picture, on the other hand, the primary replacements of "x" in this form are "he," "that person," etc., and its use with "I" is secondary, peculiar, not a true ascriptive use. But it is essential to the character of these predicates that they have both first-and third-person ascriptive uses, that they are both self-ascribable otherwise than on the basis of observation of the behavior of the subject of them, and other-ascribable on the basis of behavior criteria. To learn their use is to learn both aspects of their use. In order to *have* this type of concept, one must be both a self-ascriber and an other-ascriber of such predicates, and must see every other as a self-ascriber. And in order to *understand* this type of concept, one must acknowledge that there is a kind of predicate which is unambiguously and adequately ascribable *both* on the basis of observation of the subject of the predicate and not on this basis (independently of observation of the subject): the second case is the case where the ascriber is also the subject. If there were no concepts answering to the characterization I have just given, we should indeed have no philosophical problem about the soul; but equally we should not have our concept of a person.

To put the point—with a certain unavoidable crudity—in terms of one particular concept of this class, say, that of depression, we speak of behaving in a depressed way (of depressed behavior) and also of feeling depressed (of a feeling of depression). One is inclined to argue that feelings can be felt, but not observed, and behavior can be observed, but not felt, and that therefore there must be room here to drive in a logical wedge. But the concept of depression spans the place where one wants to drive it in. We might say, in order for there to be such a concept as that of X's depression, the depression which X has, the concept must cover both what is felt, but not observed, by X and what may be observed, but not felt, by others than X (for all values of X). But it is perhaps better to say: X's depression *is* something, one and the same thing, which is felt but not observed by X and observed but not felt by others than X. (And, of course, what can be observed can also be faked or disguised.) To refuse to accept this is to refuse to accept the structure of the language in which we talk about depression. That is, in a sense, all right. One might give up talking; or devise, perhaps, a different structure in terms of which to soliloquize. What is not all right is simultaneously to pretend to accept that structure and to refuse to accept it; i.e., to couch one's rejection in the language of that structure.

It is in this light that we must see some of the familiar philosophical difficulties in the topic of the mind. For some of them spring from just such a failure to admit, or fully appreciate, the character which I have been claiming for at least some P-predicates. It is not seen that these predicates could not have either aspect of their use (the self-ascriptive and the non-self-ascriptive) without having the other aspect. Instead, one aspect of their use is taken as self-sufficient, which it could not be, and then the other aspect appears as problematical. And so we oscillate between philosophical skepticism and philosophical behaviorism. When we take the self-ascriptive aspect of the use of some P-predicate (say, "depressed") as primary, then a logical gap seems to open between the criteria on the strength of which we say that another is depressed, and the actual state of depression. What we do not realize is that if this logical gap is allowed to open, then it swallows not only his depression, but our depression as well. For if the logical gap exists, then depressed behavior, however much there is of it, is no more than a sign of depression. And it can become a sign of depression only because of an observed correlation between it and depression. But whose depression?

Only mine, one is tempted to say. But if *only* mine, then not mine at all. The skeptical position customarily represents the crossing of the logical gap as at best a shaky inference. But the point is that not even the syntax of the premises of the inference exists if the gap exists.

If, on the other hand, we take the other-ascriptive uses of these predicates as self-sufficient, we may come to think that all there is in the meaning of these predicates, as predicates, is the criteria on the strength of which we ascribe them to others. Does this not follow from the denial of the logical gap? It does not follow. To think that it does is to forget the self-ascriptive use of these predicates, to forget that we have to do with a class of predicates to the meaning of which it is essential that they should be both self-ascribable and other-ascribable to the same individual, when self-ascriptions are not made on the observational basis on which other-ascriptions are made, but on another basis. It is not that these predicates have two kinds of meaning. Rather, it is essential to the single kind of meaning that they do have that both ways of ascribing them should be perfectly in order.

If one is playing a game of cards, the distinctive markings of a certain card constitute a logically adequate criterion for calling it, say, the Queen of Hearts; but, in calling it this, in the context of the game, one is also ascribing to it properties over and above the possession of those markings. The predicate gets its meaning from the whole structure of the game. So it is with the language which ascribes P-predicates. To say that the criteria on the strength of which we ascribe P-predicates to others are of a logically adequate kind for this ascription is not to say that all there is to the ascriptive meaning of these predicates is these criteria. To say this is to forget that they are P-predicates, to forget the rest of the language-structure to which they belong.

{ V }

Now our perplexities may take a different form, the form of the question "But how can one ascribe to oneself, not on the basis of observation, *the very same thing* that others may have, on the basis of observation, a logically adequate reason for ascribing to one?" And this question may be absorbed in a wider one, which might be phrased: "How are P-predicates possible?" or "How is the concept of a person possible?" This is the question by which we replace those two earlier questions, viz.: "Why are states of consciousness ascribed at all, ascribed to anything?" and "Why are they ascribed to the very same thing as certain corporeal characteristics, etc.?" For the answer to these two initial questions is to be found nowhere else but in the admission of the primitiveness of the concept of a person, and hence of the unique character of P-predicates. So residual perplexities have to frame themselves in this new way. For when we have acknowledged the primitiveness of the concept of a person and, with it, the unique character of P-predicates, we may still want to ask what it is in the natural facts that makes it intelligible that we should have this concept, and to ask this in the hope of a non-trivial answer.[4] I do not pretend to be able to satisfy this demand at all fully. But I may mention two very different things which might count as beginnings or fragments of an answer.

And, first, I think a beginning can be made by moving a certain class of P-predicates to a central position in the picture. They are predicates, roughly, which involve doing something, which clearly imply intention or a state of mind or at least consciousness in general, and which indicate a characteristic pattern, or range of patterns, of bodily movement, while not indicating at all precisely any very definite sensation or experience. I mean such things as "going for a walk," "furling a rope," "playing ball," "writing a letter." Such predicates have the interesting characteristic of many P-predicates that one does not, in general, ascribe them to oneself on the strength of observation, whereas one does ascribe them to others on the strength of observation. But, in the case of these predicates, one feels minimal reluctance to concede that what is ascribed in these two different ways is the same. And this is because of the marked dominance of a fairly definite pattern of bodily movement in what they ascribe, and the marked absence of any distinctive experience. They release us from the idea that the only things we can know about without observation, or inference, or both, are private experiences; we can know also, without telling by either of these means, about the present and future movements of a body. Yet bodily movements are certainly also things we can know about by observation and inference.

Among the things that we observe, as opposed to the things we know without observation, are the movements of bodies similar to that about which we have knowledge not based on observation. It is important that we understand such observed movements; they bear on and condition our own. And in fact we understand them, we interpret them, only by seeing them as elements in just such plans or schemes of action as those of which we know the present course and future development without observation of the relevant present movements. But this is to say that we see such movements (the observed movements of others) as *actions*, that we interpret them in terms of intention, that we see them as movements of individuals of a type to which also belongs that individual whose present and future movements we know about without observation; that we see others, as self-ascribers, not on the basis of observations, of what we ascribe to them on this basis.

Of course these remarks are not intended to suggest how the "problem of other minds" could be solved, or our beliefs about others given a general philosophical "justification." I have already argued that such a "solution" or "justification" is impossible, that the demand for it cannot be coherently stated. Nor are these remarks intended as a priori genetic psychology. They are simply intended to help to make it seem intelligible to us, at this stage in the history of the philosophy of this subject, that we have the conceptual scheme we have. What I am suggesting is that it is easier to understand how we can see each other (and ourselves) as persons, if we think first of the fact that we act, and act on each other, and act in accordance with a common human nature. "To see each other as persons" is a lot of things; but not a lot of separate and unconnected things. The class of P-predicates that I have moved into the center of the picture are not unconnectedly there, detached from others irrelevant to them. On the contrary, they are inextricably bound up with the others, interwoven with them. The topic of the mind does not divide into unconnected subjects.

I spoke just now of a common human nature. But there is also a sense in which a condition of the existence of the conceptual scheme we have is that human nature should not be common, should not be, that is, a community nature. Philosophers used to discuss the question of whether there was, or could be, such a thing as a "group mind." And for some the idea had a peculiar fascination, while to others it seemed utterly absurd and nonsensical and at the same time, curiously enough, pernicious. It is easy to see why these last found it pernicious: they found something horrible in the thought that people should cease to have toward individual persons the kind of attitudes that they did have, and instead have attitudes in some way analogous to those toward groups; and that they might cease to decide individual courses of action for themselves and instead merely participate in corporate activities. But their finding it pernicious showed that they understood the idea they claimed to be absurd only too well. The fact that we find it natural to individuate as persons the members of a certain class of what might also be individuated as organic bodies does not mean that such a conceptual scheme is inevitable for any class of beings not utterly unlike ourselves.

Might we not construct the idea of a special kind of social world in which the concept of an individual person has no employment, whereas an analogous concept for groups does have employment? Think, to begin with, of certain aspects of actual human existence. Think, for example, of two groups of human beings engaged in some competitive but corporate activity, such as battle, for which they have been exceedingly well trained. We may even suppose that orders are superfluous, though information is passed. It is easy to imagine that, while absorbed in such activity, the members of the groups make no references to individual persons at all, have no use for personal names or pronouns. They do, however, refer to the groups and apply to them predicates analogous to those predicates ascribing purposive activity which we normally apply to individual persons. They may, *in fact,* use in such circumstances the plural forms "we" and "they"; but these are not genuine plurals, they are plurals without a singular, such as we use in sentences like these: "We have taken the citadel," "We have lost the game." They may also refer to elements in the group, to members of the group, but exclusively in terms which get their sense from the parts played by these elements in the corporate activity. (Thus we sometimes refer to what are in fact persons as "stroke" or "tackle.")

When we think of such cases, we see that we ourselves, over a part of our social lives—not, I am thankful to say, a very large part—do operate conceptual schemes in which the idea of the individual person has no place, in which its place is taken, so to speak, by that of a group. But might we not think of communities or groups such that this part of the lives of their members was the dominant part—or was the whole? It sometimes happens, with groups of human beings, that, as we say, their members think, feel, and act "as one." The point I wish to make is that a condition for the existence, the use, of the concept of an individual person is that this should happen *only sometimes.*

It is absolutely useless to say, at this point: But all the same, even if this happened all the time, every member of the group would have an individual consciousness, would be an individual subject of experience. The point is, once more, that there is no sense in speaking of the individual consciousness just as such, of the individual subject of experience just as such: for there is no way of identifying such pure entities.[5] It is true, of course, that in suggesting this fantasy, I have taken our concept of an individual person as a starting point. It is this fact which makes the useless reaction a natural one. But suppose, instead, I had made the following suggestion: that each part of the human body, each organ and each member, had an individual consciousness, was a separate center of experiences. This, in the same way, but more obviously, would be a useless suggestion. Then imagine all the intermediate cases, for instance these. There is a class of moving natural objects, divided into groups, each group exhibiting the same characteristic pattern of activity. Within each group there are certain differentiations of appearance accompanying differentiations of function, and in particular there is one member of each group with a distinctive appearance. Cannot one imagine different sets of observations which might lead us, in the one case, to think of the particular member as the spokesman of the group, as its mouthpiece; and in the other case to think of him as its mouth, to think of the group as a single *scattered* body? The point is that as soon as we adopt the latter way of thinking then we want to drop the former; we are no longer influenced by the human analogy in its first form, but only in its second; and we no longer want to say: "Perhaps the members have consciousness." To understand the movement of our thought here, we need only remember the startling ambiguity of the phrase "a body and its members."

{ VI }

I shall not pursue this attempt at explanation any further. What I have been mainly arguing for is that we should acknowledge the logical primitiveness of the concept of a person and, with this, the unique logical character of certain predicates. Once this is acknowledged, certain traditional philosophical problems are seen not to be problems at all. In particular, the problem that seems to have perplexed Hume[6] does not exist—the problem of the principle of unity, of identity, of the particular consciousness, of the particular subject of "perceptions" (experiences) considered as a primary particular. There is no such problem and no such principle. If there were such a principle, then each of us would have to apply it in order to decide whether any contemporary experience of his was his or someone else's; and there is no sense in this suggestion. (This is not to deny, of course, that one *person* may be unsure of his own identity in some way, may be unsure, for example, whether some particular action, or series of actions, had been performed by him. Then he uses the same methods (the same in principle) to resolve the doubt about himself as anyone else uses to resolve the same doubt about him. And these methods simply involve the application of the ordinary criteria for personal identity. There remains the question of what exactly these criteria are, what their relative weights are, etc.; but, once disentangled from spurious questions, this is one of the easier problems in philosophy.)

Where Hume erred, or seems to have erred, both Kant and Wittgenstein had the better insight. Perhaps neither always expressed it in the happiest way. For Kant's doctrine that the "analytic unity of consciousness" neither requires nor entails any principle of unity is not as clear as one could wish. And Wittgenstein's remarks (at one time) to the effect that the data of consciousness are not owned, that "I" as used by Jones, in speaking of his own feelings, etc., does not refer to what "Jones" as used by another refers to, seem needlessly to flout the conceptual scheme we actually employ. It is needlessly paradoxical to deny, or seem to deny, that when Smith says "Jones has a pain" and Jones says "I have a pain," they are talking about the same entity and saying the same thing about it, needlessly paradoxical to deny that Jones can *confirm* that he has a pain. Instead of denying that self-ascribed states of consciousness are really ascribed at all, it is more in harmony with our actual ways of talking to say: For each user of the language, there is just one person in ascribing to whom states of consciousness he does not need to use the criteria of the observed behavior of that person (though he does not necessarily not do so); and that person is himself. This remark at least respects the structure of the conceptual scheme we employ, without precluding further examination of it.

NOTES

1. The evidence that Wittgenstein at one time held such a view is to be found in the third of Moore's articles in *Mind* on "Wittgenstein's Lectures in, 1930–33" (*Mind*, 1955, especially pp. 13–14). He is reported to have held that the use of "I" was utterly different in the case of "I have a tooth-ache" or "I see a red patch" from its use in the case of "I've got a bad tooth" or "I've got a matchbox." He thought that there were two uses of "I" and that in one of them "I" was replaceable by "this body." So far the view might be Cartesian. But he also said that in the other use (the use exemplified by "I have a tooth-ache" as opposed to "I have a bad tooth"), the "I" *does not denote a possessor*, and that no ego is involved in thinking or in having tooth-ache; and referred with apparent approval to Lichtenberg's dictum that, instead of saying "I think," we (or Descartes!) ought to say "There is a thought" (i.e., "Es denkt").

The attribution of such a view to Schlick would have to rest on his article "Meaning and Verification," Pt. V (*Readings in Philosophical Analysis*, H. Feigl and W. Sellars, eds.). Like Wittgenstein, Schlick quotes Lichtenberg, and then goes on to say: "Thus we see that unless we choose to call our body the owner or bearer of the data [the data of immediate experience]—which seems to be a rather misleading expression—we have to say that the data have no owner or bearer." The full import of Schlick's article is, however, obscure to me, and it is quite likely that a false impression is given by the quotation of a single sentence. I shall say merely that I have drawn on Schlick's article in constructing the case of my hypothetical "no-subject" theorist; but shall not claim to be representing his views.

Lichtenberg's anti-Cartesian dictum is, as the subsequent argument will show, one that I endorse, if properly used. But it seems to have been repeated, without being understood, by many of Descartes' critics.

The evidence that Wittgenstein and Schlick ever held a "no-subject" view seems indecisive, since it is possible that the relevant remarks are intended as criticisms of a Cartesian view rather than as expositions of the true view.

2. I can imagine an objection to the unqualified form of this statement, an objection which might be put as follows. Surely the idea of a uniquely applicable predicate (a predicate which *in fact* belongs to only one individual) is not absurd. And, if it is not, then surely the most that can be claimed is that a necessary condition of one's ascribing predicates of a certain class to one individual (oneself) is that one should be prepared, or ready, on appropriate occasions, to ascribe them to other individuals, and hence that one should have a conception of what those appropriate occasions for ascribing them would be; but not, necessarily, that one should actually do so on any occasion.

The shortest way with the objection is to admit it, or at least to refrain from disputing it; for the lesser claim is all that the argument strictly requires, though it is slightly simpler to conduct it on the basis of the larger claim. But it is well to point out further that we are not speaking of a single predicate, or merely of some group or other of predicates, but of the whole of an enormous class of predicates such that the applicability of those predicates or their negations determines a major logical type or category of individuals. To insist, at this level, on the distinction between the lesser and the larger claims is to carry the distinction over from a level at which it is clearly correct to a level at which it may well appear idle or, possibly, senseless.

The main point here is a purely logical one: the idea of a predicate is correlative with that of a range of distinguishable individuals of which the predicate can be significantly, though not necessarily truly, affirmed.

3. A little further thought will show how limited this concession is. But I shall not discuss the question now.

4. I mean, in the hope of an answer which does not merely say: Well, there are people in the world.

5. More accurately: their identification is necessarily secondary to the identification of persons.

6. Cf. the Appendix to the *Treatise of Human Nature*.

Real Selves

Persons as a Substantial Kind

E. J. Lowe

I. Introduction

Are persons substances or modes? (The terminology may seem archaic, but the issue is a live one.) Two currently dominant views may be characterized as giving the following rival answers to this question. According to the first view, persons are just *biological substances*. According to the second, persons are *psychological modes* of substances which, as far as human beings are concerned, happen to be biological substances, but which could in principle be non-biological. There is; however, also a third possible answer, and this is that persons are *psychological substances*. Such a view is inevitably associated with the name of Descartes, and this helps to explain its current unpopularity, since substantial dualism of his sort is now widely rejected as "unscientific." But one may, as I hope to show, espouse the view that persons are psychological substances without endorsing Cartesianism. This is because one may reject certain features of Descartes's conception of substance. Consequently, one may also espouse a version of substantial dualism which is distinctly non-Cartesian. One may hold that a person, being a psychological substance, is an entity distinct from the biological substance that is (in the human case) his or her body, and yet still be prepared to ascribe corporeal characteristics to this psychological substance.[1] By this account, a human person is to be thought of neither as a non-corporeal mental substance (a Cartesian mind), nor as the product of a mysterious "union" between such a substance and a physical, biological substance (a Cartesian animal body). This is not to deny that the mind—body problem is a serious and difficult one, but it is to imply that there is a version of substantial dualism which does not involve regarding the "mind" as a distinct substance in its own right.

II. What Is a Substance?

But what do we—or, more to the point, what *should* we—mean by a "substance"? I am prepared to defend what I take to be a more or less Aristotelian conception of this notion. That is, I shall follow the Aristotle of the *Categories* in taking a "primary" substance to be a concrete individual *thing*, or "particular," or "continuant."[2] Paradigm examples are such entities as an individual horse (say, Eclipse) and an individual house (say, the one I live in). (If, as some commentators believe,[3] Aristotle changed his mind about this between composing the *Categories* and the *Metaphysics*, then so be it; I am really only interested in the doctrine, not in whether or when Aristotle held it.)

Such substances (henceforth I shall drop the word "primary") belong to kinds, that is, to species and genera (which Aristotle, in the *Categories* but not elsewhere, called "secondary" substances). The kinds to which substances belong I shall call *substantial* kinds. Not *all* kinds are substantial kinds, of course, since there are kinds of non-substantial individuals: for example, kinds of events and kinds of numbers. Events, though concrete individuals, are not substances by the "Aristotelian" account because they are not entities capable of persisting through qualitative change—indeed, they just *are*, broadly speaking, the changes which substances undergo. Numbers are not substances because—assuming indeed that they really exist at all—they are purely abstract entities.

Substantial kinds may be *natural* (like the kind *horse*) or they may be *artefactual* (like the kind *house*). This distinction is mutually exclusive and perhaps also exhaustive—though arguably there genuinely exist substantial kinds, like perhaps the culinary kind *vegetable*, which are neither natural nor artefactual.[4] But to call a substantial kind "natural" is not to imply that individual exemplars of it could not be artificially synthesized. Rather, the characteristic feature of natural substantial kinds (henceforth, simply "natural kinds") is that they are *subjects of natural law*. This requires some expansion. Obviously, it is not that an artefact, such as a watch, is not subject *to* natural law: if a watch is dropped, its fall will be governed by the law of gravity, quite as much as will the fall of a tree. The point rather is that there are no natural laws that are distinctively *about* watches or artefacts of any other kind: artefactual kinds are not subjects *of* natural law. By contrast, there *are* laws about plants and animals and stars and atoms and all other such natural kinds. The laws in question belong to the various special sciences: biology, astronomy, nuclear physics, and so forth. Each of these sciences is about substances of certain appropriate natural kinds. The kinds that are proper to one science are not, in general, proper to another: thus astronomy has something to say about stars but not about starfish, while the reverse is true of biology. Furthermore, I see no good reason to believe that all laws about natural kinds are even "in principle" reducible to, or wholly explicable in terms of, laws about some privileged set of "basic" or "fundamental" natural kinds—such as sub-atomic particles. That is to say, I consider the various special sciences to be for the most part relatively autonomous, despite numerous theoretical interconnections between them.

One reason why I reject reductionism about laws is that I reject it about substantial individuals of the kinds which are the subjects of laws. For instance, I reject the view that a biological entity such as a tree can simply be regarded as being nothing over and above an assemblage of sub-atomic particles, even though we now believe that the ultimate constituents of trees (and of everything else material) are indeed such particles. It may perhaps be true that the existence of the tree in some sense "supervenes" upon that of its constituent particles at any given time (though saying this is no clearer than the somewhat obscure notion of supervenience permits it to be). But that these particles constitute a *tree* rather than an entity of some quite different non-biological kind crucially depends upon their organization (that is, in Aristotelian terms, upon their realizing the "form" of a tree). And this organization can only be appropriately described (I would contend) in distinctively *biological* terms. Thus, what is crucial as far as the presence or absence of a *tree* is concerned, is that the particles in question should be so organized as to subserve the characteristic life-sustaining functions of the various typical parts of a tree—respiration, photosynthesis, nutrition, and so forth. (By a tree's "typical" parts I mean such parts as its leaves, branches, roots and so on, all of which play distinctive biological roles in its overall structure and economy.) Saying what these typical parts and characteristic functions are, and explaining their proper interrelationships, are precisely matters for the science of biology, and will involve the recognition of various distinctively biological laws. Biological laws are laws about living organisms *qua* living organisms (rather than, for example, *qua* material bodies), and since talk of living organisms is not reducible to talk of assemblages of sub-atomic particles, neither are biological laws reducible to the laws of nuclear physics.

III. Persons as Biological Substances

Having explained what I mean by "substance" and "substantial kind," I can return now to my main theme: the ontological status of persons. According to the first view mentioned in my opening section, persons are biological substances—that is, they are members of a substantial kind which is a kind of living organism. Briefly: persons are a kind of animal. This seems to have been Aristotle's own view, and in modern times it is well represented in the work of David Wiggins.[5]

One striking feature of this view is that it threatens either to promote a (to my mind) ethically dubious anthropomorphic "speciesism" or else to play havoc with zoological taxonomies.[6] To see this, it should be noted that it is normally the case in zoology that, if a species a is subordinate to both of two distinct genera b and c, then either b is subordinate to c or c is subordinate to b. (I use the term "genus" here in a broad sense just to mean a higher kind than another, relative to which the latter is correspondingly a "species.") Formally, we may state this principle as follows (where "/" symbolizes the subordinancy relation):

$P.\ a/b\ \&\ a/c \to b = c \lor b/c \lor c/b.$

For instance, goats are both ruminants and ungulates—and, as it turns out, ruminants are (i.e. are subordinate to) ungulates, in accordance with the requirements of principle P. Consequently, if two distinct species a and a' are both subordinate to a genus b, while a is also subordinate to a genus c and a' is subordinate to a genus c', then (by our principle P) it is *both* the case that either b is subordinate to c or c is subordinate to b, *and* the case that either b is subordinate to c' or c' is subordinate to b. It follows (assuming that our principle P also applies to the genera and that the subordinancy relation is transitive) that in such a case either c is subordinate to c', or c' is subordinate to c, or else c and c' are both subordinate to b. Now, an adherent of the view that persons are a kind of animal will doubtless want to say that *humans* (i.e. members of the species *homo sapiens*) are *persons* and are also (for example) *mammals*. But could an adherent of this view also accept the possibility of there being a hitherto unknown species of *amphibians* (say), call them *bolgs*, which were likewise *persons*? Not if our taxonomic principle P is correct, for this would commit them to the proposition that either mammals are amphibians, or amphibians are mammals, or else both mammals and amphibians are persons—and none of these disjuncts is true. (The last disjunct is of course false because if amphibians are—i.e. are subordinate to—persons then, since frogs are amphibians, frogs would have to be persons, by virtue of the transitivity of the subordinacy relation. But frogs are not persons, outside the realms of fairy tale.) So either a widely applicable taxonomic principle must be rejected or else it must be claimed that creatures such as our imagined bolgs cannot be persons—which seems to require an intolerable degree of anthropocentric prejudice.

Perhaps, however, all that this shows is that our principle P should indeed be rejected in favour of a weaker one, expressible formally as follows:[7]

$P'. a/b \& a/c \rightarrow b = c \vee b/c \vee c/b \vee (\exists x)(b/x \& c/x).$

Appealing to this principle, an adherent of the biological substance view of persons could hold that both humans and bolgs are indeed persons, even though humans are mammals and bolgs are amphibians. For the only constraint that P' imposes here is that mammals, amphibians, and persons should all be subordinate to some one higher genus—and an adherent of the biological substance view will of course be quite happy to allow this, seeing the genus *animal* as occupying precisely such a role. The proposed set of relationships is displayed in Figure 1.

Such a taxonomic structure cannot, I think, be ruled out *a priori*, since I am certainly prepared to allow that structures isomorphic with it may obtain amongst artefactual kinds. However, amongst *natural* (and more specifically *biological*) kinds this seems most improbable. This is connected with the fact that natural kinds are subjects of natural law. If persons are a natural, biological kind, as is now being proposed, then one would expect there to be distinctive biological laws relating to personkind—laws intimately linked to the evolution

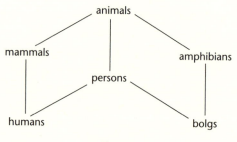

Figure 1

of persons as a biological kind. Such laws would have to be applicable to both humans and bolgs, these both being *ex hypothesi* species of person. However, humans and bolgs, being mammals and amphibians respectively, must be presumed to have had quite different evolutionary histories, tenuously linked only by a very remote common ancestor species: and this seems to make it little short of miraculous that they should none the less *both* have evolved to be governed by the *same* distinctive network of biological laws, even to the extent of qualifying them as species of a single biological kind, personkind. It is rather as if we were to discover that although all the frogs we have hitherto encountered are amphibians, there is in fact also a mammalian species of frogs, exhibiting many of the features we are familiar with in frogs and yet warm-blooded and given to suckling their young. As an imaginary contribution to biological science, the theory of persons just adumbrated is no less incredible.

At this point various responses are available to my opponent. One is to remark that in fact evolution *has* thrown up species sharing many morphological features despite their having no close common antecedent, a phenomenon which is often reflected in the popular names of these species: for instance, *wolves* and *marsupial wolves*.[8] But such examples do not really help my opponent, since biological science does *not* in fact classify such species as genuinely falling under the same genus by virtue of the shared morphological features in question. Marsupial wolves are *not* regarded by zoologists as a species of dog, unlike true wolves (*canis lupus*). However, to this my opponent may respond that I have unfairly stacked the cards against him by taking zoological species as my paradigm of biological kinds.[9] "Obviously," he may say, "persons can't be regarded as a zoological species on a par with *canis lupus* or *homo sapiens*, and so can't be expected to fit in neatly with zoological taxonomies; but this doesn't mean that they can't constitute a biological kind—a kind of animal—which finds a place in some alternative (though not for that reason *rival*) taxonomic scheme."

My reply to this suggestion is that it is threatened by the following dilemma. Either it will be compelled to regard persons as constituting a purely "nominal" (as opposed to a "real") kind—and this will undermine the supposedly biological status of persons. Or else it will have difficulty in establishing compatibility between the zoological taxonomy and the proposed alternative biological taxonomy in which persons are supposed to find a place. To see this, we must recall that an adherent of the suggestion will want to claim that individual human beings are *both* members of the zoological species *homo sapiens* and *also* members of the allegedly biological kind *person*. Now, if *person* is regarded as a purely nominal kind—that is, as a "kind" membership of which is secured merely by possession of some set of "defining characteristics" (so that, in my view, it deserves the name "kind" by courtesy only)—then the claim in question is not threatened by inconsistency. However, it does now appear obscure in what sense it could still be insisted that the concept of a person is essentially a *biological* one. For if personhood is determined by the satisfaction of a set of defining characteristics, it seems clear that the favoured candidates for such characteristics would have to be broadly *psychological* ones: an ability to reason, the possession of consciousness, a capacity to perceive and to engage in intentional activity, and so forth.[10] It certainly is not clear why we should have to include amongst these characteristics any mention of a biological substrate or of distinctively biological functions. There seems to be no good reason, either *a priori* or *a posteriori*, to suppose that the psychological capacities mentioned earlier could not in principle be associated with an inorganic body, and indeed even with a wholly artefactual one.[11]

So let us turn to the other horn of the dilemma, by supposing that persons are to be regarded as a *real* biological kind. My point now is that it is difficult to see how this can be consistent with regarding individual members of the species *Homo sapiens* as also being instances of the kind *person*, given the relative independence of the two taxonomic schemes within which these kinds are supposed to find their places. The reason for this is as follows. Specifying what real or substantial kind(s) a particular belongs to is, in Aristotelian terms, tantamount to determining its *essence*. Thus, bound up with such a specification will be an account of the particular's *persistence conditions*; that is, an account of the sorts of admissible changes it can undergo while yet surviving as a particular of that kind. Changes that are admissible for particulars of one kind are very often not admissible for particulars of another kind; and in general the range of admissible changes will (in the case of natural kinds) be intimately tied to the range of natural laws of which the kind in question is the subject. For example, the change from possessing gills and a tail to possessing lungs and four legs is admissible in the case of frogs but not in the case of trout, because the laws of morphological development differ for creatures of these two different kinds. Now, if *person* and *Homo sapiens* are *both* real biological kinds, then both will have associated with them a range of admissible changes determined by the developmental laws governing these kinds. However, given the relative independence of the two taxonomic schemes within which these kinds are supposed to find their places, there is no reason to suppose compatibility between these ranges of admissible changes—and indeed every reason to suppose incompatibility.[12]

For instance, suppose that our imagined bolgs are accepted as *bona fide* members of the kind *person*, and yet are also similar to their amphibian cousins the frogs in undergoing metamorphosis from a larval to an adult phase. Then bolgs *qua* amphibians can survive a change from having gills and a tail to having lungs and legs, whereas humans *qua* members of the mammalian species *Homo sapiens* cannot. But both bolgs and humans are supposedly *also* members of the allegedly biological real kind *person*, governed by its own developmental laws. Either these laws permit the change from having gills and a tail to having lungs and legs or they do not permit it. If they do, then it follows, absurdly, that an individual human being *can* survive the change *qua* person but *cannot* survive it *qua* member of *Homo sapiens*. If they do not, then it follows, equally absurdly, that an individual bolg *cannot* survive the change *qua* person but *can* survive it *qua* bolg. (If it is felt that this argument is suspect on the grounds that human beings do not have gills and a tail in the first place, or indeed on the opposing grounds that human beings do in fact undergo a metamorphosis not unlike that of amphibians but prenatally during their embryo stage, then it is easy enough to substitute for the bolgs an imagined species undergoing a metamorphosis which human beings undoubtedly *cannot* undergo despite possessing the morphological features of its initial phase—for instance, a change from having hair and arms to having feathers and wings.)

This concludes my discussion of the first view mentioned in my opening section—the view that persons are biological substances.[13] I hope I have made the unattractiveness of that view abundantly clear, and in particular I hope I have made it clear why adherents of that view are driven towards anthropocentrism. It is true that I have offered no explicit arguments against such anthropocentrism itself—against the opinion, that is, that human beings are the only persons that there could be—but this is because I find it not only morally repugnant and dangerously arrogant, but also symptomatic of a philosophically inadequate imagination. I cannot really take the suggestion seriously as one meriting detailed examination and refutation.

IV. Persons as Psychological Modes

The next view I shall consider—that of persons as psychological modes—is essentially the view of Locke and Hume; though of course Locke and Hume also had their important differences on matters to do with substance and identity. Here I should explain that by a *mode* I understand any concrete non-substantial individual, or any entity wholly constituted by concrete non-substantial individuals.

Paradigm examples of concrete non-substantial individuals are events, processes, and states. And the view of persons which we are now considering takes persons to be wholly constituted by *psychological* or *mental* events, processes, and states.

It must be conceded that Locke's adherence to the psychological mode view of persons is less clear-cut and explicit than Hume's. Hume of course quite expressly regards the self *as being* "nothing but a bundle or collection of different perceptions."[14] On the other hand, Locke's official doctrine seems to be that "person" denotes a nominal kind whose defining characteristics are all psychological in nature.[15] Even so, Locke's account of the identity conditions of persons and his concomitant treatment of the puzzle cases certainly appear to imply that, on his view, neither material nor (finite) "spiritual" *substances* can qualify as persons.[16] Furthermore, there is a passage in the *Essay* in which Locke, having claimed that the only three kinds of substance of which we have ideas are God, finite spirits, and material particles, goes on to say that "all other things [are] but modes or relations ultimately terminated in substances."[17] Given that persons (other than God, at least) are not substances, this would certainly appear to imply that for Locke they have the status of *modes*. Anyway, ignoring further exegetical complications, I shall henceforth just assume that Locke does indeed belong to the same broad camp as Hume.

In recent years, a view of persons very much like that of Locke and Hume has enjoyed a revival in the writings of such philosophers as Derek Parfit.[18] Modern adherents of the view are, however, usually concerned to represent it as a physicalist theory, or at least as being compatible with a thoroughgoing physicalism. This, they suppose, may be achieved by maintaining that mental events, processes, and states are—or at least could well be—identical with physical events, processes, and states. Such psychophysical identities may, it is further supposed, obtain either on a "type-type" or on a "token-token" basis (with the latter suggestion currently enjoying rather more popularity than the former).

How are persons supposed to be constituted by mental states? (Henceforth, for the sake of brevity, I shall use "state" in a broad way to include both events and processes.) Here theorists diverge somewhat. According to what we may call the "Lockean" school, personal identity consists in the obtaining of relationships of "co-consciousness" between mental states. That is to say, on this approach a person is constituted by a manifold of mental states by virtue of these states being connected to one another, but not to any other mental states, by relationships of co-consciousness. Just what these relationships are is a matter for further theorizing on the part of adherents of the Lockean school, but it is generally agreed that in the case of coexisting mental states they involve some sort of "unity of consciousness" condition while in the case of mental states separated by time they involve memory of a special sort (sometimes called "experiential memory" or "first person memory"). Adherents of what we may call the "Humean" school differ from those of the Lockean school chiefly in contending that the relationships between mental states which are crucial to personal identity are not so much cognitive as *causal* in character[19] (though since both schools will typically also advance causal accounts of cognitive relations like memory, the differences between the Lockean and Humean schools are more ones of emphasis than of fundamental principle). It is probably fair to say that most modern proponents of the view of persons now under consideration espouse an amalgam of neo-Lockean and neo-Humean ideas. For brevity, and in recognition of Locke's historical priority, I propose however simply to call such modern accounts collectively the *neo-Lockean theory*.

It is to the credit of the neo-Lockean theory that, unlike the neo-Aristotelian theory, it is untainted by anthropocentrism (this indeed is the lesson of Locke's story of the rational parrot). This explains, too, why the neo-Lockean theory should appeal, as it clearly does, to enthusiasts for the prospects of artificial intelligence. The existence of a neo-Lockean person is popularly likened to the running of a computer program, which is largely independent of the detailed "hardware" of the machine on which it is run. Human brains and nervous systems provide, on this view, highly efficient hardware (or "wetware") for the "running" of a person, but there is no reason in principle why the "program" should not be run on an altogether different kind of machine, constructed on electronic rather than on biological principles. This even offers human persons— albeit only in the distant future—the prospect of immortality by means of transfer to a solid state device (though equally it offers an embarrassment of riches in the form of simultaneous transfer to more than one such machine).

However, the neo-Lockean theory is untenable. Neo-Aristotelians indeed are likely to abhor it as reviving the "myth of the ghost in the machine," and as grotesquely abstracting from the bodily and social dimensions of personality. It is not clear to me that this line of criticism is at all fair, though, since it is perfectly open to the neo-Lockean to insist that persons must indeed be *embodied*, and moreover furnished with bodies apt for the performance of physical actions, including those necessary for social co-operation and communication. (After all—to pursue the computer analogy—you cannot run a program on a chunk of rock or a tin can, much less on nothing at all; nor would anyone see fit to denigrate the notion of a program as introducing the "myth" of a ghost in the hardware.) I suspect that all that this neo-Aristotelian line of criticism amounts to is once again the expression of anthropocentric prejudices. Yet for all that the neo-Lockean theory *is* untenable, and this for reasons of fundamental principle.

What is wrong with the neo-Lockean theory is that, in purporting to supply an account of the individuation and identity of persons it presupposes, untenably, that an account of the identity conditions of psychological modes can be provided which need not rely on reference to persons. But it emerges that the identity of any psychological mode turns on the identity of the person that possesses it. What this implies is that psychological modes are essentially modes *of persons*, and correspondingly that persons have to be conceived of as psychological *substances*. This is what I now hope to show.

By psychological modes I mean, as I have already explained, individual mental events, processes, and states. (It is important to emphasize that we are talking about *individual* entities here—"tokens" rather than "types.") Paradigm examples would be: a particular belief-state, a particular memory-state, a particular sensory experience, a particular sequence of thoughts constituting a particular process of reasoning, and so on. But, to repeat, such individual mental states are necessarily states *of persons*: they are necessarily "owned"—necessarily have a *subject*. The necessity in question arises from the metaphysical-cum-logical truth that such individual mental states cannot even in principle be individuated and identified without reference to the subject of which they are states. (The point has been argued before by Strawson,[20] but it is none the less worth insisting on it again since Strawson's arguments seem to have gone largely unheeded.)

Consider thus the example of a particular experience of pain, which is a 'token' mental event occurring at a specific time. (Whether it occurs at a specific *place* is more contentious. We should not confuse the phenomenological location of the pain—where it is felt "at," for instance in a certain tooth—with the place, if any, at which the token experience occurs. Physicalists would of course presume that the token experience is identifiable with a token neural event located in the brain, at least in the case of a human person; but the truth—and indeed the intelligibility—of physicalism is something that I have grave doubts about.[21]) Now, clearly, the qualitative character and time of occurrence of this token experience do not suffice to individuate it uniquely: two qualitatively indistinguishable token experiences could, logically, occur simultaneously (and quite probably often do, given the vastness of the world's population). What is additionally required to individuate the token experience, it appears, is precisely reference to its *subject*. For instance, if the pain is *mine*, then that it seems will serve to distinguish it from any other qualitatively exactly similar pain occurring at the same time.

But two questions arise here. First, can we be sure that there is no *other* way of individuating the token experience uniquely which does not require reference to its subject? And secondly, can we be sure that one and the same subject could *not* simultaneously have two qualitatively indistinguishable token experiences? Both of these questions have been interestingly addressed quite recently by Christopher Peacocke.[22] Peacocke suggests that although it is a necessary truth that one and the same subject cannot have two qualitatively indistinguishable token experiences at the same time, this is not because token experiences are individuated by reference to their qualitative character, time of occurrence, and subject: rather, the explanation is quite the reverse of this, namely, that subjects themselves are individuated by reference to token experiences in such a way that where we have evidence for the occurrence of two simultaneous and qualitatively indistinguishable token experiences, this should *ipso facto* be taken to imply the existence of two distinct subjects of experience. In support of this suggestion, Peacocke appeals to an example involving a so-called "split-brain" patient. We could, he contends, have good evidence for supposing that in the case of such a patient there might be, on a given occasion, "two distinct but qualitatively identical experiences grounded in (different) states of the same brain."[23] And, he goes on, "It seems that if we speak of two distinct minds or centres of consciousness in these circumstances, we do so because the token experiences are themselves distinct."[24] This presupposes, of course, a favourable answer to the *first* question raised a moment ago: that is, it presupposes that we can individuate token experiences independently of their subject, and hence have independent evidence, in the case of the split-brain patient, for the simultaneous occurrence of two qualitatively indistinguishable token experiences.

Now Peacocke *does* consider that a favourable (to him) answer to our first question is available. He suggests that in order to individuate token experiences it suffices, apart from referring to their qualitative character and time of occurrence, to refer to their *causes and effects*. Thus, he says,

> There is a clear motivation for saying that in the split brain there are two token experiences, a motivation which does not appeal to the identity of persons. The two experiences have different causes—for example, one results from the stimulation of one nostril, the other from the stimulation of the other nostril—and they may have different effects too.[25]

(Peacocke's example here involves, of course, olfactory experiences rather than pains, but this is beside the point.) However, I consider this line of argument to be fatally flawed. No doubt it is true that whenever two distinct token experiences occur, they will differ in respect of at least some of their causes and effects: but it is far from clear that one can effectively appeal to such causal distinctions to individuate token experiences quite independently of any reference to the subjects of those experiences. For it may be, as indeed I believe to be the case, that such causal distinctions themselves cannot be made independently of reference to subjects. But before pursuing this point it is worth remarking that to the extent that Peacocke's proposed criterion for the individuation of token experiences—sameness of causes and effects—is merely a special application of Davidson's well-known criterion for the individuation of events in general, it falls foul of the latter's fatal defect, which is a kind of circularity.[26] Briefly, the trouble with Davidson's criterion is that if (as Davidson himself presupposes) the causes and effects of events are themselves events, then the question of whether events e_1 and e_2 have the *same* causes and effects (and hence turn out to be the same event according to the criterion) is itself a question concerning the identity of events, so that in the absence of an independent criterion of event identity Davidson's criterion leaves every question of event identity unsettled: hence it is either superfluous or ineffectual. Moreover, Peacocke's special application of Davidson's criterion to mental events inherits this difficulty. For even if we suppose, for the sake of argument, that the individuation of *non*-mental events is unproblematic, it is none the less the case that no mental event has purely non-mental causes and effects: that is to say, every mental event has other mental events amongst its causes and effects. And hence the proposal to individuate mental events in terms of the sameness of their causes and effects will again presuppose answers to questions of the very sort at issue, namely, questions concerning the identity of mental events.

It will be of value to expand upon the point that mental events never have wholly non-mental causes and effects, not only in order to support a premise of the foregoing argument, but also because it will help to support the more ambitious claim I made a moment ago that causal distinctions between token experiences (and other mental states) cannot be made independently of reference to subjects. The point is that a mental event, such as a token experience, can only occur *to* a subject, and moreover only to one in a condition which involves the simultaneous possession by that same subject of a whole battery of other mental states—at least some of which will stand in causal relations to the sensory experience in question, helping to determine such features as its intensity and duration and in turn being affected by it in various ways. For instance, if one directs one's attention away from pain, its intensity may be diminished; again, if one believes that the pain is symptomatic of a serious illness, it may cause one to have fears which one would otherwise have lacked; and so on. That a pain should have such causal liaisons with other mental states of the same subject is partially constitutive of the very concept of pain. Thus we can make no sense at all of a subject undergoing a single sensory experience in the complete absence of all other mental activity, much less of a single sensory experience—a twinge of pain, say—occurring out of the blue to no subject at all. *Pace* Hume, "perceptions," even if they are "distinct," are frequently not "separable."[27] Mental events, even of the most rudimentary kinds, are only conceivable as elements within relatively well-integrated mental economies—that is, as parts of the mental lives of subjects.[28] At root, this is just a corollary of Davidson's own well-known thesis of the "holism of the mental."[29]

But let us now see how all this bears upon Peacocke's suggestion that causal distinctions can motivate a claim that two distinct token olfactory experiences occur in his imagined split-brain patient without relying on any consideration as to the number or identity of the subjects involved. What sorts of causal distinctions might be appealed to? Unfortunately, Peacocke only gestures in the direction of an answer, merely saying (as we have already seen) that "The two experiences have different causes—for example, one results from the stimulation of one nostril, the other from the stimulation of the other nostril—and they may have different effects too." But so far all we know about the imagined case is that it is one in which the *corpus callosum* of a living human brain is severed and subsequently the two nostrils neurally connected to the different hemispheres are simultaneously stimulated in the same way. Thus far, however, we have been given no reason for supposing that *either* stimulation results in an olfactory experience. For that, we need to know the answers to such questions as "Was the patient awake?", "Did he still possess a sense of smell?", "Was he paying attention to the stimulus?", and so on. But these are all questions which precisely make reference to a putative *subject* of olfactory experience. Moreover, they presume—perhaps wrongly—that there is just a *single* subject present. But how is this presumption, if mistaken, to be recognized as being in error? That is, how are we to discover that we are dealing with two subjects rather than just one? Peacocke's suggestion seems to be that we *first* determine that each stimulation results in a distinct but qualitatively exactly similar token experience, and *then* on that basis assign each to a different subject, hence concluding that we have two subjects rather than one. But we have just seen that the question

of whether a stimulation results in any olfactory experience at all is only answerable in the light of information concerning the prospective subject of that
experience (whether he is awake, and so on). So Peacocke's suggested procedure
presupposes an answer to the very question that it proposes to settle: for it presupposes, with respect to each stimulation, that we already have in view a subject to which any resulting experience may be assigned. The key point is that
whether the stimulation of a particular nostril results in an olfactory experience
depends precisely on whether that nostril is functioning as an olfactory sense
organ of a subject who is identifiable as the possessor of a suitable range of further mental states at the time of stimulation. Hence it emerges that we cannot
effectively motivate a claim that each stimulation results in a distinct token
experience without relying on presumptions concerning the existence and
identity of the prospective subject(s) of those experiences. And the more general
lesson is that one cannot reasonably form judgements about the causation of
mental events—including sensory experiences—independently of forming
judgements about the subjects of those states, and so cannot expect judgements
of the former sort to underpin the individuation of such states in a way which
makes no reference to those subjects.[30]

But what then *are* we to say about the split-brain patient? *Do* we have two
subjects here or only one? Again, is it right to dismiss (as Peacocke does) the
possibility of one and the same subject simultaneously possessing two qualitatively indistinguishable token experiences? Let me say at once that I think it is
a mistake to regard the psychological subject as a "centre of consciousness."
(Peacocke himself shifts uneasily between the terms "centre of consciousness,"
"mind," and "person"—all of which, in my view, demand quite different treatments.) The notion of the subject as a "centre of consciousness" seems to involve
precisely that Lockean conception of the self which I am now engaged in challenging: for it suggests that "unity of consciousnesses" is somehow criterial for
the identity of the self, and this I wish to deny. The case of the split-brain patient
is indeed a difficult and puzzling one: but I am strongly inclined to urge that
even in such a case we have only a single subject, albeit a subject quite possibly
suffering from a partial bifurcation of consciousness, or "divided mind." Perhaps, however, this is really no more than an extreme case of a condition to
which all psychological subjects are prone.[31] At various times we all find ourselves "dividing our attention" (as we say)—for example, engaging in conversation while negotiating busy traffic.

This being so, however, I must reject the thesis that one and the same subject
cannot possess two qualitatively indistinguishable token experiences simulta-

neously, however improbable the actual occurrence of such a state of affairs might be. And this then raises the question of how token experiences can be guaranteed to be individuated uniquely, given that reference to their qualitative character, time of occurrence, *and subject* may not suffice. But a plausible answer is that we can now appeal additionally to causal considerations. Peacocke's error (as I see it) was to suppose that we could appeal to causal considerations without needing to make reference to the subject: but in rejecting his supposition we do not have to dismiss causal considerations as irrelevant to the problem of individuation. However, the details of such a solution must await another occasion.

There remains one line of defence of the neo-Lockean theory which I have not yet tackled. The burden of my criticism of that theory has been that it fails to accommodate the fact that mental states have to be individuated as states *of persons*, for this introduces a vicious circularity into its attempt to specify the identity conditions of persons in terms of relations between mental states. But, it may be urged, the truth is only that mental states—being modes—have to be individuated as states *of something*, that is, as states of substances of *some* sort. And why, it may be asked, should not the neo-Lockean simply say that mental states are states *of the body*—allowing indeed that the body might in principle vary enormously in nature from one person to another? In fact, of course, the neo-Lockean who is also a physicalist does hold precisely this to be true. But the problem is that reference to the body is simply incapable of playing the individuative role here demanded of it. This is because by the neo-Lockean's own lights there can be no guarantee of a one-to-one correspondence between bodies (of whatever sort) and persons. Hence, in a case (however hypothetical) of co-embodiment by two distinct persons (as in the Jekyll and Hyde story), referring a mental state to a particular body will not determine to which person it belongs nor, hence, which token state it is. For persons cannot share token mental states, and so while it is left undetermined to which person a token state belongs, the identity of that token state must equally be left undetermined. For example, if the token state—say, a token belief-state—is referred to the Jekyll–Hyde body, this leaves it open whether it is Jekyll's belief-state or Hyde's belief-state: it cannot be both Jekyll's and Hyde's, but whose it is matters if we are to identify which particular belief-state it is.

Perhaps this argument will be objected to as question-begging, however. Perhaps it will be urged that reference to the Jekyll–Hyde body *will* serve to *identify* the belief-state, but merely leave undetermined whether this state belongs to Jekyll or to Hyde. But what if, as seems perfectly conceivable, Jekyll and Hyde both have token belief-states of exactly the same type? Still these token belief-states cannot be identical because, as has been remarked, token mental states are not shareable between persons. In that case there will be two exactly similar token belief-states referrable to the same body, so that reference to that body will not, after all, serve to distinguish them. The plain fact is (and we should hardly be surprised by it) that in rejecting the biological substance view of persons in favor of the psychological mode view, the neo-Lockean theory has cut itself off from any possibility of treating the *body* as the "owner" of mental states and thus as playing an essential role in their individuation. The "owner" of mental states for the neo-Lockean theory must be the person *as opposed to* the body, even though the person itself is, according to that theory, a construct of mental states—the very mental states indeed of which it is the "owner." And it is of course precisely this circularity in the theory to which I object.

V. Persons as Psychological Substances

The conclusion I draw from the preceding arguments is that a person or subject of mental states must be regarded as a *substance* of which those states are modes, and yet not as a *biological* substance (as the neo-Aristotelian theory would have it). What sort of substance, then? Clearly, a psychological substance. That is to say, a person is a substantial individual belonging to a natural kind which is the subject of distinctively psychological laws, and governed by persistence conditions which are likewise distinctively psychological in character. But thus far this is consistent with regarding a person as something like a Cartesian ego or soul, and this is a position from which I wish to distance myself. The distinctive feature of the Cartesian conception of a psychological substance is that such a substance is regarded as possessing *only* mental characteristics, not physical ones. And this is largely why it is vulnerable to certain sceptical arguments to be found in the writings of, *inter alia*, Locke and Kant. The burden of those arguments is that if psychological substances (by which the proponents of the arguments mean *immaterial* "souls" or "spirits") are the real subjects of mental states, then for all I know the substance having "my" thoughts today is not the same as the substance that had "my" thoughts yesterday: so that, on pain of having to countenance the possibility that my existence is very much more ephemeral than I care to believe, I had better not identify myself with the psychological substance (if any) currently having "my" thoughts (currently "doing the thinking in me"). But if *I* am not a psychological substance, it seems gratuitous even to suppose that such substances exist (certainly, their existence cannot be established by the Cartesian *cogito*).

But why should we suppose, with Descartes, that psychological substances must be essentially immaterial? Descartes believed this because he held a conception of substance according to which each distinct kind of substance has only one principal "attribute," which is peculiar to substances of that kind, and such that all of the states of any individual substance of this kind are modes of this unique and exclusive attribute.[32] In the case of psychological or mental substances, the attribute is Thought; whereas in the case of physical or material substance(s), the attribute is Extension. On this view, no psychological substance can possess a mode of Extension, nor any physical substance a mode of Thought. However, I am aware of no good argument, by Descartes or anyone else, in support of his doctrine of unique and exclusive attributes. Accordingly, I am perfectly ready to allow that psychological substances should possess material characteristics (that is, include physical states amongst their modes). It may be that there is no material characteristic which an individual psychological substance possesses *essentially* (in the sense that its persistence conditions preclude its surviving the loss of this characteristic). But this does not of course imply that an individual psychological substance essentially possesses *no* material characteristics (to suppose that it did imply this would be to commit a "quantifier shift fallacy" of such a blatant kind that I am loth to accuse Descartes himself of it).

How, though, does this repudiation of the Cartesian conception of psychological substance help against the skeptical arguments discussed a moment ago? Well, the main reason why those arguments seem to get any purchase is, I think, that in presupposing that psychological substances would have to be wholly non-physical, they are able to take it for granted that such substances are not possible objects of ordinary sense perception. They are represented as being invisible and intangible, and as such at best only perceptible by some mysterious faculty of introspection, and hence only by each such substance in respect of itself. But once it is allowed that psychological substances have physical characteristics and can thus be seen and touched at least as "directly" as any ordinary physical thing, the suggestion that we might be unable to detect a rapid turnover of these substances becomes as fanciful as the sceptical suggestion that the table on which I am writing might "in reality" be a succession of different but short-lived tables replacing one another undetectably. Whether one can conclusively refute such skepticism may be an open question; but I see no reason to take it seriously or to allow it to influence our choice of ontological categories.

I believe, then, that a perfectly tenable conception of psychological substance may be developed which permits us to regard such substances as the subjects of mental states: which is just to say that nothing stands in the way of our regarding *persons* precisely as being psychological substances. The detailed development of such a conception is a topic for another paper, and for now it must suffice to say that I conceive of psychological substances as the proper subject-matter of the science of psychology, which in turn I conceive to be an autonomous science whose laws are not reducible to those of biology or chemistry or physics. However, it will be appropriate to close the present paper with a few remarks on the relationship between psychological and biological substances, that is, between persons and their bodies. (I restrict myself here to the case of persons who—like human persons—have animal bodies.)

With regard to this issue I am, as I indicated at the outset, a *substantial dualist*. Persons are substances, as are their bodies. But they are not identical substances: for they have different persistence conditions, just as do their bodies and the masses of matter constituting those bodies at different times. (I should perhaps emphasize here that where a person's body is a biological substance, as in the case of human persons, the body is to be conceived of as a *living organism*, not as a mere mass of matter or assemblage of physical particles.) Clearly, though, my version of substantial dualism is quite different from Descartes's. Descartes, it seems, conceived a human person to be the product of a "substantial union" of two distinct substances: a mental but immaterial substance and a material but non-mental substance. How such a union was possible perplexed him and every subsequent philosopher who endeavoured to understand it. The chief stumbling block was, once again, Descartes's doctrine of unique and exclusive attributes. How could something essentially immaterial get to grips, causally, with something essentially material, and *vice versa*? But psychological substances as I conceive of them are *not* essentially immaterial, and thus I see no difficulty in principle about their entering into causal transactions with their physical environment. And on my view, human persons are themselves just such psychological substances, not a queer hybrid of two radically alien substances.

So, as for the relationship between a person and his or her body, I do not see that this need be more mysterious in principle than any of the other intersubstantial relationships with which the natural sciences are faced: for instance, the relationship between a biological entity such as a tree and the assemblage of physical particles that constitutes it at any given time. Most decidedly, I do not wish to minimize the scientific and metaphysical difficulties involved here. (I do not, for example, think that it would be correct to say that a person is "constituted" by his or her body in anything like the sense in which a tree is "constituted" by an assemblage of physical particles.)[33] None the less, it is my hope that by adopting a broadly Aristotelian conception of substance and by emphasizing not only the autonomy but also the continuity of the special sciences, including psychology and biology, we may see a coherent picture begin to emerge of persons as a wholly distinctive kind of being fully integrated into the natural world: a picture which simultaneously preserves the "Lockean" insight that the concept of a person is fundamentally a psychological (as opposed to a biological) one, the "Cartesian" insight that persons are a distinctive kind of substantial particulars in their own right, and the "Aristotelian" insight that persons are not essentially immaterial beings.[34]

NOTES

1. Such a view has close affinities with that advanced by P. F. Strawson, in his *Individuals: An Essay in Descriptive Metaphysics* (London: Methuen, 1959), Ch. 3.

2. See further my chapter on "Substance," in G. H. R. Parkinson (ed.), *An Encyclopaedia of Philosophy* (London: Routledge, 1988), 255–78. "Particular" is Strawson's term. The term "continuant" was coined by W. E. Johnson: see his *Logic, Part III* (Cambridge: Cambridge University Press, 1924), Ch. VII.

3. See, e.g. Alan Code, "Aristotle: Essence and Accident," in R. E. Grandy and R. Warner (eds.), *Philosophical Grounds of Rationality* (Oxford: Clarendon Press, 1986), and Michael Frede, "Substance in Aristotle's *Metaphysics*," in his *Essays in Ancient Philosophy* (Oxford: Clarendon Press, 1987).

4. See T. E. Wilkerson, "Natural Kinds," *Philosophy* 63, No. 243 (January 1988), 29–42.

5. See David Wiggins, *Sameness and Substance* (Oxford: Basil Blackwell, 1980), 187.

6. Wiggins himself (ibid. 174f.) gravitates towards the first horn of this apparent dilemma. Another recent author who gravitates towards the anthropocentric position is Kathleen Wilkes: see her *Real People: Personal Identity without Thought Experiments* (Oxford: Clarendon Press, 1988), 97ff., 230ff.

7. Cf. Wiggins, *Sameness and Substance*, 202.

8. Cf. Wiggins, ibid. 203.

9. Cf. Wiggins, ibid.

10. For a view of personhood along these lines, see Daniel C. Dennett, "Conditions of Personhood," in his *Brainstorms* (Hassocks: Harvester Press, 1979). I criticize this sort of approach in my *Kinds of Being: A Study of Individuation, Identity and the Logic of Sortal Terms* (Oxford: Basil Blackwell, 1989), 112–18. Thus I agree with Wiggins that persons constitute a real rather than a merely nominal kind, but differ from him in denying that the kind in question is a *biological* one.

11. David Wiggins challenges this view in his *Sameness and Substance*, 174–5. It has of course also been challenged, if more obliquely, by John Searle, most recently in his "Is the

Brain's Mind a Computer Program?", *Scientific American 262* (January 1990), 20–5. But I find neither challenge convincing: see my *Kinds of Being*, 111.

12. Wiggins would deny this, on the grounds that both schemes are supposedly dominated by the genus *animal*. Thus he writes. "Cross-classifications that are resolved under a higher sort do not ultimately disturb a system of natural kinds. It is always (say) animals that are under study; and different classifications will not import different identity or persistence conditions for particular animals" (*Sameness and Substance*, 204). This seems to presume that all animals, of whatever kind, are governed by the same persistence conditions. But that is patently false, at least if one means by the "persistence conditions" for a given kind of animals the range of changes which, as a matter of natural law, members of that kind can undergo. Of course, it may be *conceptually* possible for an individual member of one animal kind to survive a transmutation which renders it a member of another kind governed by persistence conditions different from those of the first. But the bare logical possibility of such fairy-tale transmogrifications obviously does nothing to lessen the tension between our two supposed taxonomic schemes, conceived as contributions to empirical biological science.

13. I raise other objections against it in my *Kinds of Being*, 108–21.

14. See David Hume, *A Treatise of Human Nature*, ed. P. H. Nidditch (Oxford: Clarendon Press, 1978), Book I, Part IV, Sect. VI, 252.

15. See John Locke, An *Essay Concerning Human Understanding*, ed. P. H. Nidditch (Oxford: Clarendon Press, 1975), Book II, Ch. XXVII, Sect. 9. Of course, Locke thought that *all* sortal terms denote merely nominal kinds, so that his classification of "person" as a nominal kind term reflects no special treatment of it.

16. See further my review of Harold W. Noonan's *Personal Identity* in *Mind 99* (1990), 477–9.

17. Locke, *Essay*, Book II, Ch. XXVII, Sect. 2.

18. See Derek Parfit, *Reasons and Persons* (Oxford: Clarendon Press, 1984), Part III.

19. Cf. Hume, *Treatise*, 261: "the true idea of the human mind, is to consider it a system of different perceptions . . . which are link'd together by the relation of cause and effect."

20. See Strawson, *Individuals*, Ch. 3.

21. See further my *Kinds of Being*, 113–14, 132–33.

22. See Christopher Peacocke, *Sense and Content: Experience, Thought and their Relations* (Oxford: Clarendon Press, 1983), 176ff.

23. Ibid. 177.

24. Ibid.

25. Ibid.

26. See Donald Davidson, "The Individuation of Events," in his *Essays on Actions and Events* (Oxford: Clarendon Press, 1980). For an exposure of the defect, see my "Impredicative Identity Criteria and Davidson's Criterion of Event Identity," *Analysis 49* (1989), 178–81.

27. Cf. Hume, *Treatise*, 233, 634.

28. This has been disputed recently by Andrew Brennan, in his "Fragmented Selves and the Problem of Ownership," *Proceedings of the Aristotelian Society XC* (1989/90), 143–58. He cites in his support clinical cases of patients suffering from Korsakov's syndrome, which involves severe amnesia. However, my thesis is not an empirical one, vulnerable to the alleged findings of such psychiatric case studies, but rather a logico-

metaphysical one which imposes an *a priori* constraint on what could *count* as an experience or as evidence for the occurrence of one.

29. See Davidson, *Essays on Actions and Events*, 217.

30. This elaborates and strengthens an argument to be found in my *Kinds of Being*, 131–33.

31. Cf. Wilkes, *Real People*, Ch. 5.

32. See Réné Descartes, *Principles of Philosophy*, Part I, Sect. 53.

33. For criticism of this suggestion, see my *Kinds of Being*, 119–20.

34. I am grateful to audiences at the Universities of Durham, Oxford, Sheffield, and York for helpful comments on earlier versions of this paper.

PERSONS AS CONSTITUTED BY BODIES

CHAPTER ELEVEN

The Ontological Status of Persons

Lynne Rudder Baker

Throughout his illustrious career, Roderick Chisholm was concerned with the nature of persons. On his view, persons are what he called *"entia per se."* They exist per se, in their own right. I too have developed an account of persons—I call it the "Constitution View"—an account that is different in important ways from Chisholm's. Here, however, I want to focus on a thesis that Chisholm and I agree on: that persons have ontological significance in virtue of being persons. Although I'll make the notion of ontological significance more precise later, the rough idea is that Fs (persons, or whatever) have ontological significance just in case a new F is a new thing and not just a change in some already-existing thing.

The Constitution View offers a way to place a traditional preoccupation of the great philosophers in the context of the "neo-Darwinian synthesis" in biology.[1] The traditional preoccupation concerns our inwardness—our abilities not just to think, but to think about our thoughts; to see ourselves and each other as subjects; to have rich inner lives. The modern synthesis in biology has made it clear that we are biological beings, continuous with the rest of the animal kingdom. The Constitution View of human persons recognizes our uniqueness even as it tries to show how we are part of the world of organisms.

On the Constitution View, something is a *person* in virtue of having a first-person perspective (or a narrowly defined capacity for one),[2] and something is a *human* person in virtue of being a person constituted by a human animal (or body).[3] Human persons are material beings, part of the natural order. As I develop the idea of constitution, this view of human persons has the consequence that although I am both a person and an animal, I am most fundamentally a person. Hence, my persistence conditions are the persistence conditions of a person (sameness of first-person perspective), not the persistence conditions of an animal (sameness of biological organism).[4] I could continue to exist without being an animal, but I could not continue to exist without being a person. If parts of my human body were replaced by synthetic parts until the body that constitutes me was no longer a human animal, then, as long as my first-person perspective remained intact, I would continue to exist and I would continue to be a person. But if nothing had my first-person perspective, then there would be no me. To put this controversial thesis in a slogan: Persons are essentially persons.[5]

I'll structure my elucidation and defense of the thesis that persons have ontological significance as follows: First, I'll explain my idea of constitution and its distinctive features. Second, I'll work out an account of ontological significance, on which both Chisholm's view and the Constitution View accord persons ontological significance. Then, I'll turn to Animalism, according to which persons are essentially animals, and show that Animalism in its several forms does not accord persons ontological significance. Finally, I'll urge—against Animalism—that what is distinctive about persons is enough to give them ontological significance.

The Idea of Constitution

The relation of constitution is exemplified all around us: Not only do human bodies constitute persons, but also DNA molecules constitute genes; pieces of plastic constitute drivers' licenses; aggregates of water molecules constitute rivers. So, constitution is a very general relation.

Several features of the idea of constitution will be important here. First, the relation of constitution, which I have discussed in elaborate detail elsewhere,[6] is in some ways like identity. However, constitution is not identity. If you wonder how a relation could be *like* identity, but not *be* identity, think of what philosophers have called "contingent identity." By "identity," I mean strict identity: $x=y \rightarrow \Box(x=y)$. The idea of constitution plays the role in my view that the idea of "contingent identity" plays in others' views. (Indeed, one advantage of my views is that I can achieve what other philosophers want when they invoke ersatz "identity," without cheapening the idea of identity.) Identity is necessary; constitution is contingent. Hence, constitution is not identity.

Behind the idea of constitution is an Aristotelian assumption. For any x, we can ask: What most fundamentally is x? The answer will be what I call x's "primary kind." Everything that exists is of exactly one primary kind—e.g., a horse or a passport or a cabbage. A thing's primary kind determines its persistence conditions. And since its primary-kind property determines what a thing most fundamentally is, a thing has its primary-kind property essentially.[7] It could not exist without having its primary-kind property.[8]

Although the idea of primary kinds is inspired by Aristotle, I differ from Aristotle in several ways: First, according to the Constitution View, there are primary kinds of artifacts, as well as of natural objects. Second, according to the Constitution View, a primary kind may be just a kind of thing; it does not have to be a kind of a broader kind (like a kind of furniture). In particular, although on my view, *person* is a primary kind, I need not say that a person is a kind *of* some further kind (such as a kind of animal).[9] Third, as we shall see in the discussion of borrowing properties, something may have a primary-kind property without having that property *as* its primary-kind property. Something may have a primary-kind property contingently when suitably related to something that has it essentially.[10]

Constitution is a relation that things have in virtue of their primary kinds. The basic idea is that when things of certain primary kinds are in certain circumstances, things of new primary kinds, with new kinds of causal powers, come into existence. For example, when a piece of marble is carved by a member of an artworld, a sculptor, to have a certain shape, a new thing of a new kind—a statue—comes into existence. If a piece of marble constitutes a statue, then the primary kind of the marble statue is *statue*. The piece of marble still exists, but the statue now has pre-eminence. What makes the difference between a sculpture and a mere piece of marble is that the existence of the sculpture requires an artworld or an artist's intention or whatever is required by the correct theory of sculptural art.

What makes the difference between a human person and a human animal is that the existence of the person requires a first-person perspective. Your persistence conditions are determined by your having a first-person perspective; your body's persistence conditions are determined by its being a human animal. The organism that constitutes you, the person, retains its persistence conditions even though you-as-constituted-by-that-organism have the persistence conditions of a person.[11]

If constitution is not identity, we need an explanation of the fact that, if x constitutes y at t, then x and y share so many properties at t. Not only are x and y at the same places at the same times (as long as one constitutes the other), but x and y have many properties in common: weighing 200 lbs., having a tooth-ache, running a 4-minute mile—properties that do not entail the existence of anything at any other time or in any other world.

There is an explanation: Even though constitution is not identity, it is a rela-tion of genuine unity. And because constitution is a relation of genuine unity, if x constitutes y at t, x may borrow properties at t from y and y may borrow properties at t from x. (Chisholm introduced me to the idea of borrowing prop-erties, but I have modified his idea quite a bit for my own purposes. On my view, if x constitutes y at t, then both x and y borrow properties at t from each other.) The intuitive idea of borrowing a property or of having a property derivatively is simple. If x constitutes y at t, then some of x's properties at t have their source (so to speak) in y, and some of y's properties at t have their source in x. I have put this less metaphorically elsewhere by defining "x has property H at t deriva-tively," but here I'll just illustrate the idea. Consider some properties of my driv-ers' license, which is constituted by a piece of plastic: My drivers' license has the property of being rectangular only because it is constituted by something that could have been rectangular even if it had constituted nothing. And the piece of plastic has the property of impressing the policeman only because it consti-tutes something that would have impressed the policeman (a valid drivers' li-cense) no matter what constituted it. The drivers' license has the property of being rectangular derivatively, and of impressing the policeman nonderivatively; the piece of plastic that constitutes my drivers' license has the property of being rectangular nonderivatively, and of impressing the policeman derivatively.

The second illustration of having a property derivatively is perhaps more controversial. Person is your primary kind. Human animal is your body's pri-mary kind. You are a person nonderivatively and a human animal derivatively; and your body is a human animal nonderivatively and a person derivatively. Although you are a person and your body is a person, there are not two per-sons where you are. This is so because constitution is a unity relation. If x con-stitutes y at t, and x is an F at t derivatively and y is an F at t nonderivatively—or vice versa—then there are not thereby two Fs.[12] Even though being a person is a primary-kind property that you have nonderivatively, your body has that property derivatively; but it (the property of being a person) is not your body's primary-kind property. Everything has its own primary-kind property essentially; but it can have a second primary-kind property contingently. For example, your body's primary-kind property is the property of being a human animal. Your body has that property essentially; although your body also has the property of being a person contingently, the property of being a person is not your body's primary-kind property. Your body is a person derivatively—solely in virtue of constituting you (who are a person nonderivatively). Your body is not a separate person from you; the fact that your body is a person is just the fact that you are a person (nonderivatively) and your body constitutes you.[13]

Not all properties may be borrowed, or had derivatively.[14] For example, although primary-kind properties—like being a person, or being a human animal—may be had derivatively, other properties—like being a person essentially, or having human animal as one's primary kind—cannot be had derivatively. So, my body has the property of being a person (derivatively), but my body does not have the property of *having being a person as its primary-kind property* at all (not derivatively, not nonderivatively). Rather, my body has the property of being a human organism as its primary-kind property. If being an F and being a G are two primary-kind properties, x may have both—one as its primary-kind property and the other derivatively—but x is not of two primary kinds.[15]

The fact that constitution is a relation of real unity has two implications for the idea of having properties derivatively: On the one hand, if x has a property derivatively, then there are not two separate exemplifications of the property: x has the property solely in virtue of its constitution-relations to something that has the property independently. On the other hand, if x has a property derivatively, x still really has it. I really am a body (derivatively); if my foot itches, then I itch. And my body is really a person (now); when I have a right to be in a certain seat, my body has a right to be in that seat. Constitution is so intimate a relation, so close to identity, that if x constitutes y at t, then—solely in virtue of the fact that x constitutes y—x has properties derivatively at t that x would not have had if x had not constituted y. (And vice versa.) The idea of having properties derivatively accounts for the otherwise strange fact that if x constitutes y at t, x and y share so many properties even though x≠y.

Before leaving the topic of constitution, I need to discuss a common criticism of the Constitution View. The criticism is that the Constitution View makes it too easy for new things to come into existence. We certainly do not want to say, for example, that at the founding of the United States a new entity, the President, came into being. But there seems to be nothing in the Constitution View to prevent taking the President to be a new entity, constituted by different people (starting with George Washington) at different times.[16]

The critic has a point. What I need is a theory of primary kinds to distinguish cases of property-acquisition (George Washington merely acquired the property of being President) from cases of constitution (a piece of clay came to constitute a statue). I do have a theory of sorts; at least it is a condition on primary kinds: A kind K is a primary kind just in case (nonderivative) members of K have their persistence conditions in virtue of being members of kind K. Although this seems fine as far as it goes, it may not fully satisfy the critic. For it provides no way to adjudicate disagreements about which properties do determine persistence conditions. For example, I include among primary kinds organisms (e.g., maggots, redwoods, dogs), artifacts (e.g., telephones, submarines, stamps), and artworks (e.g., sculptures, paintings), but not social roles (e.g., *President*). Others may disagree.

In addition to the condition on primary kinds—that primary-kind properties determine persistence conditions of their nonderivative bearers—I can offer two characteristics that distinguish constitution from property-acquisition. If x constitutes a G, as opposed to just acquiring the property of being a G, then the G has whole classes of causal properties that x would not have had if x had not constituted something. Pieces of paper constitute dollar bills, and dollar bills have a whole range of vastly different kinds of causal properties—e.g., they pay off your debts, bribe the mayor, give you peace of mind, allow you to quench your thirst by inserting them into machines—a whole range of causal properties that the constituting pieces of paper would not have had if they had not constituted anything. A second characteristic of constitution is its relative stability. For example, pieces of metal constitute keys, but if I have a metal dogtag and use it to jimmy a lock, my dogtag does not thereby constitute a key. Rather, it merely acquires the property of being used to jimmy a lock. But both of these characteristics—new causal properties and relative stability—are admittedly vague.

I am satisfied to think of the idea of constitution as offering a form of a theory that needs to be filled out by a theory of primary kinds. For purposes here, however, I only need the claim that *person* is a primary kind, and later, I'll give reasons to consider the person case to be a matter of constitution, and not mere property acquisition.

To conclude the discussion of constitution: The aim of my conception of constitution is to make sense of a relation more intimate than separate existence, but still not identity. I take identity to be necessary or strict identity: If (x=y), then □ (x=y). Many philosophers think that if x and y are not identical, then they are just two different things, like the sun and the moon. The notion of constitution offers a third position, a position intermediate between identity and separate existence. (Say that x and y have separate existence at t if and only if there is no property F such that x and y are the same F at t.) For any x and y, there are three (not two) possibilities: strict identity, constitution, and separate existence. In *Persons and Bodies*, I give a general definition of "constitution" that shows that there is "logical space" for such an intermediate position.[17] Thus, any criticism of my view that presupposes that nonidentity entails separate existence begs the question against my view.

Chisholm also uses the term "constitution," but for a relation somewhat different from the one I am trying to elucidate. On Chisholm's view, being constituted is a mark of ontological inferiority. On his view, if a table, say, is made up of boards AB on Monday and BC on Tuesday, then the table (which existed on both Monday and Tuesday) is an ontological parasite—a mere ens successivum—that does not exist in its own right.[18] Clearly, I am not using "constitution" in Chisholm's way.[19] On my view, if x constitutes y at t, then x is not just a stand-in at t for y: y exists in its own right. And not only does y borrow properties from x at t, but also x borrows properties from y at t.[20]

Here, then, is a significant contrast between Chisholm's and my conceptions of constitution. Rather than being a relation between a really existing thing and an ontological parasite, constitution on my view is a relation between really existing individuals. A world with assault weapons, fiber-optic cables, and space stations is ontologically richer than a world that contains only the particles produced by the Big Bang. A world with organisms in it is ontologically richer than a world that contains no organisms but contains all the chemicals that make up amino acids and proteins. On Chisholm's view, constitution produces ontological parasites; on my view, constitution provides a vehicle of ontological novelty.

Ontological Significance

Despite these differences between Chisholm's view and mine, Chisholm and I are allies in rejecting views that deny that persons have ontological status.[21] While disagreeing with Chisholm that a person is an *ens per se*—which cannot gain or lose parts nor come into being or pass away gradually—I heartily endorse his larger point that a person is not an ontological parasite. Moreover, Chisholm is right to hold that "person" is not a phase-sortal like "child," nor does it designate a property or an abstract entity, nor does it refer to a logical construction of nonpersonal elements, nor is it just an honorific for human animals. Persons, Chisholm and I agree, are real individuals whose appearance in the world makes an ontological difference. They have ontological significance. Now I want to try to spell out what I mean by saying that persons are ontologically significant.

Intuitively, to say that Fs (tigers, chairs, anything) have ontological significance is to say that the addition of a (nonderivative)[22] F is not just a change in something that already exists, but the coming-into-being of a new thing. The primary bearers of ontological significance are properties; things have ontological significance in virtue of having ontologically significant properties. Every individual thing that exists has ontological significance in virtue of some property or other. Ontologically significant properties must be essential to their (nonderivative) bearers. For example, being a student is not an ontologically significant property; being a water molecule is: The difference, I think, lies in the idea of persistence conditions.[23] A water molecule has its persistence conditions in virtue of being a water molecule; a student does not have her persistence conditions in virtue of being a student. To generalize:

(OS1) The property of being an F has ontological significance if and only if, necessarily, if x is an F (nonderivatively), then being an F determines x's persistence conditions.

Here is the rationale for (OS1). Suppose that the property of being an F has ontological significance. Then, the instantiation of that property brings into existence a new thing, an F. Every existing thing has persistence conditions, and has its persistence conditions essentially. Since the F has its persistence conditions essentially, instantiation of the property sufficient for bringing the F into existence must be sufficient for the F's having the persistence conditions that it has. Therefore, if the property of being an F is ontologically significant, then the property of being an F determines the (nonderivative) F's persistence conditions.

On the other hand, if the property of being an F determines the (nonderivative) F's persistence conditions, then the instantiation of the property of being an F entails that there is an F with those persistence conditions. Since things have their persistence conditions essentially, the F could not have existed before the instantiation of the property of being an F (which determines the F's persistence conditions). So, the instantiation of the property of being an F brings into existence a new entity, and the property of being an F has ontological significance. Therefore, if the property of being an F determines the (nonderivative) F's persistence conditions, the property of being an F has ontological significance. Hence, (OS1).

Ontological significance is not only a feature of properties, but also a feature of things that have those properties:

> (OS2) (Nonderivative) Fs have ontological significance in virtue of being Fs
>   if and only if the property of being an F has ontological significance.

I'll use "Fs have ontological significance" to abbreviate "(nonderivative) Fs have ontological significance in virtue of being an Fs."[24] (OS1) and (OS2) aim to explicate the basic idea of ontological significance: Being an F is an ontologically significant property if and only if the addition of a (nonderivative) F adds to the stock of what there is.[25]

Since "is a nonderivative F" in the vocabulary of the Constitution View is equivalent to "is an F" in other vocabularies, the qualification "nonderivative" in (OS1) and (OS2) is no restriction on the generality of these necessary and sufficient conditions for ontological significance. Outside the context of the Constitution View, the qualification "nonderivative" may be dropped without loss.

Now it is easy to see that on the Constitution View, persons[26] have ontological significance, given (OS1) and (OS2). Indeed, since every primary-kind property determines the persistence conditions of its (nonderivative) bearers, every primary-kind property has ontological significance—being a person, being a human animal, being a statue, being a piece of marble. So, on the Constitution View, persons and human animals both have ontological significance. Persons have ontological significance in virtue of being persons, even when they are constituted by human animals; human animals have ontological significance in virtue of being human animals, even when they constitute persons.

Likewise, on Chisholm's view, persons are ontologically significant. Indeed, Chisholm begins with the assumption that persons are *entia per se*, and the idea of an *ens per se* is formulated in terms of persistence conditions: *entia per se* cannot gain or lose parts without ceasing to exist, nor can they come into existence or pass away gradually. On one of Chisholm's definitions, a person is "that which is necessarily such that it is physically possible that there is a time at which that thing consciously thinks."[27] And he takes it that anything that instantiates this property is an *ens per se*—a being that has the persistence conditions of persons. So, according to (OS1) and (OS2), persons are ontologically significant both on my view and on Chisholm's.

Animalist Accounts of Persons

Chisholm and I not only agree that persons have ontological significance; we also agree in what we deny. Neither Chisholm nor I thinks that we persons are identical to animals or are essentially animals. With the ascendancy of biology, however, Chisholm and I may be in the minority. Many philosophers today hold that persons are most fundamentally animals. These philosophers—call them "Animalists"[28]—hold that we persons have the persistence conditions of human organisms.[29]

Suppose that Animalism is correct, and that we have the persistence conditions of human animals, and hence are essentially animals. We are also persons. How may an Animalist understand persons if persons have the persistence conditions of organisms? I'll consider two kinds of possibilities: Being a person, on an Animalist view, either concerns having psychological properties (actually or potentially) or it does not. The only way that I can think of for an Animalist to hold that being a person has nothing to do with having psychological properties, actually or potentially, is to identify the property of being a human person with the property of being a human animal.[30] (To identify the property of being a person with the property of being a human animal would be a nonstarter since it would preclude even the logical possibility of there being nonhuman persons.) Such a "property-identity" Animalist may claim that persons have ontological significance by means of the following inference:

(1) Human organisms have ontological significance;
(2) The property of being a human person = the property of being a human organism;

So, (3) Human persons have ontological significance.

The inference is valid, but the second premise is untenable for two reasons: First, there are no grounds for holding it; second, it is tantamount to eliminativism about persons.

To see that there are no grounds for the claim of identity between being a human person and being a human organism, consider: Does the assertion have any a priori or a posteriori justification? It has no a posteriori justification. Unlike the assertion of the identity of water and H_2O molecules between 0 and 100 degrees centigrade, there was no empirical discovery that would underwrite an identity of being a human person and being a human animal. Indeed, without some way to characterize the property of being a human person other than in terms of its alleged identity to the property of being a human organism it is logically impossible that there be any *discovery* that underwrites the property-identity claim.

So the justification for the property-identity claim must be a priori, based on the meanings of words. But the meanings of the words give no warrant for asserting identity. The term "person" was introduced in something like its current meaning to apply to parts of the Christian Trinity—hardly human organisms. It was given wide application by Locke, who explicitly distinguished being a person from being a "man," as he called it. Since historically, "being a human person" and "being a human organism" were not taken as denoting the same property, considerations of use or meaning do not give a priori justification for the claim of property identity. So, we are left with no justification for the claim of Animalist property-identity.

To see that the thesis of identity between the property of being a human person and the property of being a human organism is tantamount to eliminativism about persons, consider: If being a human organism is identical to being a human person, then by parity of reasoning, being an oyster is identical to being an oyster person. (At any rate, I do not believe that a property-identity Animalist has resources to make a principled objection to the thesis that being an oyster is identical to being an oyster person.) But there is no such property as being an oyster person. If there is no such property as being an oyster person, then by parity of reasoning in the other direction, there is no such property as being a human person. In that case, property-identity Animalism collapses into eliminativism about persons. Eliminativism about persons is hardly compatible with taking persons to have ontological significance. So, premise (2) is false and the argument is unsound.

So, an Animalist who takes having psychological properties to be irrelevant to being a human person does not assign ontological significance to persons. However, there are several theses available to an Animalist that construe being a person in terms of psychological properties. Consider:

(1) Necessarily, if x is a human person at t, then x has psychological properties at t.

On Animalism+(1), persons have their persistence conditions not in virtue of being persons but in virtue of being animals; nor would the property of being a person be essential to persons. *Person* would not be a substance-sortal (as it is on the Constitution View), but would be a phase-sortal like *infant* or *puppy*. In this case, being a person would be a contingent property of persons, and persons would have no ontological significance.[31] Now consider:

(2) Necessarily, if x is a human person at any time, then x has psychological properties at some time or other.

Animalism+(2) has the consequence that whether or not an embryo is a person
depends on its subsequent development. If it is miscarried or aborted before it
has psychological states, then it is not a person. If it is carried to term and is born
normally, then it was a person all along. So, on Animalism+(2), being a person
is a contingent property of persons, and persons have no ontological significance. Finally, consider the most plausible notion of personhood available to an
Animalist:

(3) Necessarily, if x is a human person at t, then x has the capacity at t to
have psychological properties.

"Capacity" is a notoriously elastic term. For purposes here, I take it that to have
a capacity at t to have F is to have an internal structure at t such that it is consistent with the laws of nature that things with that internal structure have F.
Now consider a person, Smith, who has suffered irreversible damage to the cerebral cortex, so that it is physically impossible for the brain ever to support
psychological properties again. Suppose also that Smith's lower brain that regulates animal life continues to function.[32] Does Smith still exist?

I'll consider two versions of Animalism+(3). On one, suggested by writers on
medical ethics, Smith does not still exist. On this construal, when the cerebral
cortex is destroyed, so is the human animal. So, although Smith is [identical to]
a human animal, destruction of the cerebral cortex is destruction of that human
animal and hence destruction of Smith. However, after destruction of the cerebral cortex, an animal still persists, but it is not a human animal (and thus it is
not Smith).

I do not believe that this construal is a viable option for Animalists. Here's
why. Call the animal with functioning cerebral cortex, H. Call the animal after
the cerebral cortex was destroyed, H'. Are H and H' the same animal? If so, then
being human is just a contingent property of animals. In that case, being a human animal could not furnish the persistence conditions of human animals—
since, assuming that H is the same animal as H', a human animal can lose the
property of being human without going out of existence. But if the property of
being a human animal does not provide the persistence conditions of human
animals, then Animalism is false. So, on the view that holds that a human animal cannot persist after destruction of the cerebral cortex, H and H' must not
be the same animal. But if H is not the same animal as H' and both H and H' are

animals, then H' must have replaced H.[33] What happened to H? There is no plausible answer. Without anyone's being able to detect that anything was amiss, H just disappeared. I do not believe that the persistence conditions of animals that are countenanced by biologists allow for the undetectable disappearance of one animal and its undetectable replacement by another animal. So, that version of Animalism—that takes destruction of the cerebral cortex to be destruction of the human animal—entails untenable persistence conditions for animals, and I'll not consider it further.

On the other version of Animalism+(3), the persistence conditions of human animals are determined by lower-brain functions like metabolism, digestion, respiration, and circulation.[34] On this version of Animalism, Smith still exists after destruction of his cerebral cortex. If Smith has the persistence conditions of a human animal, then Smith still exists since the lower-brain functions that regulate animal life continue to function. But since there is no longer a capacity for having psychological properties, Smith is no longer a person (according to Animalism+(3)). If Smith can exist without being a person, then being a person is irrelevant to Smith's persistence conditions. In that case, being a person is not an ontologically significant property.

We have considered two versions of Animalism coupled with (3), where (3) is the view of persons that takes personhood to be the capacity to have psychological properties. The two versions of Animalism were, first, the view that takes the destruction of the cerebral cortex to be destruction of the human animal, and, second, the view that takes the persistence conditions of the human animal to be determined by lower-brain functions. On neither of these versions of Animalism+(3) are persons ontologically significant by (OS1) and (OS2).

Notice that Animalism cannot be combined with a Chisholmian construal of a person—as being "that which is necessarily such that it is physically possible that there is a time at which that thing consciously thinks." As Chisholm would agree, human animals do not have this property. First of all, human animals come into and go out of existence gradually, but, as Chisholm argues, no person—no *ens per se*—comes into or goes out of existence gradually.[35] Putting aside that difficulty, however, there is another difficulty with attempting to combine Animalism with Chisholm's definition of a person.

Suppose that H is a human animal that comes into being in the normal way: a fertilized egg undergoes cell division, is implanted in the uterus, and approximately nine months later, a normal baby is born. Now suppose that there is another possible world in which the same egg is fertilized by the same sperm that produced H; but in this other world, the mother-to-be drinks some toxic water which results in impairment, but not destruction, of the fertilized egg just as the new animal comes into existence.[36] Given Animalism, H still comes into being in this other possible world—same egg, same sperm, same time, same uterus—but the impairment is such that there is no physical possibility that H ever consciously think. (The impairment prevents the organism from ever developing a cerebral cortex.) Nevertheless, H, the human animal, still exists in the other possible world. But since it is physically impossible for H in that other world to think, H is not a person in that other world. And, on Chisholm's definition, if H is not a person in every possible world in which H exists, then H is not a person in any possible world in which H exists. So, on Chisholm's view, H— the normal baby born in the actual world—is not and never will be a person in the actual world.

I conclude that nothing with the persistence conditions of an animal can be a person, on Chisholm's view (as Chisholm would be the first to agree). My point is to show that a hybrid position that is part-Animalist and part-Chisholmian is not available to anyone. Given Chisholm's view, it is impossible that H, the normal baby born in the actual world, is or ever will be a person—since there is a possible world in which it is physically impossible that H ever consciously think. Given an Animalist view, it is possible that H, the normal baby born in the actual world, either is or will be a person—since H is just like any other normal baby born in the actual world. It is impossible that both positions be correct.

Therefore, on none of the construals of Animalism that I can think of does Animalism accord persons ontological status. Of course, an Animalist who denies that there is a property of being a person in the first place just concurs with my point that Animalism denies that persons have ontological significance.

To sum up: On Animalism, animals have ontological significance, but persons do not. On Chisholm's view, persons have ontological significance, but animals do not. On the Constitution View, both persons have ontological significance and animals have ontological significance; and we, being essentially persons, have our persistence conditions in virtue of being persons. So, on the Constitution View and on Chisholm's view, persons have ontological significance. On the Animalist view, persons have no ontological significance.

The Upshot

The fact that on the Constitution View persons have ontological significance (in the sense defined) and on the Animalist View they do not have ontological significance has not, I think, been properly appreciated. This fact, however, does not add up to a satisfactory argument for the Constitution View over Animalism, unless persons really do have ontological significance. So, I offer the following argument:

(1) If Animalism is true, then persons do not have ontological significance.

(2) Persons do have ontological significance.

∴ (3) Animalism is not true.

I just established the first premise. Although I cannot embark on a full-scale defense of the second premise in this paper, I shall offer two considerations in favor of it.

The first consideration is this: Persons are self-conscious, and self-consciousness is unique. No other part of the animal kingdom is self-conscious in the way that we are.[37] Self-consciousness is sufficiently different from everything else known to us in the natural world that it is reasonable to say that the difference that self-consciousness makes is an ontological difference. I can almost hear the question: Why not be more Aristotelian and take the "genus and species" approach? An Aristotelian may say that we are animals who differ from other animals in being self-conscious. Then I ask: In virtue of what do I have my persistence conditions? The answer cannot be that I have my persistence conditions in virtue *both* of being a human animal and of being self-conscious. Since the animal that is supposed to be me [nonderivatively, of course] existed before it was self-conscious, I cannot be both essentially an animal and essentially self-conscious. To say that persons are essentially animals, and not essentially self-conscious, is to make properties like *wondering how one should live* irrelevant to what we most fundamentally are, and properties like *having digestion* central to what we fundamentally are. I think that what we most fundamentally are is a matter of what is distinctive about us and not what we share with nonhuman animals.

The second consideration is this: Considered in terms of genetic or morphological properties or biological functioning, there is no discontinuity between chimpanzees and human animals. In fact, human animals are biologically more closely related to certain species of chimpanzees than the chimpanzees are related to gorillas and orangutans.[38] So, biologically speaking, there's no significant difference between us and higher nonhuman animals. But all things considered, there is a huge discontinuity between us and nonhuman animals. And this discontinuity arises from the fact that we, and no other part of the animal kingdom, are self-conscious. (If I thought that chimpanzees or computers really did have first-person perspectives, I would put them in the same category that we are in—namely, persons.)

So, in biological terms, there are no significant differences between us and other higher primates, but there are enormous differences between us and non-human animals all things considered. [Only we seek to understand our place in the universe.] Biologists and biologically-oriented philosophers speak with one voice in insisting that the animal kingdom is a seamless whole in which the human animals have no special significance. This suggests that biology does not fully reveal our nature. So, perhaps we should say that biology may well reveal our animal nature, but that our animal nature does not exhaust our nature all things considered. Rather, self-consciousness distinguishes us ontologically from the rest of the animal kingdom. This is to say that self-consciousness—and thus personhood—is an ontologically significant property.

The point here concerns the status of self-consciousness. The issue is not whether or not self-consciousness is a product of evolution, or whether or not it has a neural basis. The Constitutionalist's claim is that when self-consciousness did evolve by natural selection (if it did), it was sufficiently different from every other property in the natural world that it ushered in a new kind of being.[39] Self-consciousness makes an ontological difference whether it is a product of natural selection or not. Since biologists do not recognize any ontological difference between human and nonhuman animals, we should conclude that ontology does not recapitulate biology.

In short, the uniqueness of self-conscious beings—of beings who can think of themselves as themselves, who have inner lives—makes it plausible to hold that to be a person is to be a special kind of thing—a thing that has ontological significance in virtue of being of that kind. Here again I share a Chisholmian intuition: The coming-to-be of a person is not just a change in some already existing—but theretofore nonpersonal—thing.[40] Rather, a new person is a new entity in the world.[41] If this is correct, then persons have ontological significance. And if persons have ontological significance, then Animalism is wrong.

Conclusion

What I have done here is to make precise what I mean by 'the ontological significance of persons,' and then to show that the Constitution View affirms the ontological significance of persons and that the Animalist View denies the ontological significance of persons. Finally, I offered some considerations to show that persons should be regarded as having ontological significance, and hence that the Constitution View is superior to Animalism.

The Constitution View is a materialist view that explains the sense in which we are animals—that is, biological beings, part of the seamless animal kingdom. At the same time, the Constitution View explains the sense in which we are different from other animals in a way that makes us ontologically unique. What makes us ontologically distinctive is the first-person perspective. The property of having an inner life—not just sentience—is so extraordinary, so utterly unlike any other property in the world, that beings with this property are a different kind of thing from beings without it. Only beings with first-person perspectives can write their memoirs or dread old age or discover evolution and intervene in its otherwise blind operations. And in my opinion, what something fundamentally is—its nature—is more a matter of what it can do than of what it is made of.

If the Constitution View is correct, then the property of being a person is not just a contingent property of a fundamentally nonpersonal thing like an organism. Persons have ontological significance. Although my elucidation and defense of this thesis is not very Chisholmian, I am confident that Chisholm would approve of the conclusion.[42]

NOTES

Note: This special symposium, containing this paper and two others, derives from a memorial conference in honor of Roderick M. Chisholm held at Brown University in the year 2000.

1. Variations on this term are widely used. For example, see Ernst Mayr, *Toward a New Philosophy of Biology: Observations of an Evolutionist* (Cambridge, MA: The Belknap Press of Harvard University Press, 1988); Philip Kitcher, *Abusing Science: The Case Against Creationism* (Cambridge, MA: The MIT Press, 1982); Daniel C. Dennett, *Darwin's Dangerous Idea: Evolution and the Meanings of Life* (New York: Simon and Schuster, 1995).

2. I explain what I mean by a first-person perspective in "The First-Person Perspective: A Test for Naturalism," *American Philosophical Quarterly* 35 (1998): 327–348, and in *Persons and Bodies: A Constitution View* (Cambridge, MA: Cambridge University Press, 2000): Ch. 3.

3. Unlike David Wiggins, who has a different sort of constitution view from mine, I do not distinguish between human animals and human bodies. I use the terms "human animal" and "human body" interchangeably.

4. I am aware of the controversies in biology about individuating species. But we do talk about human animals, and human animals do have persistence conditions that are different from the persistence conditions that I take persons to have. That's all I need.

5. A caveat: On my view, this slogan applies only to things that are persons nonderivatively in a sense that I shall explain.

6. See *Persons and Bodies*. For a preliminary discussion of the notion of constitution, see "Unity Without Identity: A New Look at Material Constitution," ed. Peter A. French and Howard K. Wettstein (Boston, MA: Blackwell Publishers, 1999): 144–165.

7. To borrow some paraphrases about essential properties from Chisholm, if x has the property of being a horse essentially, then "x is such that, if it were not a horse, it would not exist" or "God couldn't have created x without making it such that it is a horse": or "x is such that in every possible world in which it exists it is a horse." *Person and Object: A Metaphysical Study* (LaSalle, IL: Open Court Publishing Company, 1976), p. 25–26. Chisholm gives generalizations of these as paraphrases of the locution "x is necessarily such that it is F." But then he goes on to say, rather forlornly, that "if a person doesn't understand 'x is necessarily such that it is F', it is not likely that he will understand the expressions in terms of which we have attempted to clarify it."

8. Since a thing has the same persistence conditions in every possible world and time at which it exists, it has its persistence conditions essentially. Thus, no one who invokes persistence conditions is in a position to object to my view for invoking essential properties.

9. Gareth B. Matthews has made me realize how different my view is from Aristotle's.

10. Many properties (unrelated to this discussion) may be had essentially by some things and nonessentially by other things. A planet has the property of having a closed orbit essentially; a meteor that has a closed orbit has that property nonessentially. (This assumes that planets are planets essentially; otherwise it is only a de dicto necessity that planets have closed orbits.)

11. I have a general definition of "x constitutes y at t" that I'll not state here. The purpose of the definition is to provide assurance that the idea of constitution-without-identity is coherent; and that constitution-without-identity is not just "spatial co-location" of two otherwise separate things. See *Persons and Bodies*, Ch. 2.

12. Being a person essentially and being a person contingently are two ways of having a single property along one dimension; being a person nonderivatively and being a person derivatively are two ways of having a single property along another dimension. But if *being essentially a person* were a distinct property from *being contingently a person*, or if *being nonderivatively a person* were a distinct property from *being derivatively a person*, none of those "properties" could be borrowed. The definition of "having a property derivatively" would rule out having any of these properties derivatively. See *Persons and Bodies*, Ch. 2.

13. For further discussion of this point, see *Persons and Bodies*, Ch. 7, and "Materialism With a Human Face," in *Body, Soul, and Survival*, ed. Kevin Corcoran (Ithaca, NY: Cornell University Press, 2001): 159–180.

14. The following kinds of properties cannot be had derivatively: (1) any property expressed in English by "possibly," "necessarily," "essentially," or "primary-kind property," or variants of these terms—call these "alethic properties"; (2) any property expressed in English by "is identical to," "constitutes," "derivatively," "exists," or "is an object" or variants of these terms—call these "identity/constitution/existence properties"; (3) any property such that necessarily, x has it at t only if x exists at some time other than t—call these "properties rooted outside the times that they are had"; (4) any properties that are conjunctions of two or more properties that either entail or are entailed by two or more primary-kind properties (e.g., being a cloth flag, being a human person)—call these "hybrid properties." In *Persons and Bodies*, I amend the definition of "having a property derivatively" to accommodate having hybrid properties derivatively.

15. There may be conjunctive primary kinds. Assuming that *can-opener* is one primary kind and *corkscrew* is another, then the property of being a can-opener and a corkscrew is a primary-kind property. (I believe that Tom Nagel is responsible for a "can-opener/corkscrew" example.)

16. Dean Zimmerman, among others, has pressed this criticism on me.

17. Constitution offers the fruits of contingent identity, temporal identity, relative identity and so on without tampering with genuine identity.

18. If the boards, AB, constituted the table on Monday and the boards, BC, constituted the table on Tuesday, then what really existed on Chisholm's view were the boards, AB, which "stood in for" the table on Monday, and BC, which "stood in for" the table on Tuesday. To say that the table is an ontological parasite is to imply that all of the intrinsic, present-rooted properties of the table are borrowed (in Chisholm's sense) from the boards that constitute it.

19. I argue for my conception in "Persons in Metaphysical Perspective," in *The Philosophy of Roderick Chisholm* (Library of Living Philosophers, Vol. XXV), ed. Lewis Edwin Hahn (Chicago: Open Court Publishing Company, 1997): 433–453.

20. There are further differences between Chisholm and me here. Most important is that, on my view, constitution is a key to understanding human persons. On Chisholm's view, constitution has nothing to do with persons at all; persons exist in their own right; constituted things (on Chisholm's view) are ontological parasites.

21. On Chisholm's view, a person is either an *ens per se* or "just a *façon de parler*": "I am certain, then, that this much is true: if I'm a real thing and not just a *façon de parler*, then neither my coming into being nor my passing away is a gradual process." Roderick Chisholm, *On Metaphysics* (Minneapolis: University of Minnesota Press, 1989): 59. I think that the dichotomy—*ens per se* or "just a façon de parler"—is a false one. See my "Persons in Metaphysical Perspective."

22. A nonderivative F is a thing that is an F nonderivatively. The reason for the qualification "nonderivative" is that a derivative F may lose the property of being F without thereby going out of existence. E.g., my body is a person derivatively, but if I went out of existence while my body remained, my body would cease to be a person without ceasing to exist altogether. So, the ontological significance of a property is determined only by those things that have the property nonderivatively.

23. In "Why Constitution Is Not Identity," *Journal of Philosophy* 94 (1997): 599–621, I argued that everything that can go out of existence altogether has persistence conditions.

24. I.e., 'Fs have ontological significance' is short for: "For all x, if x is a nonderivative F, then x has ontological significance in virtue of being an F."

25. Although I avoid the "qua" locution, the way that I have elucidated "Fs have ontological significance" suggests that an alternative to that expression might be "Fs-qua-Fs have ontological significance."

26. I.e., nonderivative persons. In general, I'll drop the qualification when it seems clear that I am talking about nonderivative Fs.

27. *On Metaphysics*, 59–60. "Physically possible," Chisholm tells us, means not contrary to the laws of nature. In *Person and Object*, Chisholm says that a person is "an individual thing which is necessarily such that it is physically possible that there is something which it undertakes to bring about." Chisholm goes on to point out: "Our definition has the consequence that, if an individual thing x is a person, then in every possible world in which x exists, x is a person from the moment it comes into being until the moment it passes away." *Person and Object*, 137.

28. The term 'Animalist' comes from Paul Snowdon, who is an Animalist himself.

29. It may be reasonable to suppose that human organisms are essentially human organisms, but it is a view that Thomas Aquinas would oppose. According to Aquinas (following Aristotle), a zygote formed by a human egg and a human sperm first acquires a vegetative soul, then a sensitive soul. The organism does not become a human organism until it acquires a rational soul (at about 12 weeks). If we take it that there is a single developing organism from zygote on through birth and beyond, then on Aquinas's view, a human organism would not be essentially a human organism—since it exists before acquiring a rational soul and thus before becoming a human organism.

30. Fred Feldman takes the term "person" to be ambiguous. There are, he says, "four distinguishable concepts of personality": He claims that we have a concept of "biological personality," but he offers no warrant for using the term "personality" here; indeed, a biological person on his view is nothing other than a human organism from conception to disintegration. There is nothing particularly personal about it. However, on his view, the property of being a biological person (as opposed to the property of being a psychological person) furnishes our persistence conditions. As far as I can tell, Feldman would endorse this property identity for what he calls "biological persons." He seems to take the property of being a biological person to be the property of being a human animal. See his *Confrontations with the Reaper: A Philosophical Study of the Nature and Value of Death* (New York: Oxford University Press, 1992): 101.

31. What Feldman calls "a psychological person" conforms to Animalism+(1) (or perhaps +(2)). A psychological person on his view is just a "biological person" (a human organism) with psychological properties.

32. Similar thought experiments are used by Eric T. Olson in *The Human Animal: Personal Identity without Psychology* (New York: Oxford University Press, 1997) to illustrate Animalism. His version is the second one discussed in the text.

33. Speaking from the Constitution View, we should add another conjunct to the antecedent: ". . . and H and H' are not related by constitution."

34. See Olson's *The Human Animal*.

35. Roderick M. Chisholm, "Coming into Being and Passing Away: Can the Metaphysician Help?" in *On Metaphysics*, 49–61.

36. Whenever that is. Logically speaking, I do not believe that there could be a new individual until about two weeks after fertilization. Before that time, there is the physical possibility of "twinning." Since it is logically impossible for one thing to be identical to two things, I think that it is a logical error to hold that a new life begins at fertilization.

37. This is not to deny that there are gradations of mentality throughout the animal kingdom. My claim is that there is only one species with a first-person perspective, and that species is obviously different from all the others in what it manages to accomplish and produce.

38. Daniel C. Dennett, *Darwin's Dangerous Idea* (New York: Simon and Schuster, 1995): 336. Dennett is discussing Jared Diamond's *The Third Chimpanzee*.

39. The reason that I do not say that self-consciousness ushered in a new kind of animal is that biologists do not take self-consciousness to distinguish species, and I take the identification of new kinds of animals to be within the purview of biology.

40. Recall the arguments against identifying being a human person with being a human organism.

41. A new nonderivative person, that is. When a body comes to constitute a person, it becomes a person derivatively, but the body is not thereby a new person. The body's being a person is entirely a matter of the body's constitution-relations to a person.

42. I'd like to thank Gary Rosenkrantz, my commentator at the Chisholm Memorial Conference at Brown University, November 10–11, 2000, for helpful comments. Also, thanks are due to Gareth B. Matthews for reading many drafts of this paper and to Katherine A. Sonderegger for searching discussions of these matters.

PERSONS AS RELATIONAL BEINGS

Selections from Part III of *Mind, Self, and Society from the Standpoint of a Social Behaviorist*

G. H. Mead

21. The Self and the Subjective

The process out of which the self arises is a social process which implies interaction of individuals in the group, implies the pre-existence of the group.[1] It implies also certain co-operative activities in which the different members of the group are involved. It implies, further, that out of this process there may in turn develop a more elaborate organization than that out of which the self has arisen, and that the selves may be the organs, the essential parts at least, of this more elaborate social organization within which these selves arise and exist. Thus, there is a social process out of which selves arise and within which further differentiation, further evolution, further organization, take place.

It has been the tendency of psychology to deal with the self as a more or less isolated and independent element, a sort of entity, that could conceivably exist by itself. It is possible that there might be a single self in the universe if we start off by identifying the self with a certain feeling-consciousness. If we speak of this feeling as objective, then we can think of that self as existing by itself. We can think of a separate physical body existing by itself, we can assume that it has these feelings or conscious states in question, and so we can set up that sort of a self in thought as existing simply by itself.

Then there is another use of "consciousness" with which we have been particularly occupied, denoting that which we term thinking or reflective intelligence, a use of consciousness which always has, implicitly at least, the reference to an "I" in it. This use of consciousness has no necessary connection with the other; it is an entirely different conception. One usage has to do with a certain mechanism, a certain way in which an organism acts. If an organism is endowed with sense organs then there are objects in its environment, and among those objects will be parts of its own body.2 It is true that if the organism did not have a retina and a central nervous system there would not be any objects of vision. For such objects to exist there have to be certain physiological conditions, but these objects are not in themselves necessarily related to a self. When we reach a self we reach a certain sort of conduct, a certain type of social process which involves the interaction of different individuals and yet implies individuals engaged in some sort of co-operative activity. In that process a self, as such, can arise. . . .

Emphasis should be laid on the central position of thinking when considering the nature of the self. Self-consciousness, rather than affective experience with its motor accompaniments, provides the core and primary structure of the self, which is thus essentially a cognitive rather than an emotional phenomenon. The thinking or intellectual process—the internalization and inner dramatization, by the individual, of the external conversation of significant gestures which constitutes his chief mode of interaction with other individuals belonging to the same society—is the earliest experiential phase in the genesis and development of the self. Cooley and James, it is true, endeavor to find the basis of the self in reflexive affective experiences, i.e., experiences involving "self-feeling"; but the theory that the nature of the self is to be found in such experiences does not account for the origin of the self, or of the self-feeling which is supposed to characterize such experiences. The individual need not take the attitudes of others toward himself in these experiences, since these experiences merely in themselves do not necessitate his doing so, and unless he does so, he cannot develop a self; and he will not do so in these experiences unless his self has already originated otherwise, namely, in the way we have been describing. The essence of the self, as we have said, is cognitive: it lies in the internalized conversation of gestures which constitutes thinking, or in terms of which thought or reflection proceeds. And hence the origin and foundations of the self, like those of thinking, are social. . . .

We have discussed the self from the point of view of the "I" and the "me," the "me" representing that group of attitudes which stands for others in the community, especially that organized group of responses which we have detailed in discussing the game on the one hand and social institutions on the other. In these situations there is a certain organized group of attitudes which answer to any social act on the part of the individual organism. In any cooperative process, such as the family, the individual calls out a response from the other members of the group. Now, to the extent that those responses can be called out in the individual so that he can answer to them, we have both those contents which go to make up the self, the "other" and the "I." The distinction expresses itself in our experience in what we call the recognition of others and the recognition of ourselves in the others. We cannot realize ourselves except in so far as we can recognize the other in his relationship to us. It is as he takes the attitude of the other that the individual is able to realize himself as a self.

We are referring, of course, to a social situation as distinct from such bare organic responses as reflexes of the organism, some of which we have already discussed, as in the case where a person adjusts himself unconsciously to those about him. In such an experience there is no self-consciousness. One attains self-consciousness only as he takes, or finds himself stimulated to take, the attitude of the other. . . .

26. The Realization of the Self in the Social Situation

There is still one phase in the development of the self that needs to be presented in more detail: the realization of the self in the social situation in which it arises.

I have argued that the self appears in experience essentially as a "me" with the organization of the community to which it belongs. This organization is, of course, expressed in the particular endowment and particular social situation of the individual. He is a member of the community, but he is a particular part of the community, with a particular heredity and position which distinguishes him from anybody else. He is what he is in so far as he is a member of this community, and the raw materials out of which this particular individual is born would not be a self but for his relationship to others in the community of which he is a part. Thus is he aware of himself as such, and this not only in political citizenship, or in membership in groups of which he is a part, but also from the point of view of reflective thought. He is a member of the community of the thinkers whose literature he reads and to which he may contribute by his own published thought. He belongs to a society of all rational beings, and the rationality that he identifies with himself involves a continued social interchange. The widest community in which the individual finds himself, that which is everywhere, through and for everybody, is the thought world as such. He is a member of such a community and he is what he is as such a member.

The fact that all selves are constituted by or in terms of the social process, and are individual reflections of it—or rather of this organized behavior pattern which it exhibits, and which they prehend in their respective structures— is not in the least incompatible with, or destructive of, the fact that every individual self has its own peculiar individuality, its own unique pattern; because each individual self within that process, while it reflects in its organized structure the behavior pattern of that process as a whole, does so from its own particular and unique standpoint within that process, and thus reflects in its organized structure a different aspect or perspective of this whole social behavior pattern from that which is reflected in the organized structure of any other individual self within that process (just as every monad in the Leibnizian universe mirrors that universe from a different point of view, and thus mirrors a different aspect or perspective of that universe). In other words, the organized structure of every individual self within the human social process of experience and behavior reflects, and is constituted by, the organized relational pattern of that process as a whole; but each individual self-structure reflects, and is constituted by, a different aspect or perspective of this and this relational pattern, because each reflects this relational pattern from its own unique standpoint; so that the common social origin and constitution of individual selves and their structures does not preclude wide individual differences and variations among them, or contradict the peculiar and more or less distinctive individuality which each of them in fact possesses. Every individual self within a given society or social community reflects in its organized structure the whole relational pattern of organized social behavior which that society or community exhibits or is carrying on, and its organized structure is constituted by this pattern; but since each of these individual selves reflects a uniquely different aspect or perspective of this pattern in its structure, from its own particular and unique place or standpoint within the whole process of organized social behavior which exhibits this pattern—since, that is, each is differently or uniquely related to that whole process, and occupies its own essentially unique focus of relations therein—the structure of each is differently constituted by this pattern from the way in which the structure of any other is so constituted. . . .

29. A Contrast of Individualistic and Social Theories of the Self

The differences between the type of social psychology which derives the selves of individuals from the social process in which they are implicated and in which they empirically interact with one another, and the type of social psychology which instead derives that process from the selves of the individuals involved in it, are clear. The first type assumes a social process or social order as the logical and biological precondition of the appearance of the selves of the individual organisms involved in that process or belonging to that order. The other type, on the contrary, assumes individual selves as the presuppositions, logically and biologically, of the social process or order within which they interact.

The difference between the social and the individual theories of the development of mind, self, and the social process of experience or behavior is analogous to the difference between the evolutionary and the contract theories of the state as held in the past by both rationalists and empiricists.[3] The latter theory takes individuals and their individual experiencing—individual minds and selves—as logically prior to the social process in which they are involved, and explains the existence of that social process in terms of them; whereas the former takes the social process of experience or behavior as logically prior to the individuals and their individual experiencing which are involved in it, and explains their existence in terms of that social process. But the latter type of theory cannot explain that which is taken as logically prior at all, cannot explain the existence of minds and selves; whereas the former type of theory can explain that which it takes as logically prior, namely, the existence of the social process of behavior, in terms of such fundamental biological or physiological relations and interactions as reproduction, or the co-operation of individuals for mutual protection or for the securing of food.

Our contention is that mind can never find expression, and could never have come into existence at all, except in terms of a social environment; that, an organized set or pattern of social relations and interactions (especially those of communication by means of gestures functioning as significant symbols and thus creating a universe of discourse) is necessarily presupposed by it and involved in its nature. And this entirely social theory or interpretation of mind[4]— this contention that mind develops and has its being only in and by virtue of the social process of experience and activity, which it hence presupposes, and that in no other way can it develop and have its being—must be clearly distinguished from the partially (but only partially) social view of mind. On this view, though

mind can get expression only within or in terms of the environment of an organized social group, yet it is nevertheless in some sense a native endowment—
a congenital or hereditary biological attribute—of the individual organism, and
could not otherwise exist or manifest itself in the social process at all; so that it
is not itself essentially a social phenomenon, but rather is biological both in its
nature and in its origin, and is social only in its characteristic manifestations or
expressions. According to this latter view, moreover, the social process presupposes, and in a sense is a product of, mind; in direct contrast is our opposite
view that mind presupposes and is a product of, the social process. The advantage of our view is that it enables us to give a detailed account and actually to
explain the genesis and development of mind; whereas the view that mind is a
congenital biological endowment of the individual organism does not really
enable us to explain its nature and origin at all: neither what sort of biological
endowment it is, nor how organisms at a certain level of evolutionary progress
come to possess it.[5] Furthermore, the supposition that the social process presupposes, and is in some sense a product of, mind seems to be contradicted by the
existence of the social communities of certain of the lower animals, especially
the highly complex social organizations of bees and ants, which apparently
operate on a purely instinctive or reflex basis, and do not in the least involve the
existence of mind or consciousness in the individual organisms which form or
constitute them. And even if this contradiction is avoided by the admission that
only at its higher levels—only at the levels represented by the social relations
and interactions of human beings—does the social process of experience and
behavior presuppose the existence of mind or become necessarily a product of
mind, still it is hardly plausible to suppose that this already ongoing and developing process should suddenly, at a particular stage in its evolution, become
dependent for its further continuance upon an entirely extraneous factor, introduced into it, so to speak, from without.

   The individual enters as such into his own experience only as an object, not
as a subject; and he can enter as an object only on the basis of social relations
and interactions, only by means of his experiential transactions with other individuals in an organized social environment. It is true that certain contents of
experience (particularly kinesthetic) are accessible only to the given individual
organism and not to any others; and that these private or "subjective," as opposed to public or "objective," contents of experience are usually regarded as
being peculiarly and intimately connected with the individual's self, or as being
in a special sense self-experiences. But this accessibility solely to the given individual organism of certain contents of its experience does not affect, nor in any

way conflict with, the theory as to the social nature and origin of the self that we are presenting; the existence of private or "subjective" contents of experience does not alter the fact that self-consciousness involves the individual's becoming an object to himself by taking the attitudes of other individuals toward himself within an organized setting of social relationships, and that unless the individual had thus become an object to himself he would not be self-conscious or have a self at all. Apart from his social interactions with other individuals, he would not relate the private or "subjective" contents of his experience to himself, and he could not become aware of himself as such, that is, as an individual, a person, merely by means or in terms of these contents of his experience; for in order to become aware of himself as such he must, to repeat, become an object to himself, or enter his own experience as an object, and only by social means—only by taking the attitudes of others toward himself—is he able to become an object to himself.[6]

It is true, of course, that once mind has arisen in the social process it makes possible the development of that process into much more complex forms of social interaction among the component individuals than was possible before it had arisen. But there is nothing odd about a product of a given process contributing to, or becoming an essential factor in, the further development of that process. The social process, then, does not depend for its origin or initial existence upon the existence and interactions of selves; though it does depend upon the latter for the higher stages of complexity and organization which it reaches after selves have arisen within it.

NOTES

1. The relation of individual organisms to the social whole of which they are members is analogous to the relation of the individual cells of a multi-cellular organism to the organism as a whole.

2. Our constructive selection of our environment is what we term "consciousness," in the first sense of the term. The organism does not project sensuous qualities—colors, for example—into the environment to which it responds; but it endows this environment with such qualities, in a sense similar to that in which an ox endows grass with the quality of being food, or in which—speaking more generally—the relation between biological organisms and certain environmental contents give rise to food objects. If there were no organisms with particular sense organs there would be no environment, in the proper or usual sense of the term. An organism constructs (in the selective sense) its environment; and consciousness often refers to the character of the environment in so far as it is determined or constructively selected by our human organisms, and depends upon the relationship between the former (as thus selected or constructed) and the latter.

3. Historically, both the rationalist and the empiricist are committed to the interpretation of experience in terms of the individual (1931).

Other people are there as much as we are there; to be a self requires other selves (1924).

In our experience the thing is there as much as we are here. Our experience is in the thing as much as it is in us (MS).

4. In defending a social theory of mind we are defending a functional, as opposed to any form of substantive or entitive, view as to its nature. And in particular, we are opposing all intracranial or intra-epidermal views as to its character and locus. For it follows from our social theory of mind that the field of mind must be co-extensive with, and include all the components of, the field of the social process of experience and behavior, i.e., the matrix of social relations and interactions among individuals, which is presupposed by it, and out of which it arises or comes into being. If mind is socially constituted, then the field or locus of any given individual mind must extend as far as the social activity or apparatus of social relations which constitutes it extends; and hence that field cannot be bounded by the skin of the individual organism to which it belongs.

5. According to the traditional assumption of psychology, the content of experience is entirely individual and not in any measure to be primarily accounted for in social terms, even though its setting or context is a social one. And for a social psychology like Cooley's—which is founded on precisely this same assumption—all social interactions depend upon the imaginations of the individuals involved, and take place in terms of their direct conscious influences upon one another in the processes of social experience. Cooley's social psychology, as found in his *Human Nature and the Social Order,* is hence inevitably introspective, and his psychological method carries with it the implication of complete solipsism: society really has no existence except in the individual's mind, and the concept of the self as in any sense intrinsically social is a product of imagination. Even for Cooley the self presupposes experience, and experience is a process within which selves arise; but since that process is for him primarily internal and individual rather than external and social, he is committed in his psychology to a subjectivistic and idealistic, rather than an objectivistic and naturalistic, metaphysical position.

6. The human being's physiological capacity for developing mind or intelligence is a product of the process of biological evolution, just as is his whole organism; but the actual development of his mind or intelligence itself, given that capacity, must proceed in terms of the social situations wherein it gets its expression and import; and hence it itself is a product of the process of social evolution, the process of social experience and behavior.

CHAPTER THIRTEEN

The Impact of the Concept of Culture on the Concept of Man

Clifford Geertz

{ I }

Toward the end of his recent study of the ideas used by tribal peoples, *La Pensée Sauvage*, the French anthropologist Lévi-Strauss remarks that scientific explanation does not consist, as we have been led to imagine, in the reduction of the complex to the simple. Rather, it consists, he says, in a substitution of a complexity more intelligible for one which is less. So far as the study of man is concerned, one may go even further, I think, and argue that explanation often consists of substituting complex pictures for simple ones while striving somehow to retain the persuasive clarity that went with the simple ones.

Elegance remains, I suppose, a general scientific ideal; but in the social sciences, it is very often in departures from that ideal that truly creative developments occur. Scientific advancement commonly consists in a progressive complication of what once seemed a beautifully simple set of notions but now seems an unbearably simplistic one. It is after this sort of disenchantment occurs that intelligibility, and thus explanatory power, comes to rest on the possibility of substituting the involved but comprehensible for the involved but incomprehensible to which Lévi-Strauss refers. Whitehead once offered to the natural sciences the maxim "Seek simplicity and distrust it"; to the social sciences he might well have offered "Seek complexity and order it."

Certainly the study of culture has developed as though this maxim were being followed. The rise of a scientific concept of culture amounted to, or at least was connected with, the overthrow of the view of human nature dominant in the Enlightenment—a view that, whatever else may be said for or against it, was both clear and simple—and its replacement by a view not only more complicated but enormously less clear. The attempt to clarify it, to reconstruct an intelligible account of what man is, has underlain scientific thinking about culture ever since. Having sought complexity and, on a scale grander than they ever imagined, found it, anthropologists became entangled in a tortuous effort to order it. And the end is not yet in sight.

The Enlightenment view of man was, of course, that he was wholly of a piece with nature and shared in the general uniformity of composition which natural science, under Bacon's urging and Newton's guidance, had discovered there. There is, in brief, a human nature as regularly organized, as thoroughly invariant, and as marvelously simple as Newton's universe. Perhaps some of its laws are different, but there *are* laws; perhaps some of its immutability is obscured by the trappings of local fashion, but it *is* immutable.

A quotation that Lovejoy (whose magisterial analysis I am following here) gives from an Enlightenment historian, Mascou, presents the position with the useful bluntness one often finds in a minor writer:

> The stage setting [in different times and places] is, indeed, altered, the actors change their garb and their appearance; but their inward motions arise from the same desires and passions of men, and produce their effects in the vicissitudes of kingdoms and peoples.[1]

Now, this view is hardly one to be despised; nor, despite my easy references a moment ago to "overthrow," can it be said to have disappeared from contemporary anthropological thought. The notion that men are men under whatever guise and against whatever backdrop has not been replaced by "other mores, other beasts."

Yet, cast as it was, the Enlightenment concept of the nature of human nature had some much less acceptable implications, the main one being that, to quote Lovejoy himself this time, "anything of which the intelligibility, verifiability, or actual affirmation is limited to men of a special age, race, temperament, tradition or condition is [in and of itself] without truth or value, or at all events without importance to a reasonable man."[2] The great, vast variety of differences among men, in beliefs and values, in customs and institutions, both over time and from place to place, is essentially without significance in defining his nature. It consists of mere accretions, distortions even, overlaying and obscuring what is truly human—the constant, the general, the universal—in man.

Thus, in a passage now notorious, Dr. Johnson saw Shakespeare's genius to lie in the fact that "his characters are not modified by the customs of particular places, unpractised by the rest of the world; by the peculiarities of studies or professions, which can operate upon but small numbers; or by the accidents of transient fashions or temporary opinions."[3] And Racine regarded the success of his plays on classical themes as proof that "the taste of Paris . . . conforms to that of Athens; my spectators have been moved by the same things which, in other times, brought tears to the eyes of the most cultivated classes of Greece."[4]

The trouble with this kind of view, aside from the fact that it sounds comic coming from someone as profoundly English as Johnson or as French as Racine, is that the image of a constant human nature independent of time, place, and circumstance, of studies and professions, transient fashions and temporary opinions, may be an illusion, that what man is may be so entangled with where he is, who he is, and what he believes that it is inseparable from them. It is precisely the consideration of such a possibility that led to the rise of the concept of culture and the decline of the uniformitarian view of man. Whatever else modern anthropology asserts—and it seems to have asserted almost everything at one time or another—it is firm in the conviction that men unmodified by the customs of particular places do not in fact exist, have never existed, and most important, could not in the very nature of the case exist. There is, there can be, no backstage where we can go to catch a glimpse of Mascou's actors as "real persons" lounging about in street clothes, disengaged from their profession, displaying with artless candor their spontaneous desires and unprompted passions. They may change their roles, their styles of acting, even the dramas in which they play; but—as Shakespeare himself of course remarked—they are always performing.

This circumstance makes the drawing of a line between what is natural, universal, and constant in man and what is conventional, local, and variable extraordinarily difficult. In fact, it suggests that to draw such a line is to falsify the human situation, or at least to misrender it seriously.

Consider Balinese trance. The Balinese fall into extreme dissociated states in which they perform all sorts of spectacular activities—biting off the heads of living chickens, stabbing themselves with daggers, throwing themselves wildly about, speaking with tongues, performing miraculous feats of equilibration, mimicking sexual intercourse, eating feces, and so on—rather more easily and much more suddenly than most of us fall asleep. Trance states are a crucial part of every ceremony. In some, fifty or sixty people may fall, one after the other ("like a string of firecrackers going off," as one observer puts it), emerging anywhere from five minutes to several hours later, totally unaware of what they have been doing and convinced, despite the amnesia, that they have had the most extraordinary and deeply satisfying experience a man can have. What does one learn about human nature from this sort of thing and from the thousand similarly peculiar things anthropologists discover, investigate, and describe? That the Balinese are peculiar sorts of beings, South Sea Martians? That they are just the same as we at base, but with some peculiar, but really incidental, customs we do not happen to have gone in for? That they are innately gifted or even instinctively driven in certain directions rather than others? Or that human nature does not exist and men are pure and simply what their culture makes them?

It is among such interpretations as these, all unsatisfactory, that anthropology has attempted to find its way to a more viable concept of man, one in which culture, and the variability of culture, would be taken into account rather than written off as caprice and prejudice, and yet, at the same time, one in which the governing principle of the field, "the basic unity of mankind," would not be turned into an empty phrase. To take the giant step away from the uniformitarian view of human nature is, so far as the study of man is concerned, to leave the Garden. To entertain the idea that the diversity of custom across time and over space is not a mere matter of garb and appearance, of stage settings and comedic masques, is to entertain also the idea that humanity is as various in its essence as it is in its expression. And with that reflection some well-fastened philosophical moorings are loosed and an uneasy drifting into perilous waters begins.

Perilous, because if one discards the notion that Man with a capital "M," is to be looked for "behind," "under," or "beyond" his customs and replaces it with the notion that man, uncapitalized, is to be looked for "in" them, one is in some danger of losing sight of him altogether. Either he dissolves, without residue, into his time and place, a child and a perfect captive of his age, or he becomes a conscripted soldier in a vast Tolstoian army, engulfed in one or another of the terrible historical determinisms with which we have been plagued from Hegel forward. We have had, and to some extent still have, both of these aberrations in the social sciences—one marching under the banner of cultural relativism, the other under that of cultural evolution. But we also have had, and more commonly, attempts to avoid them by seeking in culture patterns themselves the defining elements of a human existence which, although not constant in expression, are yet distinctive in character.

{ II }

Attempts to locate man amid the body of his customs have taken several directions, adopted diverse tactics; but they have all, or virtually all, proceeded in terms of a single overall intellectual strategy: what I will call, so as to have a stick to beat it with, the "stratigraphic" conception of the relations between biological, psychological, social, and cultural factors in human life. In this conception, man is a composite of "levels," each superimposed upon those beneath it and underpinning those above it. As one analyzes man, one peels off layer after layer, each such layer being complete and irreducible in itself, revealing another, quite different sort of layer underneath. Strip off the motley forms of culture and one finds the structural and functional regularities of social organization. Peel off these in turn and one finds the underlying psychological factors— "basic needs" or what-have-you—that support and make them possible. Peel off psychological factors and one is left with the biological foundations—anatomical, physiological, neurological—of the whole edifice of human life.

The attraction of this sort of conceptualization, aside from the fact that it guaranteed the established academic disciplines their independence and sovereignty, was that it seemed to make it possible to have one's cake and eat it. One did not have to assert that man's culture was all there was to him in order to claim that it was, nonetheless, an essential and irreducible, even a paramount ingredient in his nature. Cultural facts could be interpreted against the background of noncultural facts without dissolving them into that background or dissolving that background into them. Man was a hierarchically stratified animal, a sort of evolutionary deposit, in whose definition each level—organic, psychological, social, and cultural—had an assigned and incontestable place. To see what he really was, we had to superimpose findings from the various relevant sciences—anthropology, sociology, psychology, biology—upon one another like so many patterns in a *moiré;* and when that was done, the cardinal importance of the cultural level, the only one distinctive to man, would naturally appear, as would what it had to tell us, in its own right, about what he really was. For the eighteenth century image of man as the naked reasoner that appeared when he took his cultural costumes off, the anthropology of the late nineteenth and early twentieth centuries substituted the image of man as the transfigured animal that appeared when he put them on.

At the level of concrete research and specific analysis, this grand strategy came down, first, to a hunt for universals in culture, for empirical uniformities that, in the face of the diversity of customs around the world and over time, could be found everywhere in about the same form, and, second, to an effort to relate such universals, once found, to the established constants of human biology, psychology, and social organization. If some customs could be ferreted out of the cluttered catalogue of world culture as common to all local variants of it, and if these could then be connected in a determinate manner with certain invariant points of reference on the subcultural levels, then at least some progress might be made toward specifying which cultural traits are essential to human existence and which merely adventitious, peripheral, or ornamental. In such a way, anthropology could determine cultural dimensions of a concept of man commensurate with the dimensions provided, in a similar way, by biology, psychology, or sociology.

In essence, this is not altogether a new idea. The notion of a *consensus gentium* (a consensus of all mankind)—the notion that there are some things that all men will be found to agree upon as right, real, just, or attractive and that these things are, therefore, in fact right, real, just, or attractive—was present in the Enlightenment and probably has been present in some form or another in all ages and climes. It is one of those ideas that occur to almost anyone sooner or later. Its development in modern anthropology, however—beginning with Clark Wissler's elaboration in the 1920s of what he called "the universal cultural pattern," through Bronislaw Malinowski's presentation of a list of "universal institutional types" in the early forties, up to G. P. Murdock's elaboration of a set of "common-denominators of culture" during and since World War II—added something new. It added the notion that, to quote Clyde Kluckhohn, perhaps the most persuasive of the *consensus gentium* theorists, "some aspects of culture take their specific forms solely as a result of historical accidents; others are tailored by forces which can properly be designated as universal."[5] With this, man's cultural life is split in two: part of it is, like Mascou's actors' garb, independent of men's Newtonian "inward motions"; part is an emanation of those motions themselves. The question that then arises is: Can this halfway house between the eighteenth and twentieth centuries really stand?

Whether it can or not depends on whether the dualism between empirically universal aspects of culture rooted in subcultural realities and empirically variable aspects not so rooted can be established and sustained. And this, in turn, demands (1) that the universals proposed be substantial ones and not empty categories; (2) that they be specifically grounded in particular biological, psychological, or sociological processes, not just vaguely associated with "underlying realities"; and (3) that they can convincingly be defended as core elements in a definition of humanity in comparison with which the much more numerous cultural particularities are of clearly secondary importance. On all three of these counts it seems to me that the *consensus gentium* approach fails; rather than moving toward the essentials of the human situation it moves away from them.

The reason the first of these requirements—that the proposed universals be substantial ones and not empty or near-empty categories—has not been met is that it cannot be. There is a logical conflict between asserting that, say, "religion," "marriage," or "property" are empirical universals and giving them very much in the way of specific content, for to say that they are empirical universals is to say that they have the same content, and to say they have the same content is to fly in the face of the undeniable fact that they do not. If one defines religion generally and indeterminately—as man's most fundamental orientation to reality, for example—then one cannot at the same time assign to that orientation a highly circumstantial content; for clearly what composes the most fundamental orientation to reality among the transported Aztecs, lifting pulsing hearts torn live from the chests of human sacrifices toward the heavens, is not what comprises it among the stolid Zuñi, dancing their great mass supplications to the benevolent gods of rain. The obsessive ritualism and unbuttoned polytheism of the Hindus express a rather different view of what the "really real" is really like from the uncompromising monotheism and austere legalism of Sunni Islam. Even if one does try to get down to less abstract levels and assert, as Kluckhohn did, that a concept of the afterlife is universal, or as Malinowski did, that a sense of Providence is universal, the same contradiction haunts one. To make the generalization about an afterlife stand up alike for the Confucians and the Calvinists, the Zen Buddhists and the Tibetan Buddhists, one has to define it in most general terms, indeed—so general, in fact, that whatever force it seems to have virtually evaporates. So, too, with any notion of a sense of Providence, which can include under its wing both Navajo notions about the relations of gods to men and Trobriand ones. And as with religion, so with "marriage," "trade," and all the rest of what A. L. Kroeber aptly called "fake universals," down to so seemingly tangible a matter as "shelter." That everywhere people mate and produce children, have some sense of mine and thine, and protect themselves in one fashion or another from rain and sun are neither false nor, from some points of view, unimportant; but they are hardly very much help in drawing a portrait of man that will be a true and honest likeness and not an untenered "John Q. Public" sort of cartoon.

My point, which should be clear and I hope will become even clearer in a moment, is not that there are no generalizations that can be made about man as man, save that he is a most various animal, or that the study of culture has nothing to contribute toward the uncovering of such generalizations. My point is that such generalizations are not to be discovered through a Baconian search for cultural universals, a kind of public-opinion polling of the world's peoples in search of *a consensus gentium* that does not in fact exist, and, further, that the attempt to do so leads to precisely the sort of relativism the whole approach was expressly designed to avoid. "Zuñi culture prizes restraint," Kluckhohn writes; "Kwakiutl culture encourages exhibitionism on the part of the individual. These are contrasting values, but in adhering to them the Zuñi and Kwakiutl show their allegiance to a universal value; the prizing of the distinctive norms of one's culture."[6] This is sheer evasion, but it is only more apparent, not more evasive, than discussions of cultural universals in general. What, after all, does it avail us to say, with Herskovits, that "morality is a universal, and so is enjoyment of beauty, and some standard for truth," if we are forced in the very next sentence, as he is, to add that "the many forms these concepts take are but products of the particular historical experience of the societies that manifest them"?[7] Once one abandons uniformitarianism, even if, like the *consensus gentium* theorists, only partially and uncertainly, relativism is a genuine danger; but it can be warded off only by facing directly and fully the diversities of human culture, the Zuñi's restraint and the Kwakiutl's exhibitionism, and embracing them within the body of one's concept of man, not by gliding past them with vague tautologies and forceless banalities.

Of course, the difficulty of stating cultural universals which are at the same time substantial also hinders fulfillment of the second requirement facing the *consensus gentium* approach, that of grounding such universals in particular biological, psychological, or sociological processes. But there is more to it than that: the "stratigraphic" conceptualization of the relationships between cultural and noncultural factors hinders such a grounding even more effectively. Once culture, psyche, society, and organism have been converted into separate scientific "levels," complete and autonomous in themselves, it is very hard to bring them back together again.

The most common way of trying to do so is through the utilization of what are called "invariant points of reference." These points are to be found, to quote one of the most famous statements of this strategy—the "Toward a Common Language for the Areas of the Social Sciences" memorandum produced by Talcott Parsons, Kluckhohn, O. H. Taylor, and others in the early forties—

in the nature of social systems, in the biological and psychological nature of the component individuals, in the external situations in which they live and act, in the necessity of coordination in social systems. In [culture] . . . these "foci" of structure are never ignored. They must in some way be "adapted to" or "taken account of."

Cultural universals are conceived to be crystallized responses to these unevadable realities, institutionalized ways of coming to terms with them.

Analysis consists, then, of matching assumed universals to postulated underlying necessities, attempting to show there is some goodness of fit between the two. On the social level, reference is made to such irrefragable facts as that all societies, in order to persist, must reproduce their membership or allocate goods and services, hence the universality of some form of family or some form of trade. On the psychological level, recourse is had to basic needs like personal growth—hence the ubiquity of educational institutions—or to panhuman problems, like the Oedipal predicament—hence the ubiquity of punishing gods and nurturant goddesses. Biologically, there is metabolism and health; culturally, dining customs and curing procedures. And so on. The tack is to look at underlying human requirements of some sort or other and then to try to show that those aspects of culture that are universal are, to use Kluckhohn's figure again, "tailored" by these requirements.

The problem here is, again, not so much whether in a general way this sort of congruence exists, but whether it is more than a loose and indeterminate one. It is not difficult to relate some human institutions to what science (or common sense) tells us are requirements for human existence, but it is very much more difficult to state this relationship in an unequivocal form. Not only does almost any institution serve a multiplicity of social, psychological, and organic needs (so that to say marriage is a mere reflex of the social need to reproduce, or that dining customs are a reflex of metabolic necessities, is to court parody), but there is no way to state in any precise and testable way the interlevel relationships that are conceived to hold. Despite first appearances, there is no serious attempt here to apply the concepts and theories of biology, psychology, or even sociology to the analysis of culture (and, of course, not even a suggestion of the reverse exchange) but merely a placing of supposed facts from the cultural and subcultural levels side by side so as to induce a vague sense that some kind of relationship between them—an obscure sort of "tailoring"—obtains. There is no theoretical integration here at all but a mere correlation, and that intuitive, of separate findings. With the levels approach, we can never, even by invoking "invariant points of reference," construct genuine functional interconnections between cultural and noncultural factors, only more or less persuasive analogies, parallelisms, suggestions, and affinities.

However, even if I am wrong (as, admittedly, many anthropologists would hold) in claiming that the *consensus gentium* approach can produce neither substantial universals nor specific connections between cultural and noncultural phenomena to explain them, the question still remains whether such universals should be taken as the central elements in the definition of man, whether a lowest-common-denominator view of humanity is what we want anyway. This is, of course, now a philosophical question, not as such a scientific one; but the notion that the essence of what it means to be human is most clearly revealed in those features of human culture that are universal rather than in those that are distinctive to this people or that is a prejudice we are not necessarily obliged to share. Is it in grasping such general facts—that man has everywhere some sort of "religion"—or in grasping the richness of this religious phenomenon or that—Balinese trance or Indian ritualism, Aztec human sacrifice or Zuñi raindancing—that we grasp him? Is the fact that "marriage" is universal (if it is) as penetrating a comment on what we are as the facts concerning Himalayan polyandry, or those fantastic Australian marriage rules, or the elaborate bride-price systems of Bantu Africa? The comment that Cromwell was the most typical Englishman of his time precisely in that he was the oddest may be relevant in this connection, too: it may be in the cultural particularities of people—in their oddities—that some of the most instructive revelations of what it is to be generically human are to be found; and the main contribution of the science of anthropology to the construction—or reconstruction—of a concept of man may then lie in showing us how to find them.

{ III }

The major reason why anthropologists have shied away from cultural particularities when it came to a question of defining man and have taken refuge instead in bloodless universals is that, faced as they are with the enormous variation in human behavior, they are haunted by a fear of historicism, of becoming lost in a whirl of cultural relativism so convulsive as to deprive them of any fixed bearings at all. Nor has there not been some occasion for such a fear: Ruth Benedict's *Patterns of Culture*, probably the most popular book in anthropology ever published in this country, with its strange conclusion that anything one group of people is inclined toward doing is worthy of respect by another, is perhaps only the most outstanding example of the awkward positions one can get into by giving oneself over rather too completely to what Marc Bloch called "the thrill of learning singular things." Yet the fear is a bogey. The notion that unless a cultural phenomenon is empirically universal it cannot reflect anything about the nature of man is about as logical as the notion that because sickle-cell anemia is, fortunately, not universal, it cannot tell us anything about human genetic processes. It is not whether phenomena are empirically common that is critical in science—else why should Becquerel have been so interested in the peculiar behavior of uranium?—but whether they can be made to reveal the enduring natural processes that underly them. Seeing heaven in a grain of sand is not a trick only poets can accomplish.

In short, we need to look for systematic relationships among diverse phenomena, not for substantive identities among similar ones. And to do that with any effectiveness, we need to replace the "stratigraphic" conception of the relations between the various aspects of human existence with a synthetic one; that is, one in which biological, psychological, sociological, and cultural factors can be treated as variables within unitary systems of analysis. The establishment of a common language in the social sciences is not a matter of mere coordination of terminologies or, worse yet, of coining artificial new ones; nor is it a matter of imposing a single set of categories upon the area as a whole. It is a matter of integrating different types of theories and concepts in such a way that one can formulate meaningful propositions embodying findings now sequestered in separate fields of study.

In attempting to launch such an integration from the anthropological side and to reach, thereby, a more exact image of man, I want to propose two ideas. The first of these is that culture is best seen not as complexes of concrete behavior patterns—customs, usages, traditions, habit clusters—as has, by and large, been the case up to now, but as a set of control mechanisms—plans, recipes, rules, instructions (what computer engineers call "programs")—for the governing of behavior. The second idea is that man is precisely the animal most desperately dependent upon such extragenetic, outside-the-skin control mechanisms, such cultural programs, for ordering his behavior.

Neither of these ideas is entirely new, but a number of recent developments, both within anthropology and in other sciences (cybernetics, information theory, neurology, molecular genetics) have made them susceptible of more precise statement as well as lending them a degree of empirical support they did not previously have. And out of such reformulations of the concept of culture and of the role of culture in human life comes, in turn, a definition of man stressing not so much the empirical commonalities in his behavior, from place to place and time to time, but rather the mechanisms by whose agency the breadth and indeterminateness of his inherent capacities are reduced to the narrowness and specificity of his actual accomplishments. One of the most significant facts about us may finally be that we all begin with the natural equipment to live a thousand kinds of life but end in the end having lived only one.

The "control mechanism" view of culture begins with the assumption that human thought is basically both social and public—that its natural habitat is the house yard, the marketplace, and the town square. Thinking consists not of "happenings in the head" (though happenings there and elsewhere are necessary for it to occur) but of a traffic in what have been called, by G. H. Mead and others, significant symbols—words for the most part but also gestures, drawings, musical sounds, mechanical devices like clocks, or natural objects like jewels—anything, in fact, that is disengaged from its mere actuality and used to impose meaning upon experience. From the point of view of any particular individual, such symbols are largely given. He finds them already current in the community when he is born, and they remain, with some additions, subtractions, and partial alterations he may or may not have had a hand in, in circulation after he dies. While he lives he uses them, or some of them, sometimes deliberately and with care, most often spontaneously and with ease, but always with the same end in view: to put a construction upon the events through which he lives, to orient himself within "the ongoing course of experienced things," to adopt a vivid phrase of John Dewey's.

Man is so in need of such symbolic sources of illumination to find his bearings in the world because the nonsymbolic sort that are constitutionally ingrained in his body cast so diffused a light. The behavior patterns of lower animals are, at least to a much greater extent, given to them with their physical structure; genetic sources of information order their actions within much narrower ranges of variation, the narrower and more thoroughgoing the lower the animal. For man, what are innately given are extremely general response capacities, which, although they make possible far greater plasticity, complexity, and, on the scattered occasions when everything works as it should, effectiveness of behavior, leave it much less precisely regulated. This, then, is the second face of our argument: Undirected by culture patterns—organized systems of significant symbols—man's behavior would be virtually ungovernable, a mere chaos of pointless acts and exploding emotions, his experience virtually shapeless. Culture, the accumulated totality of such patterns, is not just an ornament of human existence but—the principal basis of its specificity—an essential condition for it.

Within anthropology some of the most telling evidence in support of such a position comes from recent advances in our understanding of what used to be called the descent of man: the emergence of *Homo sapiens* out of his general primate background. Of these advances three are of critical importance: (1) the discarding of a sequential view of the relations between the physical evolution and the cultural development of man in favor of an overlap or interactive view; (2) the discovery that the bulk of the biological changes that produced modern man out of his most immediate progenitors took place in the central nervous system and most especially in the brain; (3) the realization that man is, in physical terms, an incomplete, an unfinished, animal; that what sets him off most graphically from nonmen is less his sheer ability to learn (great as that is) than how much and what particular sorts of things he *has* to learn before he is able to function at all. Let me take each of these points in turn.

The traditional view of the relations between the biological and the cultural advance of man was that the former, the biological, was for all intents and purposes completed before the latter, the cultural, began. That is to say, it was again stratigraphic: Man's physical being evolved, through the usual mechanisms of genetic variation and natural selection, up to the point where his anatomical structure had arrived at more or less the status at which we find it today; then cultural development got under way. At some particular stage in his phylogenetic history, a marginal genetic change of some sort rendered him capable of producing and carrying culture, and thenceforth his form of adaptive response to environmental pressures was almost exclusively cultural rather than genetic. As he spread over the globe, he wore furs in cold climates and loin cloths (or nothing at all) in warm ones; he didn't alter his innate mode of response to environmental temperature. He made weapons to extend his inherited predatory powers and cooked foods to render a wider range of them digestible. Man became man, the story continues, when, having crossed some mental Rubicon, he became able to transmit "knowledge, belief, law, morals, custom" (to quote the items of Sir Edward Tylor's classical definition of culture) to his descendants and his neighbors through teaching and to acquire them from his ancestors and his neighbors through learning. After that magical moment, the advance of the hominids depended almost entirely on cultural accumulation, on the slow growth of conventional practices, rather than, as it had for ages past, on physical organic change.

The only trouble is that such a moment does not seem to have existed. By the most recent estimates the transition to the cultural mode of life took the genus *Homo* several million years to accomplish; and stretched out in such a manner, it involved not one or a handful of marginal genetic changes but a long, complex, and closely ordered sequence of them.

In the current view, the evolution of *Homo sapiens*—modern man—out of his immediate pre-*sapiens* background got definitely under way nearly four million years ago with the appearance of the now famous Australopithecines—the so-called ape men of southern and eastern Africa—and culminated with the emergence of *sapiens* himself only some one to two or three hundred thousand years ago. Thus, as at least elemental forms of cultural, or if you wish protocultural, activity (simple toolmaking, hunting, and so on) seem to have been present among some of the Australopithecines, there was an overlap of, as I say, well over a million years between the beginning of culture and the appearance of man as we know him today. The precise dates—which are tentative and which further research may later alter in one direction or another—are not critical; what is critical is that there was an overlap and that it was a very extended one. The final phases (final to date, at any rate) of the phylogenetic history of man took place in the same grand geological era—the so-called Ice Age—as the initial phases of his cultural history. Men have birthdays, but man does not.

What this means is that culture, rather than being added on, so to speak, to a finished or virtually finished animal, was ingredient, and centrally ingredient, in the production of that animal itself. The slow, steady, almost glacial growth of culture through the Ice Age altered the balance of selection pressures for the evolving *Homo* in such a way as to play a major directive role in his evolution. The perfection of tools, the adoption of organized hunting and gathering practices, the beginnings of true family organization, the discovery of fire, and, most critically, though it is as yet extremely difficult to trace it out in any detail, the increasing reliance upon systems of significant symbols (language, art, myth, ritual) for orientation, communication, and self-control all created for man a new environment to which he was then obliged to adapt. As culture, step by infinitesimal step, accumulated and developed, a selective advantage was given to those individuals in the population most able to take advantage of it—the effective hunter, the persistent gatherer, the adept toolmaker, the resourceful leader—until what had been a small-brained, protohuman *Australopithecus* became the large-brained fully human *Homo sapiens*. Between the cultural pattern, the body, and the brain, a positive feedback system was created in which each shaped the progress of the other, a system in which the interaction among increasing tool use, the changing anatomy of the hand, and the expanding representation of the thumb on the cortex is only one of the more graphic examples. By submitting himself to governance by symbolically mediated programs for producing artifacts, organizing social life, or expressing emotions, man determined, if unwittingly, the culminating stages of his own biological destiny. Quite literally, though quite inadvertently, he created himself.

Though, as I mentioned, there were a number of important changes in the gross anatomy of genus *Homo* during this period of his crystallization—in skull shape, dentition, thumb size, and so on—by far the most important and dramatic were those that evidently took place in the central nervous system; for this was the period when the human brain, and most particularly the forebrain, ballooned into its present top-heavy proportions. The technical problems are complicated and controversial here; but the main point is that though the Australopithecines had a torso and arm configuration not drastically different from our own, and a pelvis and leg formation at least well-launched toward our own, they had cranial capacities hardly larger than those of the living apes—that is to say, about a third to a half of our own. What sets true men off most distinctly from protomen is apparently not overall bodily form but complexity of nervous organization. The overlap period of cultural and biological change seems to have consisted in an intense concentration on neural development and perhaps associated refinements of various behaviors—of the hands, bipedal locomotion, and so on—for which the basic anatomical foundations—mobile shoulders and wrists, a broadened ilium, and so on—had already been securely laid. In itself, this is perhaps not altogether startling; but, combined with what I have already said, it suggests some conclusions about what sort of animal man is that are, I think, rather far not only from those of the eighteenth century but from those of the anthropology of only ten or fifteen years ago.

Most bluntly, it suggests that there is no such thing as a human nature independent of culture. Men without culture would not be the clever savages of Golding's *Lord of the Flies* thrown back upon the cruel wisdom of their animal instincts; nor would they be the nature's noblemen of Enlightenment primitivism or even, as classical anthropological theory would imply, intrinsically talented apes who had somehow failed to find themselves. They would be unworkable monstrosities with very few useful instincts, fewer recognizable sentiments, and no intellect: mental basket cases. As our central nervous system—and most particularly its crowning curse and glory, the neocortex—grew up in great part in interaction with culture, it is incapable of directing our behavior or organizing our experience without the guidance provided by systems of significant symbols. What happened to us in the Ice Age is that we were obliged to abandon the regularity and precision of detailed genetic control over our conduct for the flexibility and adaptability of a more generalized, though of course no less real, genetic control over it. To supply the additional information necessary to be able to act, we were forced, in turn, to rely more and more heavily on cultural sources—the accumulated fund of significant symbols. Such symbols are thus not mere expressions, instrumentalities, or correlates of our biological, psychological, and social existence; they are prerequisites of it. Without men, no culture, certainly; but equally, and more significantly, without culture, no men.

We are, in sum, incomplete or unfinished animals who complete or finish ourselves through culture—and not through culture in general but through highly particular forms of it: Dobuan and Javanese, Hopi and Italian, upper-class and lower-class, academic and commercial. Man's great capacity for learning, his plasticity, has often been remarked, but what is even more critical is his extreme dependence upon a certain sort of learning: the attainment of concepts, the apprehension and application of specific systems of symbolic meaning. Beavers build dams, birds build nests, bees locate food, baboons organize social groups, and mice mate on the basis of forms of learning that rest predominantly on the instructions encoded in their genes and evoked by appropriate patterns of external stimuli: physical keys inserted into organic locks. But men build dams or shelters, locate food, organize their social groups, or find sexual partners under the guidance of instructions encoded in flow charts and blueprints, hunting lore, moral systems and aesthetic judgments: conceptual structures molding formless talents.

We live, as one writer has neatly put it, in an "information gap." Between what our body tells us and what we have to know in order to function, there is a vacuum we must fill ourselves, and we fill it with information (or misinformation) provided by our culture. The boundary between what is innately controlled and what is culturally controlled in human behavior is an ill-defined and wavering one. Some things are, for all intents and purposes, entirely controlled intrinsically: we need no more cultural guidance to learn how to breathe than a fish needs to learn how to swim. Others are almost certainly largely cultural; we do not attempt to explain on a genetic basis why some men put their trust in centralized planning and others in the free market, though it might be an amusing exercise. Almost all complex human behavior is, of course, the interactive, nonadditive outcome of the two. Our capacity to speak is surely innate; our capacity to speak English is surely cultural. Smiling at pleasing stimuli and frowning at unpleasing ones are surely in some degree genetically determined (even apes screw up their faces at noxious odors); but sardonic smiling and burlesque frowning are equally surely predominantly cultural, as is perhaps demonstrated by the Balinese definition of a madman as someone who, like an American, smiles when there is nothing to laugh at. Between the basic ground plans for our life that our genes lay down—the capacity to speak or to smile— and the precise behavior we in fact execute—speaking English in a certain tone of voice, smiling enigmatically in a delicate social situation—lies a complex set of significant symbols under whose direction we transform the first into the second, the ground plans into the activity.

Our ideas, our values, our acts, even our emotions, are, like our nervous system itself, cultural products—products manufactured, indeed, out of tendencies, capacities, and dispositions with which we were born, but manufactured nonetheless. Chartres is made of stone and glass. But it is not just stone and glass; it is a cathedral, and not only a cathedral, but a particular cathedral built at a particular time by certain members of a particular society. To understand what it means, to perceive it for what it is, you need to know rather more than the generic properties of stone and glass and rather more than what is common to all cathedrals. You need to understand also—and, in my opinion, most critically—the specific concepts of the relations among God, man, and architecture that, since they have governed its creation, it consequently embodies. It is no different with men: they, too, every last one of them, are cultural artifacts.

{ IV }

Whatever differences they may show, the approaches to the definition of human nature adopted by the Enlightenment and by classical anthropology have one thing in common: they are both basically typological. They endeavor to construct an image of man as a model, an archetype, a Platonic idea or an Aristotelian form, with respect to which actual men—you, me, Churchill, Hitler, and the Bornean headhunter—are but reflections, distortions, approximations. In the Enlightenment case, the elements of this essential type were to be uncovered by stripping the trappings of culture away from actual men and seeing what then was left—natural man. In classical anthropology, it was to be uncovered by factoring out the commonalities in culture and seeing what then appeared—consensual man. In either case, the result is the same as that which tends to emerge in all typological approaches to scientific problems generally: the differences among individuals and among groups of individuals are rendered secondary. Individuality comes to be seen as eccentricity, distinctiveness as accidental deviation from the only legitimate object of study for the true scientist: the underlying, unchanging, normative type. In such an approach, however elaborately formulated and resourcefully defended, living detail is drowned in dead stereotype: we are in quest of a metaphysical entity, Man with a capital "M," in the interests of which we sacrifice the empirical entity we in fact encounter, man with a small "m."

The sacrifice is, however, as unnecessary as it is unavailing. There is no opposition between general theoretical understanding and circumstantial understanding, between synoptic vision and a fine eye for detail. It is, in fact, by its power to draw general propositions out of particular phenomena that a scientific theory—indeed, science itself—is to be judged. If we want to discover what man amounts to, we can only find it in what men are: and what men are, above all other things, is various. It is in understanding that variousness—its range, its nature, its basis, and its implications—that we shall come to construct a concept of human nature that, more than a statistical shadow and less than a primitivist dream, has both substance and truth.

It is here, to come round finally to my title, that the concept of culture has its impact on the concept of man. When seen as a set of symbolic devices for controlling behavior, extrasomatic sources of information, culture provides the link between what men are intrinsically capable of becoming and what they actually, one by one, in fact become. Becoming human is becoming individual, and we become individual under the guidance of cultural patterns, historically created systems of meaning in terms of which we give form, order, point, and direction to our lives. And the cultural patterns involved are not general but specific—not just "marriage" but a particular set of notions about what men and women are like, how spouses should treat one another, or who should properly marry whom; not just "religion" but belief in the wheel of karma, the observance of a month of fasting, or the practice of cattle sacrifice. Man is to be defined neither by his innate capacities alone, as the Enlightenment sought to do, nor by his actual behaviors alone, as much of contemporary social science seeks to do, but rather by the link between them, by the way in which the first is transformed into the second, his generic potentialities focused into his specific performances. It is in man's *career*, in its characteristic course, that we can discern, however dimly, his nature, and though culture is but one element in determining that course, it is hardly the least important. As culture shaped us as a single species—and is no doubt still shaping us—so too it shapes us as separate individuals. This, neither an unchanging subcultural self nor an established cross-cultural consensus, is what we really have in common.

Oddly enough—though on second thought, perhaps not so oddly—many of our subjects seem to realize this more clearly than we anthropologists ourselves. In Java, for example, where I have done much of my work, the people quite flatly say, "To be human is to be Javanese." Small children, boors, simpletons, the insane, the flagrantly immoral, are said to be *ndurung djawa*, "not yet Javanese." A "normal" adult capable of acting in terms of the highly elaborate system of etiquette, possessed of the delicate aesthetic perceptions associated with music, dance, drama, and textile design, responsive to the subtle promptings of the divine residing in the stillnesses of each individual's inward-turning conscious-ness, is *sampun djawa*, "already Javanese," that is, already human. To be human is not just to breathe; it is to control one's breathing, by yogalike techniques, so as to hear in inhalation and exhalation the literal voice of God pronouncing His own name—"hu Allah." It is not just to talk, it is to utter the appropriate words and phrases in the appropriate social situations in the appropriate tone of voice and with the appropriate evasive indirection. It is not just to eat; it is to prefer certain foods cooked in certain ways and to follow a rigid table etiquette in consuming them. It is not even just to feel but to feel certain quite distinctively Javanese (and essentially untranslatable) emotions—"patience," "detachment," "resignation," "respect."

To be human here is thus not to be Everyman; it is to be a particular kind of man, and of course men differ: "Other fields," the Javanese say, "other grasshop-pers." Within the society, differences are recognized, too—the way a rice peas-ant becomes human and Javanese differs from the way a civil servant does. This is not a matter of tolerance and ethical relativism, for not all ways of being hu-man are regarded as equally admirable by far; the way the local Chinese go about it is, for example, intensely dispraised. The point is that there are different ways; and to shift to the anthropologist's perspective now, it is in a systematic review and analysis of these—of the Plains Indian's bravura, the Hindu's obses-siveness, the Frenchman's rationalism, the Berber's anarchism, the American's optimism (to list a series of tags I should not like to have to defend as such)—that we shall find out what it is, or can be, to be a man.

We must, in short, descend into detail, past the misleading tags, past the metaphysical types, past the empty similarities to grasp firmly the essential character of not only the various cultures but the various sorts of individuals within each culture, if we wish to encounter humanity face to face. In this area, the road to the general, to the revelatory simplicities of science, lies through a concern with the particular, the circumstantial, the concrete, but a concern or-ganized and directed in terms of the sort of theoretical analyses that I have touched upon—analyses of physical evolution, of the functioning of the nervous system, of social organization, of psychological process, of cultural patterning, and so on—and, most especially, in terms of the interplay among them. That is to say, the road lies, like any genuine Quest, through a terrifying complexity.

"Leave him alone for a moment or two," Robert Lowell writes, not as one might suspect of the anthropologist but of that other eccentric inquirer into the nature of man, Nathaniel Hawthorne.

> Leave him alone for a moment or two,
> and you'll see him with his head
> bent down, brooding, brooding,
> eyes fixed on some chip,
> some stone, some common plant,
> the commonest thing,
> as if it were the clue.
> The disturbed eyes rise,
> furtive, foiled, dissatisfied
> from meditation on the true
> and insignificant.[8]

Bent over his own chips, stones, and common plants, the anthropologist broods, too, upon the true and insignificant, glimpsing in it, or so he thinks, fleetingly and insecurely, the disturbing, changeful image of himself.

NOTES

1. A. O. Lovejoy, *Essays in the History of Ideas* (New York, 1960), p. 173.
2. Ibid., p. 80.
3. "Preface to Shakespeare," *Johnson on Shakespeare* (London, 1931), pp. 11–12.
4. From the Preface to *Iphigénie*.
5. A. L. Kroeber, ed., *Anthropology Today* (Chicago, 1953), p. 516.
6. C. Kluckhohn, *Culture and Behavior* (New York, 1962), p. 280.
7. M. J. Herskovits, *Cultural Anthropology* (New York, 1955), p. 364.
8. Reprinted with permission of Farrar, Straus & Giroux, Inc., and Faber & Faber, Ltd., from "Hawthorne," in *For the Union Dead*, p. 39. Copyright © 1964 by Robert Lowell.

CHAPTER FOURTEEN

Selection from *Personal Being*

Rom Harré

3. Sense of Identity

To explore the sense we have of our own identity in any disciplined fashion one must avoid vague discussions of what it feels like to be "myself." We can follow an alternative route by exploring the idea of a criterion of personal identity: a criterion I might be imagined to employ to decide about myself. What can be made of the questions "Who am I?" and statements like "I'm not myself today"? Does the former represent a genuine puzzle, and is the latter an expression of a discovery about personal identity? To answer this one must ask what conditions have to be met for there to be a criterion, for an entity to be judged to be this or that kind of thing (*see* Shoemaker, *Self-knowledge and self-identity*). Clearly, one important condition must be that we admit the possibility of the criterion not being met and candidates being rejected. In attempting to answer the question "Who am I?," could I make the discovery that I am not, after all, myself? Could I, for example, find out I was someone else? It is intuitively obvious, I think, that these considerations are nonsensical. They are nonsensical because, to query one's own personal, as contrasted with one's social identity undermines one of the very presuppositions that are required for first person utterances to make sense, namely that they are the utterances of an individual person. In short, to have just this sense of any individuality, to treat myself as a possible subject of predication as I treat others, is a necessary part of what it is to be a person. When I ask, "Who am I," the most I could mean would be "Which of various possible social identities, publicly identified, is legitimately or properly mine." Amnesia is not a loss of the sense of identity, but rather involves the inaccessibility of various items of knowledge about my public and social being, my past history. The fact that some of the loss concerns private—individual matters shows that the ability to *maintain* a continuous autobiography is secondary. The joint unities, point of view and point of action, make autobiographies possible. The statement "I am not myself today" can only mean that I do not feel the same as I did yesterday, which presupposes a conserved sense of identity. Since, then, I cannot doubt that I am the author, as it were, of my own speech, the very idea of a criterion for my sense of my own identity is empty.

Philosophers have made this point in various ways. Butler, "Of personal identity," for example, argued that memory cannot be the basis of a sense of identity since the very notion of memory presupposes that identity. For instance, it is empty to ask whether these memories I am remembering are mine. I can ask only whether what I take to be a memory is an accurate recollection of what happened to me or of what I did. To ponder on whether my recollections are another's memories is at most to ask whether I could perhaps be recollecting someone else's experience. Whatsoever they were, they must, as recollections, be my experiences since I am now experiencing them. At best I can be amazed that my imaginings are like your rememberings, so alike as to be qualitatively identical with your recollections in so far as we can make comparisons. But even in that case, my discovery that you and I have identical, i.e. very similar, recollections of a great many events is no ground whatever for the hypothesis that I am you.

What, then, are the origins of this strong sense of identity? I propose to show that the best hypothesis is that, though the sense of identity is conceptually and logically distinct from the fact of personal identity, nevertheless the former, in the course of human development, derives from the latter. Adequate empirical studies of this matter have yet to be made, but there are pieces of work which can be treated as the first step in a program of research into the psychological foundations of personal being. The very first step in devising such a program must be the classification of the relevant features of the notion of identity, brought out by philosophical analysis, features that could serve as the basis of hypotheses to be explored by developmental psychologists. Bruner's work on "peek-a-boo" games in "Early rule structure" would make a good beginning.

The arguments of philosophers such as Hampshire, *Thought and action*, concerning the role of bodily identity in personhood lead, as I have pointed out, to the idea that a person experiences the world from a particular here and now, that is, has a point of view, which is coordinated in the spatiotemporal system with their point of action. This doctrine derives from the necessary conditions for the referential uses of words. If I am to be able to refer to something, to point to it, in the world, I must know from where I am pointing as well as to what. That is, I must anchor my frame of reference to the corporeal here and now. Ordinarily, this is done through the indexical presuppositions of the uses of the word "I," presuppositions which embody the very idea that I am here and speaking now. One might wish to argue that having acquired a language and in so doing grasped the indexicality of referential expressions, a human being is in possession of the concept of numerical identity in space and time, since experience soon provides that person with the idea of a trajectory through a spatiotemporal system which is the locus of their coordinated points of view and points of action.

However, in order to achieve this happy coincidence, the actor must be in possession of the system of personal pronouns and know-how to use them. The indexicality of "I" depends, it might be argued, upon the grasp of the simple referential function of "you." Since "myself" is not a thing I could discover, it seems I cannot first experience myself and then attach the personal pronoun "I" to that experience. I must be learning the pronoun system as a whole through the ways in which and the means by which I am treated as a person by others. So that, by being treated as "you," or as a member of "we," I am now in a position to add "I" to my vocabulary, to show where, in the array of persons, speaking, thinking, feeling, promising and so on, is happening. In order to be addressed as "you," I must be being perceived as a definite embodied person, that is, as a distinct human but material individual by others. This unity of pronoun system might be one of the things that is meant by the social construction of the self. But it depends upon the recognizable bodily identity that I have even as an infant. I have identified these as the indexical uses of "I."

I am also treated by other people as having a distinct point of view and being the locus of exercises of agency. So that these very conditions of bodily identity, identified by Hampshire, *Thought and action,* as necessary conditions for having the idea of myself as a person, are also, it seems, to be taken as presumptions that are embedded in all kinds of social practices. For example, the idea that a person has a distinct point of action is embedded in such practices as moral praise and blame. That kind of talk makes sense only upon the presupposition that one has a point of action through which one's intentions and so on can be realized.

So the acquisition of the idea of personal identity for oneself, through which one develops a sense of identity, is at least in part a consequence of social practices which derive from the fact of identity as it is conceived in a culture. Our first preliminary conclusion, then, must be that a human being learns that he or she is a person from others and in discovering a sphere of action the source of which is treated by others as the very person they identify as having spatiotemporal identity. Thus, a human being does not learn that he or she is a person by the empirical disclosure of an experiential fact. Personal identity is symbolic of social practices not of empirical experiences. It has the status of a theory.

However, there is a great deal more to the sense of personal identity than the realization that one has a point of view and can act upon the world at certain places. We must now turn to what I shall call transcendental conditions. These require certain features of personhood as necessary conditions for the possibility of certain kinds of human activities. Philosophers have insisted, and rightly, since the days of David Hume, that in an important sense the self is not experienced. As Hume pointed out, "I never can catch *myself* at any time without a perception, and never can observe anything but the perception" (*A treatise of human nature*, book 1, pt. 4, s. 4).

4. Summary of the Argument

The first step towards identifying transcendental features of selfhood involved in the sense of identity was to notice that the considerations advanced above and the analysis based upon them depend upon the assumption of the existence of two kinds of unities.

There is a unity of the realm of consciousness in that, for instance, the experiences I have as a being, spatiotemporally and socially located, and acting where I am, are coordinated in one realm of experience. Consciousness is not divided, and hence does not have to be combined. But this is not to say that that of which I am conscious is not ordered. Clearly, there is an indefinite potential hierarchy of "knowings" which is given by the possibility of reflexive consciousness. Thus, I can become aware of an orange, pay attention to it, and perhaps, if suitably prompted, can know that I am attending to it, and so on. One of the commonplace techniques of dealing with pain is to attend not so much to the pain but to the relation in which I, as experiencer, stand to that pain.

This leads to a second kind of unity. The hierarchy of experience is paralleled for human beings by a hierarchy of action. I can act upon the things in the world, for instance tennis balls, and I can act upon my actions upon the things in the world, for instance I can improve my forehand style. It would not be unreasonable to say that the hierarchies of awareness and of action involve a regress of the very same self; that the centre of consciousness and the source of action are one self. I act according to a rule; I adopt the rule according to some principle; I accept a principle according to some theory, and so on. It would not be unreasonable to argue that it is the very same "I" who is aware of the peeling of an orange, who knows that he is aware of peeling an orange, and so on.

It is now clear, I hope, where the need for a transcendental hypothesis comes from. These coordinated unified hierarchies are unified via the self which is presupposed in them. Each time that an individual is able to make a start up the hierarchy of action and hopes, naïvely, to experience the self which makes that step and which is, as it were, the origin of the sphere of experience, that self must remove itself from the realm of experience. The sense I have of myself, then, must include the very complex idea of something not experienced but presupposed as a necessary condition for the form that experience takes; in particular, its unified and hierarchical form. The fine structure of this kind of hierarchy has been perceptively explored by Langford in "Persons as necessarily social." From the point of view of the philosophy of science, "the self" is a theoretical concept, and the sense of self derives from the way we experience our experiences as unified, but is not reducible to it. From the point of view of the philosophy of psychology, that unification is an achievement, made possible by the possession of the chief unifying concept, "myself." The "now" and "what" of all this will occupy us in the chapters to come.

These matters need to be further elaborated: the idea of an array of persons as the moral order that forms the background of all thought and action; the uses of personal pronouns as a key to the understanding of the structuring of experience; the identification of a mother—infant interaction pattern from which personal being emerges.

5. Autobiography as Self-knowledge

Presented in the course of development with a sense of self, a human being can undertake the organization of memories and beliefs into a narrative of which he or she is the central character. However, autobiography is not just a chronicle of episodes, whether private or public. It has also to do with a growing grasp of capabilities and potentials. As such it involves the exploitation of the conditions for both consciousness and agency. For expository purposes, the structure of the argument of this work can be reflected in three aspects of autobiography.

Consciousness, I have argued, is not some unique state, but is the possession of certain grammatical models for the presentation to oneself and others of what one knows by inter- and intrapersonal perception. These models provide the structures by which I can know that which *I* am currently feeling, thinking, suffering, doing and so on, that is, they provide the wherewithal for an organization of knowledge as mine.

Agency, likewise, is an endowment from theory, permitting the formulation of hypotheses about what I was, am or could be capable. Through this my history is enriched by reference to possibilities of thought and action and so finds a continuous link with the moral orders through which I have lived my life.

To create autobiography out of this some of my beliefs about myself must stand as memories, of what I have at other times thought, done, felt and enjoyed. But as we have seen there is nothing in the phenomenal quality of experiences which authenticates them as true recollections. The category of belief-as-recollection is socially constructed and hierarchically organized. Autobiography involves the social conditions of the confirmation of recollections. The systematic exploitation of this feature of autobiographical work is the foundation of De Waele's "assisted construction" method in "Autobiography as a scientific method," for the development of a self-history (*see* research menu 8).

6. Speculation: The Breakdown of Transcendental Unities

I have argued that what makes a being a person is the possession and use of a certain theory, in terms of which that being constructs and orders its beliefs, plans, feelings and actions. I have suggested that the acquisition of the person-engendering theory occurs, and indeed must occur, in the course of changing responsibilities within relationships of psychological symbiosis.

One of the learning progressions which contributes most to the capacity to grasp oneself as a being who perceives the world from a certain point of view is the acquisition of the capacity to use the personal pronouns. With this goes a practical understanding of indexicality, the technique of displaying where in an array of persons something personal is happening. At the same time a nascent person is receiving praise, blame, exhortation, prohibition and so on for what he or she is doing or trying to do. Through these language games a being is acquiring the idea that it can be an actor, with a point of action, that is, has leverage within the world, and with the idea comes the capacity.

The theory I have used to illustrate the social constructivist thesis identifies consciousness and agency, point of view and point of action as one and as mine through the theoretical concept of "self." I follow Kant in calling this a transcendental unity, not given in experience, but rather the means by which experience is ordered. There may be cultures where the unity of experience and the unity of action are not unified in a higher order singular conception.

What might be expected to happen to people built up in our way if the unity between point of view and point of action begins to break down? Remember this is not the idea of there being an awareness of some phenomenological disaster, but rather the lapsing of a theoretical standpoint, like ceasing to believe in the unity of electricities.

Failure of memory might make it impossible to order one's experience around the idea of a continuous trajectory of point of view, while one may continue to deploy moment by moment the idea that one acts more or less where one is currently located and in accordance with what one is momentarily intending. This possibility could be realized in some forms of senility. Only against the background of a general belief in the unity of unities does senility appear as a deficit, as opposed to just another form of life.

Another theoretical possibility is that the sense of agency, of being in control of one's actions, may dissolve while one retains a continuous sense of self as a being experiencing the world and one's own states from a continuously developing trajectory of space—time locations and relationships with other people. Certain kinds of schizophrenia seem to have this general character. This is not intended as any kind of rough sketch of a theory of schizophrenia, rather a speculation as to one of the cognitive deficits that might enter into the condition. Then there are cases where, though point of view and point of action are both maintained, they are not unified, but if both dissolve the person has ceased to be.

RESEARCH MENU 8

All the necessary techniques for research into the autobiographies of individual human beings are already available in the work of J.-P. de Waele (see De Waele and Harré, "Autobiography as a scientific method"). Whenever this method has been put to work, the results have been very encouraging; see, for example, work of Debi Stec on the autobiographies of the obese currently under way at SUNY, Binghamton. Of course, an autobiographical study takes time and trouble.

BIBLIOGRAPHICAL NOTES

From the huge body of literature on personal identity I select the following: S. H. Ampshire, *Thought and action* (London: Chatto and Windus, 1959), B. A. O. Williams, *Problems of the self* (Cambridge: Cambridge University Press, 1973), M. Prince, *The dissociation of personality* (London: Kegan Paul, Truscott and Shrubner, 1905), I. Helling, "Autobiography as self-presentation" (in *Life sentences*, ed. R. Harré, London: John Wiley and Sons, 1976), S. Shoemaker, *Self-knowledge and self-identity* (Ithaca: Cornell University Press, 1963), an excellent work. Much of our modern way of looking at the problems of identity of persons comes from J. Butler, "Of personal identity" (in *The works of Bishop Butler*, ed. J. H. Bernard, London: 1900).

For the hierarchical nature of the sense of identity see G. Langford, "Persons as necessarily social" (*Journal for the Theory of Social Behaviour*, 8, 1978, 263–83).

Additional works cited in the text are J. Bruner, "Early rule structure: the case of peek-a-boo" (in *Life sentences*, ed. R. Harré, Chichester: John Wiley and Sons, 1976); J. Canfield, *Wittgenstein, language and world* (Amherst: University of Massachusetts Press, 1981); J.-P. De Waele and R. Harré, "Autobiography as a scientific method" (in *Emerging strategies in social scientific research*, ed. G. P. Ginsburg, Chichester: John Wiley and Sons, 1979, ch. 8); D. Hume, *A treatise of human nature* (1739, ed. D. G. C. Macnabb, London: Fontana, Collins, 1962).

CHAPTER FIFTEEN

Selection from *Dementia Reconsidered: The Person Comes First*

Tom Kitwood

The Concept of Personhood

The term *personhood*, together with its synonyms and parallels, can be found in three main types of discourse: those of transcendence, those of ethics and those of social psychology. The functions of the term are different in these three contexts, but there is a core of meaning that provides a basic conceptual unity.

Discourses of transcendence make their appeal to a very powerful sense, held in almost every cultural setting, that being-in-itself is sacred, and that life is to be revered. Theistic religions capture something of this in their doctrines of divine creation; in eastern traditions of Christianity, for example, there is the idea that each human being is an "Ikon of God." Some forms of Buddhism, and other non-theistic spiritual paths, believe in an essential, inner nature: always present, always perfect, and waiting to be discovered through enlightenment. Secular humanism makes no metaphysical assumptions about the essence of our nature, but still often asserts, on the basis of direct experience, that "the ultimate is persona."

In the main ethical discourses of Western philosophy one primary theme has been the idea that each person has absolute value. We thus have an obligation to treat each other with deep respect; as ends, and never as means towards some other end. The principle of respect for persons, it was argued by Kant and those who followed in his footsteps, requires no theological justification; it is the only assumption on which our life as social beings makes sense. There are parallels to this kind of thinking in the doctrine of human rights, and this has been used rhetorically in many different contexts, including that of dementia (King's Fund 1986). One problem here, however, is that in declarations of rights the person is framed primarily as a separate individual; there is a failure to see human life as interdependent and interconnected.

In social psychology the term personhood has had a rather flexible and varied use. Its primary associations are with self-esteem and its basis; with the place of an individual in a social group; with the performance of given roles; and with the integrity, continuity and stability of the sense of self. Themes such as these have been explored, for example, by Tobin (1991) in his work on later life, and by Barham and Hayward (1991) in their study of ex-mental patients living in the community. Social psychology, as an empirical discipline, seeks to ground its discourses in evidence, even while recognizing that some of this may consist of pointers and allusions. Robust measures such as those valued by the traditional natural sciences usually cannot be obtained, even if an illusion is created that they can.

Thus we arrive at a definition of personhood, as I shall use the term in this book. It is a standing or status that is bestowed upon one human being, by others, in the context of relationship and social being. It implies recognition, respect and trust. Both the according of personhood, and the failure to do so, have consequences that are empirically testable.

The Issue of Inclusion

As soon as personhood is made into a central category, some crucial questions arise. Who is to be viewed and treated as a person? What are the grounds for inclusion and exclusion, since "person" is clearly not a mere synonym for "human being"? Is the concept of personhood absolute, or can it be attenuated?

Such questions have been examined many times, particularly in Western moral philosophy. In one of the best-known discussions Quinton (1973) suggests five criteria. The first is consciousness, whose normal accompaniment is consciousness of self. The second is rationality, which in its most developed form includes the capacity for abstract reasoning. The third is agency: being able to form intentions, to consider alternatives, and to direct action accordingly.

The fourth is morality, which in its strongest form means living according to principle, and being accountable for one's actions. The fifth is the capacity to form and hold relationships; essential here is the ability to understand and identify with the interests, desires and needs of others. Quinton suggests that each criterion can be taken in a stronger or a weaker sense. We can make the distinction, for example, between someone who has all the capabilities of a moral agent, and someone who does not, but who is nevertheless the proper subject for moral concern.

With the arrival of computers and the creation of systems with artificial intelligence, doubts began to be raised about whether the concept of personhood is still valid (Dennett 1975). The central argument is as follows. In computers we have machines which mimic certain aspects of human mental function. We can (and often do) describe and explain the "behavior" of computers as if they were intentional beings, with thoughts, wishes, plans and so on. However, there is no necessity to do this; it is simply an anthropomorphism—a convenient short cut. In fact the behavior of computers can be completely described and explained in physical terms. It is then argued that the same is possible, in principle, with human beings, although the details are more complex. Thus an intentional frame is not strictly necessary; and the category of personhood, to which it is so strongly tied, becomes redundant.

Behind such debates a vague shadow can be discerned. It is that of the liberal academic of former times: kind, considerate, honest, fair, and above all else an intellectual. Emotion and feeling have only a minor part in the scheme of things; autonomy is given supremacy over relationship and commitment; passion has no place at all. Moreover the problems seem to center on how to describe and explain, which already presupposes an existential stance of detachment. So long as we stay on this ground the category of personhood is indeed in danger of being undermined, and with it the moral recognition of people with mental impairments. At a popularistic level, matters are more simple. Under the influence of the extreme individualism that has dominated Western societies in recent years, criteria such as those set out by Quinton have been reduced to two: autonomy and rationality. Now the shadowy figure in the background is the devotee of "business culture." Once this move is made, there is a perfect justification for excluding people with serious disabilities from the "personhood club."

Both the mainstream philosophical debate and its popularistic reductions have been radically questioned by Stephen Post, in his book *The Moral Challenge of Alzheimer's Disease* (1995). Here he argues that it has been a grave error to place such great emphasis on autonomy and rational capability; this is part of the imbalance of our cultural tradition. Personhood, he suggests, should be linked far more strongly to feeling, emotion and the ability to live in relationships, and here people with dementia are often highly competent—sometimes more so than their carers.

Post also suggests a principle of *moral solidarity:* a recognition of the essential unity of all human beings, despite whatever differences there may be in their mental capabilities as conventionally determined. Thus we are all, so to speak, in the same boat; and there can be no empirically determined point at which it is justifiable to throw some people into the sea. The radical broadening of moral awareness that Post commends has many applications in the context of dementia: for example to how diagnostic information is handled, to the negotiation of issues such as driving or self-care, and ultimately to the most difficult questions of all, concerning the preservation of life.

Personhood and Relationship

There is another approach to the question of what it means to be a person, which gives priority to experience, and relegates analytic discussion to a very minor place. One of its principal exponents was Martin Buber, whose small book *Ich und Du* was first published in 1922, and later appeared in an English translation, with the title *I and Thou*, in 1937. It is significant that this work was written during that very period when the forces of modernization had caused enormous turmoil throughout the world, and in the aftermath of the horrific brutalities of the First World War.

Buber's work centers on a contrast between two ways of being in the world; two ways of living in relationship. The first he terms I–It, and the second I–Thou. In his treatment of Thou he has abstracted one of many meanings; making it so to speak, into a jewel. In older usage it is clear that a person could be addressed as Thou in many forms of "strong recognition": command, accusation, insult and threat, as well as the special form of intimacy that Buber portrays. Relating in the I–It mode implies coolness, detachment, instrumentality. It is a way of maintaining a safe distance, of avoiding risks; there is no danger of vulnerabilities being exposed. The I–Thou mode, on the other hand, implies going out towards the other; self-disclosure, spontaneity—a journey into uncharted territory. Relationships of the I–It kind can never rise beyond the banal and trivial. Daring to relate to another as Thou may involve anxiety or even suffering, but Buber sees it also as the path to fulfilment and joy. "The primary word I–Thou can only be spoken with the whole being. The primary Word I–It can never be spoken with the whole being" (1937: 2).

Buber's starting point then, is different from that of Western individualism. He does not assume the existence of ready-made monads, and then inquire into their attributes. His central assertion is that relationship is primary; to be a person is to be addressed as Thou. There is no implication here that there are two different kinds of objects in the world: Thous and Its. The difference lies in the manner of relating. Thus it is possible (and, sad to say, all too common) for one human being to engage with another in the I–It mode. Also it is possible, at least to some degree, to engage with a non-human being as Thou. We might think, for example, of a woman in her 80s whose dog is her constant and beloved companion, or of a Japanese man who faithfully attends his bonsai tree each day.

In the English language we have now almost lost the word Thou. Once it was part of everyday speech, corresponding to the life of face-to-face communities. Its traces remain in just a few places still; for example in North country dialects, and in old folk songs such as one about welcoming a guest, which has the heart-warming refrain:

Draw chair raight up to t'table;
Stay as long as Thou art able;
I'm always glad to see a man like Thee.

Among minority groups in Britain, the Quakers were the last to give up the use of Thou in daily conversation, and they did so with regret. Their sense of the sacredness of every person was embedded in their traditional form of speech.

One of the most famous of all Buber's sayings is "All real living is meeting" (1937: 11). Clearly it is not a matter of committees or business meetings, or even a meeting to plan the management of care. It is not the meeting of one intellectual with another, exchanging their ideas but revealing almost nothing of their feelings. It is not the meeting between a rescuer and a victim, the one intent on helping or "saving" the other. It is not necessarily the meeting that occurs during a sexual embrace. In the meeting of which Buber speaks there is no ulterior purpose, no hidden agenda. The ideas to be associated with this are openness, tenderness, presence (present-ness), awareness. More than any of these, the word that captures the essence of such meeting is *grace*. Grace implies something not sought or bought, not earned or deserved. It is simply that life has mysteriously revealed itself in the manner of a gift.

For Buber, to become a person also implies the possibility of freedom. "So long as the heaven of Thou is spread out over me, the wind of causality cowers at my heels, and the whirlwind of fate stays its course" (1937: 9). Here, in poetic language, is a challenge to all determinism, all mechanical theories of action. In that meeting where there is full acceptance, with no attempt to manipulate or utilize, there is a sense of expansiveness and new possibility, as if all chains have been removed. Some might claim that this is simply an illusion, and that no human being can escape from the power of heredity and conditioning. Buber, however, challenges the assumption that there is no freedom by making a direct appeal to the experience of the deepest form of relating. It is here that we gain intuitions of our ability to determine who we are, and to choose the path that we will take. This experience is to be taken far more seriously than any theory that extinguishes the idea of freedom.

Buber's work provides a link between the three types of discourse in which the concept of personhood is found: transcendental, ethical and social-psychological. His account is transcendental, in that he portrays human relationship as the only valid route to what some would describe as an encounter with the divine. His account is ethical, in that it emphasizes so strongly the value of persons. It is not, however, a contribution to analytic debate. For Buber cuts through all argumentation conducted from a detached and intellectualized standpoint, and gives absolute priority to engagement and commitment. Against those who might undermine the concept of personhood through analogies from artificial intelligence, Buber might simply assert that no one has yet engaged with a computer as Thou.

In relation to social psychology, we have here the foundation for an empirical inquiry in which the human being is taken as a person rather than as an object. There is, of course, no way of proving—either through observation or experiment—whether Buber's fundamental assertions are true or false. Any attempt to do so would make them trivial, and statements that appeal through their poetic power would lose their meaning. (It would be equally foolish, for example, to set about verifying the statement "My love is like a red, red rose, that's newly sprung in June.") The key point is this. Before any kind of inquiry can get under way in a discipline that draws on evidence, assumptions have to be made. Popper (1959) likened these to stakes, driven into a swamp, so that a stable building can be constructed. These assumptions are metaphysical, beyond the possibility of testing. Thus, in creating a social psychology, we can choose (or not) to accept these particular assumptions, according to whether they help to make sense of everyday experience and whether they correspond to our moral convictions (Kitwood and Bredin 1992).

To see personhood in relational terms is, I suggest, essential if we are to understand dementia. Even when cognitive impairment is very severe, an I–Thou form of meeting and relating is often possible. There is, however, a very somber point to consider about contemporary practice. It is that a man or woman could be given the most accurate diagnosis, subjected to the most thorough assessment, provided with a highly detailed care plan and given a place in the most pleasant surroundings—without any meeting of the I–Thou kind ever having taken place.

The Psychodynamics of Exclusion

Many cultures have shown a tendency to depersonalize those who have some form of serious disability, whether of a physical or a psychological kind. A consensus is created, established in tradition and embedded in social practices, that those affected are not real persons. The rationalizations follow on. If people show bizarre behavior "they are possessed by devils"; "they are being punished for the sins of a former life"; "the head is rotten"; "there is a mental disorder whose symptoms are exactly described in the new diagnostic manual."

Several factors come together to cause this dehumanization. In part, no doubt, it corresponds to characteristics of the culture as a whole; where personhood is widely disregarded, those who are powerless are liable to be particularly devalued. Many societies, including our own, are permeated by an ageism which categorizes older people as incompetent, ugly and burdensome, and which discriminates against them at both a personal and a structural level (Bytheway 1995). Those who have dementia are often subjected to ageism in its most extreme form; and, paradoxically, even people who are affected at a relatively young age are often treated as if they were "senile." In financial terms, far too few resources have been allocated to the provision of the necessary services. There is also the fact that very little attention has been given to developing the attitudes and skills that are necessary for good psychological care. In the case of dementia, until very recently this was not even recognized as an issue, with the consequence that many people working in this field have had no proper preparation for their work.

Behind these more obvious reasons, there may be another dynamic which excludes those who have dementia from the world of persons. There seems to be something special about the dementing conditions—almost as if they attract to themselves a particular kind of inhumanity: a social psychology that is malignant in its effects, even when it proceeds from people who are kind and well-intentioned (Kitwood 1990). This might be seen as a defensive reaction, a response to anxieties held in part at an unconscious level.

The anxieties seem to be of two main kinds. First, and naturally enough, every human being is afraid of becoming frail and highly dependent; these fears are liable to be particularly strong in any society where the sense of community is weak or non-existent. Added to that, there is the fear of a long drawn-out process of dying, and of death itself. Contact with those who are elderly, weak and vulnerable is liable to activate these fears, and threaten our basic sense of security (Stevenson 1989). Second, we carry fears about mental instability. The thought of being insane, deranged, lost forever in confusion, is terrifying. Many people have come close to this at some point, perhaps in times of great stress, or grief, or personal catastrophe, or while suffering from a disease that has affected mental functioning. At the most dreadful end of these experiences lies the realm of "unbeing," where even the sense of self is undermined.

Dementia in another person has the power to activate fears of both kinds: those concerned with dependence and frailty, and those concerned with going insane. Moreover, there is no real consolation in saying "it won't happen to me," which can be done with many other anxiety-provoking conditions. Dementia is present in almost every street, and discussed repeatedly in the media. We know also that people from all kinds of background are affected, and that among those over 80 the proportion may be as high as one in five. So in being close to a person with dementia we may be seeing some terrifying anticipation of how we might become.

It is not surprising, then, if sensitivity has caused many people to shrink from such a prospect. Some way has to be found for making the anxieties bearable. The highly defensive tactic is to turn those who have dementia into a different species, not persons in the full sense. The principal problem, then, is not that of changing people with dementia, or of "managing" their behavior; it is that of moving beyond our own anxieties and defenses, so that true meeting can occur, and life-giving relationships can grow.

The Uniqueness of Persons

At a commonsensical level it is obvious that each person is profoundly different from all others. It is easy to list some of the dimensions of that difference: culture, gender, temperament, social class, lifestyle, outlook, beliefs, values, commitments, tastes, interests—and so on. Added to this is the matter of personal history. Each person has come to be who they are by a route that is uniquely their own; every stage of the journey has left its mark.

In most of the contexts of everyday life, perhaps this kind of perception will suffice. There are times, however, when it is essential to penetrate the veil of common sense and use theory to develop a deeper understanding. It is not that theory is important in itself, but that it can challenge popular misconceptions; and it helps to generate sensitivity to areas of need, giving caring actions a clearer direction (Kitwood 1997).

Within conventional psychology the main attempt to make sense of the differences between persons has been through the concept of personality, which may roughly be defined as "a set of widely generalized dispositions to act in certain kinds of way" (Alston 1976). The concept of personality, in itself, is rich enough to provide many therapeutic insights. However, by far the greatest amount of effort in psychology has been spent in attempts to "measure" it in terms of a few dimensions (extraversion, neuroticism, and so on), using standard questionnaires—personality inventories, as they are often called. The questions tend to be simplistic and are usually answered through self-report. This approach does have some value, perhaps, in helping to create a general picture, and it has been used in this way in the context of dementia. The main use of personality measurement, however, has been in classifying and selecting people for purposes that were not their own. Psychometric methodology is, essentially, a servant of the I–It mode.

There is another approach within psychology, whose central assumption is that each person is a meaning-maker and an originating source of action (Harré and Secord 1972, Harré 1993). Because of its special interest in everyday life it is sometimes described as being ethogenic, by analogy with the ethological study of animals in their natural habitats. Social life can be considered to consist of a series of episodes, each with certain overriding characteristics (buying a pot plant, sharing a meal, and so on). In each episode the participants make their "definitions of the situation" usually at a level just below conscious awareness, and then bring more or less ready-made action schemata into play. Interaction occurs as each interprets the meaning of the others' actions. Personality here is viewed as an individual's stock of learned resources for action. It is recognized that one person may have a richer set of resources than another, and in that sense have a more highly developed personality. A full "personality inventory" would consist of the complete list of such resources, together with the types of situation in which each item is typically deployed.

This view can be taken further by assimilating to it some ideas that are central to depth psychology and psychotherapeutic work. The resources are of two main kinds, which we might term *adaptive* and *experiential*. The first of these consists of learned ways of responding "appropriately" to other people's demands (both hidden and explicit), to social situations, and to the requirements of given roles. The process of learning is relatively straightforward, and is sometimes portrayed as involving imitation, identification and internalization (Danziger 1978). The second kind of resource relates to a person's capacity to experience what he or she is actually undergoing. Development here occurs primarily when there is an abundance of comfort, pleasure, security and freedom. In Jungian theory the adaptive resources correspond roughly to the ego, and the experiential resources to the Self (Jung 1934). The term that I shall use for the latter is "experiential self."

In an ideal world, both kinds of personal resource would grow together. The consequence would be an adult who was highly competent in many areas of life, and who had a well-developed subjectivity. He or she would be "congruent," in the sense used by Rogers (1961): that is, there would be a close correspondence between what the person was undergoing, experiencing, and communicating to others. In fact, however, this is very rarely the case. The development of adaptive resources is often blocked by lack of opportunity, by the requirements of survival, and sometimes by the naked imposition of power. The growth of an experiential self is impeded where there is cruelty or a lack of love, or where the demands of others are overwhelming. Many people have been subjected to some form of childhood abuse: physical, sexual, emotional, commercial, spiritual. Areas of pain and inner conflict are hidden away, and the accompanying anxiety is sealed off by psychological defenses. According to the theorists of Transactional Analysis, this is the context in which each person acquires a "script"—a way of "getting by" that makes it possible to function in difficult circumstances (Stewart and Joines 1987). As a result of extreme overadaptation, so Winnicott suggested, a person acquires a "false self," a "front" that is radically out of touch with experience and masks an inner chaos (Davis and Wallbridge 1981).

These ideas, which I have sketched here in only the barest outline, can be developed into a many-sided view or model of personal being. As we shall see, it can shed much light on the predicament of men and women who have dementia. Where resources have been lost, we might ask some very searching questions about what has happened and why. If personhood appears to have been undermined, is any of that a consequence of the ineptitude of others, who have all their cognitive powers intact? If uniqueness has faded into a grey oblivion, how far is it because those around have not developed the empathy that is necessary, or their ability to relate in a truly personal way? Thus we are invited to look carefully at ourselves, and ponder on how we have developed as persons; where we are indeed strong and capable, but also where we are damaged and deficient. In particular, we might reflect on whether our own experiential resources are sufficiently well developed for us to be able to help other people in their need.

Personhood and Embodiment

Thus far in this chapter we have looked at issues related to personhood almost totally from the standpoint of the human sciences. The study of dementia, however, has been dominated by work in such disciplines as anatomy, physiology, biochemistry, pathology and genetics. If our account of personhood is to be complete, then, we must find a way of bringing the discourses of the human and natural sciences together.

There is a long-standing debate within philosophy concerning the problem of how the mind is related to the body, and to matter itself. The debate first took on a clear form with the work of Descartes in the seventeenth century, and since that time several distinct positions have emerged. I am going to set out one of these, drawing to some extent on the work of the philosopher Donald Davidson (1970), and the brain scientists Steven Rose (1984) and Antonio Damasio (1995). The starting point is to reject the assumption with which Descartes began: that there are two fundamentally different substances, matter and mind. Instead, we postulate a single (exceedingly complex) reality; it can be termed "material," so long as it is clear that "matter" does not consist of the little solid particles that atoms were once taken to be.

We can never grasp this reality, as it really is, because of the limitations of our nervous system, but we can talk about it in several different ways. Often we use an intentional kind of language, with phrases such as "I feel happy," "I believe that you are telling the truth," "I ought to go and visit my aunt." Through this kind of language we can describe our feelings, draw up plans, ask people to give reasons for their actions, and so on. Often when we speak and think along these lines we have a sense of freedom, as if we are genuinely making choices, taking decisions, and making things happen in the world.

The natural sciences operate on very different lines. Here the aim is to be rigorously objective, using systematic observation and experiment. Within any one science regularities are discovered, and processes are seen in terms of causal relationships. People who work as scientists sometimes have a sense of absolute determinism. The determinism is actually built in from the start; it is part of the "grammar." We know no other way of doing the thing called natural science.

Each type of discourse has its particular uses. One of the greatest and commonest mistakes is to take the descriptions and explanations given in language as if these were the reality itself. Once that is done, many false problems arise; for example, whether or not we really have free will, whether the mind is inside the brain, whether the emotions are merely biochemical, and so on. There are strong reasons for believing that the reality itself, whatever it may be, is far too complex to be caught fully in any of our human nets of language.

Moving on now to the topic of mind and brain, the basic assumption is that any psychological event (such as deciding to go for a walk) or state (such as feeling hungry) is also a brain event or state. It is not that the psychological experience (ψ) is causing the brain activity (**b**) or vice versa; it is simply that some aspect of the true reality is being described in two different ways.

Hence in any individual, $\psi \equiv \mathbf{b}$

The "equation" simply serves to emphasize the assumption that psychology and neurology are, in truth, inseparable.

It is not known how far experiences which two different individuals describe in the same way have parallel counterparts in brain function; scanning methods which look at brain metabolism do, however, suggest broad similarities (Fischbach 1992).

Now the brain events or states occur within an "apparatus" that has a structure, an architecture. The key functioning part is a system of around ten thousand million (10^{10}) neurons, with their myriads of branches and connections, or synapses. A synapse is the point at which a "message" can pass from one neurone to another, thus creating the possibility of very complex "circuits." So far as is known, the basic elements of this system, some general features of its development, and most of the "deeper" forms of circuitry (older in evolutionary terms), are genetically "given." On the other hand the elaboration of the whole structure, and particularly the cerebral cortex, is unique to each individual and not pregiven. The elaboration, then, is epigenetic: subject to processes of learning that occur after the genes have had their say. Each human face is unique; so also is each human brain.

It is probable that there are at least two basic types of learning: explicit and implicit (Kandel and Hawkins 1992). The former involves, for example, remembering faces and places, facts and theories. The latter involves acquiring skills that have a strong physical component; for example learning to walk, to swim or to play the piano. In both cases, learning is thought to proceed by stages. First, over a period of minutes or hours, existing neuron circuits are modified, by the strengthening and weakening of synaptic connections that already exist. Then, and much more slowly—over days, weeks and months—new synaptic connections are formed.

> The design of brain circuits continues to change. The circuits are not only receptive to the results of first experiences, but repeatedly pliable and modifiable by continued experience. Some circuits are remodelled over and over throughout the life span, according to the changes that the organism undergoes.
>
> (Damasio 1995: 112)

The brain is a "plastic" organ. The continuing developmental aspect of its structure can be symbolized as B^d.

In dementia there is usually a loss of neurons and synaptic connections, making it impossible for the brain to carry out its full set of functions (Terry 1992). Some of this occurs slowly, and is a "normal" part of aging. It probably arises from the accumulation of errors in the reproduction of biological materials over a long period, and chemical processes such as oxidation. The more serious and rapid losses, however, appear to be the consequence of disease or degenerative processes, and these may be symbolized as B_p (brain pathology). So, very crudely, the situation within an individual can be represented thus:

$$\frac{\psi \equiv \mathbf{b}}{(B^d, B_p)}$$

(Any psychological event or state is also a brain event or state, "carried" by a brain whose structure has been determined by both developmental and pathological factors.)

If this view is correct in principle, it shows how the issues related to personhood are also those of brain and body. Here, there is one particularly important point to note. It is that the developmental, epigenetic aspects of brain structure have been grossly neglected in recent biomedical research on dementia; moreover, there is scarcely a hint of interest in this topic in contemporary psychiatry and clinical psychology. Yet neuroscience now suggests that there may be very great differences between human beings in the degree to which nerve architecture has developed as a result of learning and experience. It follows that individuals may vary considerably in the extent to which they are able to withstand processes in the brain that destroy synapses, and hence in their resistance to dementia.

In this kind of way we move towards a "neurology of personhood." All events in human interaction—great and small—have their counterpart at a neurological level. The sense of freedom which Buber associates with I–Thou relating may correspond to a biochemical environment that is particularly conducive to nerve growth. A malignant social psychology may actually be damaging to nerve tissue. Dementia may be induced in part, by the stresses of life. Thus anyone who envisages the effects of care as being "purely psychological," independent of what is happening in the nervous system, is perpetuating the error of Descartes in trying to separate mind from body. Maintaining personhood is both a psychological and a neurological task.

REFERENCES

Alston, W. P. 1976. Traits, consistency and conceptual alternatives for personality theory. In R. Harré (ed.), *Personality*. Oxford: Blackwell.
Barham, P., and Hayward, R. 1991. *From the Mental Patient*. London: Routledge.
Buber, M. 1937. *I and Thou* (trans. by R. Gregor Smith). Edinburgh: Clark.
Bytheway, B. 1995. *Ageism*. Buckingham: Open University Press.
Damasio, A. R. 1995. *Descartes' Error*. London: Picador.
Danziger, K. 1978. *Socialization*. Harmondsworth: Penguin.
Davidson, D. 1970. Mental events. In L. Foster and J. W. Swanson (eds.), *Experience and Theory*. Boston, MA: University of Massachusetts Press.
Davis, M., and Wallbridge, D. 1981. *Boundary and Space*. Harmondsworth: Penguin.
Dennett, D. C. 1975. *Brainstorms: Philosophical Essays on Mind and Psychology*. Brighton: Harvester.
Fischbach, G. D. 1992. Mind and brain. *Scientific American, Special Issue,* September: 24–33.
Harré, R. 1993. Rules, roles and rhetoric. *Psychologist*, 16(1): 24–8.
Harré, R., and Secord, P. F. 1972. *The Explanation of Social Behaviour*. Oxford: Blackwell.
Jung, C. G. 1934. The stages of life. In *Modern Man in Search of a Soul*. London: Routledge and Kegan Paul.
Kandel, E. R., and Hawkins, R. D. 1992. The biological basis of learning and individuality. *Scientific American, Special Issue,* September: 53–60.
King's Fund. 1986. *Living Well into Old Age: Applying Principles of Good Practice to Services for Elderly People with Severe Mental Disabilities*. London: The King's Fund.
Kitwood, T. 1990. The dialectics of dementia: With particular reference to Alzheimer's disease. *Ageing and Society*, 10: 177–96.
Kitwood, T. 1997. The uniqueness of persons in dementia. In M. Marshall (ed.), *The State of the Art in Dementia Care*. London: Centre for Policy on Ageing Publications.
Kitwood, T., and Bredin, K. 1992. Towards a theory of dementia care: personhood and well-being. *Ageing and Society*, 12: 269–87.

Popper, K. 1959. *The Logic of Scientific Discovery.* London: Hutchinson.

Post, S. 1995. *The Moral Challenge of Alzheimer's Disease.* Baltimore, MD: Johns Hopkins University Press.

Quinton, A. 1973. *The Nature of Things.* London: Routledge.

Rogers, C. R. 1961. *On Becoming a Person.* Boston, MA: Houghton Mifflin.

Rose, S. P. R. 1984. Disordered molecules and diseased minds. *Journal of Psychiatric Research,* 4: 357–60.

Stevenson, O. 1989. *Age and Vulnerability.* London: Edward Arnold.

Stewart, I., and Joines, V. 1987. *TA Today.* Nottingham: Lifespan Publications.

Terry, R. D. 1992. The pathogenesis of Alzheimer's disease: What causes dementia? In Y. Chisten and P. Churchland (eds.), *Neurophilosophy and Alzheimer's Disease.* Berlin: Springer Verlag.

Tobin, S. S. 1991. *Personhood in Advanced Old Age.* New York: Springer.

PERSONS AS SELF-CONSCIOUS BEINGS

CHAPTER SIXTEEN

Freedom of the Will and the Concept of a Person

Harry G. Frankfurt

What philosophers have lately come to accept as analysis of the concept of a person is not actually analysis of *that* concept at all. Strawson, whose usage represents the current standard, identifies the concept of a person as "the concept of a type of entity such that *both* predicates ascribing states of consciousness *and* predicates ascribing corporeal characteristics . . . are equally applicable to a single individual of that single type."[1] But there are many entities besides persons that have both mental and physical properties. As it happens—though it seems extraordinary that this should be so—there is no common English word for the type of entity Strawson has in mind, a type that includes not only human beings but animals of various lesser species as well. Still, this hardly justifies the misappropriation of a valuable philosophical term.

Whether the members of some animal species are persons is surely not to be settled merely by determining whether it is correct to apply to them, in addition to predicates ascribing corporeal characteristics, predicates that ascribe states of consciousness. It does violence to our language to endorse the application of the term "person" to those numerous creatures which do have both psychological and material properties but which are manifestly not persons in any normal sense of the word. This misuse of language is doubtless innocent of any theoretical error. But although the offense is "merely verbal," it does significant harm. For it gratuitously diminishes our philosophical vocabulary, and it increases the likelihood that we will overlook the important area of inquiry with which the term "person" is most naturally associated. It might have been expected that no problem would be of more central and persistent concern to philosophers than that of understanding what we ourselves essentially are. Yet this problem is so generally neglected that it has been possible to make off with its very name almost without being noticed and, evidently, without evoking any widespread feeling of loss.

There is a sense in which the word "person" is merely the singular form of "people" and in which both terms connote no more than membership in a certain biological species. In those senses of the word which are of greater philosophical interest, however, the criteria for being a person do not serve primarily to distinguish the members of our own species from the members of other species. Rather, they are designed to capture those attributes which are the subject of our most humane concern with ourselves and the source of what we regard as most important and most problematical in our lives. Now these attributes would be of equal significance to us even if they were not in fact peculiar and common to the members of our own species. What interests us most in the human condition would not interest us less if it were also a feature of the condition of other creatures as well.

Our concept of ourselves as persons is not to be understood, therefore, as a concept of attributes that are necessarily species-specific. It is conceptually possible that members of novel or even of familiar nonhuman species should be persons; and it is also conceptually possible that some members of the human species are not persons. We do in fact assume, on the other hand, that no member of another species is a person. Accordingly, there is a presumption that what is essential to persons is a set of characteristics that we generally suppose—whether rightly or wrongly—to be uniquely human.

It is my view that one essential difference between persons and other creatures is to be found in the structure of a person's will. Human beings are not alone in having desires and motives, or in making choices. They share these things with the members of certain other species, some of whom even appear to engage in deliberation and to make decisions based upon prior thought. It seems to be peculiarly characteristic of humans, however, that they are able to form what I shall call "second-order desires" or "desires of the second order."

Besides wanting and choosing and being moved *to do* this or that, men may also want to have (or not to have) certain desires and motives. They are capable of wanting to be different, in their preferences and purposes, from what they are. Many animals appear to have the capacity for what I shall call "first-order desires" or "desires of the first order," which are simply desires to do or not to do one thing or another. No animal other than man, however, appears to have the capacity for reflective self-evaluation that is manifested in the formation of second-order desires.[2]

{ I }

The concept designated by the verb "to want" is extraordinarily elusive. A statement of the form "*A* wants to *X*"—taken by itself, apart from a context that serves to amplify or to specify its meaning—conveys remarkably little information. Such a statement may be consistent, for example, with each of the following statements: (a) the prospect of doing *X* elicits no sensation or introspectible emotional response in *A*; (b) *A* is unaware that he wants to *X*; (c) *A* believes that he does not want to *X*; (d) *A* wants to refrain from *X*-ing; (e) *A* wants to *Y* and believes that it is impossible for him both to *Y* and to *X*; (f) *A* does not "really" want to *X*; (g) *A* would rather die than *X*; and so on. It is therefore hardly sufficient to formulate the distinction between first-order and second-order desires, as I have done, by suggesting merely that someone has a first-order desire when he wants to do or not to do such-and-such, and that he has a second-order desire when he wants to have or not to have a certain desire of the first order.

As I shall understand them, statements of the form "*A* wants to *X*" cover a rather broad range of possibilities.[3] They may be true even when statements like (a) through (g) are true: when *A* is unaware of any feelings concerning *X*-ing, when he is unaware that he wants to *X*, when he deceives himself about what he wants and believes falsely that he does not want to *X*, when he also has other desires that conflict with his desire to *X*, or when he is ambivalent. The desires in question may be conscious or unconscious, they need not be univocal, and *A* may be mistaken about them. There is a further source of uncertainty with regard to statements that identify someone's desires, however, and here it is important for my purposes to be less permissive.

Consider first those statements of the form "*A* wants to *X*" which identify first-order desires—that is, statements in which the term "to *X*" refers to an action. A statement of this kind does not, by itself, indicate the relative strength of *A*'s desire to *X*. It does not make it clear whether this desire is at all likely to play a decisive role in what *A* actually does or tries to do. For it may correctly be said that *A* wants to *X* even when his desire to *X* is only one among his desires

and when it is far from being paramount among them. Thus, it may be true that
A wants to *X* when he strongly prefers to do something else instead; and it may
be true that he wants to *X* despite the fact that, when he acts, it is not the desire
to *X* that motivates him to do what he does. On the other hand, someone who
states that *A* wants to *X* may mean to convey that it is this desire that is motivat-
ing or moving *A* to do what he is actually doing or that *A* will in fact be moved
by this desire (unless he changes his mind) when he acts.

It is only when it is used in the second of these ways that, given the special
usage of "will" that I propose to adopt, the statement identifies *A*'s will. To identify an agent's will is either to identify the desire (or desires) by which he is
motivated in some action he performs or to identify the desire (or desires) by
which he will or would be motivated when or if he acts. An agent's will, then,
is identical with one or more of his first-order desires. But the notion of the will,
as I am employing it, is not coextensive with the notion of first-order desires. It
is not the notion of something that merely inclines an agent in some degree to
act in a certain way. Rather, it is the notion of an *effective* desire—one that
moves (or will or would move) a person all the way to action. Thus the notion
of the will is not coextensive with the notion of what an agent intends to do.
For even though someone may have a settled intention to do *X*, he may nonetheless do something else instead of doing *X* because, despite his intention, his
desire to do *X* proves to be weaker or less effective than some conflicting
desire.

Now consider those statements of the form "*A* wants to *X*" which identify
second-order desires—that is, statements in which the term "to *X*" refers to a
desire of the first order. There are also two kinds of situation in which it may be
true that *A* wants to want to *X*. In the first place, it might be true of *A* that he
wants to have a desire to *X* despite the fact that he has a univocal desire, altogether free of conflict and ambivalence, to refrain from *X*-ing. Someone might
want to have a certain desire, in other words, but univocally want that desire to
be unsatisfied.

Suppose that a physician engaged in psychotherapy with narcotics addicts
believes that his ability to help his patients would be enhanced if he understood
better what it is like for them to desire the drug to which they are addicted. Suppose that he is led in this way to want to have a desire for the drug. If it is a genuine desire that he wants, then what he wants is not merely to feel the sensations
that addicts characteristically feel when they are gripped by their desires for the
drug. What the physician wants, insofar as he wants to have a desire, is to be
inclined or moved to some extent to take the drug.

It is entirely possible, however, that, although he wants to be moved by a desire to take the drug, he does not want this desire to be effective. He may not want it to move him all the way to action. He need not be interested in finding out what it is like to take the drug. And insofar as he now wants only to *want* to take it, and not to *take* it, there is nothing in what he now wants that would be satisfied by the drug itself. He may now have, in fact, an altogether univocal desire *not* to take the drug; and he may prudently arrange to make it impossible for him to satisfy the desire he would have if his desire to want the drug should in time be satisfied.

It would thus be incorrect to infer, from the fact that the physician now wants to desire to take the drug, that he already does desire to take it. His second-order desire to be moved to take the drug does not entail that he has a first-order desire to take it. If the drug were now to be administered to him, this might satisfy no desire that is implicit in his desire to want to take it. While he wants to want to take the drug, he may have *no* desire to take it; it may be that *all* he wants is to taste the desire for it. That is, his desire to have a certain desire that he does not have may not be a desire that his will should be at all different than it is.

Someone who wants only in this truncated way to want to X stands at the margin of preciosity, and the fact that he wants to want to X is not pertinent to the identification of his will. There is, however, a second kind of situation that may be described by "*A* wants to want to X"; and when the statement is used to describe a situation of this second kind, then it does pertain to what A wants his will to be. In such cases the statement means that A wants the desire to X to be the desire that moves him effectively to act. It is not merely that he wants the desire to X to be among the desires by which, to one degree or another, he is moved or inclined to act. He wants this desire to be effective—that is, to provide the motive in what he actually does. Now when the statement that A wants to want to X is used in this way, it does entail that A already has a desire to X. It could not be true both that A wants the desire to X to move him into action and that he does not want to X. It is only if he does want to X that he can coherently want the desire to X not merely to be one of his desires but, more decisively, to be his will.[4]

Suppose a man wants to be motivated in what he does by the desire to concentrate on his work. It is necessarily true, if this supposition is correct, that he already wants to concentrate on his work. This desire is now among his desires. But the question of whether or not his second-order desire is fulfilled does not turn merely on whether the desire he wants is one of his desires. It turns on whether this desire is, as he wants it to be, his effective desire or will. If, when the chips are down, it is his desire to concentrate on his work that moves him to do what he does, then what he wants at that time is indeed (in the relevant sense) what he wants to want. If it is some other desire that actually moves him when he acts, on the other hand, then what he wants at that time is not (in the relevant sense) what he wants to want. This will be so despite the fact that the desire to concentrate on his work continues to be among his desires.

{ II }

Someone has a desire of the second order either when he wants simply to have a certain desire or when he wants a certain desire to be his will. In situations of the latter kind, I shall call his second-order desires "second-order volitions" or "volitions of the second order." Now it is having second-order volitions, and not having second-order desires generally, that I regard as essential to being a person. It is logically possible, however unlikely, that there should be an agent with second-order desires but with no volitions of the second order. Such a creature, in my view, would not be a person. I shall use the term "wanton" to refer to agents who have first-order desires but who are not persons because, whether or not they have desires of the second order, they have no second-order volitions.[5]

The essential characteristic of a wanton is that he does not care about his will. His desires move him to do certain things, without its being true of him either that he wants to be moved by those desires or that he prefers to be moved by other desires. The class of wantons includes all nonhuman animals that have desires and all very young children. Perhaps it also includes some adult human beings as well. In any case, adult humans may be more or less wanton; they may act wantonly, in response to first-order desires concerning which they have no volitions of the second order, more or less frequently.

The fact that a wanton has no second-order volitions does not mean that each of his first-order desires is translated heedlessly and at once into action. He may have no opportunity to act in accordance with some of his desires. Moreover, the translation of his desires into action may be delayed or precluded either by conflicting desires of the first order or by the intervention of deliberation. For a wanton may possess and employ rational faculties of a high order. Nothing in the concept of a wanton implies that he cannot reason or that he cannot deliberate concerning how to do what he wants to do. What distinguishes the rational wanton from other rational agents is that he is not concerned with the desirability of his desires themselves. He ignores the question of what his will is to be. Not only does he pursue whatever course of action he is most strongly inclined to pursue, but he does not care which of his inclinations is the strongest.

Thus a rational creature, who reflects upon the suitability to his desires of one course of action or another, may nonetheless be a wanton. In maintaining that the essence of being a person lies not in reason but in will, I am far from suggesting that a creature without reason may be a person. For it is only in virtue of his rational capacities that a person is capable of becoming critically aware of his own will and of forming volitions of the second order. The structure of a person's will presupposes, accordingly, that he is a rational being.

The distinction between a person and a wanton may be illustrated by the difference between two narcotics addicts. Let us suppose that the physiological condition accounting for the addiction is the same in both men, and that both succumb inevitably to their periodic desires for the drug to which they are addicted. One of the addicts hates his addiction and always struggles desperately, although to no avail, against its thrust. He tries everything that he thinks might enable him to overcome his desires for the drug. But these desires are too powerful for him to withstand, and invariably, in the end, they conquer him. He is an unwilling addict, helplessly violated by his own desires.

The unwilling addict has conflicting first-order desires: he wants to take the drug, and he also wants to refrain from taking it. In addition to these first-order desires, however, he has a volition of the second order. He is not a neutral with regard to the conflict between his desire to take the drug and his desire to refrain from taking it. It is the latter desire, and not the former, that he wants to constitute his will; it is the latter desire, rather than the former, that he wants to be effective and to provide the purpose that he will seek to realize in what he actually does.

The other addict is a wanton. His actions reflect the economy of his first-order desires, without his being concerned whether the desires that move him to act are desires by which he wants to be moved to act. If he encounters problems in obtaining the drug or in administering it to himself, his responses to his urges to take it may involve deliberation. But it never occurs to him to consider whether he wants the relations among his desires to result in his having the will he has. The wanton addict may be an animal, and thus incapable of being concerned about his will. In any event he is, in respect of his wanton lack of concern, no different from an animal.

The second of these addicts may suffer a first-order conflict similar to the first-order conflict suffered by the first. Whether he is human or not, the wanton may (perhaps due to conditioning) both want to take the drug and want to refrain from taking it. Unlike the unwilling addict, however, he does not prefer that one of his conflicting desires should be paramount over the other; he does not prefer that one first-order desire rather than the other should constitute his will. It would be misleading to say that he is neutral as to the conflict between his desires, since this would suggest that he regards them as equally acceptable. Since he has no identity apart from his first-order desires, it is true neither that he prefers one to the other nor that he prefers not to take sides.

It makes a difference to the unwilling addict, who is a person, which of his conflicting first-order desires wins out. Both desires are his, to be sure; and whether he finally takes the drug or finally succeeds in refraining from taking it, he acts to satisfy what is in a literal sense his own desire. In either case he does something he himself wants to do, and he does it not because of some external influence whose aim happens to coincide with his own but because of his desire to do it. The unwilling addict identifies himself, however, through the formation of a second-order volition, with one rather than with the other of his conflicting first-order desires. He makes one of them more truly his own and, in so doing, he withdraws himself from the other. It is in virtue of this identification and withdrawal, accomplished through the formation of a second-order volition, that the unwilling addict may meaningfully make the analytically puzzling statements that the force moving him to take the drug is a force other than his own, and that it is not of his own free will but rather against his will that this force moves him to take it.

The wanton addict cannot or does not care which of his conflicting first-order desires wins out. His lack of concern is not due to his inability to find a convincing basis for preference. It is due either to his lack of the capacity for reflection or to his mindless indifference to the enterprise of evaluating his own desires and motives.[6] There is only one issue in the struggle to which his first-order conflict may lead: whether the one or the other of his conflicting desires is the stronger. Since he is moved by both desires, he will not be altogether satisfied by what he does no matter which of them is effective. But it makes no difference *to him* whether his craving or his aversion gets the upper hand. He has no stake in the conflict between them and so, unlike the unwilling addict, he can neither win nor lose the struggle in which he is engaged. When a *person* acts, the desire by which he is moved is either the will he wants or a will he wants to be without. When a *wanton* acts, it is neither.

{ III }

There is a very close relationship between the capacity for forming second-order volitions and another capacity that is essential to persons—one that has often been considered a distinguishing mark of the human condition. It is only because a person has volitions of the second order that he is capable both of enjoying and of lacking freedom of the will. The concept of a person is not only, then, the concept of a type of entity that has both first-order desires and volitions of the second order. It can also be construed as the concept of a type of entity for whom the freedom of its will may be a problem. This concept excludes all wantons, both infrahuman and human, since they fail to satisfy an essential condition for the enjoyment of freedom of the will. And it excludes those suprahuman beings, if any, whose wills are necessarily free.

Just what kind of freedom is the freedom of the will? This question calls for an identification of the special area of human experience to which the concept of freedom of the will, as distinct from the concepts of other sorts of freedom, is particularly germane. In dealing with it, my aim will be primarily to locate the problem with which a person is most immediately concerned when he is concerned with the freedom of his will.

According to one familiar philosophical tradition, being free is fundamentally a matter of doing what one wants to do. Now the notion of an agent who does what he wants to do is by no means an altogether clear one: both the doing and the wanting, and the appropriate relation between them as well, require elucidation. But although its focus needs to be sharpened and its formulation refined, I believe that this notion does capture at least part of what is implicit in the idea of an agent who *acts* freely. It misses entirely, however, the peculiar content of the quite different idea of an agent whose *will* is free.

We do not suppose that animals enjoy freedom of the will, although we recognize that an animal may be free to run in whatever direction it wants. Thus, having the freedom to do what one wants to do is not a sufficient condition of having a free will. It is not a necessary condition either. For to deprive someone of his freedom of action is not necessarily to undermine the freedom of his will. When an agent is aware that there are certain things he is not free to do, this doubtless affects his desires and limits the range of choices he can make. But suppose that someone, without being aware of it, has in fact lost or been deprived of his freedom of action. Even though he is no longer free to do what he wants to do, his will may remain as free as it was before. Despite the fact that he is not free to translate his desires into actions or to act according to the determinations of his will, he may still form those desires and make those determinations as freely as if his freedom of action had not been impaired.

When we ask whether a person's will is free we are not asking whether he is in a position to translate his first-order desires into actions. That is the question of whether he is free to do as he pleases. The question of the freedom of his will does not concern the relation between what he does and what he wants to do. Rather, it concerns his desires themselves. But what question about them is it?

It seems to me both natural and useful to construe the question of whether a person's will is free in close analogy to the question of whether an agent enjoys freedom of action. Now freedom of action is (roughly, at least) the freedom to do what one wants to do. Analogously, then, the statement that a person enjoys freedom of the will means (also roughly) that he is free to want what he wants to want. More precisely, it means that he is free to will what he wants to will, or to have the will he wants. Just as the question about the freedom of an agent's action has to do with whether it is the action he wants to perform, so the question about the freedom of his will has to do with whether it is the will he wants to have.

It is in securing the conformity of his will to his second-order volitions, then, that a person exercises freedom of the will. And it is in the discrepancy between his will and his second-order volitions, or in his awareness that their coincidence is not his own doing but only a happy chance, that a person who does not have this freedom feels its lack. The unwilling addict's will is not free. This is shown by the fact that it is not the will he wants. It is also true, though in a different way, that the will of the wanton addict is not free. The wanton addict neither has the will he wants nor has a will that differs from the will he wants. Since he has no volitions of the second order, the freedom of his will cannot be a problem for him. He lacks it, so to speak, by default.

People are generally far more complicated than my sketchy account of the structure of a person's will may suggest. There is as much opportunity for ambivalence, conflict, and self-deception with regard to desires of the second order, for example, as there is with regard to first-order desires. If there is an unresolved conflict among someone's second-order desires, then he is in danger of having no second-order volition; for unless this conflict is resolved, he has no preference concerning which of his first-order desires is to be his will. This condition, if it is so severe that it prevents him from identifying himself in a sufficiently decisive way with *any* of his conflicting first-order desires, destroys him as a person. For it either tends to paralyze his will and to keep him from acting at all, or it tends to remove him from his will so that his will operates without his participation. In both cases he becomes, like the unwilling addict though in a different way, a helpless bystander to the forces that move him.

Another complexity is that a person may have, especially if his second-order desires are in conflict, desires and volitions of a higher order than the second. There is no theoretical limit to the length of the series of desires of higher and higher orders; nothing except common sense and, perhaps, a saving fatigue prevents an individual from obsessively refusing to identify himself with any of his desires until he forms a desire of the next higher order. The tendency to generate such a series of acts of forming desires, which would be a case of humanization run wild, also leads toward the destruction of a person.

It is possible, however, to terminate such a series of acts without cutting it off arbitrarily. When a person identifies himself *decisively* with one of his first-order desires, this commitment "resounds" throughout the potentially endless array of higher orders. Consider a person who, without reservation or conflict, wants to be motivated by the desire to concentrate on his work. The fact that his second-order volition to be moved by this desire is a decisive one means that there is no room for questions concerning the pertinence of desires or volitions of higher orders. Suppose the person is asked whether he wants to want to want to concentrate on his work. He can properly insist that this question concerning a third-order desire does not arise. It would be a mistake to claim that, because he has not considered whether he wants the second-order volition he has formed, he is indifferent to the question of whether it is with this volition or with some other that he wants his will to accord. The decisiveness of the commitment he has made means that he has decided that no further question about his second-order volition, at any higher order, remains to be asked. It is relatively unimportant whether we explain this by saying that this commitment implicitly generates an endless series of confirming desires of higher orders, or by saying that the commitment is tantamount to a dissolution of the pointedness of all questions concerning higher orders of desire.

Examples such as the one concerning the unwilling addict may suggest that volitions of the second order, or of higher orders, must be formed deliberately and that a person characteristically struggles to ensure that they are satisfied. But the conformity of a person's will to his higher-order volitions may be far more thoughtless and spontaneous than this. Some people are naturally moved by kindness when they want to be kind, and by nastiness when they want to be nasty, without any explicit forethought and without any need for energetic self-control. Others are moved by nastiness when they want to be kind and by kindness when they intend to be nasty, equally without forethought and without active resistance to these violations of their higher-order desires. The enjoyment of freedom comes easily to some. Others must struggle to achieve it.

{ IV }

My theory concerning the freedom of the will accounts easily for our disinclination to allow that this freedom is enjoyed by the members of any species inferior to our own. It also satisfies another condition that must be met by any such theory, by making it apparent why the freedom of the will should be regarded as desirable. The enjoyment of a free will means the satisfaction of certain desires—desires of the second or of higher orders—whereas its absence means their frustration. The satisfactions at stake are those which accrue to a person of whom it may be said that his will is his own. The corresponding frustrations are those suffered by a person of whom it may be said that he is estranged from himself, or that he finds himself a helpless or a passive bystander to the forces that move him.

A person who is free to do what he wants to do may yet not be in a position to have the will he wants. Suppose, however, that he enjoys both freedom of action and freedom of the will. Then he is not only free to do what he wants to do; he is also free to want what he wants to want. It seems to me that he has, in that case, all the freedom it is possible to desire or to conceive. There are other good things in life, and he may not possess some of them. But there is nothing in the way of freedom that he lacks.

It is far from clear that certain other theories of the freedom of the will meet these elementary but essential conditions: that it be understandable why we desire this freedom and why we refuse to ascribe it to animals. Consider, for example, Roderick Chisholm's quaint version of the doctrine that human freedom entails an absence of causal determination.[7] Whenever a person performs a free action, according to Chisholm, it's a miracle. The motion of a person's hand, when the person moves it, is the outcome of a series of physical causes; but some event in this series, "and presumably one of those that took place within the brain, was caused by the agent and not by any other events" (18). A free agent has, therefore, "a prerogative which some would attribute only to God: each of us, when we act, is a prime mover unmoved" (23).

This account fails to provide any basis for doubting that animals of subhuman species enjoy the freedom it defines. Chisholm says nothing that makes it seem less likely that a rabbit performs a miracle when it moves its leg than that a man does so when he moves his hand. But why, in any case, should anyone *care* whether he can interrupt the natural order of causes in the way Chisholm describes? Chisholm offers no reason for believing that there is a discernible difference between the experience of a man who miraculously initiates a series of causes when he moves his hand and a man who moves his hand without any such breach of the normal causal sequence. There appears to be no concrete basis for preferring to be involved in the one state of affairs rather than in the other.[8]

It is generally supposed that, in addition to satisfying the two conditions I have mentioned, a satisfactory theory of the freedom of the will necessarily provides an analysis of one of the conditions of moral responsibility. The most common recent approach to the problem of understanding the freedom of the will has been, indeed, to inquire what is entailed by the assumption that someone is morally responsible for what he has done. In my view, however, the relation between moral responsibility and the freedom of the will has been very widely misunderstood. It is not true that a person is morally responsible for what he has done only if his will was free when he did it. He may be morally responsible for having done it even though his will was not free at all.

A person's will is free only if he is free to have the will he wants. This means that, with regard to any of his first-order desires, he is free either to make that desire his will or to make some other first-order desire his will instead. Whatever his will, then, the will of the person whose will is free could have been otherwise; he could have done otherwise than to constitute his will as he did. It is a vexed question just how "he could have done otherwise" is to be understood in contexts such as this one. But although this question is important to the theory of freedom, it has no bearing on the theory of moral responsibility. For the assumption that a person is morally responsible for what he has done does not entail that the person was in a position to have whatever will he wanted.

This assumption *does* entail that the person did what he did freely, or that he did it of his own free will. It is a mistake, however, to believe that someone acts freely only when he is free to do whatever he wants or that he acts of his own free will only if his will is free. Suppose that a person has done what he wanted to do, that he did it because he wanted to do it, and that the will by which he was moved when he did it was his will because it was the will he wanted. Then he did it freely and of his own free will. Even supposing that he could have done otherwise, he would not have done otherwise; and even supposing that he could have had a different will, he would not have wanted his will to differ from what it was. Moreover, since the will that moved him when he acted was his will because he wanted it to be, he cannot claim that his will was forced upon him or that he was a passive bystander to its constitution. Under these conditions, it is quite irrelevant to the evaluation of his moral responsibility to inquire whether the alternatives that he opted against were actually available to him.[9]

In illustration, consider a third kind of addict. Suppose that his addiction has the same physiological basis and the same irresistible thrust as the addictions of the unwilling and wanton addicts, but that he is altogether delighted with his condition. He is a willing addict, who would not have things any other way. If the grip of his addiction should somehow weaken, he would do whatever he could to reinstate it; if his desire for the drug should begin to fade, he would take steps to renew its intensity.

The willing addict's will is not free, for his desire to take the drug will be effective regardless of whether or not he wants this desire to constitute his will. But when he takes the drug, he takes it freely and of his own free will. I am inclined to understand his situation as involving the overdetermination of his first-order desire to take the drug. This desire is his effective desire because he is physiologically addicted. But it is his effective desire also because he wants it to be. His will is outside his control, but, by his second-order desire that his desire for the drug should be effective, he has made this will his own. Given that it is therefore not only because of his addiction that his desire for the drug is effective, he may be morally responsible for taking the drug.

My conception of the freedom of the will appears to be neutral with regard to the problem of determinism. It seems conceivable that it should be causally determined that a person is free to want what he wants to want. If this is conceivable, then it might be causally determined that a person enjoys a free will. There is no more than an innocuous appearance of paradox in the proposition that it is determined, ineluctably and by forces beyond their control, that certain people have free wills and that others do not. There is no incoherence in the proposition that some agency other than a person's own is responsible (even *morally* responsible) for the fact that he enjoys or fails to enjoy freedom of the will. It is possible that a person should be morally responsible for what he does of his own free will and that some other person should also be morally responsible for his having done it.[10]

On the other hand, it seems conceivable that it should come about by chance that a person is free to have the will he wants. If this is conceivable, then it might be a matter of chance that certain people enjoy freedom of the will and that certain others do not. Perhaps it is also conceivable, as a number of philosophers believe, for states of affairs to come about in a way other than by chance or as the outcome of a sequence of natural causes. If it is indeed conceivable for the relevant states of affairs to come about in some third way, then it is also possible that a person should in that third way come to enjoy the freedom of the will.

NOTES

1. P. F. Strawson, *Individuals* (London: Methuen, 1959), pp. 101–102. Ayer's usage of "person" is similar: "it is characteristic of persons in this sense that besides having various physical properties . . . they are also credited with various forms of consciousness" [A. J. Ayer, *The Concept of a Person* (New York: St. Martin's, 1963), p. 82]. What concerns Strawson and Ayer is the problem of understanding the relation between mind and body, rather than the quite different problem of understanding what it is to be a creature that not only has a mind and a body but is also a person.

2. For the sake of simplicity, I shall deal only with what someone wants or desires, neglecting related phenomena such as choices and decisions. I propose to use the verbs "to want" and "to desire" interchangeably, although they are by no means perfect synonyms. My motive in forsaking the established nuances of these words arises from the fact that the verb "to want," which suits my purposes better so far as its meaning is concerned, does not lend itself so readily to the formation of nouns as does the verb "to desire." It is perhaps acceptable, albeit graceless, to speak in the plural of someone's "wants." But to speak in the singular of someone's "want" would be an abomination.

3. What I say in this paragraph applies not only to cases in which "to X" refers to a possible action or inaction. It also applies to cases in which "to X" refers to a first-order desire and in which the statement that "*A* wants to X" is therefore a shortened version of a statement—"*A* wants to want to X"—that identifies a desire of the second order.

4. It is not so clear that the entailment relation described here holds in certain kinds of cases, which I think may fairly be regarded as nonstandard, where the essential difference between the standard and the nonstandard cases lies in the kind of description by which the first-order desire in question is identified. Thus, suppose that *A* admires *B* so fulsomely that, even though he does not know what *B* wants to do, he wants to be effectively moved by whatever desire effectively moves *B*; without knowing what *B*'s will is, in other words, *A* wants his own will to be the same. It certainly does not follow that *A* already has, among his desires, a desire like the one that constitutes *B*'s will. I shall not pursue here the questions of whether there are genuine counterexamples to the claim made in the text or of how, if there are, that claim should be altered.

5. Creatures with second-order desires but no second-order volitions differ significantly from brute animals, and, for some purposes, it would be desirable to regard them as persons. My usage, which withholds the designation "person" from them, is thus somewhat arbitrary. I adopt it largely because it facilitates the formulation of some of the points I wish to make. Hereafter, whenever I consider statements of the form "*A* wants to want to X," I shall have in mind statements identifying second-order volitions and not statements identifying second-order desires that are not second-order volitions.

6. In speaking of the evaluation of his own desires and motives as being characteristic of a person, I do not mean to suggest that a person's second-order volitions necessarily manifest a *moral* stance on his part toward his first-order desires. It may not be from the

278   *Harry G. Frankfurt*

point of view of morality that the person evaluates his first-order desires. Moreover, a person may be capricious and irresponsible in forming his second-order volitions and give no serious consideration to what is at stake. Second-order volitions express evaluations only in the sense that they are preferences. There is no essential restriction on the kind of basis, if any, upon which they are formed.

7. "Freedom and Action," in K. Lehrer, ed., *Freedom and Determinism* (New York: Random House, 1966), pp. 11–44.

8. I am not suggesting that the alleged difference between these two states of affairs is unverifiable. On the contrary, physiologists might well be able to show that Chisholm's conditions for a free action are not satisfied, by establishing that there is no relevant brain event for which a sufficient physical cause cannot be found.

9. For another discussion of the considerations that cast doubt on the principle that a person is morally responsible for what he has done only if he could have done otherwise, see my "Alternate Possibilities and Moral Responsibility," *Journal of Philosophy*, LXVI, 23 (Dec 4, 1969): 829–839.

10. There is a difference between being *fully* responsible and being *solely* responsible. Suppose that the willing addict has been made an addict by the deliberate and calculated work of another. Then it may be that both the addict and this other person are fully responsible for the addict's taking the drug, while neither of them is solely responsible for it. That there is a distinction between full moral responsibility and sole moral responsibility is apparent in the following example. A certain light can be turned on or off by flicking either of two switches, and each of these switches is simultaneously flicked to the "on" position by a different person, neither of whom is aware of the other. Neither person is solely responsible for the light's going on, nor do they share the responsibility in the sense that each is partially responsible; rather, each of them is fully responsible.

Part II / Persons at the Beginning of Life

CHAPTER SEVENTEEN

Jewish Perspectives on Abortion

Aaron L. Mackler

Jewish tradition holds that the fetus has value and that elective abortion generally is wrong.[1] However, if there is a conflict between the life of the fetus and
the life of the woman, the imperative to protect the woman's life takes precedence. Jewish writers express diverse views about whether and to what extent
the woman's health and well-being also could justify abortion. This essay will
sketch the historical development of Jewish perspectives and then will examine
contemporary views, first briefly regarding the status of the fetus or unborn
child and then more extensively concerning the acceptability of abortion in
various circumstances.

Historical Development

Judaism has roots in the Hebrew Bible (also known as Tanakh, or Old Testa-
ment). For traditional Judaism, the Torah (first five books of the Bible) represents
the paradigmatic revelation of God's will and serves as the foundational text for
ascertaining concrete moral responsibilities. The Hebrew Bible does not directly
discuss the issue of abortion but does provide values and concepts that help to
shape later deliberation. These values include human life, compassion, healing,

and procreation.² One precedent that becomes influential in the Jewish tradition is provided in the Book of Exodus (21:22–23): "When men fight, and one of them pushes a pregnant woman and a miscarriage results, but no other damage ensues, the one responsible shall be fined according as the woman's husband may exact from him, the payment to be based on reckoning. But if other damage ensues, the penalty shall be life for life."³ The Hebrew Bible also contains passages that reflect the value of the unborn child and God's relationship with individuals before birth. Thus, Jeremiah is addressed by God: "Before I created you in the womb, I selected you; before you were born, I consecrated you" (Jeremiah 1:5). In ascertaining concrete responsibilities, however, the clear distinction between the status of woman and fetus in Exodus 21 exerted greater influence and provides a touchstone for the later development of Jewish law and ethics.

A central text in rabbinic deliberations about abortion is found in the Mishnah, compiled around 200.

> If a woman is having [life-threatening] difficulty giving birth, one dismembers the fetus within her and brings it forth limb by limb, because her life comes before its life. Once the greater part has emerged, one may not touch it, for one may not set aside one life (*nefesh*) to save another.⁴

All Jewish authorities agree that the fetus has a lesser status than that of the woman, though there is debate as to whether this status is virtually equivalent to hers, or significantly lower, according greater scope for permissible abortions. All Jewish authorities agree that abortion is permitted to save the woman's life, though the permissibility of abortion for other reasons is contested.

The Talmud, compiled in the sixth and seventh centuries, includes passages of both *halakhah* (Jewish law) and *aggadah* ("narrative," denoting nonlegal literature) about the fetus and abortion.⁵ In the realm of narrative, we are told that Rabbi Judah Hanasi had a discussion with the Roman emperor Antoninus about when a soul enters the body of a fetus. Antoninus persuaded the rabbi that a soul must be present from conception.⁶ Another passage states that a light burns above the head of the fetus that enables it to see from one end of the world to the other. The fetus learns the entire Torah, which it is caused to forget when it is born.⁷

Sources of *halakhah*, or Jewish law, had a stronger influence on later developments in Jewish law and ethics. Three *halakhic* passages from the Talmud are noteworthy. One (from the tractate *Sanhedrin*) presents the opinion of Rav Huna that a minor may be considered a pursuer, or material aggressor, whose life may be taken in self-defense. Rav Hisda posed a question on the basis of the Mishnah. "We learned, 'once his head has come forth, he may not be harmed, for one may not set aside one life to save another.' But why so; is he not a pursuer?" The response: "There it is different, for she is pursued by heaven." A second passage (from *Arakhin*) discusses a situation that strikes modern readers as bizarre, and most likely was never followed in practice. While Talmudic authorities accepted capital punishment in principle, they believed that a delay between the imposition of a death sentence and the execution would represent cruel and unusual punishment for the guilty party. Accordingly, the Mishnah reports that if a pregnant woman is sentenced to death, she is executed immediately. The Talmud reports the view of Samuel, as quoted by Rav Judah, that the fetus is killed before the execution "so that she will not be subject to disgrace (*nivul*)." While today this ruling has no direct practical application, some authorities have cited this precedent to allow abortion in order to prevent anguish or shame. A third passage (again from *Sanhedrin*) presents the midrash (creative exegesis) of Rabbi Ishmael on Genesis 9:6. This passage is generally understood to mean, "Whoever sheds the blood of man, by man shall his blood be shed." The Hebrew also could be read, "Whoever sheds the blood of man in man, his blood shall be shed." The "man in man" is identified as the fetus in the mother's womb. Accordingly, abortion would be (at least generally and in principle) a capital offense.[8]

Two passages from medieval authorities generally have been understood to pull in opposite directions in the abortion debate. The first is from the commentary of Rashi (eleventh century), explaining the rulings of the first Talmudic passage concerning innocent aggressors: "For as long as it has not come into the world it is not a living person (*nefesh*) and it is permissible to take its life in order to save its mother. Once the head has come forth one may not touch it to kill it, for then it is considered born, and one life may not be taken to save another."[9] This passage would tend to support an understanding of a lesser status for the fetus. Another passage is found in the legal code of Rabbi Moses Maimonides (twelfth century), the *Mishneh Torah*:

This is, moreover, a *mitzvah* [commandment], not to take pity on the life of a pursuer. Therefore, the sages have ruled that if a woman has difficulty giving birth, one dismembers the fetus within her womb, either by drugs or by surgery, because it is like a pursuer seeking to kill her. Once its head has emerged, it may not be touched, for we do not set aside one life for another; this is the natural course of the world.[10]

This passage is understood by many to reflect a status for the fetus virtually equivalent to that of the mother, with relatively restrictive implications for abortion.

As summarized by Rabbi David Feldman, later authorities generally may be categorized into two groups, both agreeing that while abortion is generally prohibited, it does not constitute homicide, and that it is permitted to save the woman's life. One group follows Maimonides, viewing the fetus as having almost the full status of a human person and abortion as akin to homicide. These authorities may "build down" from this position, ruling leniently by construing threats to the woman's life in a broad manner. The other group follows Rashi, emphasizing the subordinate status of the fetus, but then "builds up" to avoid indiscriminate abortion.[11]

Rabbi Joseph Trani (seventeenth century) was responsible for perhaps the first responsum dealing with elective abortion. He held that the fetus is not a *nefesh*, and so abortion does not constitute homicide, but that abortion represents a generally impermissible wounding of the woman. Abortion is permitted "for need" or for the mother's healing. Rabbi Yair Bachrach (seventeenth century) understood abortion to violate a prohibition against contraception (or "wasting seed").[12] While this could allow room for exceptions for compelling reasons, Bachrach refused permission for a woman experiencing remorse after adultery, in order not to condone and foster immorality. Rabbi Jacob Emden (eighteenth century) also understood abortion to violate a prohibition against contraception. He cautiously found room to permit abortion in a case of a woman pregnant from an adulterous relationship. "There is room for leniency for great need, as long as the birth process has not started, even if it is not to save the life of the mother, but to save her from the evil of great pain." For authorities such as Rabbi Ezekiel Landau (eighteenth century) and Rabbi Hayim Soloveitchik (nineteenth century), however, the status of the fetus is virtually equal to that of the mother. Abortion is only permitted to save her life, justified only by the pursuer argument in conjunction with the slightly lesser status of the fetus. Abortion in other cases would violate the prohibition against homicide.[13]

The Status of the Fetus or Unborn Child

No Jewish authority views the status of the fetus as fully equal to that of the mother, even at the end of gestation. Even an opponent of abortion such as Rabbi Immanuel Jakobovits will acknowledge, "Jewish law assumes that the full title to life arises only at birth."[14] This appears to be motivated in part by the traditional authority of the Mishnah text, and in part by the dominant value of saving life (the woman's) reflected in that text. Some Jewish thinkers do accord the fetus the value of a person, virtually equivalent (though not quite fully equal) to that of the mother. Rabbis Hayim Soloveitchik and Mosheh Feinstein rule that the fetus is a person (*nefesh*), though not yet fully so (*nefesh gamur*). Because of this status, and because the fetus's future viability is less certain than that of the mother, abortion would be permitted when that is the only way to save the mother's life. Otherwise, though, abortion would represent the killing of a person, and hence would be prohibited as homicide.[15] Some contemporary Jewish writers argue that current scientific understanding supports a higher status for the fetus than that found in some traditional sources, close to if not quite equal to personhood.[16]

While Jewish writers agree that the fetus does not fully acquire the status of personhood until birth, they hold nevertheless that the fetus does have a significant status that generally would prohibit abortion, albeit with exceptions in appropriate cases. Variation can be seen generally among writers in different movements (denominations) of Judaism: from right to left, Orthodox, Conservative, and Reform.[17] Conservative rabbis Ben Zion Bokser and Kassel Abelson write that throughout gestation, "the fetus is a life in the process of development, and the decision to abort it should never be taken lightly."[18] Others emphasize that abortion destroys "potential life," prevents the development of a personal life of observing *mitzvot* (commandments), and contradicts the creative work of God.[19]

Some authorities have suggested various stages as representing change in the fetus's status, rendering abortion somewhat easier to justify early in gestation and more difficult to justify in later stages. The Talmud refers to the embryo before forty days of development as "mere liquid" (corresponding roughly with much ancient and medieval thought).[20] For some authorities, this suggests greater leeway for abortion in the earliest stages. Some authorities also postulate a significant change at the end of gestation. Throughout pregnancy, the fetus is considered as part of the mother's body; in the Talmud's phrase, *ubar yerekh imo*, "the fetus is the thigh of its mother." Once the birth process begins, the fetus is considered a distinct body, *gufa ahrina*.[21]

Some writers note other markers. Perceptible fetal movement is understood to occur after about three months of gestation. One recent authority refers to viability, at about six months, as a significant marker. Generally, though, these stages are understood to represent quantitative change, somewhat altering the strength of reasons needed to justify abortion, but not decisively altering fetal status. Even at the earliest stages, fetal status is significant, requiring compelling reasons to justify abortion. Even at the last stages before birth, the fetus does not have an equal status to the mother.[22]

The Prohibition of Abortion and Possible Exceptions
Abortion to Save the Mother's Life

All Jewish thinkers would accept abortion if it were required to save the mother's life. This permission reflects in part Jewish understandings regarding the status of the fetus, allowing for greater leniency with regard to ending its life. This also reflects the power of the imperative to preserve life, entailing stringency in this regard.[23] For example, Orthodox rabbi Immanuel Jakobovits condemns abortion as "an appurtenance of murder," and argues against abortion in cases involving rape or likely birth defects. He advocates national laws restricting abortion, even if these impose suffering in some cases. Nevertheless, abortion to prevent a threat to the mother's life is mandated. Indeed,

> such a threat to the mother need not be either immediate or absolutely certain. Even a remote risk of life invokes all the life-saving concessions of Jewish law, provided the fear of such a risk is genuine and confirmed by the most competent medical opinions. Hence, Jewish law would regard it as an indefensible desecration of human life to allow a mother to perish in order to save her unborn child.[24]

Some other Jewish thinkers would agree that abortion is permitted only in order to save the mother's life. Abortion for any other reason would be condemned as unjustifiable homicide.[25]

Abortion to Avoid Serious Threats to Health

Most Jewish writers would accept abortion in some cases that do not involve an immediate threat to the woman's life. Reflecting the values and precedents of the tradition, they tend to do so by expansively construing the mandate to prevent threats to life. Most authorities consider severe psychiatric illness as potentially representing a danger to life, and so even authorities generally opposed to abortion would authorize it in some cases to avoid such dangers.[26] Many would allow abortion to avoid a severe threat to the woman's health, even when her life is not endangered; they argue that abortion does not represent homicide, nor is it biblically forbidden, and so the prohibition of abortion may be superseded by the imperative of healing.[27] A consensus statement of the Conservative movement's Committee on Jewish Law and Standards holds that "abortion is justifiable if a continuation of the pregnancy might cause the mother severe physical or psychological harm."[28]

Orthodox rabbi Ben Zion Uziel allowed abortion in a case in which the woman was threatened by deafness from a continuation of the pregnancy. While this case involves medical risk, Uziel offers a more general rationale for permissible abortion. He cites the Talmud's authorization of fetal death to save a woman from emotional anguish (in connection with capital punishment), and Emden's acceptance of abortion following adultery for "great need" and in order to save the woman from "great pain." Uziel continues: "It is clear that abortion is not permitted unless there is a need, even a slim need (*tzorekh kalush*) such as avoiding dishonor for the mother, but it is certain that if there is no need it is forbidden, because of destruction and the prevention of the possibility of life."[29] Writing about this opinion, Feldman observes: "The law of Israel, just as it requires that the foetus be sacrificed to save the mother's physical life, likewise requires that it be sacrificed to save her spirit from torture and suffering."[30]

Abortion for Other Reasons

Uziel's argument for abortion to avoid deafness suggests a broader range of reasons that might be invoked to justify abortion. Abortion could be justified for great need, and in order to avoid suffering and shame, even without invoking medical threat.

Many Jewish authorities accept abortion in some circumstances to avoid the woman's suffering, even when her health is not directly threatened. The abortion of a fetus with a serious genetic disease, such as Tay-Sachs disease, is often approached in these terms. Jewish writers typically do not claim that the future suffering of the child after birth would make his or her life not worth living, but rather they justify such abortion when it would save the woman from anguish that she would find unbearable. Orthodox rabbi Eliezer Yehudah Waldenberg, for example, appeals to Emden's acceptance of abortion for great need and to avoid great pain. "If so, ask yourself if there is need, suffering, and pain greater than that of our case" involving prenatal diagnosis of Tay-Sachs; as the child suffered on the way to certain death within a number of years, the parents would suffer the anguish of observing without being able to help. This would represent a clear case of allowing abortion for great need and to avoid suffering. Waldenberg expresses greater hesitancy about aborting a fetus with less severe problems. Generally, a fetus with Down syndrome should not be aborted. Indeed,

Waldenberg urges a questioner to avoid amniocentesis to test for this condition, since that procedure would entail unnecessary wounding to the woman and risk fetal death. Amniocentesis would only be appropriate in extreme situations, as when the husband or wife are consumed with worry, unable to sleep day or night. Similarly, aborting a fetus with Down syndrome could be acceptable only in exceptional circumstances, when there is great need because giving birth to a child with this condition would lead to anguish, illness, and harm to the marriage. Such permission could only be given cautiously and on a case-by-case basis, with the authorization of a rabbi familiar with the specific circumstances involved.[31]

Other rabbis, arguing along similar lines, are somewhat more ready to accept abortion in cases of fetal deformity. Conservative rabbi Kassel Abelson writes: "If the tests indicate that the child will be born with major defects that would preclude a normal life and that make the mother and the family anxious about the future, it is permitted to abort the fetus."[32] Reform rabbi Solomon Freehof similarly asserts that in a case in which a pregnant woman had been exposed to rubella, entailing a likelihood of physical and mental deformity, "then for the mother's sake (i.e., her mental anguish now and in the future)" abortion may be performed.[33]

Blu Greenberg is willing to stretch the rubric of therapeutic abortion yet further; though an Orthodox layperson, her views differ markedly from those of Orthodox rabbinic authorities. She acknowledges *halakhic* precedent restricting abortion, as well as dangers of abuse and the devaluation of life, but also notes competing values: "Unless one is physically and emotionally unable to cope, not yet settled in marriage, etc., abortion should be avoided." Precedents allowing abortion to guard the woman's psychological health could be expanded to "encompass such variables as physical strength, stress, even delay in child-raising for purposes of family planning or a career." Greenberg understands herself as a feminist who is part of the Jewish religious community and informed by traditional values; she advocates allowing women to choose abortion when compelled by personal needs and concern for family relationships.[34]

Reform rabbi Balfour Brickner advocates a broad scope for a woman's right to choose abortion, expressing less hesitancy and ambivalence than does Greenberg. He emphasizes that the tradition does not consider the fetus a person, and so the value of the woman's autonomy is decisive. Brickner understands this stance to support women's rights to choose abortion without restrictions as a matter of U.S. law and deference to individual conscience and women's choices as a matter of morality.

It is precisely because of this regard for that sanctity [of human life] that we see as most desirable the right of any couple to be free to produce only that number of children whom they felt they could feed and clothe and educate properly: only that number to whom they could devote themselves as real parents, as creative partners with God. It is precisely this traditional Jewish respect for the sanctity of human life that moves us now to support that legislation which would help all women to be free to choose when and under what circumstances they would elect to bring life into the world.[35]

Even Brickner, at the pro-choice extreme on the spectrum of Jewish writers, acknowledges a need for thoughtfulness in making moral decisions about abortion. "Jewish law teaches a reverent and responsible attitude to the question of abortion."[36] "Judaism looks on abortion with distaste, discourages and tries to restrict it, but it clearly permits it."[37] Other writers, Reform and Conservative as well as Orthodox, give greater emphasis to moral concerns weighing against abortion. Many take care to distinguish their liberal stance from simple abortion on demand. As one Reform responsum concludes: "We do not encourage abortion, nor favor it for trivial reasons, or sanction it 'on demand.' "[38] Likewise, a consensus statement from the Conservative Rabbinical Assembly proclaims: "Jewish tradition is sensitive to the sanctity of life and does not permit abortion on demand."[39]

Jewish writers devote some discussion to the causes leading to abortion. Poverty and sexism should be fought. Greater support should be given to women, children, and families. Attitudes and practices reflecting respect for human life and sexual responsibility should be fostered. Jakobovits criticizes sexual irresponsibility. He also insists that society do more "to assume the burdens which the individual family can no longer bear."[40] Blu Greenberg advocates greater sexual responsibility and worries about "the devaluation of human life": "Abortion is really a symptom of a larger problem. Ours is a society which establishes the value of goods over relationships, or possessions over people, or ease and comfort over labor and a life of giving. . . . As a result, contemporary society borders on the selfish."[41]

Conclusion

For Judaism, the fetus must be respected as potential personal life but does not have the full status of a person at any stage of gestation. All Jewish writers would permit abortion when necessary to save the mother's life. Most Jewish authorities would permit abortion to avoid a serious threat to the mother's health. Many Jewish thinkers would accept abortion in some other circumstances to avoid significant personal suffering for the mother.

A perspective on abortion may be provided by framing the issue in terms of the intrinsic dignity and value of human life, sometimes expressed as the sanctity of life. All Jewish authorities are committed to this principle but specify and balance this principle and others differently. For Jewish thinkers, the life of the fetus or unborn child has value and deserves respect, but somewhat less so than the woman. According to some authorities, the status of the fetus is virtually equal to that of the mother; commitment to the sanctity of life demands abortion to save the woman's life but condemns abortion in any other circumstance. For other Jewish thinkers, the imperative to preserve the life of the woman is more broadly construed, entailing a commitment to preserve health. This approach reflects leniency with regard to fetal life but also the stringency to preserve the woman's life and health.[42] Yet other Jewish writers emphasize that the sanctity of life and respect for human dignity involve more than safeguarding biological existence. There are limits to the sacrifice and suffering a pregnant woman is obligated to undergo, even to preserve the life of the fetus.

Diverse Jewish writers would agree on the important value of reverence for human life. One clear implication of this value is that, as a moral matter, abortion is at least prima facie wrong; that is, the moral prohibition against abortion is binding unless outweighed by competing ethical considerations. As well, reverence for human life supports attention to problems of poverty and attitudes of selfishness, which contribute to the prevalence of abortion and harm human well-being in many other ways.

NOTES

1. This essay draws extensively on my *Introduction to Jewish and Catholic Bioethics: A Comparative Analysis* (Washington, DC: Georgetown University Press, 2003), especially chapter 5, "Abortion," 120–55.

2. See ibid., chapter 1, 1–24.

3. Translations from the Hebrew Bible generally follow NJPS, *Tanakh* (Philadelphia: Jewish Publication Society, 1999). A significant variation is found in the Septuagint, the ancient Greek translation that became influential for Christianity, but not for rabbinic Judaism: "If two men strive and smite a woman, and her child is imperfectly formed, he shall be forced to pay a penalty. . . . But if he be perfectly formed, he shall give life for life. . . ." In John Connery, *Abortion: The Development of the Roman Catholic Perspective*

(Chicago: Loyola University Press, 1977), 17; see also David M. Feldman, *Birth Control in Jewish Law*, rev. ed. (Northvale, NJ: Jason Aronson, 1998), 257–58.

4. Mishnah *Oholot* 7:6.

5. On *halakhah* and *aggadah*, see Mackler, *Introduction to Jewish and Catholic Bioethics*, 45–46.

6. Talmud *Sanhedrin* 91b; Feldman, *Birth Control*, 271. The word translated as "soul" (*neshamah*) does not have all the connotations of "soul" in contemporary English, or in Christianity. It may refer to what in Aristotelian terms might be considered the sensitive (or animalistic) soul; see Aristotle, *De Anima* (*On the Soul*).

7. Talmud *Niddah* 30b.

8. Talmud *Sanhedrin* 72b, *Arakhin* 7a, *Sanhedrin* 57b.

9. Rashi, commentary to *Sanhedrin* 72b.

10. Maimonides, *Mishneh Torah*, "Laws of Murder and the Preservation of Life," 1:9.

11. Feldman, *Birth Control*, 284.

12. See also Avraham Steinberg, *Encyclopedia of Jewish Medical Ethics* (Jerusalem: Schlesinger Institute, 1988), s.v. "Abortion," 2:77; Feldman, *Birth Control*, 251–53. The dominant Jewish position has been that contraception is discouraged, but that sexual relations within marriage are normative and contraception is mandated when needed to protect the life or health of a woman; see Feldman, *Birth Control*. The paradigm of contraception thus would provide support for a general prohibition of abortion that allows exceptions.

13. Soloveitchik, *Hiddushei R. Hayim Halevi al HaRambam* (Israel: n.p., 1992), commentary to Maimonides, *Mishneh Torah*, "Laws of Murder and the Preservation of Life," 1:9, pp. 266–67; Trani, *Resp. Maharit*, No. 99; Bachrach, *Resp. Havot Ya'ir*, No. 31; Emden, *Resp. Sh'elat Ya'avetz*, No. 43; Landau, *Resp. Noda Bi'Yehudah, Mahadura Tinyana, Hoshen Mishpat*, No. 59; all discussed by Feldman, *Birth Control*, 256–89; J. David Bleich, "Abortion in Halakhic Literature," in *Contemporary Halakhic Problems*, vol. 1 (New York: Ktav, 1977), 327–65; and Basil F. Herring, *Jewish Ethics and Halakhah for Our Time* (New York: Ktav and Yeshiva University Press, 1984), 31–43.

14. Immanuel Jakobovits, "Jewish Views on Abortion," in *Abortion and the Law*, ed. David T. Smith (Cleveland: Western Reserve University Press, 1967), 129.

15. Soloveitchik, *Hiddushei R. Hayim Halevi al Ha Rambam*; Feinstein, *Iggerot Moshe*, vol. 7 (Bnei Berak, Israel: Ohel Yosef, 1985), *Hoshen Mishpat* 2, No. 69, p. 296; and sources cited in Steinberg, *Encyclopedia*, 2:78–80.

16. David Novak, *Law and Theology in Judaism* (New York: Ktav, 1974), 123; Richard Alan Block, "The Right to Do Wrong: Reform Judaism and Abortion," *Journal of Reform Judaism* 28, No. 2 (1981): 9–12.

17. See Mackler, *Introduction to Jewish and Catholic Bioethics*, 46–48.

18. Ben Zion Bokser and Kassel Abelson, "A Statement on the Permissibility of Abortion," in *Life and Death Responsibilities in Jewish Biomedical Ethics*, ed. Aaron L. Mackler (New York: Jewish Theological Seminary of America, Finkelstein Institute, 2000), 195.

19. Isaac Klein, "A Teshuvah on Abortion," in *Life and Death Responsibilities in Jewish Biomedical Ethics* (see note 18), 208; Steinberg, *Encyclopedia*, 76–78.

20. Talmud *Yevamot* 69b; Feldman, *Birth Control*, 266. Some have applied the concept of "mere liquid" (*maya be'alma*) to the early preembryo, especially one existing in vitro: Aaron L. Mackler, "In Vitro Fertilization," in *Life and Death Responsibilities in Jewish Biomedical Ethics* (see note 18), 118n42; Elliot N. Dorff, "Stem Cell Research," 2002, http:// www.rabbinicalassembly.org/teshuvot/docs/19912000/dorff_stemcell.pdf (accessed May 29, 2008) at note 18.

21. Feldman, *Birth Control*, 253, 265; Talmud *Hullin* 58a.

22. See Feldman, *Birth Control*, 265–67; Herring, *Jewish Ethics*, 36–38; Eliezer Yehudah Waldenberg, *Tzitz Eliezer* (Jerusalem: n.p., 1985), Vol. 9, No. 51, sec. 3, p. 239; Vol. 14, No. 100, p. 186.

23. See Mackler, *Introduction to Jewish and Catholic Bioethics*, 4–5.

24. Jakobovits, "Jewish Views on Abortion," 143, 124–43.

25. Feinstein (who would only allow abortion if the threat to the mother's life were certain), *Iggerot Moshe*; Bleich, "Abortion," 356; and others cited by Steinberg, *Encyclopedia*, 80–86. Rabbi Issar Unterman considers abortion to be an appurtenance of murder, based partly on Rabbi Ishmael's midrashic reading of Genesis 9:6, noted above; because it is not fully considered murder, abortion is permitted when necessary to save life ("On the Matter of Saving of the Life of a Fetus," *Noam* 6 [1963]: 5, 1–11). Moshe Tendler writes similarly that "abortion is tantamount to murder and can be sanctioned only when the life of the gestating mother is in danger" ("On the Interface of Religion and Medical Science: The Judeo-Biblical Perspective," in *Jewish and Catholic Bioethics: An Ecumenical Dialogue*, ed. Edmund D. Pellegrino and Alan I. Faden [Washington, DC: Georgetown University Press, 1999], 108). Abortion in such cases is traditionally justified by viewing the fetus as a *rodeif*, or (material) aggressor. Catholic writer Lisa Sowle Cahill observes: "Such analogies to assault serve simultaneously to protect the mother and the fetus. As David Novak illustrates by the Jewish comparison of a fetus to a 'pursuer,' references to a victim-aggressor conflict imply that the fetus is to be killed if and only if there exists the gravest reason, i.e., threat to the mother's life" ("Abortion and Argument by Analogy," *Horizons* 9, no. 2 [1982]: 277–78; citing David Novak, "Judaism and Contemporary Bioethics," *Journal of Medicine and Philosophy* 4 [1979]: 357).

26. See Feldman, *Birth Control*, 284–86; Bleich, "Abortion," 362–63; Steinberg, *Encyclopedia*, 85.

27. Steinberg, *Encyclopedia*, 85–86; Bleich, "Abortion," 354–56; Herring, *Jewish Ethics*, 40–42. Some, such as the classical authority Joseph Trani, understand the basic reason for the prohibition of abortion to be that it would represent impermissible self-injury for the woman. As the self-injury of amputation is allowed when it is required to improve health, so abortion would be permitted for this purpose.

28. Bokser and Abelson, "Statement," 195.

29. Ben Zion Uziel, *Mishpetei Uziel* 3, Hoshen Mishpat, No. 46 (Jerusalem: Va'ad L'hotza'at Kitvei Harav, 1995), 224, 221–26; and discussion in Feldman, *Birth Control*, 289–91; Herring, *Jewish Ethics*, 41; Bleich, "Abortion," 355.

30. Feldman, *Birth Control*, 290, attributing this observation to Viktor Aptowitzer.

31. Waldenberg, Vol. 13, No. 102, p. 209; Vol. 14, Nos. 100–102, pp. 183–92. Waldenberg's primary concerns are with preventing anguish for the woman and harm to the marital relationship. In the extreme case of Tay-Sachs, he presents, as a supplementary reason warranting abortion, concern to avoid suffering of the child in the future. Waldenberg emphasizes the need for seriousness and caution in all cases concerning abortion (Vol. 9, No. 51, sec. 3, p. 240; Vol. 14, No. 100, p. 186).

32. Kassel Abelson, "Prenatal Testing and Abortion," in *Life and Death Responsibilities in Jewish Biomedical Ethics*, 219.

33. Solomon Freehof, "Abortion," in *American Reform Responsa*, ed. Walter Jacob (New York: Central Conference of American Rabbis, 1983), No. 171, p. 543.

34. Blu Greenberg, "Abortion: A Challenge to Halakhah," *Judaism* 25 (1976): 202–6.

35. Balfour Brickner, "Judaism and Abortion," in *Contemporary Jewish Ethics*, ed. Menachem Marc Kellner (New York: Sanhedrin, 1978), 282–83.

36. Ibid., 282.

37. Balfour Brickner, "A Critique of Bleich on Abortion," *Sh'ma* 5, No. 85 (1975): 200.

38. Walter Jacob, "When Is Abortion Permitted?" in *Contemporary American Reform Responsa*, ed. Walter Jacob (New York: Central Conference of American Rabbis, 1987), No. 16, p. 27. Reform thinker Mark Washofsky writes: "Two broad conclusions emerge from this picture of a conversation between *halakhic* positions. The first is that a woman would not be entitled to abortion on demand; there must exist a warrant, a sufficient and carefully-reasoned justification for the procedure. The second is that the definition of 'sufficient' will differ from case to individual case" ("Abortion and the Halakhic Conversation: A Liberal Perspective," in *The Fetus and Fertility*, ed. Walter Jacob and Moshe Zemer [Pittsburgh: Rodef Shalom Press, 1995], 75).

39. Bokser and Abelson, "Statement," 195. While supporting abortion for compelling reasons, and advocating generally permissive laws, Conservative rabbi Robert Gordis likewise condemns abortion on demand as immoral: "Abortion on demand is a threat to a basic ethical principle" of reverence for life. "When an embryo is aborted, we are, in the fine rabbinic phrase, 'diminishing the divine image in which man is fashioned'" ("Abortion: Major Wrong or Basic Right?" in *Life and Death Responsibilities* [see note 18], 228).

40. Jakobovits, "Jewish Views on Abortion," 142, 139.

41. Greenberg, "Abortion," 204–207. See also Gordis, "Abortion," 228–29.

42. See Mackler, *Introduction to Jewish and Catholic Bioethics*, 4–5, 8–10, 89–101.

When Do People Begin?

Germain Grisez

"People" here does not refer to God or angels. However, it refers not only to human persons but to beings like E.T., for if such beings arrived on earth, we surely would consider them people like ourselves.

In a 1970 book on abortion, I treated three questions about people's beginnings. When do human individuals begin? In moral reflection, which human individuals should count as persons? And, which for legal purposes? I concluded that most human individuals begin at fertilization and that both morality and law should consider all of them persons.[1] I still think that. But to remedy defects in my treatment and to deal with two decades of development in both embryology and the debate, the questions need fresh treatment, which this paper only sketches out. I hope it will encourage and help someone to write a book on the subject.

To those who are persons, personhood is either accidental or essential. If accidental, it is either bestowed by others or acquired naturally. If essential, persons are either nonbodily substances or bodily. If bodily, either they come to be by substantial change after the biological beginning of new human individuals or every new human individual is a person. And new human individuals come to be either after or at fertilization. Thus, there are six answers to our question.

I. Some think that personhood is a status bestowed by others. On this notion, people begin when others accept them as persons.
II. Others think that personhood is an attribute that some entities develop by a natural process. On this notion, people begin when nonpersonal entities become able to behave as persons.
III. Others think that only certain nonbodily substances—for example, souls or minds—are persons. On this notion, the beginning of a bodily individual need not be the beginning of a person.
IV. Others think that only human bodies with the organic basis for intellectual acts can receive personal souls. On this notion, prepersonal human organisms substantially change into persons.
V. Others think that all whole, human individuals are persons, but that none of them begins until the primitive streak stage. On this notion, people begin two to three weeks after fertilization.
VI. I think that all whole, bodily, substantial individuals of any species having a rational nature are persons, and that most human individuals begin at fertilization. On this notion, most human people begin when a human sperm and ovum fuse.

I shall first dispose of objections against the sixth position by criticizing the other five. Then I shall sketch out the proper rationale of the sixth position.

I. Personhood: A Status Bestowed

Pierre de Locht, a Belgian theologian, having suggested that abortion involves a conflict of rights, formulated one line of argument for the notion that personhood is a status bestowed by others:

> But it seems to me useful to pose a preliminary question: How is one constituted a human person? Is it by a merely biological act? It seems to me astonishing that a spiritual being be constituted by a solely biological act. Does not the fact that the parents *perceive* the fetus as a human person make any difference in its constitution as a human being, as a spiritual being? Is it not necessary that there be established a relation of person to person, a relation of generators with the fetus, for it to become a human person?[2]

On this proposal, parents confer personhood on a fetus by perceiving it as a *thou*, and so giving it a place in the human community.

I suggest arguments along the following lines against this view.

Suppose a pregnant woman does not perceive the fetus as a person, but her husband does. Is that fetus a person or not?

Underlying de Locht's proposal, undoubtedly, is the fact that human meaning-giving constitutes social and cultural realities. But unlike such realities, people are principles of society and culture. So, human meaning-giving presupposes rather than constitutes people.

Also underlying his proposal is the insight that persons are beings who exist only in interpersonal communion. But granting this, one can argue, even without invoking faith, that human individuals are constituted persons not by their parents' perception of them but by God's creative knowledge and love of them.[3]

Mary Warnock, who thinks one can handle relevant moral issues without settling the question of personhood, offers another line of argument for the notion that personhood is a status which others bestow:

> The philosopher John Locke understood that, as he put it, the word "person" (which he distinguished from the word "man") is not a biological but a *forensic* term. That is as much as to say that whether or not someone, or some corporate body, is to be deemed a person is something that must be *decided*. To settle it, we need to know the criteria that have been established for settling such cases, or else we must establish new criteria for ourselves.[4]

She adds that there can be bad criteria for making such designations, and rejects as not generally applicable a criterion for personhood some apply to neonates, namely, whether they are wanted.

I suggest arguments along the following lines against this view.

Warnock is right in rejecting wantedness as a criterion for personhood. But can she reject it because of its lack of general applicability? To do so is to apply something like the Golden Rule, and to apply such a principle is to presuppose that one can pick out the *others* whom one should do unto as one would be done unto. But Warnock denies that there is any determinate class of relevant others prior to the decision about criteria.

Admittedly, biologists can do without the word "person," and the law does bestow personhood on corporations, seagoing ships, and so on, as well as on some human individuals, while denying it to others. For instance, Chief Standing Bear of the Poncas became a person in April 1879 by a court decision rejecting the U.S. district attorney's contention that the Chief was not a person "within the meaning of the law." The following month, when Standing Bear's brother, Big Snake, tried to leave the reservation, General Sherman pointed out that the decision about Standing Bear applied only to him, and Big Snake was shot to death while resisting arrest.[5] To those who decided criteria for his personhood, Big Snake was not a person, and so the Golden Rule did not apply to him.

The argument I shall sketch out against the second notion of personhood also tells against any version of this first one.

II. Personhood: An Attribute Acquired by Development

Michael Tooley is the leading proponent of this notion of personhood. Like Warnock, he denies that personhood is reducible to membership in the biological species *homo sapiens*[6] and thinks that he can resolve relevant-moral issues without settling the definition of "person." But unlike Warnock, Tooley thinks he can settle the definition of "person" by rational inquiry.[7] His strategy is to begin from ethical judgments:

> . . . one can first determine what properties, other than potentialities, suffice to endow an entity with a right to life. Then one can define the term "person" as applying to all and only those things that have at least one of the relevant properties.[8]

To determine what properties suffice to endow an entity with the right to life, Tooley treats rights in general. He assumes that nothing which lacks desires can have rights.[9] On this assumption he argues:

> The non-potential property that makes an individual a person—that is, that makes the destruction of something intrinsically wrong, and seriously so, and that does so independently of the individual's value—is the property of being an enduring subject of non-momentary interests.[10]

Tooley includes the phrase "and that does so independently of the individual's value" to distinguish people from objects such as works of art whose destruction also might be considered intrinsically and seriously wrong.[11] He understands "being an enduring subject of non-momentary interests" in a way that requires "possession, either now or at some time in the past, of a sense of time, of a concept of a continuing subject of mental states, and of a capacity for thought episodes."[12]

Thus, in specifying that personhood be defined by a "non-potential property," Tooley wishes to exclude its definition by an operative potency, such as reason. He does not justify this restriction, but simply stipulates that the defining property may not be potential.[13] He thus excludes not only unborn but newborn babies from personhood.

Tooley also assumes that the morality of acts which bear on others depends on how those acts affect their getting what they want. His metaethics provides no direct support for this ethics; indeed, in discussing metaethics, Tooley claims that he rests nothing important on his view of it.[14] Since he criticizes people who hold ethical theories at odds with his, Tooley perhaps feels that he indirectly establishes his ethical theory. But he does not, because in many cases his criticisms do not concern his opponents' ethical theories. Thus, Tooley provides no grounds, direct or indirect, for accepting the ethical theory he presupposes.[15]

It follows that Tooley's affirmative argument as a whole is question begging against most who disagree with his views on abortion and infanticide.[16]

Against the notion that personhood is an acquired attribute, I suggest the following line of argument.

Both this notion of personhood and the previous one miss what "people" usually means in ordinary language. True, personhood has ethical implications, adult human beings are paradigmatic instances of the concept of *person*, and the word "person" does not mean the same thing as the phrase "member of the species *homo sapiens*." Still, in ordinary language "person" refers to newborn babies as well as to grown men and women.[17] And we can see why "person" is used in this way precisely by beginning from paradigmatic instances of the concept of *person*.

Adults regularly speak of themselves as persons—for example, when they use personal pronouns—in ways which show that they think of their personhood, not as an acquired trait, but as an aspect of their very being. When one says "I cannot remember that far back; my earliest memory is . . . ," one assumes that one already existed before one had that experience; when one says "I was born at such and such a time and place," one takes the word "I" to refer to the same person one now is.

To put the point in logical language: "person" connotes a *substance sortal*. But a substance sortal is an essential property, which implies that whatever has it necessarily has it and never exists without it: individual persons come to be and become persons at the same time, and they cannot cease to be persons without ceasing to be the individuals they are.[18]

Now, a sound, nonstipulative definition of anything must begin by picking out what is to be defined, and this picking out must employ a concept underlying ordinary language. In forming the definition, one can refine this concept and adjust its extension. But no sound nonstipulative definition can set aside the logic of the concept from which the inquiry began insofar as that logic is evident in the use of the word to refer to the concept's paradigmatic instances. It follows that notions of personhood as a bestowed status or an acquired trait involve stipulative definitions, and that no such notion can ground a satisfactory answer to the question "When do people begin?" if that question is understood as people in general understand and wonder about it.[19]

III. Personhood: Limited to Nonbodily Substances

If personhood is limited to nonbodily substances, we bodily individuals are persons only because our bodies are associated with the nonbodily entities that we really are. Such a view is dualism, whether cast in terms of soul and body, mind and body, or noumenal self and phenomenal self.

Classical arguments for dualism—for example, those involving the thesis that thought and extension are incompatible properties—were based on the irreducibility to bodily functioning of acts of inquiry, free choice, and purposeful use.[20] Today, hardly anyone argues for dualism, but many assume it. For example, Joseph Fletcher thinks the solution to questions about abortion would be to deny that a fetus is a personal being. He holds that the body is not part of the person, and that persons are to their bodies as artists are to their materials.[21]

Although Tooley mainly defends the second notion of personhood, he also slips into dualism. For example, he says that if a human being irreparably loses cerebral functioning, "it seems plausible to hold that although a human organism lingers on, the conscious individual once associated with that body no longer exists."[22] Again, he argues that a person would be destroyed but no biological organism would be killed if the brain of an adult human were completely reprogrammed with totally different "memories," beliefs, attitudes, and personality traits—for instance, "The pope is reprogrammed, say, on the model of David Hume."[23]

Against the notion of personhood which limits it to nonbodily substances, I know of only the following line of argument.

Every dualism sets out to be a theory of one's personal identity as a unitary and subsisting self—a self always organically living, but only discontinuously conscious, and now and then inquiring, choice-making, and using means to achieve purposes. But every form of dualism renders inexplicable the unity in complexity which we experience in every act we consciously do. For instance, as I write this, I am the unitary subject of *my* fingers hitting the keys, the sensations *I* feel in them, the thought *I* am expressing, *my* commitment to do this paper, and *my* use of the computer to express *myself.* So, in me thought and extension (thinking and moving my fingers) coexist, and dualism starts out to explain me. But every dualism ends by denying that there is any *one* something of which to be the theory. It does not explain me; it tells me about two things, one a nonbodily person and the other a nonpersonal body, neither of which I can recognize as myself. Therefore, whatever persons are, personhood cannot be limited to nonbodily substances.[24]

If the views considered thus far are excluded, it follows that human persons come to be when their personal bodies come to be and cease to be when their personal bodies die.[25]

IV. Personhood: Dependent on Sense Organs and a Brain

Proponents of the theory of delayed hominization reject dualism but hold that an early embryo cannot be a personal body, since, they say, personhood depends on sense organs and a brain. Unlike Tooley, they think that personhood is an essential property. But like him, they think that personhood requires a certain level of organic development. They hold that the early embryo really is a prepersonal entity, which substantially changes into a person when the sense organs and brain develop. Joseph F. Donceel, S.J., argued for this view.[26]

Relying on Aristotle's biology, St. Thomas thought that an active power in semen gradually forms a new living individual out of *nonliving* matter (the menstrual blood) and that the developing body is not ready to receive a personal soul until at least forty days after conception. Donceel rejects Aristotle's biology but thinks that modern biology together with the hylemorphic theory still requires delayed hominization.

Donceel's argument for delayed hominization is that since the soul is the substantial form of the body, and a substantial form can exist only in matter able to receive it, the personal soul can exist only in a highly organized body.[27] Donceel notes, "Philosophically speaking, we can be certain that an organism is a human person only from its activities." But that would delay hominization until long after birth. So, he concludes:

> The least we may ask before admitting the presence of a human soul is the availability of these organs: the senses, the nervous system, the brain, and especially the cortex. Since these organs are not ready during early pregnancy, I feel certain that there is no human person until several weeks have elapsed.[28]

In a footnote to this passage, Donceel clearly excludes personhood during the first two or three months after conception.

Against the notion that personhood is delayed until the brain and sense organs develop, I suggest the following line of argument.

Substantial changes are radical, and in typical instances—such as death, digestion of food, and chemical reactions—their occurrence is dearly marked. But nothing in the nervous system's development clearly marks any substantial change. Hence, everything depends on Donceel's interpretation of the hylemorphic theory.

Donceel plainly realizes it would be ludicrous to say that babies substantially change into persons some time after they are born. So he settles for hominization when the brain *first* begins to develop. However, this beginning of the brain's development is not the bodily basis for intellectual activities but only its precursor. Now, if this precursor satisfies the requirement of the hylemorphic theory, there is no reason why earlier precursors should fail to satisfy it. But each embryonic individual has from the outset its specific developmental tendency, which includes the epigenetic primordia of all its organs. Therefore, the hylemorphic theory does not preclude a human zygote's having a personal soul.[29]

It follows that neither the facts nor the theory establishes the substantial change which delayed hominization involves.[30] Thus, that substantial change and the multiplication of entities it involves are unnecessary. Now, entities are not to be multiplied without necessity. Consequently, delayed hominization is to be rejected.[31]

Besides Donceel's argument based on hylemorphism, people sometimes offer other arguments to support a theory somewhat like his.

One is the argument that since brain death is sufficient to mark the death of the person, the onset of brain function is necessary to mark the beginning of the person.[32] This argument fails for two reasons.

First, "brain death" means an irreversible loss of function. But the early embryo only temporarily lacks brain functions. So, the two cases are not alike.

Second, "brain death" has two meanings. In one sense, it refers to the irreversible loss of cerebral functions; in another, it refers to the irreversible loss of all functioning of the whole brain. If the argument from brain death is based on the former, it is likely to be question begging, since those who reject delayed hominization generally also deny that a person who loses only cerebral functions is dead. But if the argument is based on the latter, the assumed correspondence between life's beginning and its end does not obtain.

For when the whole brain is dead, nothing remains to integrate the functioning of the organism, and so the organism has ceased to be, and, therefore, the person is dead. By contrast, before the brain develops—even in the zygote—something (some "primary organ" in a broad sense) integrates the whole embryo's organic functioning, and a unified, whole, human individual is developing. As the development of the whole goes on, so does the development of its integrating principles, until, finally, the mature brain integrates the mature individual's functioning.

Another sort of argument for delayed hominization is drawn from common sense. Someone indicates some clear and striking difference between the early embryo and any experientially typical person, even a newborn—for example, "The fertilized egg is much smaller than the period at the end of this sentence," or "It has no eyes, no ears, no mouth, no brain, and like a parasite draws its nourishment from the pregnant woman's blood." Pictures or drawings of very early embryos support such statements, and many people think that this evidence shows that hominization is delayed until the embryo's eighth to twelfth week of development.

Such arguments are rhetorically powerful because they use imagery and directly affect feelings. Usually, in judging whether or not to apply a predicate to an experienced entity, we do not examine it to see whether it meets a set of intelligible criteria. We judge by appearances, using as our guide past experience of individuals of that sort. The early embryo, usually never experienced, falls far outside the range of sensory standards for recognizing people. Images of early embryos do not *fit;* the test of appearances indicates that these strange entities are not persons. The impression is like that of someone who never saw anyone of a different race: those strangers surely are not people.

One can answer this argument only by dealing with its instances: in each case one must point out that while the difference to which attention is called is striking because of our limited experience, entities which are different in that way can meet the intelligible criteria for personhood.[33]

V. Personal Individuals; Formed Two Weeks after Fertilization

This is the view of those who hold that all whole human individuals are persons but maintain that no human individual *ever* begins before the stage of early development after which no individual *can* begin. Norman M. Ford, S.D.B., makes the fullest case I know of for this position.

Ford grants that the zygote "shows all the signs of a single living individual since its activities are all directed from within in an orderly fashion."[34] He also reports the finding of a Royal Commission, which took evidence from "eminent scientists from all over the world. None of them suggested that human life begins at any time other than at conception." Ford adds: "Most embryologists and biologists would appear to agree."[35]

Yet, Ford thinks that persons begin more than two weeks *after* fertilization.[36] Why? Unlike Tooley and others, Ford does not argue that the zygote is only a potential human individual. He acknowledges that the zygote is a real, biologically human individual, but maintains that it is not "ontologically" the same individual as the eventual baby. To prove this, Ford offers arguments to show that there are philosophically significant discontinuities of existence that most scientists overlook.[37]

Ford bases one of his arguments on the fact that, until the primitive streak stage, identical twins can develop from a single zygote. He says that this shows that the zygote has an inherent *active* potentiality to become one or more human beings. And because all the cells into which a zygote divides in the first few cell divisions could, if separated, develop into complete individuals, Ford thinks that every zygote has the capacity for twinning. This leads to a dilemma. If the zygote is a human individual because it can develop into an adult, its openness to becoming one or more adults implies the absurdity that it is at once both one individual and many.[38] But if the zygote *already* is a human individual in its own right, when twinning occurs, that individual either begets its own sibling or ceases to be without dying, leaving behind two new human individuals as its remains. If the former, Ford argues, there would be nothing to determine which twin had been the zygote, since the two would be identical in every way: "Both would be identical indiscernibles, except for their separate concrete existences."[39] But if the latter, both identical twins would be the grandchildren of their putative parents.[40]

Animal experiments also show that genetically distinct embryonic cells or groups of cells can be joined together to develop into one chimeric individual. Ford says that this fact shows that the zygote and the cells into which it divides in the very early stages are too indeterminate to constitute a real ongoing human individual.[41]

Moreover, the zygote's development does not at once differentiate the cells which form the embryo proper from those which form the placenta and other accessory tissues. Ford thinks that this temporary indeterminacy shows that the zygote cannot already be the ontological human individual.[42] He acknowledges that some biologists say that the accessory tissues are an organ of the baby until it is born. But he argues that these tissues cannot be part of the individual: identical twins can share them, fertilization involving only male chromosomes sometimes develops into placental tissue without an embryo (hydatidiform mole), and chimeras can be formed of cells sufficiently differentiated that the embryo proper and the accessory tissues differ genetically from each other.[43]

In some species, ova can develop parthenogenetically—without any sperm. Such development has been induced in mice, but never goes beyond the early stages. Ford thinks that those who hold that the human individual begins before implantation also must hold that a parthenogenetic human embryo would be a human individual.[44]

Ford's main argument—the one he offers for his position that the human individual begins precisely at the primitive streak stage—is that only then does a tiny individual take definite shape with recognizable boundaries, a front and back, a right and left, a head end and lower end. He considers this decisive:

> The unity of the individual human organism would imply a characteristic minimal specific heterogeneity of quantitative parts arranged to provide determinate sites for the co-ordinated development of structures, tissues and organs along a primordial body axis.[45]

Ford supports this point by invoking the testimony of a biologist, a physician, and two theologians who agree that individuality begins at the primitive streak stage.[46]

Besides his direct arguments, Ford argues for his position indirectly by giving an account of the discontinuity he asserts between the zygote (which he admits is a *biologically* human, new individual) and the "ontologically" human individual which he thinks begins at the primitive streak stage. When the first cell division occurs, he says, the individual which was the zygote ceases to be. From then until the primitive streak stage, each of the multiplying cells is a distinct individual. Thus, the true human individual emerges from "a few thousand" distinct individuals.[47]

Against the notion that personhood never begins until about two weeks after fertilization, I suggest the following line of argument.

Despite the facts about twinning, chimeras, and so on, most unborn babies with their accessory tissues develop from a single zygote and are alone in developing from that zygote. Unless the facts support Ford's theory that the baby is formed at the primitive streak stage from a few thousand distinct individuals (the "mass" of cells), in most cases individuality will have to be admitted *to appear* to be continuous, and there will be no reason to deny it, unless the arguments from twinning, chimeras, and so on *by themselves* plainly show that a substantial change is absolutely required—for example, at the primitive streak stage.[48]

Now, the evidence does not support Ford's theory that cell division gives rise to really distinct individuals until a small army of them form the true human individual. It would be interesting to review the facts. But it is enough to notice that if they supported Ford's theory, most biologists would not think: "Fertilization in mammals normally represents the beginning of life for a new individual."[49]

Ford tries to minimize the evidence for the functional unity of the developing "mass" of cells.[50] He also argues that to use this evidence to establish individuality is to beg the question, because distinct individuals—the male and female, and also the sperm and ovum—likewise function toward a common end. Of course, Ford is right that groups of individuals can function toward one end, but he ignores a fact about such a group which prevents us from regarding it as an individual: it is not even a *physical* whole, undivided in itself.

Moreover, the coordinated functioning of male and female, sperm and ovum, can be explained, but Ford has trouble explaining why a few thousand distinct individuals work together in embryogenesis to make themselves into one individual. Finally, he says:

> Prior to this [primitive streak] stage we do not have a living individual human body, but a mass of pre-programmed loosely organized developing cells and heterogeneous tissues until their "clock" mechanisms become synchronized and triggered to harmoniously organize, differentiate and grow as heterogeneous parts of a single whole human organism.[51]

However, Ford's own summary of the scientific literature indicates that the synchronization and triggering essential to his account are a construct that he imposes on the data. For he says that embryologists

> ... suggest that the timing of early differentiation at the blastocyst stage is governed by some "clock" mechanism inbuilt into the DNA of the chromosomes of each cell of the embryo. It seems to be set from the time of fertilization, with each cell's "clock" running in dependence on, and in co-ordination with, what is happening in its surrounding cells.[52]

If so, the cells and tissues do not need to have their "clock" mechanisms synchronized and triggered, because they always are working together harmoniously, which is to be expected if they are, not a mass of distinct individuals, but integral parts of one developing *individual.*

It follows that most unborn babies with their accessory tissues appear to be individuals continuous with the biologically human, new individuals formed at fertilization. Thus, the question is: Do twinning and so on *by themselves* show that the "ontological" human individual comes to be by a substantial change at the primitive streak stage?

The phenomena of twinning and chimeras do not. Even Ford does not suggest that all zygotes have an active tendency to become parts of chimeras. If all zygotes had an active potentiality to become twins, they would do so unless some accident prevented it. Thus, contrary to what Ford asserts (without argument), in those zygotes which develop continuously as individuals, the facts do not evidence an *active* potentiality to develop otherwise. Rather, at most the facts show that all early embryos could *passively* undergo division or combination.

Nor is it evidence of substantial change that the zygote will develop not only into the embryo proper but into the accessory tissues which will be discarded as afterbirth. The accessory tissues are an organ of the unborn baby. Identical twins can share this organ until birth just as Siamese twins can share other organs at birth. Hydatidiform mole, an abnormal development, will be considered below. That chimeras can be formed with accessory tissues from one contributor and an embryo proper from another does not show that the accessory tissues are not an organ of the embryo, for chimeras also can be formed in which the embryo proper includes genetically different contributions.

Nor does the fact that the embryo proper first becomes recognizable at the primitive streak stage show that a substantial change brings the person into being at this stage. For once one sets aside Ford's hypothesis that many distinct individuals form one individual, his main argument comes down to an appeal to common sense: all the people we know have at least a recognizable, definitely shaped body; prior to the primitive streak stage there is no recognizable embryo proper; so, prior to this stage there is no "ontological" human individual. Like all appeals to common sense, this argument is based on appearances. It does not show that a substantial change occurs at the primitive streak stage, for it does not show that either new individuals or the epigenetic primordia of a developed human person come to be only at this stage.

A hydatidiform mole is a new organic individual, genetically both human and unique, but it is not a new human being. Why not? A sperm and an ovum are two distinct organisms, each an individual cell with its own membrane. A sperm loses its membrane when it enters the ovum; the ovum quickly reacts; the two cells fuse into one, and the process of development begins.[53] The sperm and the ovum no longer exist as distinct entities; the activated ovum is a new, biologically human individual.[54] If it has in itself the epigenetic primordia of a human body normal enough to be the organic basis of at least some intellectual act, this new individual is a person. But the activated ovum lacks these epigenetic primordia if it includes *in itself* anything which predetermines it, genetically or otherwise, to develop only into accessory tissues. That is the case with the activated ovum which develops into a hydatidiform mole.[55]

There are no logical or biological problems if identical twins come about by the division of a previous individual and if chimeric individuals are formed from previously distinct individuals.[56] Ford virtually admits as much when he is reduced to saying that such an account "has little appeal" and that "it would be more plausible to argue that an ontological human individual had not yet begun to exist."[57] It does offend common sense to say that a couple's identical twins are really their grandchildren. But common sense simply cannot be trusted when the subject matter is unfamiliar. Moreover, the twins are not grandchildren in the familiar sense, but descendants mediated in an unfamiliar way.[58]

In sum, Ford's supposedly inductive philosophical reasoning actually proceeds from judgments of common sense, based on appearances. None of his arguments shows that scientists overlook philosophically significant discontinuities in development.

Many, especially of a theological bent, deny the personhood of the zygote with an argument which Ford satisfactorily answers. Donceel, for example, cites a theological opinion which questions basing moral norms on the supposition that hominization occurs at conception, inasmuch as "50% of the 'human beings'—real human beings with an 'immortal' soul and an eternal destiny—do not, from the very start, get beyond this first stage of a human existence."[59] As Ford points out, many natural pregnancy losses are due to severe chromosomal defects (and so as explained above are not losses of human beings). Moreover, for most of human history the infant mortality rate was very high. And, theologically, the argument is presumptuous, since we know nothing about how God provides for those who never come to the use of reason.[60]

VI. Persons: All Whole, Bodily Individuals with a Rational Nature

According to this notion, what is necessary and sufficient to be a human person is to be a whole, bodily individual with a human nature. On this notion, if a human activated ovum has in itself the epigenetic primordia of a human body normal enough to be the organic basis of some intellectual act, that activated ovum is a person. But some activated ova are too abnormal to be people, and some people, including some or all identical twins, never were activated ova. Thus, most human persons begin at fertilization, although some begin during the next two or three weeks by others' dividing and perhaps also by others' combining.

The argument that a normal human zygote is a person is *not* that it is a *potential* person, which will develop into an actual person if all goes well. The argument, rather, is that the activated ovum which has suitable epigenetic primordia is an *actual* human individual which—unless he or she ceases to be, which can happen to anyone—will remain the same individual while developing continuously into a grown man or woman. Now, whatever, remaining the same individual, will develop into a paradigmatic instance of a substantial kind already is an actual instance of that kind.

Thus, to deny that the activated ovum is a person is either to deny that any bodily human individual is a person or to posit a substantial change between the zygote and the adult. Arguments against the fourth and fifth notions of personhood exclude substantial change, and the argument against dualism excludes denying personhood to bodily individuals.

A unique, human genome is neither necessary nor sufficient to constitute a person. It is not necessary, since someone like E.T. would be a person without a human genome and identical twins are persons with the same genome. It is not sufficient, since a unique, human genome is present in tissues surviving from people who have died as well as in hydatidiform moles and other biologically human entities which lack the epigenetic primordia that make normal human zygotes persons.

Persons are whole bodily individuals. The human body is personal through and through: if others harm my body, they harm me, for my body is I. Yet persons are more than their bodies; we subsist in our bodies but transcend them. So, although I am my body, I am not my body in the *same sense* that my body is I. I am the subject of my bodily properties, processes, sensations, and feelings, but I also am the subject of my nonbodily intellectual knowledge and chokes, and my more-than-bodily use of things to achieve my purposes.

Tooley raises an important question: How can personhood defined in terms of *rational nature* account for the ethical significance that each individual's personhood has for others' moral responsibilities?[61] For instance, why should newborn babies' personhood require their parents and others not to kill them? The answer is that all moral responsibilities toward others arise, not from their desires and interests, as Tooley assumes, but from moral truth, beginning with the first principles of practical reason, which direct deliberation and freely chosen acts toward the fulfillment of persons—of the agent and of others as well—in interpersonal communion. Precisely because the goods which are objects of these principles are aspects of what unborn and newborn babies *can* be as persons, these goods generate responsibilities toward these persons, not on the basis of anything actual about them beyond their being persons, but precisely on the basis of their potentialities and needs, whose fulfillment depends as much on the love and care of their parents and others as on their own eventual desires for goods and efforts to attain them.[62]

Tooley's work also shows that if one defends the sixth notion of the person, one must carefully handle the metaphysical and logical concepts involved. One must explain and defend *substance, individual*, and so on.[63]

If the preceding lines of argument were developed fully, would there remain any room for questions about whether normal human zygotes are people? Perhaps room for theoretical questions—which always can be raised—but not for practical doubt. There is a very strong factual and theoretical ground for thinking that almost all of us once were zygotes. The counter-positions are weak. To be willing to kill what for all one knows is a person is to be willing to kill a person. Hence, in making moral judgments the unborn should be considered persons from the beginning—their lives instances of innocent human life.[64]

Some argue that a notion of personhood like Warnock's is sufficient at least for legal purposes. I still consider sound the case I made against that position in my book on abortion. That case is complex, but its central idea is simple:

> The law with all its fictions and devices exists to serve persons, to protect them, to guide them in fulfilling their duties, to assist them in vindicating their rights. People are not for the law; the law is for people. Thus the person in a sense stands outside the legal system and above it. Hence the law cannot dispose of persons by its own fiat, any more than action upon a stage can make non-entities of the producer, the stage crew, and the audience.[65]

Thus, when fundamental rights are at stake, just law may not stipulate who are persons but must recognize as persons all who really are persons.

NOTES

1. *Abortion: The Myths, the Realities, and the Arguments* (New York: Corpus, 1970), pp. 11–33, 273–307, 361–410.

2. Pierre de Locht, "Discussion," in *L'Avortement: Actes du Xème Colleque International de Sexologie* (Louvain: Centre International Cardinal Suenens, 1968), 2:155 (my translation). Also see: Louis Beirnaert, S. J., "L'avortement: est-il un infanticide?" *Études* 333 (1970):520–523.

3. Stanislaw Grygiel developed this argument in a lecture, "The Identity of the Unborn Human Person," at a conference, *Marriage and Family in Modern Culture*, 17–20 March 1988, Franciscan University of Steubenville (Ohio). Dr. Grygiel's address: John Paul II Institute for Studies on Marriage and Family; Pontifical Lateran University; Piazza S. Giovanni in Laterano, 4; 00120 Vatican City.

4. "Do Human Cells Have Rights?" *Bioethics* 1 (1987):2.

5. Dee Brown, *Bury My Heart at Wounded Knee* (New York: Holt, Rinehart and Winston, 1970), pp. 351–366.

6. Tooley argues this point at length: *Abortion and Infanticide* (Oxford: Clarendon Press, 1983), pp. 50–86.

7. Ibid., pp. 33–39.

8. Ibid., p. 35. Tooley here states his strategy only in a provisional way; he later dispenses with "right to life" and finally holds (p. 419) "that it is being a subject of non-momentary interests that makes something a person." My criticism will not depend on the difference between his formulations.

9. See ibid., pp. 95–123, where Tooley undertakes to argue for this view, but begs the question by assuming what he needs to prove (p. 101). A telling critique of this element of Tooley's position: Michael Wreen, "Whatever Happened to Baby Jane?" *Nous* 23 (1989):690–696.

10. Ibid., p. 303.

11. Ibid., pp. 53–54.

12. Ibid., pp. 419–420.

13. Ibid., pp. 34–35. Because normal adults are paradigmatic instances of the concept of *person* and because Tooley argues at length against restricting personhood to human beings, his stipulation might seem to him reasonable. But granting those points, one can hold a principle such as Jane Beer Blumenfeld proposes: "It is morally wrong to intentionally kill an innocent individual belonging to a species whose members typically are rational beings, unless at least one of the following conditions obtains: . . ." But Tooley also rejects (ibid., pp. 69–72) this proposal, and in doing so he simply assumes that individuals who have not manifested rationality can at most have a potentiality for it (rather than have it as a capacity, which will be exercised under suitable conditions).

14. Ibid., p. 24.

15. That ethical theory—which is consequentislist—is shared by many others who defend this notion of personhood. For example, Daniel Callahan, *Abortion: Law, Choice and Morality* (New York: Macmillan, 1970), embraces it (although without facing its

implications for infanticide): "Abortion is an act of killing, the violent, direct destruction of potential human life, already in the process of development. That fact should not be disguised, or glossed over by euphemism and circumlocution. It is not the destruction of a human person—for at no stage of its development does the conceptus fulfill the definition of a person, which implies a developed capacity for reasoning, willing, desiring and relating to others—but it is the destruction of an important and valuable form of human life" (pp. 497–498; cf. 384–389, where he first adopts the "developmental" notion of personhood). Callahan likes this view partly for the precise reason that it "provides a way of weighing the comparative value of the lives at stake" (p. 396). As usual, the consequentialist who provides the scales determines the outcome of the weighing: the "body-life" of the potential person is easily outweighed by the "person-life" of the pregnant woman in "a huge number of situations" (p. 496; cf. pp. 398, 498). Like Tooley, Callahan gives no argument whatever for adopting the ethical theory he assumes.

16. Tooley considers some arguments involving other notions of personhood when he deals with potential persons; he also criticizes a "metaphysical" argument (which he constructs but insinuates is Thomistic) for the personhood of neonates: Tooley, *Abortion and Infanticide*, pp. 169–241 and 332–347. Rosalind Hursthouse, *Beginning Lives* (Oxford: Basil Blackwell/Open University, 1987), pp. 107–117, also criticizes the circularity of Tooley's argument.

17. Both *Webster's Third New International Dictionary* and the *Oxford English Dictionary* say that a standard use of "person" is to refer to *a living, human individual*.

18. To develop this argument: David Wiggins, "Locke, Butler and the Stream of Consciousness: And Men as a Natural Kind," *Philosophy* 51 (1976):131–158, and the works Wiggins cites in his note 33; James W. Anderson, "Three Abortion Theorists: A Critical Appraisal" (Ph.D. diss., Georgetown University, 1985), pp. 176–201; Michael Lockwood, "Warnock versus Powell (and Harradine): When Does Potentiality Count?" *Bioethics* 2 (1988):187–213; "Hare on Potentiality: A Rejoinder," *Bioethics* 2 (1988):343–352.

19. Stephen D. Schwarz, *The Moral Question of Abortion* (forthcoming), chapter seven, develops some other promising lines of argument against a position like Tooley's. One of them is based on the implications of using for personhood criteria which are subject to degree. On this, also see Germain Grisez and Joseph M. Boyle, Jr., *Life and Death with Liberty and Justice* (Notre Dame, Ind.: University of Notre Dame, 1979), pp. 229–236. Two criticisms of the earlier version of Tooley's argument will repay study: James G. Hanink, "Persons, Rights, and the Problem of Abortion" (Ph.D. diss., Michigan State University, 1975), pp. 42–172; Gary M. Atkinson, "Persons in the Whole Sense," *American Journal of Jurisprudence* 22 (1977):86–117.

20. A nondualistic theory can account for the irreducibility to bodily functioning of spiritual acts: Germain Grisez, *Beyond the New Theism: A Philosophy of Religion* (Notre Dame, Ind.: University of Notre Dame Press, 1975), pp. 343–353.

21. *Morals and Medicine* (Boston: Beacon Press, 1954), pp. 152, 211–213.

22. Tooley, *Abortion and Infanticide*, p. 64.

23. Ibid., p. 103. Tooley often uses this notion of person-as-software (see pp. 154–155, 163–164, 175–176); he even asks (p. 130) "whether the desires before and after reprogramming belong to the same mental substance."

24. Some articulations of this line of argument: B. A. O. Williams, "Are Persons Bodies?" in *The Philosophy of the Body: Rejections of Cartesian Dualism*, ed. Stuart F. Spicker (New York: Quadrangle/New York Times Books, 1970), pp. 137–156; Gabriel Marcel,

The Mystery of Being, vol. I, *Reflection and Mystery* (Chicago: Henry Regnery, 1960), pp. 127–153; Grisez and Boyle, *Life and Death with Liberty and Justice*, pp. 70–71, 375–379, 402; J. M. Cameron, "Bodily Existence," *Proceedings of the American Catholic Philosophical Association* 53 (1979):59–70. On Kant's form of dualism and some related theories: Joseph M. Boyle, Jr., Germain Grisez, and Olaf Tollefsen, *Free Choice: A Self-Referential Argument* (Notre Dame, Ind.: University of Notre Dame Press, 1976), pp. 110–121. If no dualism can explain me, much less can the sorts of dualism usually assumed today explain people with amnesia and other abnormal mental states: Kathleen V. Wilkes, *Real People: Personal Identity without Thought Experiments* (Oxford: Clarendon Press, 1988), pp. 100–131.

25. When human persons die, there may be not only bodily but spiritual remains: St. Thomas, *Super priman epistolam ad Corinthios lecture*, XV, lec. ii: "We naturally desire salvation for our very selves, but since the soul is part of the human body, it is not the whole person; therefore, even if the soul attains salvation in another life, still I am not saved, nor anyone else."

26. "Immediate Animation and Delayed Hominization," *Theological Studies* 31 (1970): 76–105.

27. Ibid., pp. 79–83.

28. Ibid., p. 101.

29. Benedict Ashley, O.P., makes a cogent case against delayed hominization: "A Critique of the Theory of Delayed Hominization," in *An Ethical Evaluation of Fetal Experimentation: An Interdisciplinary Study*, ed. Donald G. McCarthy and Albert S. Moraczewski, O.P. (St. Louis, Missouri: Pope John XXIII Medical-Moral Research and Education Center, 1976), pp. 113–133. Ashley points out that Donceel drastically understates the case when he says that St. Thomas knew well that the early embryo was not yet a fully organized body. In fact, following Aristotle, Thomas thought that life originates from the semen and the menstrual blood, that neither is alive, and that the very limited, active instrumental power in the semen only gradually organizes the blood into a body which can begin to grow and nourish itself. But Thomas also held that God's infinite power accomplished instantaneously in the conception of Jesus what the semen's power normally takes forty or eighty days to do. Thus, it seems that Thomas accepted Aristotle's theory of hominization, not because he thought that matter cannot receive a personal soul until it has the *organs* required for the sensory basis of spiritual activities, but only because he thought that the semen does not bring about the epigenetic *primordium* of the personal body until forty or eighty days.

30. Moreover, to maintain this hypothesis, Donceel is forced to add another. He stresses ("Immediate Animation," p. 85) that the soul, as form, cannot be the efficient cause of the development of the embryo; rather, the soul is the term of the generative process. St. Thomas thought that the father imparted instrumental efficacy to the semen, and that it remained present as the active principle of development. Since that hypothesis plainly is mistaken, Donceel offers another: Somewhat as in evolutionary development of humans from lower forms of life, God is the proper efficient cause of embryonic development, creatively transforming the parents' contributions until the material is ready to receive a personal soul, which he then also creates.

31. Donceel also claims (ibid., pp. 92–96) that historical evidence shows that delayed hominization was given up under the influence both of the erroneous biological theory of preformation and of Cartesian dualisms. On this, see my *Abortion*, pp. 171–172.

32. The clearest statement of this argument I know of: Robert M. Veatch, "Definitions of Life and Death: Should There Be Consistency?" in *Defining Human Life: Medical, Legal,*

and *Ethical Implications*, ed. Margery W. Shaw and A. Edward Dondera (Ann Arbor, Michigan: AUPHA Press, 1983), pp. 99–113.

33. Stephen D. Schwarz, *The Moral Question of Abortion* (forthcoming), chapter six, skillfully treats numerous versions of the common sense argument, and in doing so provide an excellent model for treating many others.

34. *When Did I Begin? Conception of the Human Individual in History, Philosophy and Science* (Cambridge: Cambridge University Press, 1988), p. 108.

35. Ibid., p. 115.

36. Ibid., pp. 168–170.

37. Ibid., p. 129.

38. Ibid., pp. 119–120; cf. pp. 121–122, 135, 170–172.

39. Ibid., p. 122. Sentences like this make it hard to interpret Ford's argument in a way that allows it coherence and plausibility. But I have done my best.

40. Ibid., p. 136.

41. Ibid., pp. 139–145.

42. Ibid., p. 124; cf. pp. 117–118, 133, 157.

43. Ibid., pp. 133, 159. He also relies heavily on arguments based on common sense, e.g. (p. 157): "But the placenta has no nerves, is insentient and has always been regarded as extraembryonic tissue. While respect and grief have traditionally been expressed for the still-born fetus, at times giving it a burial, this has not been so for the placenta."

44. Ibid., pp. 149–151; cf. pp. 107, 119, 132.

45. Ibid., p. 162; cf. pp. 170–177.

46. Ibid., pp. 174–177. The biologist, Anne McLaren, recounts her journey to this view ("Prelude to Embryogenesis," in *Human Embryo Research: Yes or No?* [Ciba Foundation], ed. Gregory Bock and Maeve O'Connor [London: Tavistock, 1986], pp. 14–15), acknowledging that after an initial insight: "It has taken a further ten years *and some pressure from outside the scientific community* for this distinction to result in a suggested change of terminology to eliminate the ambiguity of the term 'embryo' [emphasis added]." Already at a 1964 international biomedical conference on the IUD, Christopher Tietze urged that a consensus be developed that "pregnancy, and therefore life, begins at implantation" (see my *Abortion*, pp. 111–112).

47. Ford, *When Did I Begin?*, p. 175; cf. pp. 118, 137–138, 162, 170. Ford deserves credit for *trying* to give an account of the discontinuity he posits. Most who share his view simply ignore the problem: Is it an individual all along or not? If so, why not the same individual? If not, what is it until it becomes an individual?

48. Gabriel Pastrana, O.P., "Personhood and the Beginning of Human Life," *Thomist* 41 (1977):247–294, who criticizes (pp. 252–253) my attempt—which I admit was not entirely satisfactory—in *Abortion* to show that the human individual begins at fertilization, thinks hominization occurs by a substantial change at the primitive streak stage. But he does not show (pp. 274–284) that the facts require that hypothesis, and Ashley's argument against Donceel also tells against Pastrana's understanding of the implications of the hylemorphic theory.

49. The quoted sentence opens a recent, magisterial, fifty-page summary of what is currently known about mammalian fertilization: R. Yanaginachi, "Mammalian Fertilization," in *The Physiology of Reproduction*, ed. E. Knobil, J. Neill et al. (New York: Raven Press, 1988), p. 135.

50. Ford, *When Did I Begin?*, p. 149; cf. pp. 117, 133, where he suggests that the cells formed by early divisions are identical, whereas in reality they begin at once to differ

(although at first not so much that each could not develop as a separate individual), which is why not all embryonic individuals have precisely either 2, or 4, or 8, or 16, or . . . cells; see a work that Ford himself often cites: Anne McLaren, "The Embryo," in *Reproduction in Mammals*, book 2, *Embryonic and Fetal Development*, ed. C. R. Austin and R. V. Short, 2nd ed. (Cambridge: Cambridge University Press, 1982), pp. 2–3: "Embryos with 2 and 4 cells are much more often encountered than those with 3 and 5 cells; the following day, II-cell stages predominate, but the scatter is wider; after four or five successive cleavage divisions, little synchrony remains. The first cell to divide from the 2-cell stage mouse embryo has recently been shown by Chris Graham and his colleagues in Oxford to contribute a disproportionately larger number of progeny to the inner cell mass of the blastocyst, and fewer to the outer trophectoderm." Also, Ford, *When Did I Begin?*, pp. 137–138, describes the blastomeres as if they were marbles in a bag, forgetting that in this case the bag (the zona pellucida) also is an organic *part* of the reality and that the blastomeres interact; see, for example, D. J. Hill, A. J. Strain, and R. D. G. Milner, "Growth Factors in Embryogenesis," in *Oxford Reviews of Reproductive Biology* 9 (1987), ed. J. R. Clarke (Oxford: Clarendon Press, 1987), esp. pp. 403–404 and 411, for evidence that the early embryo's cells are in constant and intense interaction, and that until implantation "the early embryo is self-sufficient with regard to the expression of intercellular messengers" (p. 411).

51. Ford, *When Did I Begin?*, p. 175.

52. Ibid., p. 155. Ford's note to this passage (p. 206 n. 36) refers to two works on embryology; neither supports Ford's fanciful notion (p. 175) that distinct, individual cells' " 'clock' mechanisms become synchronized and triggered" to form them into one new individual.

53. See ibid., pp. 102–108. If two or more sperm enter before the ovum reacts, the resultant individual, which may be a hydatidiform mole, cannot develop normally. A factual description of the fusion of sperm and ovum and the initial development of the new individual: R. G. Edwards, *Conception in the Human Female* (London: Academic Press, 1980), pp. 593–605.

54. For a detailed defense of the position that the new individual begins at this point, not at syngamy, see; St. Vincent's Bioethics Centre Working Party, "Identifying the Origin of a Human Life: The Search for a Marker Event for the Origin of Human Life," *St. Vincent's Bioethics Centre Newsletter* 5:1 (March 1987):4–6; T. V. Daly, S.J., "Individuals, Syngamy and the Origin of Human Life: A Reply to Buckle and Dawson," *St. Vincent's Bioethics Centre Newsletter* 6:4 (December 1988):1–7. The address of the St. Vincent's Bioethics Centre: St. Vincent's Hospital; 41 Victoria Parade; Melbourne, Victoria 3065; Australia.

55. An analogous account, presumably, can be given of an ovum developing parthenogenetically. However, if some parthenogenetically developing human ovum had in itself the necessary epigenetic primordia, it too would be a person. What about an anencephalic baby? In most cases the cause of anencephaly is unknown, and cases vary greatly: D. Alan Shewmon, "Anencephaly: Selected Medical Aspects," *Hastings Center Report* 18:5 (October/November 1988):11–19. Even if such a baby now lacks (but previously had the primordium of) the bodily basis of some intellectual act, he or she is a brain-damaged person, just as is the adult whose higher brain functions are irreparably lost.

56. The fact that individual plants remain individuals although they *could be* divided and grafted shows that there is nothing logically or biologically absurd in an organism remaining substantially the same although it could have been divided into two or more

individuals of the same sort or combined with another or others. On this and other facts which Ford and others use to argue against beginning at fertilization, see Thomas V. Daly, S.J., "The Status of Embryonic Human Life: A Crucial Issue in Genetic Counseling," in *Health Care Priorities in Australia: 1985 Conference Proceedings*, ed. Nicholas Tonti-Filippini (Melbourne, Australia: St. Vincent's Bioethics Centre, 1985), pp. 45–57.

57. Ford, *When Did I Begin?*, pp. 120, 136.

58. Ford offers two other arguments. First, he says (p. 118) that until the two-call and perhaps the four-call stage, the messenger RNA already in the ovum before fertilization controls events, and argues that the new human individual "could hardly be said to exist before the embryonic genome, including the paternal genes, is switched on. If the embryo's own genome is not activated or expressed, or if it is suppressed, no human individual or offspring results." But granting the factual supposition, the conclusion does not follow. For, since the ovum with its maternal RNA does nothing until the sperm penetrates it, and at that point a biologically new individual begins to be, the switching on of the embryonic genome is not necessary for the zygote's individuation. (The nonexpression or suppression of the new individual's genome can be understood as resulting in his or her early death.) Second, Ford points out (p. 168) that circulation begins around the end of the third week and argues (p. 170) that this is sufficient to show that the new individual has begun, since it is now a living body with the primordium of at least one organ formed for the benefit of the whole organism. Ford does not use this argument to deny individuality at the slightly earlier primitive streak stage. In this context, however, Ford denies (p. 170) that "the DNA of the genes of the zygote could be taken as the equivalent of an organ of a human being. The genetic instructions for the formation of the whole human being and its organs must not be confused with the actual human being and its organs." His implicit conclusion is that the zygote has no organ whatsoever, and so has no vital function at all, and therefore is not an organic individual. Both the argument based on the beginning of circulation and the assumption that the zygote has no functioning organ can be answered with the same answer: once Ford's denial that there is a continuously developing biological individual is set aside, it is clear that the individual is functioning from the start in one respect: it is growing, not in the sense of gaining mass but in the sense of multiplying and differentiating its cells. *Something* in the individual (not necessarily only the DNA) controls this process; that something is the individual's functioning organ, and the individual's development is that organ's function.

59. Donceel, "Immediate Animation," p. 100; the opinion is quoted from Karl Rahner, but many others propose the same argument.

60. Ford, *When did I Begin?*, pp. 180–181.

61. Tooley, *Abortion and Infanticide*, pp. 61–77, 231–241.

62. For the most recent refinement of several elements of this theory: German Grisez, Joseph Boyle, and John Finnis, "Practical Principles, Moral Truth, and Ultimate Ends," *American Journal of Jurisprudence* 32 (1987):99–151. We always have talked about basic *human* goods. But the principles, having been disengaged by abstraction from the specific content of human experience, actually point to the goods of bodily persons (who are the only sort of beings whose acts can be directed by these principles), whether or not of the human species. Thus, the goodness of life for bodily persons and the wrongness of choosing to violate any basic personal good entail that it would be wrong to choose to kill E.T., but do not entail that it is wrong to slaughter steers or use chimpanzees for medical experimentation.

63. See Tooley, *Abortion and Infanticide*, pp. 77–86, 146–164, 333–346. For significant help toward doing the necessary work, see Francis C. Wade, S.J., "Potentiality in the Abortion Discussion," *Review of Metaphysics* 29 (1975):239–255; John Gallagher, C.S.B., *Is the Human Embryo a Person? A Philosophical Investigation* (Toronto: Human Life Research Institute, 1985). The Human Life Research Institute's address: 240 Church Street, Toronto, Ontario M5B 1Z2.

64. While Tooley and others think otherwise, it is wrong to try to answer the question about how to treat individuals that might or might not be people before answering the question about when people begin. For if one does not answer the latter question first, one is likely to treat some individuals that should be considered persons as nonpersons— a grave injustice if they are is fact persons.

65. *Abortion*, p. 407, to be read in the context of pp. 361–429. See also Germain Grisez and Joseph M. Boyle, Jr., *Life and Death with Liberty and Justice*, pp. 68–71, 229–241, 298–313.

CHAPTER NINETEEN

Thomism and the Beginning of Personhood

Jason T. Eberl

In addressing bioethical issues at the beginning of human life, such as abortion, human embryonic stem cell research, and therapeutic cloning,[1] a primary concern is to establish when a developing human embryo or fetus can be considered a "person," for it is typically held that only persons are the subjects of moral rights, such as a "right to life."[2] The thirteenth-century philosopher and theologian Thomas Aquinas defines a person as "an individual substance of a rational nature" (ST Ia.29.1).[3] He further asserts that all human beings are persons (ST Ia.16.12 ad 1) but that an embryo or fetus is not a human being until its body is informed by a "rational soul." Aquinas's account of human embryogenesis has been generally rejected today due to its dependence upon medieval biological information. A number of scholars, however, have attempted to combine Aquinas's basic metaphysical account of human nature with current embryological data to develop a contemporary Thomistic account of a human being's beginning.[4]

Some Thomistic scholars argue that an early-term human embryo lacks the necessary intrinsic qualities for it to be rationally ensouled until it reaches a certain point in its biological development. Others contend that there is nothing about a human embryo's biological nature, from the moment the process of fertilization is complete, that disallows its being informed by a rational soul. In this paper, I will elucidate Aquinas's account of human embryogenesis and critically examine the contemporary Thomistic views that have been proposed.

Aquinas's Account of Human Embryogenesis

Aquinas understands a human being to be composed of a rational soul informing a material body (Eberl, 2004, p. 335). For a body to be rationally ensouled, it must possess the relevant *potentialities* for the soul's proper operations (SCG II.59), which requires the body to have the appropriate organic structure (QDP III.12). The appropriate organs are those associated with sensation, because it is through sense-perception of particular things that the mind comes to possess intelligible forms, which are the natures of things understood as abstracted from any particular material conditions (e.g., "humanity" as opposed to *"this* human being"). The abstraction of intelligible forms from the products of sensation is the essence of rational thought as Aquinas defines it: "Therefore, the rational soul ought to be united to a body which may be a suitable organ of sensation" (ST Ia.76.5).[5]

This understanding leads Aquinas to develop an account of successive ensoulment in a human embryo's formation. After conception occurs,[6] a material body exists that is informed by a vegetative soul (i.e., an entity that is alive at the most basic level).[7] As the early embryo develops and its organic structure increases in complexity to the point where it can support sensitive operations, the embryo's vegetative soul is annihilated and its matter is informed by a sensitive soul. Since, according to Aquinas, a living thing's identity is determined by its having the same soul (Eberl, 2004, pp. 353–359), the early vegetative embryo has ceased to exist and a new embryo has come into existence that is an animal life-form with the capacity for sensation.

The final stage of embryonic development occurs when the embryo has developed a sufficiently complex organic structure to allow for rational operations.[8] At this point, the sensitive soul is annihilated and the animal embryo ceases to exist as its matter becomes informed by a rational soul (QDA XI ad 1; QDP III.9 ad 9; ST Ia.76.3 ad 3, 118.2 ad 2; SCG II.89; CT 92; QDSC III ad 13). Since Aquinas defines a person as "an individual substance of a rational nature" and all human beings are persons, a developing embryo is neither a person nor a human being until it is informed by a rational soul.[9]

The basic metaphysical principle Aquinas employs in his account of embryogenesis is that a rational soul does not inform a physical body unless the body is properly disposed for that type of soul. The requisite disposition is the body's having sense organs and a brain capable of processing sensory information so that the mind may abstract intelligible forms. A body disposed in such a way does not seem to exist immediately after fertilization but only after first a vegetative embryo, and then an animal embryo, has existed. Aquinas thus concludes that a living, sentient, and rational human being does not begin to exist until some point well after conception (ST Ia.118.2 ad 2).[10]

Ensoulment with Cerebral Development

In offering a contemporary interpretation of Aquinas's account of human embryogenesis, Joseph Donceel and Robert Pasnau each argue that the potentiality for rational thought is present only when a fetus has developed a functioning cerebral cortex (Donceel, 1970, p. 101; Pasnau, 2002, p. 111). This conclusion is purported to follow from the fact that a functioning cerebral cortex is required for rational thought to occur because (1) it is the organ of a human being's sensitive and imaginative capacities and (2) cerebral neural activity is correlated with rational operations. In critically analyzing this conclusion as an interpretation of Aquinas's view, we must consider carefully Aquinas's notion of "potentiality" and how it should be applied to determine when a human embryo or fetus first has the potentiality for rational thought.[11]

Aquinas distinguishes between an "active potentiality" to perform some operation and the actual operation that is brought about through some additional cause (ST Ia.48.5, 76.4 ad 1; QDP I.1; QDV V.8 ad 10; In DA II.2). In contrast to an active potentiality, something has a "passive potentiality" if it can be the subject of externally directed change such that it can become what it is not already. Active potentiality comes in two varieties. The first is what Pasnau refers to as a "capacity in hand" to perform an operation, which means that no further development or significant change is required for the potentiality to be actualized (Pasnau, 2002, p. 115). For example, I have, as an active potentiality, the capacity to speak Spanish—having majored in it in college along with philosophy. It just happens to be the case at this moment that I am not using this capacity and so it is not in actual operation, which it would be if I were actually speaking Spanish right now. The second is what Norman Kretzmann refers to as a substance's "natural potentiality" to develop a capacity to perform an operation (Kretzmann, 1999, p. 39). For example, before I learned to speak Spanish and thus developed a capacity to do so, I had a natural potentiality to develop this capacity. I have numerous other natural potentialities, some of which I have developed into capacities in hand, such as my capacity to play chess, and others that I have left undeveloped, such as my potentiality to learn to read Sanskrit.

In applying these concepts, Aquinas contends that all that is required for something to be rationally ensouled is for it to have an active potentiality to perform rational operations. The actual performance of such operations is accidental to a rational being's existence (ST Ia.118.1 ad 4; QDA XII; Kretzmann, 1999, p. 379 n. 27). A developing human being—even while still *in utero*—has an active potentiality for rational thought, although it cannot yet actually think rationally (SCG II.59). By contrast, sperm and ova do not have such an active potentiality. Rather, sperm and ova are best understood as having a passive potentiality to become a living, sentient, and rational human being (In M IX.6.1837). Each must undergo a change brought about by an extrinsic principle: Sperm must be changed through union with an ovum and vice versa, which transforms them into a substance with active potentialities for a human being's definitive operations. Once this "substantial change" occurs, a human being exists even if it is not actually exercising all of its definitive operations.

The change required for something to actualize an active or passive potentiality is brought about by its "proper active principle." An active principle is required because a potentiality can be actualized only by something that is already in a state of actuality. Something can be moved from a state of potentiality to a state of actuality only by some active principle that is either internal or external to it. A sufficient condition for something's having an active potentiality is if it can actualize the potentiality by some active principle *internal* to it. As will be discussed below, Benedict Ashley and others contend that, from conception onward, a human embryo has a complete human genome and other material factors that are sufficient—given a nutritive uterine environment—for it to develop a functioning cerebral cortex supportive of sensation and rational operations. One can thus infer that a human embryo, well before it forms a functioning cerebral cortex, has an active potentiality for rational thought insofar as it has a natural potentiality to develop a capacity in hand for such operations.

While the interpretations offered by Donceel and Pasnau[12] closely follow what Aquinas explicitly says concerning embryogenesis, they do not correctly take account of the role Aquinas's nuanced concept of "active potentiality" plays in defining the nature of a human embryo in the light of contemporary genetic understanding. Evidence that a human embryo has an active internal principle guiding its ordered natural development into a being that actually thinks rationally is arguably sufficient to conclude that it is already a rational human being: It has an active potentiality for rational thought and is thereby informed by a rational soul.

Ensoulment at Implantation

Norman Ford argues that neither an active potentiality for rational thought, nor a human embryo's existence as an "individual substance," is possible until approximately fourteen days after fertilization is complete. At this time, the embryo implants on the wall of its mother's uterus and begins to form the "primitive streak," which is the "epigenetic primordium"[13] of the central nervous system: the brain and spinal cord. The primitive streak's formation indicates that an embryo is beginning to develop a cerebral cortex and thereby demonstrates its having an active potentiality to engage in rational operations. The occurrence of this event also signals an end to the possibility of twinning: an embryo's division into one or more genetically identical separate organisms. Ford contends that a pre-implantation embryo's intrinsic capacity to twin indicates that it is not a unified, individual substance; rather, it is a conglomeration of individual cells.[14] Once twinning is no longer possible and an embryo's cells have begun to function collectively as one organism—evidenced by the loss of cellular totipotentiality[15]—there is sufficient evidence to warrant the assertion that the embryo is informed by a rational soul. Thus, Ford concludes, a human being begins to exist approximately two weeks after conception.

Ford begins by considering the possibility that an individual human being begins to exist at conception. He asserts that, at the completion of fertilization, there exists something that has a unique genetic identity and a unique ontological identity *as a biological cell*. It does not, however, have a unique ontological identity *as a human being*. After the first mitotic event—the first division of a one-celled zygote—two cells exist that have the same *genetic* identity but are *ontologically* distinct (Ford, 2002, p. 65; 2001, p. 160; 1988, p. 117). The same follows for every event of cellular mitosis until the point is reached when mitosis that results in ontologically distinct beings can no longer occur.

The ontological uniqueness of each cell in a pre-implantation embryo is evidenced by the lack of differentiation among them. Cells remain undetermined for quite some time as to where they will go and what role they will play in the developing organism. The same indeterminism occurs in cases of twinning. A single cluster of cells is shared in the early developmental process by what will become two ontologically distinct organisms; to which organism each cell will ultimately go is largely undetermined (Ford, 1988, pp. 133–135).

Ford concludes, based on the lack of cellular differentiation and the possibility of twinning, that a pre-implantation embryo cannot be a person according to Aquinas's definition since it is not an "individual substance." The primitive streak's appearance, coincident with uterine implantation, indicates an embryo's existence as an ontologically unique organism informed by a rational soul (Ford, 1988, pp. 171–172). At the formation of the primitive streak, there exists a living biological organism, capable of nutrition and growth, developing the earliest biological tools necessary for sensation, imagination, and rational thought; all these powers are correlated with the brain and spinal cord that develop from the primitive streak. The specific powers of sensation and rational thought are not actualized until the required organs begin to function; however, a rational soul is active by informing the body in its development of the requisite organs.

Therefore, Ford concludes that a human being begins to exist as an individual biological organism with the capacities of life, sensation, and rational thought at the moment the primitive streak begins to form, twinning is no longer possible, and cells that form the embryo proper are determined to the end of constituting a human being and to no other.[16] Critics of Ford's position argue that cellular totipotentiality does not imply a lack of organic unity, organized cellular functioning to sustain the life of a single organism begins when fertilization is complete, and the possibility of a pre-implantation embryo dividing into genetically identical twins does not count against its existence as an individual substance.

"Organic" unity is often understood as a definitive sign of the "substantial" unity required in Aquinas's definition of personhood. Since, however, Aquinas holds strict criteria for something to have substantial unity, it is necessary to see if the concept of organic unity satisfies the relevant criteria. Aquinas notes various ways in which something may be considered a "unity." For example, a heap of stones is a unity in terms of the constituent stones being spatially contiguous, a house is a unity in terms of its constituent parts being functionally organized in a certain fashion, and a mover and that which it moves are a unity in terms of their agent/patient relationship (QDA X; SCG II.57). None of these types of unity count as substantial unity, though. Aquinas defines a substance as *unum simpliciter* ("one unqualifiedly"). Examples of things that are *unum simpliciter* are elemental substances, certain mixtures of elemental substances, immaterial substances, and living organisms (Pasnau, 2002, p. 88). Aquinas understands living organisms "to have a unity fundamentally different from that of nonliving aggregates" (Pasnau, 2002, p. 93).

The unity among a living organism's parts is signified by their *interdependent* functioning. Mere "functional unity" is not sufficient for substantial unity. The bricks, roof tiles, wood beams, and so on, that compose a house are functionally unified in that they must all be organized in a certain fashion relative to each other in order for the house to exist with its proper structural integrity; but a house is not *unum simpliciter*. A house's functional unity is distinguished from that of a living organism, because a living organism's parts depend on their functional relationship to each other for their very existence as the types of things they are (QDA X ad 15; SCG II.57; van Inwagen, 1990, pp. 81–97). A brick depends upon its functional relationship to the other parts of a house in order to exist "as a part of the house," but it does not depend upon that relationship in order to exist "as a brick." An organ (e.g., an eye) in an organism depends upon its functional relationship to the organism's other organs not only for its existence "as a part of the organism" but also for its existence "as an eye." Aquinas asserts that an eye that is functionally disconnected from a living organism can be called "an eye" only equivocally; it is no longer an eye in the proper sense of the term.

Hence, for Aquinas, a living organism's organic unity—defined in terms of the interdependent functional relationship among its parts (cells, tissues, organs, etc.)—is a paradigm example of substantial unity. In critically examining Ford's account, then, it is necessary to determine whether the cells composing a pre-implantation embryo are functionally interdependent. Evidence of their functional interdependence would make it reasonable to assert that a pre-implantation embryo has organic, and thus substantial, unity (Panicola, 2002, pp. 80–81; Serra and Colombo, 1998, p. 172; Lee, 1996, pp. 94–95; Flaman, 1991, p. 41).

There is evidence of an inchoate organization and intercommunication among an embryo's cells that may be indicative of their functional interdependence (Deckers, 2007, pp. 274–275). Such evidence includes the cells' coming together at implantation to form the primitive streak, as well as other embryonic and extra-embryonic tissues shortly thereafter (Lee, 1996, p. 102; Grisez, 1989, p. 37). Additionally, an embryo has an "identifiable body plan" before implantation and formation of the primitive streak: "Recent advances in embryology indicate that the 'blueprint' for the entire human body is defined within the first few hours of life, even as early as the one-cell zygotic stage of development, when the definitive axes associated with the emergence of the primitive streak appear" (Meyer, 2006, p. 213; cf. Vial Correa and Dabike, 1998, pp. 317–328; Serra and Colombo, 1998; Fisher, 1991, p. 66; Flaman, 1991, p. 46).[17]

Furthermore, Ford acknowledges that there is some sort of "clock" mechanism programmed in a zygote's DNA that guides organic development and "continues through childhood for the growth of teeth, biological changes at puberty, adulthood etc. right through to old age" (Ford, 1988, p. 155 n. 37). This clock "seems to be set from the time of fertilization, with each cell's 'clock' running in dependence on, and in co-ordination with, what is happening in its surrounding cells" (Ford, 1988, p. 155). Ford interprets this phenomenon as supporting his view that each cell constituting a pre-implantation embryo is a distinct individual organism that has its own internal clock, which is synchronized with the clocks of the other cells. Germain Grisez, though, considers such harmonious synchronization to be what one would expect if such cells "are, not a mass of distinct individuals, but integral parts of one developing *individual*" (Grisez, 1989, p. 38).

Hence, there is evidence that a pre-implantation embryo, despite the totipotentiality of its constituent cells, has an intrinsic organization grounded in its unique genetic identity to grow by cellular mitosis, implant itself in its mother's uterus, and develop into a mature human being capable of rational thought. Evidence of a pre-implantation embryo's organic unity provides a reasonable foundation for asserting its substantial unity, fulfilling Aquinas's requirement that something be *unum simpliciter* in order to count as an "individual substance."

The totipotentiality of a preimplantation embryo's constituent cells also allows for it to potentially divide into genetically identical twins. Ford argues that it is metaphysically problematic for one individual organism to give rise to two distinct organisms; especially in the case of rationally ensouled organisms.[18] The following questions arise: Does the rational soul informing the first organism divide? Do all the organisms share the same rational soul with the original? Does the original organism cease to exist, its soul separating from its matter, and two new rational souls are created to inform the divided matter? There is also a fundamental issue concerning *identity*. That something is identical to itself is necessary, and the relation of identity is transitive. Hence, a zygote is identical to itself and, if a pre-implantation embryo has the same rational soul as the zygote from which it developed, then the embryo is identical to the zygote. If the embryo divides into twins, it appears that each twin is identical to the original embryo and thus to the zygote. The twins are obviously not identical to each other, but they must be identical if they are both identical to the original embryo, because identity is transitive. Therefore, an incoherency seems to follow from the assertion that an embryo capable of dividing into twins is a substance identical with itself.

An alternative depiction of the twinning phenomenon, however, involves the original rationally ensouled embryo losing some of its matter and the matter becoming informed by a new rational soul (Klubertanz, 1953, pp. 410–411). On this construal of the twinning phenomenon, when one organism *A* divides into two organisms *B* and *C*, either *B* or *C* is identical to *A*,[19] because one of them has the same rational soul as *A*.[20] If, say, *B* is identical to *A*, then *B*'s existence can be traced back to the one-celled zygote from which *A* developed before its division. In this case, *C* is not identical to *A*, because it is informed by a new rational soul created at the moment of *A*'s division (Panicola, 2002, pp. 80–81; Finnis, 1999, p. 15; Crosby, 1993, pp. 410–411; May, 1992, pp. 80–81; Fisher, 1991, pp. 61, 67; Flaman, 1991, p. 50; Suarez, 1990, p. 631).[21] Therefore, since it is not the case that both *B* and *C* are identical to *A*, no incoherency follows from *B* and *C* not being identical to each other and *A* being a substance identical to itself.

Natural embryonic twinning would thus be akin to the artificial production of a "clone" insofar as an external agent acts upon an organism to separate some of its matter from it and the matter comes to constitute a genetically identical organism with its own substantial form (Ashley and Moraczewski, 2001, pp. 195–198). While the biological process of twinning is not fully understood, it appears to be a random event, with no apparent internal genetic factor or any clear environmental factor that causes an embryo to twin (Piontelli, 2002, p. 19). To the best scientific understanding, it is as likely that twinning is caused by factors respective of the uterine environment acting upon weak intercellular bonds to cause the embryo to lose some of its cells as it is that an embryo is genetically "programmed" to divide. If there were a genetic determiner for twinning intrinsic to an embryo, then one could argue that this factor precludes an embryo that has it from being an "individual substance" prior to its division.[22] There is, though, no conclusive evidence of an intrinsic genetic determiner for twinning (Ford, 1988, p. 119).

It would thus be misleading to equate the *biological* totipotency of the cells constituting a pre-implantation embryo with Aquinas's *metaphysical* concept of active potentiality. To say that such cells are biologically totipotent means only that they may come to constitute any of the embryo's tissues or organs, or—if a group of them were to separate from the embryo—they may constitute another embryo. No implication follows from this biological fact as to whether the cells possess an active or passive potentiality to constitute another human being. If biological totipotency entailed that each cell has an *active* potentiality to form another human being, which would certainly count against a pre-implantation embryo being *unum simpliciter,* then each cell must have a proper active principle internal to it that determines it to develop into another human being. But it is not evident that the cells constituting a pre-implantation embryo have such an intrinsic principle insofar as they do not in fact develop into another embryo while they constitute the original embryo. Nor, as noted above, do such cells have any sort of intrinsic determining factor by which some of them may be destined to separate themselves from the original embryo and form another. It is thus evident that the biological totipotency of a preimplantation embryo's cells equates with a *passive* potentiality to form another embryo if an external agent acts on the embryo to separate some of its cells from it; once separated, however, the cells would have an active potentiality to develop into a fully actualized human being.[23]

On this view, when an embryo twins, it is not the case that it is "dividing," but that it loses some of its matter. Since the separated matter is totipotent—i.e., it has an active potentiality to develop into a human being—it is immediately informed, once separated, by a rational soul. It is not necessary to accept Ford's conclusion that a pre-implantation embryo's potentiality to divide is a threat to its previous substantial unity. Furthermore, the understanding of twinning as an event in which an embryo merely loses some of its matter allows for an embryo to maintain its substantial unity through the twinning process; and thereby one of the resultant twins is identical to the original embryo: "There is one human person before twinning occurs, and that human person continues in existence after a new human person develops through parthenogenesis" (O'Rourke, 2006, p. 248).

Therefore, the possibility of a human embryo dividing into genetically identical twins does not preclude its being informed by a rational soul. Nevertheless, even if one grants that cellular totipotentiality and the possibility of twinning does not preclude a pre-implantation embryo's existence as an individual substance with organic unity, more needs to be said to support the assertion that the embryo is informed by a *rational* soul, as opposed to a merely vegetative or sensitive soul; especially given that Aquinas explicitly holds that an embryo is first informed by a vegetative soul. Responding to this issue requires providing a reason to think that a pre-implantation embryo has an active potentiality for rational thought.

Ensoulment at Conception

John Haldane and Patrick Lee interpret Aquinas as holding that only the *epigenetic primordia* for the biological structures proper to a human being are required for rational ensoulment (Haldane and Lee 2003a, p. 267). This interpretation is based, in part, on Aquinas's recognition of a prenatal human being's gradual development in terms of the actualization of its various potentialities (ST Ia.119.2; QDA XI ad 9). Benedict Ashley concurs and argues that a human zygote contains the relevant primordia by virtue of its DNA-filled nucleus, which functions as the "control center" that regulates embryonic biological functioning, such that a zygote is a unified, individual substance from fertilization onward (Ashley, 1976, p. 123; Ashley, and Moraczewski 2001, p. 197).

In line with Ashley's view, Aquinas holds that animals—human and nonhuman alike—possess a "primary organ" by which a sensitive or rational soul's power to move the various parts of its body is manifested (QDA IX ad 13, X ad 4, X ad 11, XI ad 16; In Sent I.8.v.3 ad 3).[24] Aquinas asserts that the primary organ is the foundation of an animal's unity as an organic substance and thus indicates that the animal is ensouled. In fact, all parties discussed in this debate recognize the need to define a primary organ in order to assert that a developing human embryo has a rational soul. Donceel and Pasnau contend that the primary organ is the brain with a functioning cerebral cortex, because it is directly correlated with both rational operations and metabolic regulation. Ford argues that the primitive streak is the primary organ, because it is the epigenetic primordium for the brain and nervous system. Ashley finds the zygotic nucleus to be the primary organ[25] as it is the epigenetic primordium of the primitive streak, and thus of the brain and nervous system (Ashley, 1976, p. 124).[26]

The zygotic nucleus not only functions as a pre-implantation embryo's metabolic regulator but is also the epigenetic primordium for the organ correlated with rational operations: the cerebral cortex formed out of the primitive streak. This supports the conclusion that a one-celled human zygote is informed by a rational soul (Ashley and Moraczewski, 2001, pp. 199–200).[27] It is important to note that it is not merely because of its unique genetic identity that a zygote is an individual human being, for its genetic identity will not remain unique if an identical twin or a clone is formed or be sufficient for a human being to develop if a hydatidiform mole is produced.[28] A zygote must also have a primary organ and any other intrinsic biological factors necessary for its unilateral development into an actually thinking rational human being.[29] In normal cases, a human zygote has an active potentiality to be, through development, an actually thinking rational human being; and this is sufficient to conclude that it is informed by a rational soul.[30] By applying Aquinas's metaphysical principles to contemporary embryological data, Ashley, as well as Haldane and Lee, concludes that a human being begins to exist at conception.[31]

Embryos and Clones

A key first step in addressing the moral permissibility of human embryonic stem cell [hESC] research is to establish the metaphysical nature of a human embryo prior to uterine implantation.[32] Is it a human being or is it merely a conglomeration of cells with human DNA? Arguments for the latter position consist of claims that an unimplanted embryo is only a "potential" human being insofar as, if it is placed in a uterus and not disturbed, it will develop into such a being, but it is not yet such a being. Donceel, Pasnau, and Ford defend this view from a Thomistic perspective.[33] Prior to uterine implantation or the formation of the cerebral cortex, a human being does not exist because the embryo is not informed by a rational soul. By contrast, Haldane, Lee, and Ashley argue that a human embryo is a human being because it requires only a supportive uterine environment to develop into an actually thinking rational being. It is informed from conception by a rational soul that is the metaphysical blueprint for embryonic and fetal development, which is an extended process of actualizing a human being's vegetative, sensitive, and rational capacities. Therefore, to disaggregate a human embryo in order to derive hESCs involves causing a human being's death.

The conclusion is no different if a *cloned* embryo is produced through either blastomere separation (Hall, Engel, Gindoff, Motta, and Stillman, 1993) or somatic cell nuclear transfer (Cibelli, Lanza, West, and Ezzell, 2002; Wilmut, Schnieke, McWhir, Kind, and Campbell, 1997). So long as a cloned embryo has everything *in itself,* other than a supportive environment, required to develop into a being that actually thinks rationally, it is regarded as informed by a rational soul insofar as it has an active potentiality for rational thought. There is no apparent reason to deny that a cloned embryo fulfills this criterion for rational ensoulment once it is "conceived."

The President's Council on Bioethics notes the argument that, though a cloned embryo is a potential human being, its potential is not sufficient for it to already be a human being:

> But the *potential* to become something (or someone) is hardly the same as *being* something (or someone), any more than a pile of building materials is the same as

a house. A cloned embryo's potential to become a human person can be realized, if at all, only by the further human act of implanting the cloned blastocyst into the uterus of a woman. (President's Council on Bioethics [PCB], 2002, 48)

This assessment of a cloned embryo's potentiality, however, neglects Aquinas's distinction between active and passive potentiality. A cloned embryo has an active potentiality to be an actually thinking rational human being, because it has everything internally required for its *ordered natural development* toward such a state of actuality. A cloned embryo's potentiality is not akin to the potentiality of a pile of building materials to be a house. Such materials have merely a passive potentiality to be a house, because they require an external agent to organize them into the structure of a house (Eberl, 2006, pp. 30–31). A cloned embryo with a complete human genome directs its own organized development from a single-celled zygote into a fully developed human being who actually thinks rationally.

A cloned embryo in a petri dish, though, does require external aid if its development is to continue beyond the earliest stages: It must be implanted in a supportive uterine environment. R. Alta Charo thus asserts:

A fertilized egg or early embryo in a petri dish most certainly has an intrinsic tendency to continue growing and dividing. Without the provision of an artificial culture medium, however, it will never grow and divide more than about 1 week. If the provision of such a medium is considered a form of external assistance akin to that at issue in passive potentiality, then the fertilized egg is a potential week-old embryo, not a potential baby. (Charo, 2001, p. 86)

Contra Charo, an embryo's requirement of a supportive uterine environment does not preclude its possessing an active potentiality to develop itself into an actually thinking rational being (Deckers, 2007, p. 273). A uterus provides a supportive environment for an embryo to exercise *its own* developmental capacity. Uterine implantation does not alter an embryo's intrinsic nature or bestow upon it more inherent potentialities than it already possesses.

The form of external assistance a uterus provides is analogous to an astronaut's spacesuit or an underwater explorer's submarine. Each provides what the person needs to exercise her vital metabolic capacities; but the lack of such support does not entail that she lacks those capacities. If an astronaut's spacesuit malfunctions and stops supplying oxygen, her vital metabolic functions will cease shortly thereafter. If, however, a fellow astronaut fixes her suit in a timely fashion and restores the flow of oxygen, her vital metabolic functions will resume. This indicates that the astronaut's *intrinsic capacity* for such functions remained despite the loss of the requisite supportive environment.[34] Another relevant example is the incubator most prematurely born infants require to continue their postnatal development. Although such infants cannot survive without the incubator's assistance, their dependence on it does not entail that their potentiality for full development is merely passive and not self-directed. Thus, a cloned—or any *in vitro*—embryo's potentiality for development into an actually thinking rational human being does not preclude its existence as a human being already. This is because the potentiality at issue is an *active* potentiality that is part of the embryo's intrinsic nature, defined by its being informed by a rational soul.

Conclusion

Establishing a proper Thomistic understanding of the beginning of a human being's life involves determining when one can assert that a rational soul informs a human body. The evidence required to support such an assertion is a body's having, at minimum, active potentialities for vegetative, sensitive, and rational operations. I have described more extensively various interpretive issues with the view proffered by Donceel and Pasnau (Eberl, 2005a). And while I have previously advocated Ford's account (Eberl, 2000) and continue to consider it a metaphysically coherent and plausible position, I agree with the critics who conclude that Ford does not offer a sufficiently compelling argument to deny that a pre-implantation embryo may be an individual human organism informed by a rational soul (Eberl, 2007). I thus conclude in agreement with Haldane, Lee, and Ashley that the active potentialities definitive of rational ensoulment are present when an organism with human DNA comes into existence with some sort of primary organ—or "control center"—through which integrative organic functioning is exercised; such functioning indicates an organism's substantial unity. At the very beginning of human life, the primary organ seems to be the nucleus of a one-celled human zygote, which provides the epigenetic primordium of a human being's brain and nervous system. Once it develops, the brain is the integrative foundation for a human being's sensitive and vegetative operations and is correlated with rational operations (Eberl, 2005b). The presence of the brain's epigenetic primordium is thus sufficient for a human zygote to have the active potentialities relative to a rational soul's proper operations, since the zygote's ordered natural development will result in an actually thinking rational human being. Therefore, it is reasonable to conclude that a human zygote is informed by a rational soul and is thus a human being—a person.

This metaphysical conclusion provides a foundation from which to argue that a human embryo enjoys the full moral status that a fully actualized human being is recognized to possess. Formulating such an argument, however, requires invoking a particular ethical theory and taking various values into account, which is outside the scope of this paper.[35] Nevertheless, it appears *prima facie* that, despite the potentially significant benefits of hESC research and therapeutic cloning, both are morally problematic from a Thomistic perspective because they unavoidably involve the directly intended death of human embryos. An alternative avenue worth exploring involves the creation of "nonviable embryo-like artifacts" that lack the biological status of an organism—and hence the ontological status of a human being—but yet provide a source for deriving functional hESCs (PCB, 2004, pp. 90–93; Hurlbut in PCB, 2002, pp. 274–276). Lacking an active potentiality for rational thought, such entities would not share the moral status of rationally ensouled human embryos; but further biological, metaphysical, and ethical analysis is warranted.

NOTES

A more extensive version of this essay appears in Eberl (2006), chap. 2. I have used this opportunity, however, to incorporate more recent research into the current essay.

1. "Therapeutic cloning" refers to the production of cloned human embryos that are not destined to be implanted for reproductive purposes but from which human embryonic stem cells may be derived or other research performed.

2. It is arguable that some species of nonpersons, such as sentient animals capable of feeling pleasure and pain, also bear certain moral rights. While this may very well be the case, the rights of persons are still generally held to trump those of nonpersons in cases of conflict. For elaboration of a Thomistic account of animal rights, see Barad (1988).

3. Aquinas adopts this definition first made in the early sixth century by Boethius (*Contra Eutychen et Nestorium* III). All translations of Aquinas's texts are my own.

4. Since Aquinas holds that all "human beings" are "persons," I will use these terms interchangeably. However, as noted below (see nn. 10 and 31), there may be entities—for example, some anencephalic infants—who are biologically members of the species *Homo sapiens* but, ontologically speaking, are not human beings.

5. This section is derived from Eberl (2005a).

6. Aquinas, following Aristotle, understands conception to involve male semen acting upon female menstrual blood to form an embryo (ST Ia.118.1 ad 4; DGA II.3.736a24–737b6). Neither Aristotle nor Aquinas had knowledge of sperm, ova, and DNA.

7. Following Aristotle, Aquinas defines a "rational soul" as a soul that has the relevant capacities for life, sensation, and rational thought and as the type of soul proper to the human species. A "sensitive soul," on the other hand, has the relevant capacities for only

life and sensation and is the type of soul proper to all nonhuman species of the animal genus. A "vegetative soul" has the relevant capacities for life alone and is proper to all non-animal living organisms (In DA II.3.414a30–415a14).

8. Since Aquinas holds that rational operations do not require the use of a bodily organ (QDA II), the requisite "organic complexity" here is that which supports the operations of sensation that allow for the mind to abstract intelligible forms. For a discussion of Aquinas's account of sensory and intellective cognition, see Stump (2003, chap. 8).

9. This allows for the possibility that not all members of the biological species *Homo sapiens* are "human beings" as Aquinas defines the term; for there may be entities that are biologically "human" but are not rationally ensouled. A relevant example may be some anencephalic infants whose anencephaly results from a genetic anomaly present from conception that precludes their possessing the intrinsic capacity to develop a cerebral cortex supportive of sensation and rational operations.

10. Aquinas contends, following Aristotle, that a developing embryo is first informed by a rational soul at the time of "quickening," which occurs forty days after conception if it is male and ninety days after conception if it is female (In Sent, III.3.v.2; HA VII.3.583b3–5). This, of course, is one of Aquinas's "empirical" conclusions we may happily jettison while maintaining the validity of his overall *metaphysical* viewpoint.

11. This section is derived from Eberl (2005a).

12. For further discussion of Pasnau's view, see Haldane and Lee (2003a) and the subsequent responses: Pasnau (2003); Haldane and Lee (2003b).

13. An "epigenetic primordium" is that from which a particular tissue, organ, or organ system will naturally develop if unimpeded. The tissue, organ, or organ system does not exist actually, but virtually, in its epigenetic primordium insofar as a developmental continuity can be traced from one to the other. See Haldane and Lee (2003b, p. 537).

14. The cells in this conglomeration are individual living substances, each informed by a vegetative soul (Eberl, 2000, pp. 151–152).

15. "Totipotentiality" refers to the capacity of each of a pre-implantation embryo's cells to divide and form any tissue or organ of a human body or even a whole other body.

16. For additional arguments supportive of Ford's conclusion from a Thomistic metaphysical perspective, see Kenny (2006); Eberl (2000); Wallace (1995); Bole (1990); Smith (1983); and Diamond (1975). For arguments supportive of Ford's conclusion, but not from an explicitly Thomistic perspective, see Smith and Brogaard (2003); Olson (1997, pp. 89–93); Shannon (1996); Lockwood (1995); Porter (1995); McCormick (1991); van Inwagen (1990, pp. 152–154); Shannon and Wolter (1990); and Grobstein (1988).

17. Meyer cites embryological evidence from Pearson (2002) and Beddington and Robertson (1999). See also PCB (2004, Appendix A).

18. Unlike the vegetative soul of, say, a flatworm, which may be divisible if the worm's body is divided into two distinct living worms (QDP III.12 ad 5; QDSC IV ad 19; In M VII.16.1635; In DA II.4), Aquinas argues that a rational soul is indivisible, simple, and one (QDP V.10 ad 6; QDSC IV ad 9; QDA X ad 15; SCG II.86).

19. This way of construing the twinning phenomenon makes the case that the proximate progenitor of one of the twins, B or C, is A; whereas the proximate progenitor of A and the other twin is A's mother and father. This conclusion may be technically true, but unproblematic, because, for all practical purposes and due to the epistemic uncertainty regarding which of the twins is identical to A, A's mother and father can be considered as the parents of both B and C.

20. I do not see any possible epistemic criterion for determining which of the twins, *B* or *C*, has the same rational soul as *A* and which is the new organism generated by a new rational soul informing matter that previously composed *A*. Epistemic uncertainty regarding which twin is identical to *A*, however, does not preclude the metaphysical claim that one of the twins is identical to *A* while the other is not.

21. Kevin Flannery offers a different proposal, in which the first ensouled embryo goes out of existence when twinning occurs and thus both of the resulting twins are numerically distinct human beings from the original. The picture that Flannery depicts, however, is ontologically onerous compared to the view presented here (Flannery, 2003, p. 277).

22. This conclusion may apply only in cases in which an embryo is genetically programmed to twin. If an embryo is not so programmed, then it would be an individual substance at conception. Alternatively, an embryo that is programmed to twin may compose *two* individual human beings at conception who are later separated from each other when twinning occurs (Deckers, 2007, p. 279; Koch-Hershenov, 2006, pp. 157–160); this view is problematic, however, from a Thomistic metaphysical perspective (Eberl, 2007, pp. 286–287).

23. I am grateful to John Lizza for raising the issue addressed in this paragraph.

24. Aquinas, following Aristotle, understands the primary organ to be the heart, though contemporary science understands it to be the brain. For further discussion, see Eberl (2005b, p. 32).

25. It may be problematic to refer to the zygotic nucleus as an "organ" (Shannon, 1996, p. 732), and so the term "control center" or "primary organizer"—the latter is Ashley's term—is probably more appropriate.

26. Nicanor Austriaco disagrees with Ashley's assertion that the zygotic nucleus functions as the primary organ for a developing embryo, but nonetheless agrees that rational ensoulment occurs at conception due to the *systemic* functioning of the embryo as a whole guiding its own epigenetic development (Austriaco, 2004, pp. 735–736).

27. Juan Vélez contends that it is preferable to consider the rational soul as informing the matter of the conjoined *gametes* in order to bring a zygote into existence, rather than informing the already formed *zygote* (Vélez, 2005, p. 21). To clarify the issue at hand, a rational soul immediately informs what Aquinas terms "prime matter" to compose a human being. Such matter, as Vélez notes, previously composed the gametes, but the gametes cease to exist as individual substances at the completion of the fertilization process when *syngamy*—the fusion of the gametes' chromosomes—occurs. At this point, a new substance—the zygote—comes into existence. Rational ensoulment thus occurs in the moment of *transition* when the gametes cease to exist and the zygote begins to exist.

28. A hydatidiform mole is a mass of placental tissue with the same genetic identity as an embryo. What separates a hydatidiform mole and a developing embryo is that the former can never, despite its intrinsic genetic structure and even if it is placed in a supportive uterine environment, develop into an organism with a functioning cerebral cortex; the latter can. For discussion of the importance of hydatidiform moles to the question of whether a human embryo possesses the intrinsic biological factors sufficient for it to be a human being, see Bedate and Cefalo (1989) and Suarez (1990).

29. A zygote's "unilateral" development into a mature human being presumes that it is in a supportive environment—first the fallopian tube and then the uterus—and no external factors impede its development.

30. A relevant "abnormal" case would be some anencephalic infants whose anencephaly results from a genetic anomaly present from conception that precludes their possessing

334 Jason T. Eberl

the intrinsic capacity to develop a cerebral cortex supportive of sensation and rational operations. Such entities, despite appearing quite human, would evidently not be informed by a rational soul.

31. For similar arguments for this conclusion, see Koch-Hershenov (2006); Bracken (2001); Mirkes (2001); De Koninck (1999); Johnson (1995); Heaney (1992); Wade (1985); Pastrana (1977); and Gerber (1966).

32. This section is derived from Eberl (2006, pp. 66–68, 80–86).

33. Ford's argument from twinning in particular has been utilized to support hESC research. See Green (2002, p. 22); McCartney (2002, pp. 604–608); Shannon (2001, p. 178); Eberl (2000); Lanza (2000); and Robertson (1999, p. 117).

34. Does the astronaut's dependence on her fellow astronaut's assistance in restoring her supportive environment imply that her potentiality for being alive is merely *passive*? No, because the assistance provided does nothing to alter or replace the astronaut's organic structure by which she is able to breathe in and circulate oxygen once it is made available to her again.

35. For discussion of specific issues at the beginning of human life, from a Thomistic metaphysical and ethical perspective, see Eberl (2006, chap. 4).

REFERENCES

Aquinas, T. *Compendium theologiae* [CT]. In Commissio Leonina (ed.), *S. Thomae Aquinatis Doctoris Angelici Opera Omnia*. Rome: Vatican Polyglot Press, 1882–.
———. *Sententia libri De anima* [In DA]. In Commissio Leonina (ed.), *S. Thomae Aquinatis Doctoris Angelici Opera Omnia*. Rome: Vatican Polyglot Press, 1882–.
———. *In duodecim libros metaphysicorum Aristotelis expositio* [In M]. R. Cathala and R. Spiazzi (eds.). Turin: Marietti, 1950.
———. *Scriptum super sententiis magistri Petri Lombardi* [In Sent]. P. Mandonnet and M. Moos (eds.). Paris: Lethielleux, 1929–1947.
———. *Quaestio disputata de anima* [QDA]. In Commissio Leonina (ed.), *S. Thomae Aquinatis Doctoris Angelici Opera Omnia*. Rome: Vatican Polyglot Press, 1882–.
———. *Quaestiones disputatae de potentia* [QDP]. In R. Spiazzi (ed.), *Quaestiones disputatae*, vol. 2. Turin: Marietti, 1949.
———. *Quaestio disputata de spiritualibus creaturis* [QDSC]. In R. Spiazzi (ed.), *Quaestiones disputatae*, vol. 2. Turin: Marietti, 1949.
———. *Quaestiones disputatae de veritate* [QDV]. In Commissio Leonina (ed.), *S. Thomae Aquinatis Doctoris Angelici Opera Omnia*. Rome: Vatican Polyglot Press, 1882–.
———. *Summa contra gentiles* [SCG]. In Commissio Leonina (ed.), *S. Thomae Aquinatis Doctoris Angelici Opera Omnia*. Rome: Vatican Polyglot Press, 1882–.
———. *Summa theologiae* [ST]. In Commissio Leonina (ed.), *S. Thomae Aquinatis Doctoris Angelici Opera Omnia*. Rome: Vatican Polyglot Press, 1882–.
Aristotle. *De anima* [DA]. In J. Barnes (ed.), *The Complete Works of Aristotle*, vol. 1. Princeton, NJ: Princeton University Press, 1984.
———. *De generatione animalium* [DGA]. In J. Barnes (ed.), *The Complete Works of Aristotle*, vol. 1. Princeton, NJ: Princeton University Press, 1984.
———. *Historia animalium* [HA]. In J. Barnes (ed.), *The Complete Works of Aristotle*, vol. 1. Princeton, NJ: Princeton University Press, 1984.

Ashley, B. 1976. A critique of the theory of delayed hominization. In D. McCarthy and A. Moraczewski (eds.), *An Ethical Evaluation of Fetal Experimentation: An Interdisciplinary Study.* St. Louis: Pope John XXIII Center.

Ashley, B., and Moraczewski, A. 2001. Cloning, Aquinas, and the embryonic person. *The National Catholic Bioethics Quarterly* 1: 189–201.

Austriaco, N. 2004. Immediate hominization from the systems perspective. *The National Catholic Bioethics Quarterly* 4: 719–738.

Barad, J. 1988. Aquinas's inconsistency on the nature and the treatment of animals. *Between the Species* 4: 102–111.

Bedate, C., and Cefalo, R. 1989. The zygote: To be or not be a person. *The Journal of Medicine and Philosophy* 14: 641–645.

Beddington, R., and Robertson, E. 1999. Axis development and early asymmetry in mammals. *Cell* 96: 195–209.

Boethius. *Contra Eutychen et Nestorium.* In H. F. Stewart, E. K. Rand, and S. J. Tester (trans.), *Tractates and the Consolation of Philosophy.* Cambridge, MA: Harvard University Press, 1918.

Bole, T. J., III. 1990. Zygotes, souls, substances, and persons. *Journal of Medicine and Philosophy* 15: 637–652.

Bracken, W. J. 2001. Is the early embryo a person? *Linacre Quarterly* 68: 49–70.

Charo, R. A. 2001. Every cell is sacred: Logical consequences of the argument from potential in the age of cloning. In P. Lauritzen (ed.), *Cloning and the Future of Human Embryo Research.* New York: Oxford University Press.

Cibelli, J. B., Lanza, R. P., West, M. D., and Ezzell, C. 2002. The first human cloned embryo. *Scientific American* 286(1): 44–51.

Crosby, J. 1993. The personhood of the human embryo. *The Journal of Medicine and Philosophy* 18: 399–418.

Deckers, J. 2007. Why Eberl is wrong: Reflections on the beginning of personhood. *Bioethics* 21: 270–282.

De Koninck, T. 1999. Persons and things. In T. Hibbs and J. O'Callaghan (eds.), *Recovering Nature: Essays in Natural Philosophy, Ethics, and Metaphysics in Honor of Ralph McInerny.* Notre Dame: University of Notre Dame Press.

Diamond, J. J. 1975. Abortion, animation, and biological hominization. *Theological Studies* 36: 305–324.

Donceel, J. 1970. Immediate animation and delayed hominization. *Theological Studies* 31: 76–105.

Eberl, J. T. 2000. The beginning of personhood: A Thomistic biological analysis. *Bioethics* 14: 134–157.

———. 2004. Aquinas on the nature of human beings. *Review of Metaphysics* 58: 333–365.

———. 2005a. Aquinas's account of human embryogenesis and recent interpretations. *Journal of Medicine and Philosophy* 30: 379–394.

———. 2005b. A Thomistic understanding of human death. *Bioethics* 19: 29–48.

———. 2006. *Thomistic Principles and Bioethics.* New York: Routledge.

———. 2007. A Thomistic perspective on the beginning of personhood: Redux. *Bioethics* 21: 283–289.

Finnis, J. 1999. Abortion and health care ethics. In H. Kuhse and P. Singer (eds.), *Bioethics: An Anthology.* Oxford: Blackwell.

Fisher, A. 1991. "When did I begin?" revisited. *Linacre Quarterly* 58: 59–68.

Flaman, P. 1991. When did I begin? Another critical response to Norman Ford. *Linacre Quarterly* 58: 39–55.

Flannery, K. L. 2003. Applying Aristotle in contemporary embryology. *The Thomist* 67: 249–278.

Ford, N. M. 1988. *When Did I Begin? Conception of the Human Individual in History, Philosophy and Science.* New York: Cambridge University Press.

———. 2001. The human embryo as person in Catholic teaching. *The National Catholic Bioethics Quarterly* 1: 155–160.

———. 2002. *The Prenatal Person: Ethics from Conception to Birth.* Oxford: Blackwell.

Gerber, R. 1966. When is the human soul infused? *Laval Theologique et Philosophique* 22: 234–247.

Green, R. M. 2002. Determining moral status. *American Journal of Bioethics* 2(1): 20–30.

Grisez, G. 1989. When do people begin? *Proceedings of the American Catholic Philosophical Association* 63: 27–47.

Grobstein, C. 1988. *Science and the Unborn: Choosing Human Futures.* New York: Basic Books.

Haldane, J., and Lee, P. 2003a. Aquinas on human ensoulment, abortion and the value of life. *Philosophy* 78: 255–278.

———. 2003b. Rational souls and the beginning of life: A reply to Robert Pasnau. *Philosophy* 78: 532–540.

Hall, J. L., Engel, D., Gindoff, P. R., Motta, G. L., and Stillman, R. J. 1993. Experimental cloning of human polypoid embryos using an artificial zona pellucida. Paper presented at the American Fertility Society conjointly with the Canadian Fertility and Andrology Society.

Heaney, S. 1992. Aquinas on the presence of the human rational soul in the early embryo. *The Thomist* 56: 19–48.

Johnson, M. 1995. Delayed hominization: Reflections on some recent Catholic claims for delayed hominization. *Theological Studies* 56: 743–763.

Kenny, A. 2006. The beginning of individual human life. *Proceedings of the American Catholic Philosophical Association* 80: 29–38.

Klubertanz, G. 1953. *The Philosophy of Human Nature.* New York: Appleton-Century-Crofts.

Koch-Hershenov, R. 2006. Totipotency, twinning, and ensoulment at fertilization. *Journal of Medicine and Philosophy* 31: 139–164.

Kretzmann, N. 1999. *The Metaphysics of Creation: Aquinas's Natural Theology in Summa Contra Gentiles II.* Oxford: Clarendon Press.

Lanza, R. P., Caplan, A. L., Silver, L. M., Cibelli, J. B., West, M. D., and Green, R. M. 2000. The ethical validity of using nuclear transfer in human transplantation. *Journal of the American Medical Association* 284: 3175–3179.

Lee, P. 1996. *Abortion and Unborn Human Life.* Washington, DC: Catholic University of America Press.

Lockwood, M. 1995. Human identity and the primitive streak. *Hastings Center Report* 25: 45.

May, W. E. 1992. The moral status of the embryo. *Linacre Quarterly* 59: 76–83.

McCartney, J. J. 2002. Embryonic stem cell research and respect for human life: Philosophical and legal reflections. *Albany Law Review* 65: 597–624.

McCormick, R. A. 1991. Who or what is the preembryo? *Kennedy Institute of Ethics Journal* 1: 1–15.

Meyer, J. R. 2006. Embryonic personhood, human nature, and rational ensoulment. *The Heythrop Journal* 47: 206–225.

Mirkes, R. 2001. NBAC and embryo ethics. *The National Catholic Bioethics Quarterly* 1: 163–187.

Olson, E. 1997. *The Human Animal: Personal Identity without Psychology*. New York: Oxford University Press.

O'Rourke, K. D. 2006. The embryo as person. *The National Catholic Bioethics Quarterly* 6: 241–251.

Panicola, M. 2002. Three views on the preimplantation embryo. *The National Catholic Bioethics Quarterly* 2: 69–97.

Pasnau, R. 2002. *Thomas Aquinas on Human Nature*. New York: Cambridge University Press.

———. 2003. Souls and the beginning of life: A reply to Haldane and Lee. *Philosophy* 78: 521–531.

Pastrana, G. 1977. Personhood and the beginning of human life. *The Thomist* 41: 247–294.

Pearson, H. 2002. Your destiny, from day one. *Nature* 418(6893): 14–15.

Piontelli, A. 2002. *Twins: From Fetus to Child*. New York: Routledge.

Porter, J. 1995. Individuality, personal identity, and the moral status of the preembryo: A response to Mark Johnson. *Theological Studies* 56: 763–770.

President's Council on Bioethics [PCB]. 2002. *Human Cloning and Human Dignity: An Ethical Inquiry*. http://bioethics.gov/reports/cloningreport/index.html.

———. 2004. *Monitoring Stem Cell Research*. http://bioethics.gov/reports/stemcell/index.html.

Robertson, J. A. 1999. Ethics and policy in embryonic stem cell research. *Kennedy Institute of Ethics Journal* 9: 109–136.

Serra, A., and Colombo, R. 1998. Identity and status of the human embryo: The contribution of biology. In J. Vial Correa and E. Sgreccia (eds.), *Identity and Statute of Human Embryo*. Vatican City: Libreria Editrice Vaticana.

Shannon, T. 1996. Delayed hominization: A response to Mark Johnson. *Theological Studies* 57: 731–734.

———. 2001. From the micro to the macro. In S. Holland, K. Lebacqz, and L. Zoloth (eds.), *The Human Embryonic Stem Cell Debate: Science, Ethics, and Public Policy*. Cambridge, MA: MIT Press.

Shannon, T., and Wolter, A. 1990. Reflections on the moral status of the pre-embryo. *Theological Studies* 51: 603–626.

Smith, B., and Brogaard, B. 2003. Sixteen days. *Journal of Medicine and Philosophy* 28: 45–78.

Smith, P. 1983. The beginning of personhood: A Thomistic perspective. *Laval Theologique et Philosophique* 39: 195–214.

Stump, E. 2003. *Aquinas*. New York: Routledge.

Suarez, A. 1990. Hydatidiform moles and teratomas confirm the human identity of the preimplantation embryo. *Journal of Medicine and Philosophy* 15: 627–635.

van Inwagen, P. 1990. *Material Beings*. Ithaca: Cornell University Press.

Vélez, J. R. 2005. Immediate animation: Thomistic principles applied to Norman Ford's objections. *Ethics and Medicine* 21: 11–28.

Vial Correa, J., and Dabike, M. 1998. The embryo as an organism. In J. Vial Correa and E. Sgreccia (eds.), *Identity and Statute of Human Embryo*. Vatican City: Libreria Editrice Vaticana.

Wade, F. 1985. The beginning of individual human life from a philosophical perspective. In J. Bopp, Jr. (ed.), *Human Life and Health Care Ethics*. Frederick, MD: University Publications of America.

Wallace, W. A. 1995. St. Thomas on the beginning and ending of human life. In D. Ols (ed.), *Sanctus Thomas de Aquino Doctor Hodiernae Humanitatis*. Vatican City: Libreria Editrice Vaticana.

Wilmut, I., Schnieke, A. E., McWhir, J., Kind, A. J., and Campbell, K. H. S. 1997. Viable offspring derived from fetal and adult mammalian cells. *Nature* 385: 810–813.

Individuals, Humans, and Persons

The Issue of Moral Status

Helga Kuhse and Peter Singer

Some well-known arguments against non-therapeutic embryo research rest on the premise that fertilization marks the beginning of "genetically new human life organized as a distinct entity oriented towards further development,"[1] and the additional premise that it is wrong to destroy such life, either because of what it currently is, or because of what it has the potential to become. This type of argument, put forward in the majority report of the Australian Senate Select Committee on the Human Experimentation Bill 1985,[2] can also be found in the Vatican's *Instruction on Respect for Human Life*.[3]

We believe there are good reasons for rejecting this type of argument. In Section I of this chapter we outline the reasons why we should reject the view that a zygote or early human embryo is a distinct human individual;[4] in Section II, we argue against the common view that an early embryo has a right to life because it is an innocent human being; in Section III, we put the argument that experimentation on early human embryos is no harder to justify than various other reproductive choices; and finally, in Section IV, we shall sketch a positive account of how we should think about embryo research.

{ I }

It is often assumed that the answer to the question: "When does a particular human life begin?" will also provide the answer to the question of how that life ought, morally, to be treated. We shall, however, set the moral question aside for the moment and instead focus on some prior issues that must be faced by anyone who wants to claim that fertilization marks the time when a particular human life or "I" began to exist.[5]

What this claim amounts to is that the newly fertilized egg, the early embryo and I are, in some sense of the term, the same individual. Now, in one very obvious sense, the zygote that gave rise to me and I, the adult, are not the same individual—the former is a unicellular being totally devoid of consciousness, whereas I am a conscious being consisting of many millions of cells. So the claim that the zygote and I are the same individual must rely on a different sense of "individual." And so it does.

It is usually thought that the zygote and I are the same individual in one or both of the following two senses: first, that there is a genetic continuity between the zygote and me (we share the same genetic code); and, second, that there is what, for want of a better term, one might call "numerical continuity" between us (we are the same single thing). In other words, the zygote does not just have the potential to produce an as-yet-unidentifiable individual, rather the zygote is, from the first moment of its existence, already a particular individual—Tom, or Dick, or Harry. But, as we shall see, this view, which we shall call the "identity thesis," faces some very serious problems. For, contrary to what is often believed, recent scientific findings do not support the view that fertilization marks the event when a particular, identifiable individual begins to exist.

It is true that the life of the fertilized ovum is a genetically new life in the sense that it is neither genetically nor numerically continuous with the life of the egg or the sperm before fertilization. Before fertilization, there were two genetically distinct entities, the egg and the sperm; now there is only one entity, the fertilized egg or zygote, with a new and unique genetic code. It is also true that the zygote will—other things being equal—develop into an embryo, fetus, and baby with the same genetic code.

But, as we shall see, things are not always equal and some serious problems are raised for supporters of the identity thesis.

Here are two scenarios of what might happen during early human development.

In the first scenario, a man and a woman have intercourse, fertilization takes place, and a genetically new zygote, let's call it Tom, is formed. Tom has a specific genetic identity—a genetic blueprint—that will be repeated in every cell once the first cell begins to split, first into two, then into four cells, and so on. On day 8, however, the group of cells which is Tom divides into two separate identical cell groups. These two separate cell groups continue to develop and, some nine months later, identical twins are born. Now, which one, if either of them, is Tom? There are no obvious grounds for thinking of one of the twins as Tom and the other as Not-Tom; the twinning process is quite symmetrical and both twins have the same genetic blueprint as the original Tom. But to suggest that both of them are Tom does, of course, conflict with numerical continuity: there was one zygote and now there are two babies.

People have thought in various ways about this: for example, that when the original cell split, Tom ceased to exist and that two new individuals, Dick and Harry, came into existence. But if that were conceded then it would, of course, no longer be true that the existence of the babies Dick and Harry began at fertilization: their existence did not begin until eight days *after* fertilization. Moreover (and we shall come back to this in a moment) if Tom died on day 8, how is it that he left no earthly remains?

Now consider the second scenario. A man and a woman have intercourse and fertilization takes place. But this time, two eggs are fertilized and two zygotes come into existence—Mary and Jane. The zygotes begin to divide, first into two, then into four cells, and so on. But, then, on day 6, the two embryos combine, forming what is known as a chimera, and continue to develop as a single organism, which will eventually become a baby. Now, who is the baby—Mary or Jane, both Mary and Jane, or somebody else—Nancy?

In one plausible sense of the term, there is genetic continuity between Mary, Jane, and the baby. Because the baby is a chimera, she carries the unique genetic code of both Mary and Jane. Some of the millions of cells that make up her body contain the genetic code of Mary, others the genetic code of Jane. So in that sense the baby would seem to be both Mary and Jane. But in terms of numerical continuity, this poses a problem. There is now only one individual where there were formerly two. Does this mean that Mary or Jane, or both of them, have ceased to exist? But to suggest that one of them has ceased to exist poses the problem of explaining why one and not the other should have ceased to exist. Moreover, to say that anyone has ceased to exist will put one in the difficult position (already encountered in the previous example of Tom) of having to explain how it can be that a human individual has ceased to exist when nothing has been lost or has perished—in other words, when there has been a death but there is no corpse.

We could sketch other scenarios to show further complexities, but enough has been said to demonstrate that even before the advent of new reproductive technologies serious problems were raised for the "identity thesis." As we shall see, these problems have been compounded by new scientific findings.

It is now believed that early embryonic cells are totipotent; that is, that, contrary to the "identity thesis," an early human embryo is not one particular individual, but rather has the potential to become one or more different individuals. Up to the 8-cell stage, each single embryonic cell is a distinct entity in the sense that there is no fusion between the individual cells; rather, the embryo is a loose collection of distinct cells, held together by the zona pellucida, the outer membrane of the egg. Animal studies on four-cell embryos indicate that each one of these cells has the potential to produce at least one fetus or baby.

Take a human embryo consisting of four cells. On the assumption that this embryo is a particular human individual, we shall call it Adam. Because each of Adam's four cells is totipotent, any three cells could be removed from the zona pellucida and the remaining cell would still have the potential to develop into a perfect fetus or baby. Now, it might be thought that this baby is Adam, the same baby that would have resulted had all four cells continued to develop jointly. But this poses a problem because we could have left any one of the other three cells in the zona pellucida, each with the potential to develop into a baby. The same baby—Adam? Things are not made any easier by the recognition that the three "surplus" cells, each placed into an empty zona pellucida, would also have the potential to develop into babies. We now have four distinct human individuals with the potential to develop into four babies. Because it does not make good sense to identify any one particular individual as Adam, let's call them Bill, Charles, David and Eddy.

This example shows that there are not only problems regarding individual identity, but also closely related problems regarding the early embryo's potential to produce one or more human individuals. In the above example, the zygote had the potential to produce either one individual, Adam, or four individuals—Bill, Charles, David and Eddy. But this is not where its potential ends. Had we waited until the embryo had cleaved one more time in its petri dish, there would have been not four, but eight, totipotent cells—that is, eight distinct individual entities oriented towards further development and hence eight potential babies: Fred, Graeme, Harry, Ivan and so on. Moreover, since these individual cells also have the potential to recombine to form, say, just one or two distinct individuals, fertilization cannot be regarded as the beginning of a particular human life.

Those who want to object to embryo experimentation because it destroys a particular or identifiable human life would be on much safer ground were they to argue that a particular human life begins not at fertilization but at around day 14 after fertilization. By that time, totipotency has been lost, and the development of the primitive streak precludes the embryo from becoming two or more different individuals through twinning. Once the primitive streak has formed, it would thus be much easier to argue that it is Adam, Bill or Charles that is developing, or all three of them, but as distinct individuals.

{ II }

Next we want to raise the moral question that we set aside at the beginning of this chapter. Let us assume that we have settled the issue of when a particular individual's life begins—and for the moment it doesn't matter whether this happens at around day 14 or at fertilization. All that we need to assume for our present purposes is that there is such a marker event, that we have identified it and that the entity we are talking about has crossed this particular developmental hurdle.

Now what is it about the new human entity that could raise moral questions about destructive embryo experimentation? Many people believe that it is wrong to use human embryos in research because these embryos are human beings, and all human beings have a right to life. The syllogism goes like this:

Every human being has a right to life.
A human embryo is a human being.
Therefore the human embryo has a right to life.

In case anyone is worrying about issues like capital punishment, or killing in self-defence, we should perhaps add that the term "innocent" is here and henceforth assumed whenever we are talking of human beings and their rights.

The standard argument has a standard response: to accept the first premise—that all human beings have a right to life—but to deny the second premise, that the human embryo is a human being. This standard response, however, runs into difficulties, because the embryo is clearly a being, of some sort, and it can't possibly be of any other species than *Homo sapiens*. Thus it seems to follow that it must be a human being.

Questioning the First Premise

So the standard argument for attributing a right to life to the embryo can withstand the standard response. It is not easy to challenge directly the claim that
the embryo is a human being. What the standard argument cannot withstand,
however, is a more critical examination of its first premise: that every human
being has a right to life. At first glance, this seems the stronger premise. Do we
really want to deny that every (innocent) human being has a right to life? Are
we about to condone murder? No wonder it is on the second premise that most
of the fire has been directed. But the surprising vulnerability of the first premise
becomes apparent as soon as we cease to take "Every human being has a right
to life" as an unquestionable moral axiom, and instead inquire into the moral
basis for our particular objection to killing human beings.

By "our particular objection to killing human beings," we mean the objection we have to killing human beings, over and above any objection we have to
killing other living beings, such as pigs and cows and dogs and cats, and even
trees and lettuces. Why do we think killing human beings is so much more serious than killing these other beings?

The obvious answer is that human beings are different from other animals,
and the greater seriousness of killing them is a result of these differences. But
which of the many differences between humans and other animals justify such
a distinction? Again, the obvious response is that the morally relevant differences are those based on our superior mental powers—our self-awareness, our
rationality, our moral sense, our autonomy, or some combination of these. They
are the kinds of thing, we are inclined to say, which make us "uniquely human."
To be more precise, they are the kinds of thing which make us persons.

That the particular objection to killing human beings rests on such qualities
is very plausible. To take the most extreme of the differences between living
things, consider a person who is enjoying life, is part of a network of relationships with other people, is looking forward to what tomorrow may bring, and is
freely choosing the course her or his life will take for the years to come. Now
think about a lettuce, which, we can safely assume, knows and feels nothing at
all. One would have to be quite mad, or morally blind, or warped, not to see that
killing the person is far more serious than killing the lettuce.

We shall postpone asking which mental qualities make it more morally serious
to kill a person than to kill a lettuce. For our immediate purposes, we will merely
note that the plausibility of the assertion that human beings have a right to life
depends on the fact that human beings generally possess mental qualities that

other living beings do not possess. So should we accept the premise that every human being has a right to life? We may do so, but only if we bear in mind that by "human being" here we refer to those beings who have the mental qualities which generally distinguish members of our species from members of other species.

If this is the sense in which we can accept the first premise, however, what of the second premise? It is immediately clear that in the sense of the term "human being" which is required to make the first premise acceptable, the second premise is false. The embryo, especially the early embryo, is obviously not a being with the mental qualities that generally distinguish members of our species from members of other species. The early embryo has no brain, no nervous system. It is reasonable to assume that, so far as its mental life goes, it has no more awareness than a lettuce.

It is still true that the human embryo is a member of the species *Homo sapiens*. That is why it is difficult to deny that the human embryo is a human being. But we can now see that this is not the sense of "human being" needed to make the standard argument work. A valid argument cannot equivocate on the meanings of its central terms. If the first premise is true when "human" means "a being with certain mental qualities" and the second premise is true when "human" means "member of the species *Homo sapiens*," the argument is based on a slide between the two meanings, and is invalid.

Can the argument be rescued? It obviously can't be rescued by claiming that the embryo is a being with the requisite mental qualities. That might be arguable only for some later stage of the development of the fetus. If the second premise cannot be reconciled with the first, then, can the first perhaps be defended in a form which makes it compatible with the second? Can it be argued that human beings have a right to life, not because of any moral qualities they may possess, but because they—unlike pigs, cows, dogs or lettuces—are members of the species *Homo sapiens*?

This is a desperate move. Those who make it find themselves having to defend the claim that species membership is in itself morally relevant to the wrongness of killing a being. But why should that be so? If we are considering whether it is wrong to destroy something, surely we must look at its actual characteristics, not just the species to which it belongs. If visitors from other planets turn out to be sensitive, thinking, planning beings, who form deep and lasting relationships just like we do, would it be acceptable to kill them simply because they are not members of our species? What if we substituted "race" for "species" in the question? If we reject the claim that membership of a particular race is in itself morally relevant to the wrongness of killing a being, it is not easy to see how we could accept the same claim when based on species membership. The fact that other races, like our own, can feel, think and plan for the future is not relevant to this question, for we are considering membership in a particular group—whether race or species—as the sole basis for determining the wrongness of killing members of one group or another. It seems clear that neither race nor species can, in itself, provide any justifiable basis for such a distinction.

So the standard argument fails. It does so not because the embryo is not a human being, but because the sense in which the embryo is a human being is not the sense in which we should accept that every human being has a right to life.

{ III }

We have now seen the inadequacies of arguing that the human zygote or early embryo is a distinct human individual, and that destructive embryo experimentation is wrong because the zygote or embryo is a member of the human species. But there are other reasons why one might consider embryo experimentation wrong. Since the early embryo, devoid of a nervous system or a brain, can neither experience pain or pleasure, nor any of the things occurring in the world, the most important thing about it is that it is a potential baby or person, a person just like us. In other words, when we destroy an early human embryo in research, a potential baby or person will now not exist.

Why is this fact morally significant? One plausible answer is provided by R. M. Hare when he appeals, in a well-known article on abortion, to a type of formal argument, captured in the ancient Christian and pre-Christian Golden Rule, that has been the basis of almost all theories of moral reasoning: that we should do to others as we wish them to do to us.[6] In other words, given that we are glad that nobody destroyed us when we were embryos, we should, other things being equal, not destroy an embryo that would have a life like us.

It might seem that the Golden Rule applied to embryo experimentation would impose on us an extremely conservative position, for it would seem to rule out the destruction of all but the most seriously abnormal zygote or embryo. But before we too readily embrace that conclusion, we should also note something already pointed out by Hare in the abortion context: when you are glad that you exist, you do not confine this gladness to gladness that you were not aborted when an embryo or fetus. Rather, you are also glad that you were brought into existence in the first place—that your parents had intercourse without contraception when they did.[7]

Let us apply this sort of thinking to our present context—that of the IVF embryo—and assume that, at some time between the beginning of the process of fertilization and the formation of the primitive streak, the existence of an identifiable individual began. Let us also assume that you developed from that individual. Now, it will immediately become apparent that regardless of what event marked the beginning of your life as an identifiable entity, none of the other events that preceded it were any less important for your present existence. Just as you would not have existed had a scientist performed a destructive experiment on the embryo from which you developed when it was 14 days old, so you would not have existed had she or he performed it on the zygote when it was one day old. Similarly, you would not have existed had your mother's egg with your father's sperm already inside it been destroyed just before syngamy had occurred, or just after that event. Nor, we should hasten to add, would you have existed had the scientist, instead of using one particular egg, used another egg or had a different sperm fertilized the egg, and so on.

The upshot is that the marker event for the beginning of a human individual, on whose identification so much time and energy is being expended, is of no importance so far as the existence of a particular person is concerned. If it is the existence of a particular person that is relevant—a Tom, a Dick, or a Harry—who would treasure his life in much the same way as we do, then it does not matter whether his existence was thwarted before or after fertilization, or the formation of the primitive streak, had occurred.

We should also note that there are numerous ways in which the existence of particular individuals can be thwarted. A totipotent IVF embryo, for example, is not, as we saw, one particular individual, but rather an entity with the potential to become one or more different individuals, because each cell is a distinct entity with the potential for further development. What are we doing, then, when we refrain from separating the cells, leaving all four or eight of them together? And what are we doing when we extract and destroy a single cell for gene-typing of the embryo? We believe we should, in consistency, say that we are depriving a number of human individuals of their chance of existence.

This is one important point. The other important point is this: our reproductive choices almost invariably constitute an explicit or implicit choice between different individuals. We said a moment ago that had the scientist who assisted your imaginary IVF conception used a different sperm or a different egg, you would not have existed, and the same thing applies, of course, to other scenarios in natural reproduction as well. But—and this is the morally important point—seeing that your parents wanted to raise a child of their own, it is likely that another child would have been born. While this person would not have been you, it would have been a person just like you in the morally relevant sense that she or he would now, presumably, be just as glad to exist as you are glad to exist.

But if our reproductive choices typically constitute a choice between different individuals, then the destruction of early human embryos—particularly if it makes possible improved IVF techniques and, therefore, the existence of IVF children who would not otherwise have existed—is no harder to justify than many of our other reproductive choices: for example, when and with whom, to have intercourse, without contraception, to have the two or three children we are going to have.

{ IV }

We have now seen that some of the most common objections to destructive experimentation on early human embryos are seriously flawed. But when, in its development from zygote to baby, does the embryo acquire any rights or interests? We believe the minimal characteristic needed to give the embryo a claim to consideration is sentience, or the capacity to feel pleasure or pain. Until that point is reached, the embryo does not have any interests and, like other non-sentient organisms (a human egg, for example), cannot be harmed—in a morally relevant sense—by anything we do. We can, of course, damage the embryo in such a way as to cause harm to the sentient being it will become, if it lives, but if it never becomes a sentient being, the embryo has not been harmed, because its total lack of awareness means that it never has had any interests at all.

The fact that the early embryo has no interests is also relevant to a distinction embodied in the *Infertility (Medical Procedures) Act* 1984 (Vic.) between "spare" embryos left over from infertility treatments (which may be used in experimentation), and the creation of embryos especially for research (which is prohibited).[8] The report of the Waller Committee, on which the legislation is based, speaks of such a creation as using a human being as a means rather than as an end.[9] This is a principle of Kantian ethics that makes some sense when applied to rational, autonomous beings—or perhaps even, though more controversially, when applied to sentient beings who, though not rational or autonomous, may have ends of their own. There is no basis at all, however, for applying it to a totally non-sentient embryo, which can have no ends of its own.

Finally, we point to a curious consequence of restrictive legislation on embryo research. In sharp contrast to the human embryo at this early stage of its existence, non-human animals such as primates, dogs, rabbits, guinea pigs, rats and mice clearly can feel pain, and thus often are harmed by what is done to them in the course of scientific research. We have already suggested that the species of a being is not, in itself, relevant to its ethical status. Why, then, is it considered acceptable to poison conscious rabbits in order to test the safety of drugs and household chemicals, but not considered acceptable to carry out tests on totally non-sentient human embryos? It is only when an embryo reaches the stage at which it may be capable of feeling pain that we need to control the experimentation which can be done with it. At this point the embryo ranks, morally, with those non-human animals we have mentioned. These animals have often been unjustifiably made to suffer in scientific research. We should have stringent controls over research to ensure that this cannot happen to embryos, just as we should have stringent controls to ensure that it cannot happen to animals.

At what point, then, does the embryo develop a capacity to feel pain? Though we are not experts in this field, from our reading of the literature, we would say that it cannot possibly be earlier than six weeks, and it may well be as late as 18 or 20 weeks.[10] While we think we should err on the side of caution, it seems to us that the 14-day limit suggested by both the Waller and Warnock committees is too conservative.[11] There is no doubt that the embryo is not sentient for some time after this date. Even if we were to be very, very cautious in erring on the safe side, a 28-day limit would provide sufficient protection against the possibility of an embryo suffering during experimentation.

NOTES

1. Senate Select Committee on the Human Embryo Experimentation Bill 1985, *Human Embryo Experimentation in Australia* (Senator Michael Tate, chairman), (AGPS, Canberra, 1986), p. 13.

2. Ibid.

3. Congregation for the Doctrine of the Faith, *Instruction on Respect for Human Life in its Origin and on the Dignity of Procreation—Replies to Certain Questions of the Day* (Vatican City, 1987).

4. Section I of this chapter was inspired by Michael Coughlan's "'From the Moment of Conception . . .': The Vatican Instruction on Artificial Procreation Techniques," *Bioethics* II, 3 (July 1988).

5. For a more detailed discussion of this issue, see Norman Ford, *When did I begin?* (Cambridge University Press, Cambridge, 1988).

6. Hare, R. M., "Abortion and the golden rule," *Philosophy and Public Affairs* 4:3 (1975), 201–22.

7. Ibid., p. 212.

8. *Infertility (Medical Procedures) Act* 1984 (Vic.).

9. Committee to Consider the Social, Ethical and Legal Issues Arising from In Vitro Fertilization, *Report on the Disposition of Embryos Produced by In Vitro Fertilization* (Prof. Louis Waller, chairman), (Victorian Government Printer, Melbourne, 1984), para. 3.27.

10. For an expert opinion on when a fetus may begin to be capable of feeling pain, see the report of the British Government's Advisory Group on Fetal Research, *The Use of Foetuses and Foetal Material for Research* (Sir John Peel, chairman), (HMSO, London, 1972). A clear summary of some relevant scientific evidence, with further references, can be found in M. Tooley, *Abortion and Infanticide* (Clarendon Press, Oxford, 1983), pp. 347–407.

11. Waller, *Report on the Disposition of Embryos*, para. 3.29; and *Report of the Committee of Inquiry into Human Fertilization and Embryology* (Mary Warnock, chair), (HMSO, London, 1984), pars. 11.19–11.22.

CHAPTER TWENTY-ONE

On the Moral and Legal Status of Abortion

Mary Anne Warren

We will be concerned with both the moral status of abortion, which for our purposes we may define as the act which a woman performs in voluntarily terminating, or allowing another person to terminate, her pregnancy, and the legal status which is appropriate for this act. I will argue that, while it is not possible to produce a satisfactory defense of a woman's right to obtain an abortion without showing that a fetus is not a human being, in the morally relevant sense of that term, we ought not to conclude that the difficulties involved in determining whether or not a fetus is human make it impossible to produce any satisfactory solution to the problem of the moral status of abortion. For it is possible to show that, on the basis of intuitions which we may expect even the opponents of abortion to share, a fetus is not a person, and hence not the sort of entity to which it is proper to ascribe full moral rights.

Of course, while some philosophers would deny the possibility of any such proof,[1] others will deny that there is any need for it, since the moral permissibility of abortion appears to them to be too obvious to require proof. But the inadequacy of this attitude should be evident from the fact that both the friends and the foes of abortion consider their position to be morally self-evident. Because pro-abortionists have never adequately come to grips with the conceptual issues surrounding abortion, most if not all, of the arguments which they advance in opposition to laws restricting access to abortion fail to refute or even weaken the traditional antiabortion argument, i.e., that a fetus is a human being, and therefore abortion is murder.

These arguments are typically of one of two sorts. Either they point to the terrible side effects of the restrictive laws, e.g., the deaths due to illegal abortions, and the fact that it is poor women who suffer the most as a result of these laws, or else they state that to deny a woman access to abortion is to deprive her of her right to control her own body. Unfortunately, however, the fact that restricting access to abortion has tragic side effects does not, in itself, show that the restrictions are unjustified, since murder is wrong regardless of the consequences of prohibiting it; and the appeal to the right to control one's body, which is generally construed as a property right, is at best a rather feeble argument for the permissibility of abortion. Mere ownership does not give me the right to kill innocent people whom I find on my property, and indeed I am apt to be held responsible if such people injure themselves while on my property. It is equally unclear that I have any moral right to expel an innocent person from my property when I know that doing so will result in his death.

Furthermore, it is probably inappropriate to describe a woman's body as her property, since it seems natural to hold that a person is something distinct from her property, but not from her body. Even those who would object to the identification of a person with his body, or with the conjunction of his body and his mind, must admit that it would be very odd to describe, say, breaking a leg, as damaging one's property, and much more appropriate to describe it as injuring one*self.* Thus it is probably a mistake to argue that the right to obtain an abortion is in any way derived from the right to own and regulate property.

But however we wish to construe the right to abortion, we cannot hope to convince those who consider abortion a form of murder of the existence of any such right unless we are able to produce a clear and convincing refutation of the traditional antiabortion argument, and this has not, to my knowledge, been done. With respect to the two most vital issues which that argument involves, i.e., the humanity of the fetus and its implication for the moral status of abortion, confusion has prevailed on both sides of the dispute.

Thus, both proabortionists and antiabortionists have tended to abstract the question of whether abortion is wrong to that of whether it is wrong to destroy a fetus, just as though the rights of another person were not necessarily involved. This mistaken abstraction has led to the almost universal assumption that if a fetus is a human being, with a right to life, then it follows immediately that abortion is wrong (except perhaps when necessary to save the woman's life), and that it ought to be prohibited. It has also been generally assumed that unless the question about the status of the fetus is answered, the moral status of abortion cannot possibly be determined.

Two recent papers, one by B. A. Brody,[2] and one by Judith Thomson,[3] have attempted to settle the question of whether abortion ought to be prohibited apart from the question of whether or not the fetus is human. Brody examines the possibility that the following two statements are compatible: (1) that abortion is the taking of innocent human life, and therefore wrong; and (2) that nevertheless it ought not to be prohibited by law, at least under the present circumstances.[4] Not surprisingly, Brody finds it impossible to reconcile these two statements, since, as he rightly argues, none of the unfortunate side effects of the prohibition of abortion is bad enough to justify legalizing the *wrongful* taking of human life. He is mistaken, however, in concluding that the incompatibility of (1) and (2), in itself, shows that "the legal problem about abortion cannot be resolved independently of the status of the fetus problem" (p. 369).

What Brody fails to realize is that (1) embodies the questionable assumption that if a fetus is a human being, then of course abortion is morally wrong, and that an attack on *this* assumption is more promising, as a way of reconciling the humanity of the fetus with the claim that laws prohibiting abortion are unjustified, than is an attack on the assumption that if abortion is the wrongful killing of innocent human beings then it ought to be prohibited. He thus overlooks the possibility that a fetus may have a right to life and abortion still be morally permissible, in that the right of a woman to terminate an unwanted pregnancy might override the right of the fetus to be kept alive. The immorality of abortion is no more demonstrated by the humanity of the fetus, in itself, than the immorality of killing in self-defense is demonstrated by the fact that the assailant is a human being. Neither is it demonstrated by the *innocence* of the fetus, since there may be situations in which the killing of innocent human beings is justified.

It is perhaps not surprising that Brody fails to spot this assumption, since it has been accepted with little or no argument by nearly everyone who has written on the morality of abortion. John Noonan is correct in saying that "the fundamental question in the long history of abortion is, How do you determine the humanity of a being?"[5] He summarizes his own antiabortion argument, which is a version of the official position of the Catholic Church, as follows:

> ... it is wrong to kill humans, however poor, weak, defenseless, and lacking in op-
> portunity to develop their potential they may be. It is therefore morally wrong to
> kill Biafrans. Similarly, it is morally wrong to kill embryos.[6]

Noonan bases his claim that fetuses are human upon what he calls the theologians' criterion of humanity: that whoever is conceived of human beings is
human. But although he argues at length for the appropriateness of this criterion, he never questions the assumption that if a fetus is human then abortion
is wrong for exactly the same reason that murder is wrong.

Judith Thomson is, in fact, the only writer I am aware of who has seriously
questioned this assumption; she has argued that, even if we grant the antiabortionist his claim that a fetus is a human being, with the same right to life as any
other human being, we can still demonstrate that, in at least some and perhaps
most cases, a woman is under no moral obligation to complete an unwanted
pregnancy.[7] Her argument is worth examining, since if it holds up it may enable
us to establish the moral permissibility of abortion without becoming involved
in problems about what entitles an entity to be considered human, and accorded full moral rights. To be able to do this would be a great gain in the power
and simplicity of the proabortion position, since, although I will argue that
these problems can be solved at least as decisively as can any other moral problem, we should certainly be pleased to be able to avoid having to solve them as
part of the justification of abortion.

On the other hand, even if Thomson's argument does not hold up, her insight, i.e., that it requires *argument* to show that if fetuses are human then abortion is properly classified as murder, is an extremely valuable one. The assumption she attacks is particularly invidious, for it amounts to the decision that it is
appropriate, in deciding the moral status of abortion, to leave the rights of the
pregnant woman out of consideration entirely, except possibly when her life is
threatened. Obviously, this will not do; determining what moral rights, if any,
a fetus possesses is only the first step in determining the moral status of abortion. Step two, which is at least equally essential, is finding a just solution to the
conflict between whatever rights the fetus may have, and the rights of the
woman who is unwillingly pregnant. While the historical error has been to pay
far too little attention to the second step, Ms. Thomson's suggestion is that if we
look at the second step first we may find that a woman has a right to obtain an
abortion *regardless* of what rights the fetus has.

Our own inquiry will also have two stages. In Section I, we will consider
whether or not it is possible to establish that abortion is morally permissible

even on the assumption that a fetus is an entity with a full-fledged right to life. I will argue that in fact this cannot be established, at least not with the conclusiveness which is essential to our hopes of convincing those who are skeptical about the morality of abortion, and that we therefore cannot avoid dealing with the question of whether or not a fetus really does have the same right to life as a (more fully developed) human being.

In Section II, I will propose an answer to this question, namely, that a fetus cannot be considered a member of the moral community, the set of beings with full and equal moral rights, for the simple reason that it is not a person, and that it is personhood, and not genetic humanity, i.e., humanity as defined by Noonan, which is the basis for membership in this community. I will argue that a fetus, whatever its stage of development, satisfies none of the basic criteria of personhood, and is not even enough *like* a person to be accorded even some of the same rights on the basis of this resemblance. Nor, as we will see, is a fetus's *potential* personhood a threat to the morality of abortion, since, whatever the rights of potential people may be, they are invariably overridden in any conflict with the moral rights of actual people.

{ I }

We turn now to Professor Thomson's case for the claim that even if a fetus has full moral rights, abortion is still morally permissible, at least sometimes, and for some reasons other than to save the woman's life. Her argument is based upon a clever, but I think faulty, analogy. She asks us to picture ourselves waking up one day, in bed with a famous violinist. Imagine that you have been kidnapped, and your bloodstream hooked up to that of the violinist, who happens to have an ailment which will certainly kill him unless he is permitted to share your kidneys for a period of nine months. No one else can save him, since you alone have the right type of blood. He will be unconscious all that time, and you will have to stay in bed with him, but after the nine months are over he may be unplugged, completely cured, that is provided that you have cooperated.

Now then, she continues, what are your obligations in this situation? The antiabortionist, if he is consistent, will have to say that you are obligated to stay in bed with the violinist: for all people have a right to life, and violinists are people, and therefore it would be murder for you to disconnect yourself from him and let him die (p. 49). But this is outrageous, and so there must be something wrong with the same argument when it is applied to abortion. It would certainly be commendable of you to agree to save the violinist, but it is absurd to suggest that your refusal to do so would be murder. His right to life does not obligate you to do whatever is required to keep him alive; nor does it justify anyone else in forcing you to do so. A law which required you to stay in bed with the violinist would clearly be an unjust law, since it is no proper function of the law to force unwilling people to make huge sacrifices for the sake of other people toward whom they have no such prior obligation.

Thomson concludes that, if this analogy is an apt one, then we can grant the antiabortionist his claim that a fetus is a human being, and still hold that it is at least sometimes the case that a pregnant woman has the right to refuse to be a Good Samaritan towards the fetus, i.e., to obtain an abortion. For there is a great gap between the claim that x has a right to life, and the claim that y is obligated to do whatever is necessary to keep x alive, let alone that he ought to be forced to do so. It is y's duty to keep x alive only if he has somehow contracted a *special* obligation to do so; and a woman who is unwillingly pregnant, e.g., who was raped, has done nothing which obligates her to make the enormous sacrifice which is necessary to preserve the conceptus.

This argument is initially quite plausible, and in the extreme case of pregnancy due to rape it is probably conclusive. Difficulties arise, however, when we try to specify more exactly the range of cases in which abortion is clearly justifiable even on the assumption that the fetus is human. Professor Thomson considers it a virtue of her argument that it does not enable us to conclude that abortion is *always* permissible. It would, she says, be "indecent" for a woman in her seventh month to obtain an abortion just to avoid having to postpone a trip to Europe. On the other hand, her argument enables us to see that "a sick and desperately frightened schoolgirl pregnant due to rape may *of course* choose abortion, and that any law which rules this out is an insane law" (p. 65). So far, so good; but what are we to say about the woman who becomes pregnant not through rape but as a result of her own carelessness, or because of contraceptive failure, or who gets pregnant intentionally and then changes her mind about wanting a child? With respect to such cases, the violinist analogy is of much less use to the defender of the woman's right to obtain an abortion.

Indeed, the choice of a pregnancy due to rape, as an example of a case in which abortion is permissible even if a fetus is considered a human being, is extremely significant; for it is only in the case of pregnancy due to rape that the woman's situation is adequately analogous to the violinist case for our intuitions about the latter to transfer convincingly. The crucial difference between a pregnancy due to rape and the *normal* case of an unwanted pregnancy is that in the normal case we cannot claim that the woman is in no way responsible for her predicament; she could have remained chaste, or taken her pills more faithfully, or abstained on dangerous days, and so on. If, on the other hand, you are kidnapped by strangers, and hooked up to a strange violinist, then you are free of any shred of responsibility for the situation, on the basis of which it could be argued that you are obligated to keep the violinist alive. Only when her pregnancy is due to rape is a woman clearly just as nonresponsible.[8]

Consequently, there is room for the antiabortionist to argue that in the normal case of unwanted pregnancy a woman has, by her own actions, assumed responsibility for the fetus. For if x behaves in a way which he could have avoided, and which he knows involves, let us say, a 1 percent chance of bringing into existence a human being, with a right to life, and does so knowing that if this should happen then that human being will perish unless x does certain things to keep him alive, then it is by no means clear that when it does happen x is free of any obligation to what he knew in advance would be required to keep that human being alive.

The plausibility of such an argument is enough to show that the Thomson analogy can provide a clear and persuasive defense of a woman's right to obtain an abortion only with respect to those cases in which the woman is in no way responsible for her pregnancy, e.g., where it is due to rape. In all other cases, we would almost certainly conclude that it was necessary to look carefully at the particular circumstances in order to determine the extent of the woman's responsibility, and hence the extent of her obligation. This is an extremely unsatisfactory outcome, from the viewpoint of the opponents of restrictive abortion laws, most of whom are convinced that a woman has a right to obtain an abortion regardless of how and why she got pregnant.

Of course a supporter of the violinist analogy might point out that it is absurd to suggest that forgetting her pill one day might be sufficient to obligate a woman to complete an unwanted pregnancy. And indeed it *is* absurd to suggest this. As we will see, the moral right to obtain an abortion is not in the least dependent upon the extent to which the woman is responsible for her pregnancy. But unfortunately, once we allow the assumption that a fetus has full moral rights, we cannot avoid taking this absurd suggestion seriously. Perhaps we can make this point more clear by altering the violinist story just enough to make it more analogous to a normal unwanted pregnancy and less to a pregnancy due to rape, and then seeing whether it is still obvious that you are not obligated to stay in bed with the fellow.

Suppose, then, that violinists are peculiarly prone to the sort of illness the only cure for which is the use of someone else's bloodstream for nine months, and that because of this there has been formed a society of music lovers who agree that whenever a violinist is stricken they will draw lots and the loser will, by some means, be made the one and only person capable of saving him. Now then, would you be obligated to cooperate in curing the violinist if you had voluntarily joined this society, knowing the possible consequences, and then your name had been drawn and you had been kidnapped? Admittedly, you did not promise ahead of time that you would, but you did deliberately place yourself in a position in which it might happen that a human life would be lost if you did not. Surely this is at least a prima facie reason for supposing that you have an obligation to stay in bed with the violinist. Suppose that you had gotten your name drawn deliberately; surely *that* would be quite a strong reason for thinking that you had such an obligation.

It might be suggested that there is one important disanalogy between the modified violinist case and the case of an unwanted pregnancy, which makes the woman's responsibility significantly less, namely, the fact that the fetus *comes into existence* as the result of the woman's actions. This fact might give her a right to refuse to keep it alive, whereas she would not have had this right had it existed previously, independently, and then as a result of her actions become dependent upon her for its survival.

My own intuition, however, is that x has no more right to bring into existence, either deliberately or as a foreseeable result of actions he could have avoided, a being with full moral rights (y), and then refuse to do what he knew beforehand would be required to keep that being alive, than he has to enter into an agreement with an existing person, whereby he may be called upon to save that person's life, and then refuse to do so when so called upon. Thus, x's responsibility for y's existence does not seem to lessen his obligation to keep y alive, if he is also responsible for y's being in a situation in which only he can save him.

Whether or not this intuition is entirely correct, it brings us back once again to the conclusion that once we allow the assumption that a fetus has full moral rights it becomes an extremely complex and difficult question whether and when abortion is justifiable. Thus the Thomson analogy cannot help us produce a clear and persuasive proof of the moral permissibility of abortion. Nor will the opponents of the restrictive laws thank us for anything less; for their conviction (for the most part) is that abortion is obviously *not* a morally serious and extremely unfortunate, even though sometimes justified act, comparable to killing in self-defense or to letting the violinist die, but rather is closer to being a morally neutral act, like cutting one's hair.

The basis of this conviction, I believe, is the realization that a fetus is not a person, and thus does not have a full-fledged right to life. Perhaps the reason why this claim has been so inadequately defended is that it seems self-evident to those who accept it. And so it is, insofar as it follows from what I take to be perfectly obvious claims about the nature of personhood, and about the proper grounds for ascribing moral rights, claims which ought, indeed, to be obvious to both the friends and foes of abortion. Nevertheless, it is worth examining these claims, and showing how they demonstrate the moral innocuousness of abortion, since this apparently has not been adequately done before.

{ II }

The question which we must answer in order to produce a satisfactory solution to the problem of the moral status of abortion is this: How are we to define the moral community, the set of beings with full and equal moral rights, such that we can decide whether a human fetus is a member of this community or not? What sort of entity, exactly, has the inalienable rights to life, liberty, and the pursuit of happiness? Jefferson attributed these rights to all *men,* and it may or may not be fair to suggest that he intended to attribute them *only* to men. Perhaps he ought to have attributed them to all human beings. If so, then we arrive, first, at Noonan's problem of defining what makes a being human, and, second, at the equally vital question which Noonan does not consider, namely, What reason is there for identifying the moral community with the set of all human beings, in whatever way we have chosen to define that term?

1. On the Definition of "Human"

One reason why this vital second question is so frequently overlooked in the debate over the moral status of abortion is that the term "human" has two distinct, but not often distinguished, senses. This fact results in a slide of meaning, which serves to conceal the fallaciousness of the traditional argument that since (1) it is wrong to kill innocent human beings, and (2) fetuses are innocent human beings, then (3) it is wrong to kill fetuses. For if "human" is used in the same sense in both (1) and (2) then, whichever of the two senses is meant, one of these premises is question-begging. And if it is used in two different senses then of course the conclusion doesn't follow.

Thus, (1) is a self-evident moral truth,[9] and avoids begging the question about abortion, only if "human being" is used to mean something like "a full-fledged member of the moral community." (It may or may not also be meant to refer exclusively to members of the species *Homo sapiens*.) We may call this the *moral* sense of "human." It is not to be confused with what we will call the *genetic* sense, i.e., the sense in which *any* member of the species is a human being, and no member of any other species could be. If (1) is acceptable only if the moral sense is intended, (2) is non-question-begging only if what is intended is the genetic sense.

In "Deciding Who is Human," Noonan argues for the classification of fetuses with human beings by pointing to the presence of the full genetic code, and the potential capacity for rational thought (p. 135). It is clear that what he needs to show, for his version of the traditional argument to be valid, is that fetuses are human in the moral sense, the sense in which it is analytically true that all human beings have full moral rights. But, in the absence of any argument showing that whatever is genetically human is also morally human, and he gives none, nothing more than genetic humanity can be demonstrated by the presence of the human genetic code. And, as we will see, the *potential* capacity for rational thought can at most show that an entity has the potential for *becoming* human in the moral sense.

2. Defining the Moral Community

Can it be established that genetic humanity is sufficient for moral humanity? I think that there are very good reasons for not defining the moral community in this way. I would like to suggest an alternative way of defining the moral community, which I will argue for only to the extent of explaining why it is, or should be, self-evident. The suggestion is simply that the moral community consists of all and only *people*, rather than all and only human beings;[10] and probably the best way of demonstrating its self-evidence is by considering the concept of personhood, to see what sorts of entity are and are not persons, and what the decision that a being is or is not a person implies about its moral rights.

What characteristics entitle an entity to be considered a person? This is obviously not the place to attempt a complete analysis of the concept of personhood, but we do not need such a fully adequate analysis just to determine whether and why a fetus is or isn't a person. All we need is a rough and approximate list of the most basic criteria of personhood, and some idea of which, or how many, of these an entity must satisfy in order to properly be considered a person.

In searching for such criteria, it is useful to look beyond the set of people with whom we are acquainted, and ask how we would decide whether a totally alien being was a person or not. (For we have no right to assume that genetic humanity is necessary for personhood.) Imagine a space traveler who lands on an unknown planet and encounters a race of beings utterly unlike any he has ever seen or heard of. If he wants to be sure of behaving morally toward these beings, he has to somehow decide whether they are people, and hence have full moral rights, or whether they are the sort of thing which he need not feel guilty about treating as, for example, a source of food.

How should he go about making this decision? If he has some anthropological background, he might look for such things as religion, art, and the manufacturing of tools, weapons, or shelters, since these factors have been used to distinguish our human from our prehuman ancestors, in what seems to be closer to the moral than the genetic sense of "human." And no doubt he would be right to consider the presence of such factors as good evidence that the alien beings were people, and morally human. It would, however, be overly anthropocentric of him to take the absence of these things as adequate evidence that they were not, since we can imagine people who have progressed beyond, or evolved without ever developing, these cultural characteristics.

I suggest that the traits which are most central to the concept of personhood, or humanity in the moral sense, are, very roughly, the following:

(1) consciousness (of objects and events external and/or internal to the being), and in particular the capacity to feel pain;
(2) reasoning (the *developed* capacity to solve new and relatively complex problems);
(3) self-motivated activity (activity which is relatively independent of either genetic or direct external control);
(4) the capacity to communicate, by whatever means, messages of an indefinite variety of types, that is, not just with an indefinite number of possible contents, but on indefinitely many possible topics;
(5) the presence of self-concepts, and self-awareness, either individual or racial, or both.

Admittedly, there are apt to be a great many problems involved in formulating precise definitions of these criteria, let alone in developing universally valid behavioral criteria for deciding when they apply. But I will assume that both we and our explorer know approximately what (1)–(5) mean, and that he is also able to determine whether or not they apply. How, then, should he use his findings to decide whether or not the alien beings are people? We needn't suppose that an entity must have *all* of these attributes to be properly considered a person; (1) and (2) alone may well be sufficient for personhood, and quite probably (1)–(3) are sufficient. Neither do we need to insist that any one of these criteria is *necessary* for personhood, although once again (1) and (2) look like fairly good candidates for necessary conditions, as does (3), if "activity" is construed so as to include the activity of reasoning.

All we need to claim, to demonstrate that a fetus is not a person, is that any being which satisfies *none* of (1)–(5) is certainly not a person. I consider this claim to be so obvious that I think anyone who denied it, and claimed that a being which satisfied none of (1)–(5) was a person all the same, would thereby demonstrate that he had no notion at all of what a person is—perhaps because he had confused the concept of a person with that of genetic humanity. If the opponents of abortion were to deny the appropriateness of these five criteria, I do not know what further arguments would convince them. We would probably have to admit that our conceptual schemes were indeed irreconcilably different, and that our dispute could not be settled objectively.

I do not expect this to happen, however, since I think that the concept of a person is one which is very nearly universal (to people), and that it is common to both proabortionists and antiabortionists, even though neither group has fully realized the relevance of this concept to the resolution of their dispute. Furthermore, I think that on reflection even the antiabortionists ought to agree not only that (1)–(5) are central to the concept of personhood, but also that it is a part of this concept that all and only people have full moral rights. The concept of a person is in part a moral concept; once we have admitted that *x* is a person we have recognized, even if we have not agreed to respect, *x's* right to be treated as a member of the moral community. It is true that the claim that *x* is a *human being* is more commonly voiced as part of an appeal to treat *x* decently than is the claim that *x* is a person, but this is either because "human being" is here used in the sense which implies personhood, or because the genetic and moral senses of "human" have been confused.

Now if (1)–(5) are indeed the primary criteria of personhood, then it is clear that genetic humanity is neither necessary nor sufficient for establishing that an entity is a person. Some human beings are not people, and there may well be people who are not human beings. A man or woman whose consciousness has been permanently obliterated but who remains alive is a human being which is no longer a person; defective human beings, with no appreciable mental capacity, are not and presumably never will be people; and a fetus is a human being which is not yet a person, and which therefore cannot coherently be said to have full moral rights. Citizens of the next century should be prepared to recognize highly advanced, self-aware robots or computers, should such be developed, and intelligent inhabitants of other worlds, should such be found, as people in the fullest sense, and to respect their moral rights. But to ascribe full moral rights to an entity which is not a person is as absurd as to ascribe moral obligations and responsibilities to such an entity.

3. Fetal Development and the Right to Life

Two problems arise in the application of these suggestions for the definition of the moral community to the determination of the precise moral status of a human fetus. Given that the paradigm example of a person is a normal adult human being, then (1) How like this paradigm, in particular how far advanced since conception, does a human being need to be before it begins to have a right to life by virtue, not of being fully a person as of yet, but of being *like* a person? and (2) To what extent, if any, does the fact that a fetus has the *potential* for becoming a person endow it with some of the same rights? Each of these questions requires some comment.

In answering the first question, we need not attempt a detailed consideration of the moral rights of organisms which are not developed enough, aware enough, intelligent enough, etc., to be considered people, but which resemble people in some respects. It does seem reasonable to suggest that the more like a person, in the relevant respects, a being is, the stronger is the case for regarding it as having a right to life, and indeed the stronger its right to life is. Thus we ought to take seriously the suggestion that, insofar as "the human individual develops biologically in a continuous fashion . . . the rights of a human person might develop in the same way."[11] But we must keep in mind that the attributes which are relevant in determining whether or not an entity is enough like a person to be regarded as having some of the same moral rights are no different from those which are relevant to determining whether or not it is fully a person—i.e., are no different from (1)–(5)—and that being genetically human, or having recognizably human facial and other physical features, or detectable brain activity, or the capacity to survive outside the uterus, are simply not among these relevant attributes.

Thus it is clear that even though a seven- or eight-month fetus has features which make it apt to arouse in us almost the same powerful protective instinct as is commonly aroused by a small infant, nevertheless it is not significantly more personlike than is a very small embryo. It is *somewhat* more personlike; it can apparently feel and respond to pain, and it may even have a rudimentary form of consciousness, insofar as its brain is quite active. Nevertheless, it seems safe to say that it is not fully conscious, in the way that an infant of a few months is, and that it cannot reason, or communicate messages of indefinitely many sorts, does not engage in self-motivated activity, and has no self-awareness. Thus, in the *relevant* respects, a fetus, even a fully developed one, is considerably less personlike than is the average mature mammal, indeed the average fish. And I think that a rational person must conclude that if the right to life of a fetus is to be based upon its resemblance to a person, then it cannot be said to have any more right to life than, let us say, a newborn guppy (which also seems to be capable of feeling pain), and that a right of that magnitude could never override a woman's right to obtain an abortion, at any stage of her pregnancy.

There may, of course, be other arguments in favor of placing legal limits upon the stage of pregnancy in which an abortion may be performed. Given the relative safety of the new techniques of artificially inducing labor during the third trimester, the danger to the woman's life or health is no longer such an argument. Neither is the fact that people tend to respond to the thought of abortion in the later stages of pregnancy with emotional repulsion, since mere emotional responses cannot take the place of moral reasoning in determining what ought to be permitted. Nor, finally, is the frequently heard argument that legalizing abortion, especially late in the pregnancy, may erode the level of respect for human life, leading, perhaps, to an increase in unjustified euthanasia and other crimes. For this threat, if it is a threat, can be better met by educating people to the kinds of moral distinctions which we are making here than by limiting access to abortion (which limitation may, in its disregard for the rights of women, be just as damaging to the level of respect for human rights).

Thus, since the fact that even a fully developed fetus is not personlike enough to have any significant right to life on the basis of its personlikeness shows that no legal restrictions upon the stage of pregnancy in which an abortion may be performed can be justified on the grounds that we should protect the rights of the older fetus; and since there is no other apparent justification for such restrictions, we may conclude that they are entirely unjustified. Whether or not it would be *indecent* (whatever that means) for a woman in her seventh month to obtain an abortion just to avoid having to postpone a trip to Europe, it would not, in itself, be *immoral*, and therefore it ought to be permitted.

4. Potential Personhood and the Right to Life

We have seen that a fetus does not resemble a person in any way which can support the claim that it has even some of the same rights. But what about its *potential,* the fact that if nurtured and allowed to develop naturally it will very probably become a person? Doesn't that alone give it at least some right to life? It is hard to deny that the fact that an entity is a potential person is a strong prima facie reason for not destroying it; but we need not conclude from this that a potential person has a right to life, by virtue of that potential. It may be that our feeling that it is better, other things being equal, not to destroy a potential person is better explained by the fact that potential people are still (felt to be) an invaluable resource, not to be lightly squandered. Surely, if every speck of dust were a potential person, we would be much less apt to conclude that every potential person has a right to become actual.

Still, we do not need to insist that a potential person has no right to life whatever. There may well be something immoral, and not just imprudent, about wantonly destroying potential people, when doing so isn't necessary to protect anyone's rights. But even if a potential person does have some prima facie right to life, such a right could not possibly outweigh the right of a woman to obtain an abortion, since the rights of any actual person invariably outweigh those of any potential person, whenever the two conflict. Since this may not be immediately obvious in the case of a human fetus, let us look at another case.

Suppose that our space explorer falls into the hands of an alien culture, whose scientists decide to create a few hundred thousand or more human beings, by breaking his body into its component cells, and using these to create fully developed human beings, with, of course, his genetic code. We may imagine that each of these newly created men will have all of the original man's abilities, skills, knowledge, and so on, and also have an individual self-concept, in short that each of them will be a bona fide (though hardly unique) person. Imagine that the whole project will take only seconds, and that its chances of success are extremely high, and that our explorer knows all of this, and also knows that these people will be treated fairly. I maintain that in such a situation he would have every right to escape if he could, and thus to deprive all of these potential people of their potential lives; for his right to life outweighs all of theirs together, in spite of the fact that they are all genetically human, all innocent, and all have a very high probability of becoming people very soon, if only he refrains from acting.

Indeed, I think he would have a right to escape even if it were not his life which the alien scientists planned to take, but only a year of his freedom, or, indeed, only a day. Nor would he be obligated to stay if he had gotten captured (thus bringing all these people-potentials into existence) because of his own carelessness, or even if he had done so deliberately, knowing the consequences.

Regardless of how he got captured, he is not morally obligated to remain in captivity for *any* period of time for the sake of permitting any number of potential people to come into actuality, so great is the margin by which one actual person's right to liberty outweighs whatever right to life even a hundred thousand potential people have. And it seems reasonable to conclude that the rights of a woman will outweigh by a similar margin whatever right to life a fetus may have by virtue of its potential personhood.

Thus, neither a fetus's resemblance to a person, nor its potential for becoming a person provides any basis whatever for the claim that it has any significant right to life. Consequently, a woman's right to protect her health, happiness, freedom, and even her life,[12] by terminating an unwanted pregnancy, will always override whatever right to life it may be appropriate to ascribe to a fetus, even a fully developed one. And thus, in the absence of any overwhelming social need for every possible child, the laws which restrict the right to obtain an abortion, or limit the period of pregnancy during which an abortion may be performed, are a wholly unjustified violation of a woman's most basic moral and constitutional rights.[13]

NOTES

1. For example, Roger Wertheimer, who in "Understanding the Abortion Argument" (*Philosophy and Public Affairs,* 1, No. 1 [Fall, 1971], 67–95), argues that the problem of the moral status of abortion is insoluble, in that the dispute over the status of the fetus is not a question of fact at all, but only a question of how one responds to the facts.

2. B. A. Brody, "Abortion and the Law," *The Journal of Philosophy,* 68, No. 12 (June 17, 1971), 357–69.

3. Judith Thomson, "A Defense of Abortion," *Philosophy and Public Affairs,* 1, No. 1 (Fall, 1971), 47–66.

4. I have abbreviated these statements somewhat, but not in a way which affects the argument.

5. John Noonan, "Abortion and the Catholic Church: A Summary History," *Natural Law Forum,* 12 (1967), 125.

6. John Noonan, "Deciding Who Is Human," *Natural Law Forum,* 13 (1968), 134.

7. Thomson, "A Defense of Abortion."

8. We may safely ignore the fact that she might have avoided getting raped, e.g., by carrying a gun, since by similar means you might likewise have avoided getting kidnapped, and in neither case does the victim's failure to take all possible precautions against a highly unlikely event (as opposed to reasonable precautions against a rather likely event) mean that he is morally responsible for what happens.

9. Of course, the principle that it is (always) wrong to kill innocent human beings is in need of many other modifications, e.g., that it may be permissible to do so to save a

greater number of other innocent human beings, but we may safely ignore these complications here.

10. From here on, we will use "human" to mean genetically human, since the moral sense seems closely connected to, and perhaps derived from, the assumption that genetic humanity is sufficient for membership in the moral community.

11. Thomas L. Hayes, "A Biological View," *Commonweal*, 85 (March 17, 1967), 677–78; quoted by Daniel Callahan, in *Abortion, Law, Choice, and Morality* (London: Macmillan & Co., 1970).

12. That is, insofar as the death rate, for the woman, is higher for childbirth than for early abortion.

13. My thanks to the following people, who were kind enough to read and criticize an earlier version of this paper: Herbert Gold, Gene Glass, Anne Lauterbach, Judith Thomson, Mary Mothersill, and Timothy Binkley.

Ethics and Embryos

Nicola Poplawski and Grant Gillett

We have a strong intuition that human life of whatever stage has moral significance. Some argue that this is "speciesism," in the same way that others direct
accusations of racism when the claim is made that a greater moral significance
should be placed on white human life as opposed to non-white. However, the
claim for such moral significance need not stem purely from being a member of
the species *Homo sapiens*. The claim may rest on the quality of human functioning which, in terms of conscious appreciation, interactions and behavior, has
moral weight over and above other biological life. The difficulty is that some
human beings, including fetuses and embryos, do not have these properties.

Potentiality

The standard potentiality argument argues that despite the fact that embryos
do not have the properties now, they have the potential to develop them. They
claim that if an embryo has the *potential* to be a person with "the right to life,"
the right to life should apply before the "stage" of being a person is reached.
Thus they argue *from* the premise that one type of creature will change into
something different *to* the conclusion that a creature of the first form has the

moral properties of the second form. This is a "consequentialist" view of potentiality. On this view, potential is not an inherent property of the entity. It is a projection of an anticipated future state, onto the current entity; but that future state may or may not eventuate.

But there are many problems with this view of potentiality. First, it makes little sense to give an embryo rights that it may have at a later stage unless its potential is an inherent property which confers those rights. Surely we should form attitudes to things on the basis of what they are rather than what they might be? Second, there is the distinct possibility that any given embryo will never reach the stage of having those rights. But many embryos which spontaneously abort are no different from ones that will reach the potential later stage. Why should they have different properties? Third, just how far back ought these rights to be extended; should sperm and ova be included? (If so we ban contraception.)

Clearly potentiality needs somewhat more analysis and justification or it must be discarded altogether.

We will give a more Aristotelian analysis[1] and argue that the *form* of a human being extends beyond that present at a given slice of time to take in the breadth of an entire life. There is a phase of development, a phase of moral engagement with others and a phase of dying (which may be abrupt or more drawn out). On this view, the process of becoming a person is a progression through a series of linked developmental stages. Because each stage is an essential component of the whole, the form of humanity involves a life with a characteristic longitudinal "shape."

At one stage of this whole, the individual becomes a rational social being and an inherent moral value is realized. We then take this moral value, inherent to human beings as rational social beings (persons), and attach it to the form as a whole.

To do this is to evince a feature of our general reasoning. In the main, we look at a thing not only as what it is in itself but also in view of what it is part of. For example, a gunshot has different significance as part of a clay target shoot than as part of a murder. Thus we derive the moral status of an embryo from the whole of which that embryo is a part. An embryo has present applicable rights not because some time in the future that embryo *may* become a person with rights appropriate to persons but because it is the same individual who becomes a person. We accept that the embryo *has* these rights because as a phase of the human form, it has some claim to the rights we accord to persons.

Now we must clarify when an embryo first has rights, what those rights are and how much moral weight they have, especially when they are in conflict with the rights of other persons.

Rights

What is a right? "Essentially, rights are justified claims that require action or restraint from others—that is, impose positive or negative duties on others."[2]

The debate surrounding rights concerns both natural rights, which are contentious, and constitutional/legal rights which exist (without doubt) in our society because we have created them.

At present, British and New Zealand legislation gives limited constitutional rights to embryos and fetuses. For example, a fetus is protected from abortion unless certain legal criteria are met.[3] Religious and anti-abortion groups give an embryo certain rights which they believe to be implicit in its existence. These rights, it is claimed, do not require a law or act of parliament to create them, they are therefore *natural rights*.

In the debate surrounding the status of embryos the concept of natural human rights seems, clearly, to be important and we must therefore spend some time clarifying it. Such rights could either be God-given or intrinsic to the nature of human beings. In either case, one would need to reason about the lessons to be learned (from creation/nature or from "revealed laws") to develop a substantial conception of the moral rights concerned.

John Locke and his followers espoused natural human rights on the basis of secular thought. In this tradition, Hart claims that if there are any moral rights "there is at least one natural right, the equal right of all men to be free."[4] This is close to Kant's view that all men have the right to be fully-functioning, autonomous agents. For pro-lifers, every human being also has a right to life and therefore should not be killed. Both stands appear to be based on a set of moral intuitions. However, such intuitions conflict, so they cannot provide sufficient grounds on which to assert that such rights exist.

Bentham and other utilitarians claim that natural rights are nonsense and that they exist purely as figments of our imagination.[5,6] Non-utilitarian objections to moral rights are based either on the belief that codified, and therefore non-natural *duties* alone exist, or on Skepticism, about the possible source of moral rights. The extreme skeptic denies that in a state of nature any creature has rights. Therefore, questions arise as to whether natural/moral rights have been correctly identified and where they come from. If one could find a general basis for natural rights *then* one would be able to see whether embryos or fetuses fulfilled the requisite conditions to be credited with them.

The view favored by the present authors is that natural rights arise when it goes against the intrinsic nature of moral thinking or moral agency to deprive an individual of the claim concerned. If compassion, for example, were seen to be at the heart of moral judgement in general, it follows that to act without it would be to fail in respect to one of the basic features constitutive of moral conduct.[7] We would argue that moral considerations arise in contexts where individuals interact with each other and develop reciprocal attitudes which guide their behavior. These attitudes embed a sensitivity to the needs and vulnerabilities of others and involve a kind of empathy which informs actions which impinge upon what matters to others. Therefore, we internalize the norm that we should avoid, wherever possible, harming another person.

We combine this with the view that the potential to be a person is inherent in the whole (longitudinally realized) form of a human being. This implies that a human being, simply by having a form which at some stage will participate in moral interactions, has a right not to be the subject of gratuitous insult or injury.

The Concept of Longitudinal Form

There is little doubt in most people's eyes that at some stage human beings have moral value. (We discuss this further later.) The difficulties arise when we endeavor to pinpoint when this stage is reached. However, if we look at the human form in a longitudinal way this problem becomes more tractable.

One can make an analogy with the color spectrum. It is not possible to identify the exact point where one color emerges from another because there are gradual transitions through a series of shades. Red emerges from an increasingly red shade of orange; it cannot be said to appear at a definable point. Thus, though distinctions can be made, real continuities still exist.

The adult, adolescent, child, viable fetus, pre-viable fetus, embryo, blastocyst and conceptus are similarly part of a continuum. It is not possible to determine the exact point separating adjacent stages. For this reason we cannot look at any point in the developmental process in isolation when attributing moral properties; we should look at the human being as having a single form which exists over time. Development is, therefore, a process whose overall nature may have distinct moral significance. The conceptus begins this process and the "form" which not only governs the process but also makes it morally significant, is realized as time goes by.

Note that this view may confer some moral worth on the embryo even at fertilization. If the initial stage in the human process does not occur none of the later stages can be reached and therefore this first stage is an essential component of the complex whole in the same way that the laying of foundations is the essential first stage of building a house. Who can say that any one stage of building a house is any more important than another when without all stages one has nothing? The conceptus may have moral significance because it is an essential component of the total longitudinal form of a morally signficant being (we will consider a modification of this derived status below).

The total form of a human being exists through time. We can also say that a single individual makes up that form throughout its temporal existence. Therefore, if we can justify a moral value for that individual at one point in time, that moral value ought to be conferred on the total form throughout its temporal existence. Remaining consistent to our argument we analyze problems at all phases of that form with the same moral precepts. But, even though the moral value is the same this does not entail that the moral analysis will bring about the same conclusions.

The Person as Valuable

For Kant a person has "rational willing agency as the essential characteristic"; for Locke "the ability to think combined with self-awareness over time is the essence of personhood."[8] Both formulations exclude very young infants and humans with severely damaged or defective brains from the category of persons. This exclusion seems to go against our intuitive feeling that there ought to be some value at least placed on the lives of infants.

Such feelings are admittedly not reliable indicants of moral value (remember the feelings of Americans in the "deep South" to black Africans), but they do give us a *prima facie* reason for questioning the validity of an exclusive definition of personhood. They also confirm the broadly Aristotelian view we have favored because embryos, fetuses and infants are phases of beings whose form is such that they are to be valued as persons. (In the case of the severely brain-damaged we do not have the same metaphysical support for our intuitions based on potential, indeed the intuitions themselves are less clear.)

But, when does this human form, which is to be valued, begin?

In moral history a number of beginning points for human form have been considered. *Quickening* (at approximately 20 weeks gestation) is thought by some to be the first signs of personhood. This may be because the first fetal movements felt by the mother are thought to indicate ensoulment, or because such manifestations are the first communication between the mother and fetus. *Birth* is important to others (for example, Engelhardt) for similar "interactive" reasons. Engelhardt argues that, although a newborn infant has not yet become a person (as a subject of self-awareness), he/she expresses rudiments of human nature in interpersonal interactions (which include a form of communication) and is extended the right of membership of a social group because of that interaction.[9] Perceived *membership* of a moral community, on this view, gives some rights to the infant, including the right to life. The *viability criterion* could be favoured for much the same reasons—the fetus has reached a stage in development where it could survive *ex utero* in a human environment. It therefore has the rights of any individual who can and does interact in that environment. On this basis the viable fetus is credited with certain rights because it has a capacity for what is crucial in moral communities not because it currently expresses that capacity (note that the newborn infant is still dependent for viability on the human supports around it).

Let us accept that interaction in a human context (even if it is not fully reciprocal) places moral value on the life of the subject under consideration. But perhaps that morally significant interaction occurs much earlier in the gestational process than claimed by any of the arguments above (this would imply that the interaction does not have to be of an interpersonal type).[10]

What Type of Interaction Is Significant?

We have accepted that it is the degree to which a developing embryo or fetus becomes embedded in a human community which determines moral dues or rights. (This is congenial even to Kuhse and Singer.)[11]

When the blastocyst begins to implant—approximately six days after fertilization—a physical interaction between one individual (the mother) and another (the blastocyst) begins. As development continues this physiological link becomes both stronger[12] and more obvious. First the woman realizes that she is pregnant, then the father, relatives and friends are informed, eventually even complete strangers will know of the pregnancy due to the physical appearance of the woman. As these outward changes in appearance occur, so too do inward changes. At the end of the eighth week of gestation all the major structures and organ systems are developing and electroencephalogram (EEG) activity is first detectable. At this stage a recognizable physical form has been reached. The first movement of the fetus is felt by the mother at approximately 20 weeks. This brings a special and traditional meaning to the progressing pregnancy as it

374   Nicola Poplawski and Grant Gillett

gives a sign to the mother, exclusive of medical technology, that the developing fetus is alive and growing inside her. By the 26th–28th week of gestation the lungs are sufficiently developed to be able to breathe air and the fetus would be able to survive in the external environment. (At this stage the desire of the woman to terminate her pregnancy is in practice separable from the potential for the baby to survive.)

In the usual course of events, as this fetal development occurs there is a gradual increase in the hopes and expectations of parents, relatives and friends as it becomes increasingly more certain that a baby will soon be "joining the family." Thus, a very special place is created in a community for the developing individual long before it has arrived "on the scene." This preparation of a social "niche" establishes the fetus in an interpersonal and social context and further highlights the developing interaction which is present even before birth has occurred. From the point of viability the fetus is able to be born and participate, not just as a "potential baby" but as an actual, identifiable individual in the social community.

After entering that community, at birth, the individual gradually develops the ability to communicate, conceptualize and rationalize. Thus she has a place in the moral system, based on her identity, developing personality, mental life and experiences. As a result, she shows increasing embeddedness in human interactions and takes a fully reciprocal, participating role.

So, a distinct individual enters the human community by forming interactions which are at first relatively simple and then later more complex emotional, social and moral engagements. But notice that the extended form of humanity entails that an identifiable individual who will at some stage be a rational social being with full moral rights is in existence from very early on. Thus, from implantation the individual participates in an interaction which normally leads to full moral engagement. Because that individual has moral significance at its point of full human engagement, all phases of that individual share the moral properties involved.

The individual can therefore be regarded as part of the moral community at all stages of development and as becoming increasingly embedded in a more complex and compelling way as it develops, so that at some point it realizes the mode or form of being which is the basis of its extended moral properties.

Summary of the Present Argument

We can now justify a relative sanctity for all human life. The justification is that to violate that life does violence to a basic feature of our moral attitudes.

This sanctity is attached to the human form as a whole where that form is viewed in a longitudinal sense and therefore present from conception and onwards throughout an entire life.[13] The basis of this moral value is the human ability to interact with others in those situations where moral sense and morality are grounded.[14]

All phases of the longitudinal form of a human being are aspects of the morally valued (unitary) whole and therefore all phases are morally valued in the same way. As the preimplantation period, whilst having no component of interaction, is part of that whole the preimplantation embryo is also seen to have moral value. Thus we conclude that serious consideration is due to anything which affects human life from fertilization until death because moral weight is attached to what is being destroyed whenever a human life is terminated. So, where embryonic human life is balanced against the rights of another human being, decisions should not be taken lightly. (More about this later.)

Questions and *Caveats*

In our society we draw lines. Western society says that adolescence begins with the onset of the teenage years; in the law an individual becomes a legal adult for some purposes on her eighteenth birthday and for others on her sixteenth.[15] This encourages us to appeal to more occurrently realized properties and to favor a system where moral status is seen to be derived from the individual's stage of development. But, despite claims to the contrary,[16] these lines are for convenience and, although each has a rationale, the exact points are largely arbitrary.

The development to adult form is a progression through a series of stages which merge into each other. There is a continuity of growth from blastocyst to born child, to adult and further. Because of this continuity it is impossible to identify specific points where significant change occurs. For instance, it is not possible to identify the specific point in time when the child ceases and the adolescent begins, or the adolescent ends and the adult begins. Therefore, we can see that it is more accurate (but also less convenient as far as the law is concerned) to say that form changes gradually over a period of time rather than changing suddenly. These points are familiar from arguments by Michael Tooley[17] and Bernard Williams.[18]

When we add the premise that moral value attaches to the total (longitudinal) form in virtue of its most clearly morally endowed points we can see that moral (and legal) consideration is due to a human being from the beginning of the process until the end.

Against this one could argue that mere physiological interaction is not sufficient to give moral significance. It could be said that the social or rational element must be included before significance is properly ascribed (even at a minimal level). If physical interaction alone *were* morally significant we would be faced with the dilemma of having to treat an attached parasite, such as a tapeworm, with the moral consideration given an embryo or fetus. But this neglects the longitudinal "form of a person." There is a fundamental difference in form between a tapeworm and a human organism: an internal parasite simply grows and reproduces further parasites but a human embryo becomes a person with an interactive role in a human community. This creates a moral difference.

The same applies to a blastocyst which forms a hydatidiform mole instead of an embryo; it does not have the intrinsic potential to become a human being. Of course, given present medical technology, one cannot ascertain, prospectively, which will develop to term, which will spontaneously abort and which will become hydatidiform moles. Therefore all blastocysts must be considered to have the same moral status until the time when overall longitudinal form can be determined. In some cases this will not be until after birth.

Notice that we have given a new thrust to the "potentiality argument" by relating attitudes to the individual at any given time to the attitudes to the total process of which that individual stage is an essential part. This, as we have noted, is continuous with other aspects of moral, legal, indeed general thinking. For example, taking a piece of paper from somebody's desk is much more serious if the piece of paper is a match ticket to a cricket test than if it is a nondescript scrap of notepaper. The nature of the act depends not only on the act itself but also on its role in a total human situation over time.

A "total process" approach has the right implications for other problem cases. For instance it allows us to act consistently towards individuals who are asleep, under anaesthesia or in reversible comas. Knowing that the individual has both a past ability and a potential future ability to interact in a moral and social community one can credit that individual with default intentional interests which the present circumstances do not allow her to express.[19] It also makes "moral room" for a policy of "letting die" with regard to severely malformed neonates such as anencephalics where the presence of significant interaction is impossible and the totality involved is, in important repects, very different from that in the case of a 'normal' person.

Individuals who live in isolation (for instance marooned on a desert island), and therefore in the absence of interaction, are similarly included under the present model, despite their lack of occurrent social relatedness. Their *capacity* to interact if the isolation is ended, inherent in the form of that individual, is intrinsically the same in type as that of fully moral beings and therefore they share the properties on which moral significance is grounded.

However, an excessively cognitive reading of morally significant interactions leads to problems. If one's ability to think and interact/communicate were to be graded, the individual whose form included the ability to interact on some yet to be defined "higher plane" than others would be more important than other human beings. Perhaps a person whose total form included being a university professor would be more significant than an individual who was mildly intellectually handicapped. This immediately suggests an *elitist* attitude congenial to "Ivory towered academics" but not to "normal" people. It does not seem to be a valid way to arrive at a conception of the person as the bearer of moral value. And, who is to say whether interaction with a three-month-old baby by nose-touching and noises is more or less valuable than a philosophical discussion with a twelve-year-old? We must beware of placing gratuitous value judgements on the *type* of interaction occurring. They are different types of interaction yet have both intrinsic value and value because they are parts of valued wholes, wholes which at some stage participate in moral interactions.

The moral significance of the age at which an individual dies can also be related to the natural unfolding of human form. We intuitively feel more sorrow at the death of a seven-year-old than that of a seventy-year-old, despite there being no difference in their moral value. Our different reactions are understandable. The death of a seventy-year-old is more consistent with the total form of humanity whereas the death of a seven-year-old does greater violence to the form which we value.

The question of the status of animals is also pertinent to the discussion. We see interactions between animals and humans. These are often complex and not infrequently of a similar nature to that seen between two human beings. If we are not to place value judgements on either the type of interaction or the species involved then it would seem that we have to consider animals in a similar, (potential/relational based) light to humans.

But the death of a human touches more closely the form that we value than the death of an animal. The form of an animal does not include a phase of full moral interaction, although at a minimal level some animals may interact with us as fully as do individuals with severe intellectual handicaps. Our reasoning is sensitively tied to many aspects of form, including bodily resemblance. In the case of some severely handicapped infants this inclines us to greater moral concern than, perhaps, is well grounded.[7]

However, this analysis seems to suggest that infanticide is no worse than contraception using the "morning after" pill. This is decidedly counterintuitive, and in pursuing the issue we come across an already encountered feature of human reasoning. We reason on the basis of total processes, not moments in being. It seems rational to regard a setback at an earlier, indeed vestigial stage of a process as being of much less moment than when things have developed more fully (compare a mechanical failure on the number one spot of a formula one grid as compared to the final lap of the race when one is leading). Yet this seems to counter the intuition justifying our reaction to death at different ages (see above). The "violence to overall form" argument appears to mitigate against early termination whereas the "natural investment" reasoning is more tolerant. Here it seems that we cannot easily opt for a single moral precept to capture the subtlety of our natural reasoning.

Our attitudes are based on the total form of a human being and thus our moral reactions to events at any stage take account of the relationship between that stage and the whole. But also, we take reasonable note of the extent to which a process is realized when assessing the harm done by interrupting that process. But this latter claim does not strip all value from a very early stage of the total process even if it gives it lower value than a more fully formed stage. A possible reconciling strategy would therefore be to include the "degree of realization" intuition into an understanding of our attitude to the totality of a human life.

Thus we can see that it is right that a pregnant woman has the greater claim to life because of her present ability to interact with others in the human community. There is a much more fully formed process or morally important individual "cut-off" when one kills a developed human being. This does not negate the moral weight of a fetal life but merely suggests that in certain circumstances the risk to the mother is of greater moral weight. *But*, on this view, because the embryo is morally significant the risks posed to the mother by pregnancy must be significant or else an abortion cannot be morally justified.[20]

This is not to say that a fourteen-day-old embryo has a *less human* form than a fetus of twenty weeks gestation which would thereby place different values on the individuals concerned. It is rather to acknowledge that even though moral significance is conferred on an individual at all stages of her development, it does not follow that all actions towards her, which are of the same type, have the same ethical and moral connotations at all stages.

The present "total process" view of potentiality allows us to understand the intuition that we should preserve embryonic or fetal life. Because the typical human life is part of a temporal continuum, which includes embryonic and fetal life, they are both valued as parts of the whole.

Finally the total process approach is immune to the standard objections to potentiality. Potentiality suggests that we should give ova and sperm the same moral significance as human beings. But this fails to take account of the individuals involved. Gametes do have the potential to form a person, should they be brought together under the appropriate circumstances, but their separate existences do *not* constitute part of the development of a human being. (That they could start the development of a human being is a reason, on the present account, for not regarding contraception as completely devoid of moral interest.) A pool of gametes does not yet contain identifiable human individuals in whom a morally valued form (in the longitudinal sense) has been initiated. The interaction is not between complete human individuals in a human community but an interaction of "partial individuals" in a context which differs from that discussed earlier.

"New Birth Technologies"

"New birth technologies" (NBT) form a test case for the present view.

It is now possible to use a number of techniques to bypass a woman's infertility and enable her to become pregnant, including artificial insemination with husband or donor sperm (AIH or AID), ovulation induction (OI), *in vitro* fertilization (IVF) and the newer technique of gamete intrafallopian transfer (GIFT). There has been controversy about the use of these NBTs since their creation. This is especially so with IVF because of the need for external fertilisation and the problem of "spare embryos." Certainly, to infertile couples, the use of these techniques has great value, but is this a sufficient justification?

On the one hand, it seems that the value placed on human life provides an argument in favor of NBTs: they produce something which is precious and valued. The decision to enter into such a reproductive program is rational and considered: the couple, who place high value on having a baby, are prepared to go to extraordinary lengths to do so.

On the other hand, NBTs are beset with problems. Artificial reproduction does not simply fulfil the desires of an adult, it also manufactures humans and in doing so may trivialize the ability to reproduce.[21] The ability to create human life in an artificial manner may undermine or even negate the value that the embryonic phase of the human form ought to be given. The high cost to the user of such techniques (in some countries at least) and the lengths to which one has to go to get access to them may induce the attitude that the babies produced are a commodity available to a highly motivated group of people with the ability to pay. We may come to view babies as "tailor made products" to be produced to specifications (for example, gender), when and where wanted. These possibilities and their moral implications are unsettling. In addition, NBTs carry significant risk of multiple pregnancy (see Table 1).[22] Multiple pregnancies, particularly those of quadruplet or greater (high-order), carry high risk to the health of both the fetuses and the mother. Because all these lives have moral worth it is inappropriate that such risks should be taken.

NBTs *create* the situation where multiple lives are at risk. Because of this we cannot easily assimilate the embryos to survivors in an overcrowded lifeboat. Therefore, we cannot argue that there is no problem because a hypothetical rational negotiation justifies an impartial selective reduction (the Rawlsian model)[23] and provide an ethical solution to a medically-created problem of high-order pregnancy. In the case of NBTs one has control, so to speak, over whether or not the lifeboat is set out to sea. It is clear that deliberately setting the boat adrift with prior knowledge that some of its occupants must be destroyed, if any are to reach safety at a later stage, is a morally suspect choice to make.[24]

Table 1   The risk of multiple pregnancy of varying sizes according to the type of pregnancy

Procedure	Multiple	Twin	Triplet	Quad+
Clomiphene citrate	7.2			
hCG[1]	27.9	20.4	5.3	2.1
GnRH[2]	5.7			
IVF	22.6	19.0	3.5	0.1
GIFT	33.3	21.2	9.0	3.0
Natural pregnancy	1.2	1.1	0.01	0.0001

Note: Figures shown are the percentage of term deliveries that are twin or greater (multiple), twin alone, triplet alone, or quadruplet and greater.
[1]human chorionic gonadotrophin
[2]gonadotrophin releasing hormone

But we can avoid some of these harms by controlling the aspects of NBTs which lead to the incidence of high-order multiple pregnancy (i.e., a pregnancy of four or greater). In fact there are already techniques available to achieve this control.

1. We can monitor the regimes for multiple oocyte stimulation used in the course of infertility treatments by ovulation induction. This may involve regulations controlling the situations in which the ovulating dose of human chorionic gonadotrophin (hCG) is given, restricting gonadotrophin dosage and prohibiting use in specific types of infertility.
2. We can restrict the number of embryos transferred in an IVF cycle to a maximum of three (possibly even two) to eliminate the risk of a quadruplet pregnancy.
3. We can restrict the number of oocytes transferred in a GIFT cycle to a maximum of three (or two) for the same reason.

Therefore we conclude; firstly, that we ought to pay ethical regard to *in vivo* embryos. Secondly, if NBTs are to be used to create embryos (this in itself is debated) they ought to be equally available to all. Thirdly, given that embryos are phases of that totality which is a morally significant form, there ought to be ethical guidelines and practices controlling the medical production of *in vivo* embryos through the use of NBTs.

These constraints emerge from the regard we are obliged to attach to the form of humanity and in that sense seem to justify rights for embryos which do not allow us indiscriminately to "mess around with them" without regard for ethical constraints.

Postscript: Embryos and Ethics

Since completion of this paper we have discerned a further argument about embryos and their "rights." Human beings have both general and individual properties and, in different contexts, these differentially dictate our moral choices. We can say of an identifiable human being who has her own preferences and attitudes to life events that those individual choices, that her autonomy, ought to be respected. In this sense she has individual rights. But embryos, although they may share some of the moral status that we accord to human beings because they are part of the totality which is a human being are not plausible candidates for such rights. Their rights can therefore be thought of as general, relating to nonindividuated beings of a certain type who are, in one sense, substitutable for each other. With such beings we can look at a situation in terms of its total value-outcome for beings of that type. Thus any individual of that type only has rights as an instance of the morally significant type which it is.

This allows us to defend ourselves against callous and dismissive moral attitudes to embryos in general, given that they are proper stages of morally significant beings, without defending the notion of individual and personal rights for any embryo. Any rights that an embryo has of an individual nature will attach to it only as a consequence of it having reached the stage where such attributions become intelligible.

This argument is supported by considering the indiscernability of substituting one (consanguineous) embryo for another prior to the stage of engagement with others as an identifiable individual. This cannot be materially (and therefore morally) relevant to anyone: not the mother or others because they do not and could not tell the difference; not the embryo because it cannot tell or have attitudes to anything. It is clear that the condition of substitutability and lack of individuation is steadily replaced by properties, both intrinsic and relational, which ground individual rights, as the child develops and takes its (interactive) place in a human context.

NOTES

We would like to acknowledge the support of the New Zealand Medical Research Council in undertaking this study.

1. Aristotle believed the attainment of the human form to be of great moral significance. Based on this belief, early law held the destruction of human life at any stage to be morally offensive, the penalties for such destruction being graded by the degree to which the human form had been reached.

2. Gillon, R. *Philosophical medical ethics.* Chichester: John Wiley and Sons for the *British Medical Journal,* 1985:50.

3. Skegg, P. D. G. *Law and medicine.* Oxford: Clarendon Press 1984: 1–26.

4. Hart, H. L. A. Are there any natural rights? In Waldron, J., ed. *Theories of rights.* New York: Oxford University Press, 1984: 77.

5. On the other hand, constitutional/legal rights exist as a social control to ensure that a utilitarian balance is achieved.

6. Scheffle, S., ed. *Consequentialism and its critics.* New York: Oxford University Press, 1988.

7. Gillett, G. R. Les enfant handicapes: Un defi. *Foi et vie* 1989; LXXXVIII, 6: 63–75.

8. See Gillon, *Philosophical medical ethics,* 51.

9. Engelhardt, H. T. *The foundations of bioethics.* New York: Oxford University Press, 1986: ch 4: 104 onwards.

10. Interpersonal in this context means "between two persons at a reflective level."

11. Kuhse, H., Singer, P. *Should the baby live?* Oxford: Oxford University Press, 1985.

12. A survey of the literature on pregnancy outcome reveals that for a naturally conceived pregnancy, there is an approximately 85 percent chance that the conceptus will implant and be detected as a biochemical pregnancy by beta-hCG assay, approximately 54 percent of conceptuses progress to clinical pregnancy and approximately 46 percent to term. Most clinical abortions (those losses of clinically detected pregnancies) occur in the earlier stages of pregnancy. As a pregnancy becomes later term it is less likely to terminate in spontaneous abortion.

13. It is interesting to note that such an interpretation has recently been adopted by the Danish Parliament. Law changes have led to the establishment of an ethical council whose work is to "build on the basis that human life takes its beginnings at the time of conception." Holm, S. New Danish law: Human life begins at conception. *Journal of medical ethics* 1988; 14: 77–78.

14. Wiggins, D. The person as object of science, as subject of experience, and as locus of value. In: Peacock, A. R. and Gillett, G. R.: *Persons and personality.* Oxford: Blackwell, 1987: 56–74.

15. There is no age limit below which a woman is not entitled to make decisions for her offspring. This acts to create the situation where a thirteen-year-old can decide whether or not her baby should have an operation but not that she herself should.

16. Buckle, S. Biological processes and moral events. *Journal of medical ethics* 1988; 14: 144–147.

17. Tooley, M. Abortion and infanticide. *Philosophy and public affairs* 1972: 2, 1; 37–65.

18. William, B. Which slopes are slippery? In Lockwood, M., ed. *Moral dilemmas in modern medicine.* Oxford, New York: Oxford University Press, 1985: ch. 6: 126–137.

19. Gillett, G. R. Reply to J. M. Stanley: Fiddling and clarity. *Journal of medical ethics* 1987; 13: 22–25.

20. Social policy, of course, involves factors other than morality.

21. Jones, D. G. *Manufacturing humans: the challenge of new reproductive technologies.* Leicester: Inter-varsity Press, 1987.

22. These figures are gathered from a wide range of journal sources, the data of which was combined to give overall figures.

23. Rawls, J. *A theory of justice.* Oxford: Oxford University Press, 1972.

24. Poplawski, N. K. An ethical issue for reproductive technologies. *Asia-Oceana journal of obstetrics and gynaecology* 1990; 16: 291–296.

CHAPTER TWENTY-THREE

When Does a Person Begin?

Lynne Rudder Baker

I. Introduction

The answer to the question "When does a person begin?" depends on what a
person is: If an entity is a person, what kind of being, most fundamentally, is
she? Since the persons we are familiar with are human persons—persons with
human bodies—one may simply assume that what we human persons are most
fundamentally are animals.[1] I agree that it is often useful to think of us as animals—as long as we are thinking biologically, rather than ontologically. However, on my view, our animal nature, which we share with other higher primates,
does not expose what we most fundamentally are. Ontology is not a branch of
biology.

Nevertheless, my account of human persons roots us firmly in the natural
world. Biologically, we are akin to other primates; but ontologically, we are
unique. However, we are still material beings. I believe that we are fundamentally persons who are constituted by human organisms. Since constitution is
not identity, human persons may come into existence at a different time from
the organisms that constitute them. So I shall argue.

Unfortunately, this area of inquiry is clouded with terminological difficulties. The term "human being" (as well as "human individual") is used ambiguously. Some philosophers take "human being" to be a purely biological term that refers to human organisms.[2] Others take "human being" to name a psychological kind, not a biological kind.[3] And still other philosophers seem to trade on the ambiguity when they argue that human persons are human beings and human beings are human organisms; so human persons come into existence when human organisms come into existence. This is a non sequitur: Human organisms are a biological kind; human persons cannot pretheoretically be assumed to be a biological kind. The term "human being" may be used either for human organisms or for human persons, but—in a pretheoretical context—it is tendentious to use "human being" (or "human individual") for both.

The term "human nature" inherits the ambiguity of "human being" and "human individual." "Human nature" may refer to biological characteristics (say, length of gestation period or brain size) that distinguish human organisms from nonhuman organisms. Or it may refer to rational and moral characteristics that distinguish human persons from nonpersons.[4]

Although I would prefer to use the term "human being" to refer to human persons, and "human nature" to refer to the nature of human persons (rather than of human organisms), I shall avoid these terms in order to steer clear of ambiguity. I take the term "human organism" to be interchangeable with "human animal," and I take the nature of a human organism to be whatever biologists tell us it is. I am a Darwinian about human animals. That is, I believe that there is important continuity between the most primitive organisms and us, and that we human persons have an animal nature. But I do not believe that our animal nature exhausts our nature all things considered. I shall use a biological theory of human organisms on which to build an ontological theory of human persons. Before turning to my view of persons, let us consider when a human *organism* comes into existence.

II. When Does a Human Organism Begin?

I take the question "When does a human organism begin?" to be a biological question. This empirical question stands in contrast to the philosophical question "When does a human person begin?" (Empirical data are relevant to philosophical questions, without being conclusive.) One frequently heard answer to the biological question is that a human organism comes into existence at the time of fertilization of a human egg by a sperm. (But beware: There is not an exact moment of fertilization. Fertilization itself is a process that lasts twenty-plus hours.)[5] However, the view that a human organism comes into existence at—or at the end of—fertilization is logically untenable, because a fertilized egg may split and produce twins. If it is even physically possible for a fertilized egg to produce twins (whether it actually does so or not), a fertilized egg cannot be *identical* to an organism. As long as it is possible to twin, a zygote is not *a* human anything, but a cell cluster.[6] In the case of twinning, as philosopher G. E. M. Anscombe explains: "Neither of the two humans that eventually develop can be identified as the same human as the zygote, because they can't *both* be so, as they are different humans from one another."[7] It is logically impossible for one organism to be identical to two organisms. And, of course, anything that is logically impossible is biologically impossible. In twinning, two (or more) twins come from a single fertilized egg. But neither of the twins is identical to that fertilized egg, on pain of contradiction. To see this, suppose that a zygote (a cell cluster) divides and twins result. Call the zygote "*A*," and one of the twins "*B*" and the other twin "*C*." If *A* were identical to both *B* and *C*, then—by the transitivity of identity—*B* and *C* would be identical to each other. But *B* is clearly not identical to *C*. Therefore, *A* (the zygote) cannot be identical to *B* and *C*. A human organism cannot come into existence until there is no further possibility of "twinning"—about two weeks after fertilization.

Thus, there is no new human organism until after the end of the process of implantation of a blastocyst in the wall of the womb (about fourteen days after fertilization). Even at implantation, an organism does not come into existence instantaneously. There is no sharp line demarcating the coming into existence of a new human individual organism. There is only a gradual process. But we can say this much: Soon after implantation (the primitive streak stage), the embryo is an individual, as opposed to a mass of cells.[8] At this point, there is an individual human organism that persists through fetal development, birth, maturation, adulthood, until death. There are differing views about whether the human organism ends at the time of death, but in no case does the human organism persist through the disintegration of the human body.[9]

This answers the biological question about human embryos. But there remains the ontological question—a further question that is not automatically answered by biology: Granting that a human embryo after implantation is an individual human organism, what is the relation between a human embryo and a human person? On my view, the relation is constitution: A human person is wholly constituted by a human organism, without being identical to the constituting organism. So the coming into existence of a human organism is not *ipso facto* the coming into existence of a human person. As we shall see, on my view—the constitution view—a human person is not temporally coextensive with a human organism, but is nevertheless a material being, ultimately constituted by subatomic particles. Human persons have no immaterial parts.[10]

III. What a Person Is

So, what is a person? *Person*—like *statue*—is a primary kind, one of many irreducible ontological kinds. Everything that exists is of some primary kind—the kind that determines what the thing is most fundamentally. Things have their primary-kind properties essentially. Members of the kind *organism* are organisms essentially; members of the kind *person* are persons essentially. (If x has F essentially, then there is no possible world or time at which x exists and lacks F.) Thus, when a person comes into being, a new object comes into being—an object that is a person essentially.

What distinguishes *person* from other primary kinds (like *planet* or *organism*) is that persons have first-person perspectives. Just as a statue is not a piece of clay, say, plus some other part, so too a human person is not a human organism plus some other part. The defining characteristic of a person is a first-person perspective. Human persons are beings that have first-person perspectives essentially and are constituted by human organisms (or bodies). Martian persons, if there were any, are beings that have first-person perspectives essentially and are constituted by Martian bodies. Although *person* is a psychological kind, human persons are in the domains, not only of psychology, but also of biology, on the one hand, and of the social sciences, on the other.[11] A human person, like a bronze statue, is a unified thing—but the statue is not identical to the piece of bronze that constitutes it, nor is the person identical to the body that constitutes her. Your body is a person derivatively, in virtue of constituting you, who are a person nonderivatively. You are a human organism derivatively, in virtue of being constituted by your body that is a human organism nonderivatively.

In order to understand what a person is, the property to focus on is the first-person perspective. In mature persons, to have a first-person perspective is to be able to think of oneself without the use of any name, description, or demonstrative; it is the ability to conceive of oneself as oneself, from the inside, as it were.[12]

Linguistic evidence of a first-person perspective comes from use of first-person pronouns embedded in sentences with linguistic or psychological verbs—e.g., "I wonder how I will die," or "I promise that I will stick with you."[13] The content of a thought so expressed includes ineliminable first-person reference. Call the thought expressed using "I" embedded in a sentence following a psychological or linguistic verb (e.g., "I am thinking that I am hungry now") an "I* thought."[14] What distinguishes an I* thought from a simple first-person sentence (e.g., "I am hungry now") is that in the I* thought the first-person reference is part of the content of the thought, whereas in the simple first-person sentence, the "I" could drop out: one's thought could be expressed by "hungry now." If I am wondering how I will die, then I am entertaining an I* thought; I am thinking of myself as myself, so to speak. I am not thinking of myself in any third-person way (e.g., not as Lynne Baker, nor as the person who is thinking, nor as that woman, nor as the only person in the room) at all. I could wonder how I am going to die even if I had total amnesia. I* thoughts are not expressible by any non-first-person sentences. Anything that can entertain such irreducibly first-person thoughts is a person. A being with a first-person perspective not only can have thoughts about herself, but she can also conceive of herself as the subject of such thoughts. I not only wonder how I'll die, but I realize that the bearer of that thought is myself.

A being may be conscious without having a first-person perspective. Nonhuman primates and other mammals are conscious. They have psychological states like believing, fearing, and desiring, but they do not realize that they have beliefs and desires. They have points of view (e.g., "danger in that direction"), but they cannot conceive of themselves as the subjects of such thoughts. They cannot *conceive of* themselves from the first-person. (We have every reason to think that they do not wonder how they will die.) Thus, having psychological states like beliefs and desires, and having a point of view, are necessary but not sufficient conditions for being a person. A sufficient condition for being a person—whether human, divine, ape, or silicon-based—is having a first-person perspective.[15] So, what makes something a person is not the "stuff" it is made of. It does not matter whether something is made of organic material or silicon or, in the case of God, no material "stuff" at all. If a being has a first-person perspective, it is a person.

A first-person perspective is the basis of all forms of self-consciousness. It makes possible an inner life, a life of thoughts that one realizes are her own. Although I cannot discuss it here, I believe that a first-person perspective is closely related to the acquisition of language. A first-person perspective makes possible moral agency and rational agency. We not only act on our desires (as, presumably, dogs do); we can evaluate our desires. It makes possible many new sorts of phenomena: memoirs, confessions, self-deception. It gives us the ability to assess our goals—even biologically endowed goals like survival and reproduction. And on and on.

The appearance of first-person perspectives in a world makes an ontological difference in that world: A world with beings that have inner lives is ontologically richer than a world without beings that have inner lives. But what is ontologically distinctive about being a person—namely, the capacity for a first-person perspective—does not have to be secured by an immaterial substance like a soul.[16]

IV. The Idea of a Rudimentary First-Person Perspective

What I have just described is what I shall call a *robust* first-person perspective. Now I shall distinguish a robust first-person perspective from a rudimentary first-person perspective, and then apply this distinction to the question of when a person comes into beings.[17]

Since our stereotypes of persons are of human persons, my notion of a first-person perspective is tailored to fit specifically human persons. If there are nonhuman persons, they, too, will have robust first-person perspectives, but they may not have acquired them as a development of rudimentary first-person perspectives. But human persons begin by having rudimentary first-person perspectives:

> *Rudimentary FPP.* A being has a rudimentary first-person perspective if and only if
> (i) it is conscious, a sentient being; (ii) it has a capacity to imitate; and (iii) its behavior is explainable only by attribution of beliefs, desires, and intentions.

The requirement of consciousness or sentience for a rudimentary first-person perspective rules out security cameras as conscious, even though they may be said to have a perspective on, say, a parking lot. The capacity to imitate involves differentiation of self and other. The capacity to imitate has been linked by developmental psychologists to "some form of self-recognition" that does not require a self-concept.[18] Finally, a being whose behavior is not explainable except by attribution of beliefs and desires has a perspective and can respond appropriately to changing situations. For one's behavior to be explainable only by attribution of beliefs, desires, and intentions is to be a (minimal) intentional agent. Thus, a being with a rudimentary first-person perspective is a sentient being, an imitator, and an intentional agent.[19]

Human infants have rudimentary first-person perspectives. There is empirical evidence that human infants have the three properties required for a rudimentary first-person perspective. Human infants are clearly sentient. There is abundant research to show that they are imitators from birth. For example, two well-known psychologists, Alison Gopnik and Andrew Meltzoff, tested forty newborns as young as forty-two minutes old (the average age was thirty-two hours) in 1983.[20] They wrote of the newborns' gestures of mouth opening and tongue protrusion: "These data directly demonstrate that a primitive capacity to imitate is part of the normal child's biological endowment."[21] Imitation is grounded in bodies: a newborn imitator must connect the internal feeling of his own body (kinesthesia) with the external things that he sees (and later hears).[22] (Aristotle went so far as to say, in his *Poetics*, that imitation was a distinguishing mark of human beings.) And finally, according to Ulric Neisser, "Babies are intentional agents almost from birth."[23] So human infants meet the conditions for having rudimentary first-person perspectives. Indeed, developmental psychologists agree that from birth, a first-person perspective is underway.[24]

Higher nonhuman mammals seem to meet the conditions as well. Observation of household pets like dogs and cats suggests that they have rudimentary first-person perspectives. They are sentient—they feel pain, for example. (Their brains, as well as their behavior when injured, are similar enough to ours for this to be a secure judgment.) They are imitators; even ducks, who imprint on their mothers, engage in imitative behavior. Although there is some controversy regarding the research on animal intentionality,[25] higher nonhuman mammals appear to be intentional agents. Although we have apparently successful intentional explanations of animal behavior—e.g., "Fido is digging over there because he saw you bury the bone there and he wants it"—there are no adequate nonintentional accounts of Fido's behavior. Chimpanzees that pass psychologist Gordon Gallup's famous mirror tests even more obviously have rudimentary first-person perspectives.[26]

The conclusion I draw from the work of developmental psychologists is that human infants and higher nonhuman mammals have rudimentary first-person perspectives.[27] Moreover, rudimentary first-person perspectives exhaust the first-personal resources of human infants and higher nonhuman mammals; human infants and higher nonhuman mammals exhibit no more sophisticated first-personal phenomena than what rudimentary first-person perspectives account for. Although infants differentiate themselves from others from birth, they do not pass the mirror test until they are about eighteen months old. (And chimpanzees and orangutans "show every bit as compelling evidence of self-recognition as 18- to 24-month-old human infants.")[28] According to Jerome Kagan, it is "not at all certain that [human] 12-month-olds, who experience sensations, possess any concepts about their person, and it is dubious that they are consciously aware of their intentions, feelings, appearance or actions."[29] Daniel J. Povinelli and Christopher G. Prince report that "there is little evidence that chimpanzees understand anything at all about mental states."[30] Although more evidence is needed about the cognitive development of chimpanzees, there is no clear evidence that chimpanzees have the capacity to construct higher-order representations that would allow conceptions of themselves as having pasts and futures.[31]

Another similarity between human infants and higher nonhuman mammals is that they are social creatures. There seems to be general agreement among psychologists that developmentally there is a symmetry of self and other, that humans (as well as other higher nonhuman mammals) are social creatures. Ulric Neisser puts the "interpersonal self" in which the "individual engaged in social interaction with another person" at eight weeks.[32] Philippe Rochat flatly asserts that the developmental origins of self-awareness are primarily social.[33] The idea of a first-person perspective is not Cartesian or Leibnizian: we are not monads that unfold according to an internal plan unaffected by our surroundings.

Thus, human infants and higher nonhuman mammals all have rudimentary first-person perspectives, but I hold that human infants are persons and higher nonhuman mammals are not persons (or probably not). If having a first-person perspective is what distinguishes a person from everything else, and if a human infant and a chimpanzee both have rudimentary first-person perspectives, how can a human infant be a person if a chimpanzee fails to be? What distinguishes the human infant from the chimpanzee is that the human infant's rudimentary first-person perspective is a developmental preliminary to having a robust first-person perspective, but a chimpanzee's rudimentary first-person perspective is not preliminary to anything.

By saying that a rudimentary first-person perspective is "a preliminary to a robust first-person perspective," I mean to pick out those rudimentary first-person perspectives that developmentally ground or underpin robust first-person perspectives. Unlike chimpanzees, human animals are of a kind that normally develops robust first-person perspectives. This is what makes human animals special: their rudimentary first-person perspectives are a developmental preliminary to robust first-person perspectives. A being with a rudimentary first-person perspective is a person *only if it is of a kind that normally develops robust first-person perspectives*. This is not to say that a person will develop a robust first-person perspective: perhaps severely autistic individuals, or severely retarded individuals, have only rudimentary first-person perspectives. However, they are still persons, albeit very impaired, because they have rudimentary first-person perspectives and are of a kind—human animal—that develops a robust first-person perspective. We can capture this idea by the following thesis:

> (HP) *x* constitutes a human person at *t* if and only if *x* is a human organism at *t* and *x* has a rudimentary or robust first-person perspective at *t*,

where we take "*x* constitutes a human person at *t*" as shorthand for "*x* constitutes a person at *t*, and *x* is a (nonderivative) human organism."[34] Thesis (HP) gives only a necessary and sufficient condition for there being a *human* person. There may be other kinds of persons: silicon persons (constituted by aggregates of silicon compounds) and God (not constituted by anything). (HP) is silent about other kinds of persons.

In *Persons and Bodies*, I wrote that a person comes into being when a human organism develops a robust first-person perspective or the structural capacity for one. The effect of (HP) is to push back the onset of personhood to human animals with rudimentary first-person perspectives.

In the face of (HP), someone might mount a "slippery slope" argument against it.[35] The argument would be this: "Once we introduce the notion of a preliminary, we have no reason to stop with rudimentary first-person perspectives. If we consider a being with a rudimentary first-person perspective that is preliminary to a robust first-person perspective to be a person, why not also consider a being at a prior stage that is preliminary to a rudimentary first-person perspective to be a person, and so on?" Suppose that, in place of (HP), someone proposed (HP*):

> (HP*) *x* constitutes a human person at *t* if and only if *x* is a human organism at *t* and either *x* has a robust first-person perspective or *x* has capacities that, in the normal course, produce a being with a robust first-person perspective.[36]

I reject (HP*), and with it the regress argument,[37] for the following reasons. In the first place, note that a robust first-person perspective is itself a capacity—but a capacity of a special sort. A first-person perspective (robust or rudimentary) awaits nothing for its exercise other than a subject's thinking a certain kind of thought. It is an in-hand capacity that can be exercised at will. Let us distinguish between a remote capacity and an in-hand capacity. A hammer has an in-hand capacity at *t* for driving nails whether or not it is actually driving nails; you have an in-hand capacity at *t* for digesting food whether or not you are actually digesting food. Unassembled hammer parts (a wooden handle and a metal head) have only a remote capacity at t for driving nails; an embryo has only a remote capacity at t for digesting food.[38] A remote capacity may be thought of as a second-order capacity: a capacity to develop a capacity. An in-hand capacity is a first-order capacity.

According to the constitution view—as revised to include (HP)—a first-person perspective (rudimentary as well as robust) is an in-hand capacity, not a capacity to develop a capacity. According to (HP*), a being with no in-hand capacities at all, but only with a capacity to develop a capacity, is a person. I do not believe that remote capacities suffice for making *anything* the kind of thing that it is. (HP) makes being a person depend on the more constrained notion of an in-hand capacity of a (rudimentary or robust) first-person perspective.

The second reason that I reject (HP*) is this: The properties in terms of which rudimentary first-person perspectives are specified are ones we recognize as personal: sentience, capacity to imitate, intentionality. Insofar as we think of nonhuman animals as person-like, it is precisely because they have these properties. The properties that an early-term human fetus has—say, having a heart—are not particularly associated with persons, or even with human animals. Even invertebrates have hearts. So, not just every property that is a developmental preliminary to a robust first-person perspective in humans contributes to being a person. There is a difference between those properties in virtue of which beings are person-like (the properties of rudimentary first-person perspectives) and the broader class of biological properties shared by members of many taxa. The properties in virtue of which something is a person are themselves specifically personal properties.

Given (HP), then, human infants are persons: when a human organism develops a rudimentary first-person perspective, it comes to constitute a human person. Acquisition of the properties that comprise a rudimentary first-person perspective has different ontological significance for human organisms than for nonhuman primates. Acquisition of those properties by a human organism marks the beginning of a new person. Acquisition of those properties by a nonhuman organism, however, does not mark the beginning of a new person. The rudimentary first-person perspectives of higher nonhuman mammals are not developmentally preliminary to anything further. (If nonhuman primates did develop robust first-person perspectives, then they, too, would come to constitute persons.)

According to the modern synthesis in biology, we are biological beings, continuous with the rest of the animal kingdom. The constitution view recognizes that we have animal natures. The constitution view shows how to put together Darwinian biology with a traditional concern of philosophers—our inwardness, our ability to see ourselves and each other as subjects, our ability to have rich inner lives. This first-personal aspect of us—the essential aspect, in my opinion—is of no interest to biologists. The first-person perspective may well have evolved by natural selection, but it does not stand out, biologically speaking.

On the constitution view, when a human organism acquires a rudimentary first-person perspective, a new being—a person—comes into existence. When a quantity of bronze is cast into a likeness of a man, a new thing—a statue—comes into existence. Nonderivative persons are essentially persons—just as nonderivative statues are essentially statues. (Bodies that constitute persons are persons derivatively—just as pieces of marble that constitute statues are statues derivatively.) The relation between a human person and a human animal is the same as the relation between a bronze statue and a piece of bronze: constitution. The statue is not identical to the piece of bronze, nor is the person identical to the animal. Thus, the argument for the ontological uniqueness of persons does not require any special pleading. On this view, a human person comes into existence near birth: what is born is a person constituted by an organism.

On the constitution view, as we have seen, a human person comes into existence when a human organism acquires a rudimentary first-person perspective. There is not an exact moment when this happens—just as there is not an exact moment when a human organism comes into existence. But nothing that we know of in the natural world comes into existence instantaneously.[39] When a human organism acquires a rudimentary first-person perspective, it comes to constitute a new entity: a human person. In the next two sections, I shall examine some positions that contrast with the constitution view.

V. Substance Dualism

The constitution view is materialistic: All substances in the natural world are ultimately constituted by physical particles. There are no immaterial substances in the natural world. However, the constitution view has been accused (by philosopher Dean Zimmerman) of being a terminological variant of substance dualism. The charge takes the form of a dilemma:[40] When a person thinks, "I hope that I'll be happy," there is either one thinker of the thought or two. If there are two, then there are too many thinkers. But if there is only one real bearer of the thought, the critic claims, the constitution view is indistinguishable from substance dualism of the sort that holds that immaterial souls are located in bodies that have mental states in virtue of their relations to souls. If there is only one thinker of the thought, then there are two substances (person and animal), distinguished by the fact that one of them is the thinker and the other one is not.

On the constitution view, "one thinker" would refer to the person-constituted-by-the-animal, and "two thinkers" would refer to the person (a member of one primary kind) and the constituting animal (a member of a distinct primary kind). When a person thinks, "I hope that I'll be happy," there is only one thinker that has the thought nonderivatively, the person-constituted-by-the-animal.

Thus, I take the first horn of the dilemma, but deny that it is substance dualism.[41] Zimmerman is right to say that to have a property derivatively is to be constitutionally related to something that has it nonderivatively, but he is mistaken to think that to have it derivatively is to not have it at all. I have argued at length that the constitution-relation is a relation of *unity*. If you take the constitution-relation seriously as a unity-relation, then "derivatively" is not "by courtesy." I suspect that Zimmerman's belief that to have a property derivatively is not to have it at all stems from what I take to be a metaphysical prejudice: the only properties that something *really* has are intrinsic to it. On this assumption, if *x* has a property in virtue of its relation to *y*, where *y* is nonidentical to *x*—even if the relation is as close as constitution—*x* does not *really* have the property. Since I have argued that many things have relational properties essentially, I consider it question-begging to criticize the view by assuming that to have a property in virtue of constitution-relations is not really to have it. The unity is a matter of constitution.

As I said, biologically, I'm a Darwinian: I believe that there is important continuity between the most primitive organisms and us, and that we have animal natures. But there is more to us than our animal natures. I do not believe that biological knowledge suffices for understanding our nature, all things considered. Like the substance dualist, I think that we are ontologically special: the worth or value of a person is not measured in terms of surviving offspring. But emphatically unlike the substance dualist, I do not account for what makes us special in terms of having an immaterial part.

Here are some fundamental ways that the constitution view differs from substance dualism. On the constitution view: (1) There are not just two kinds of substances—mental and physical—but indefinitely many kinds of substances. Each primary kind is ontologically special. (This is important because there is not just one big divide in nature between two disparate realms—mental and physical.) (2) The constitution relation itself is comprehensive, and is exemplified independently of any mental properties. Thus, in contrast to substance dualism, there is no special pleading for persons. (3) The derivative/nonderivative distinction is likewise comprehensive, and is exemplified independently of any mental properties.[42] So, I think that I escape the dilemma of either having to countenance too many thinkers or too many mental states or of falling into substance dualism.

According to substance dualism, there is a bifurcation within the natural world itself—not just, as traditional theists hold, a bifurcation of Creator and creation. Substance dualists take human persons to have two substantially different parts: one material (the body) and one immaterial (the mind or soul). (Whereas a substance dualist might say that we have one foot in heaven, I don't think that we have any feet in heaven.) A person comes into being, according to substance dualism, only when both the material and immaterial parts are present. Different versions of substance dualism locate the coming into being of a person at different times.

I do not believe that substance dualism is a plausible account of the natural world as we know it today. Although I reject scientism root and branch, empirical investigation of the natural world has produced an amazing body of knowledge with no end in sight.[43] Postulation of immaterial substances in the natural world should be a last resort. Since I think that we can do without postulating immaterial substances in the natural world, I think that we ought to do without them. According to the constitution view, nature itself is a unified whole with its own integrity, and human persons are a part of nature.[44] With the exception of one version (which I shall discuss in part B of Section VI), I shall put aside substance dualism.

Now let's consider two alternatives to the constitution view. Both these alternatives—which I reject—take persons to be ontologically in the same category as animals. I shall call these the "biological-animalist view" and the "Thomistic-animalist view," respectively. What I am calling the "biological-animalist view" is called simply the "animalist view" in the mainstream literature on personal identity. I am using the more awkward term, "biological animalism," in order to distinguish this view from a very different view that also takes human persons to be animals, but takes human animals to have immaterial souls. I am calling this latter view "Thomistic animalism."

VI. Persons as Animals

A. Biological Animalism

On the biological-animalist view, what we are most fundamentally are human animals, and human animals are construed as biologists construe them. The animal kingdom is a seamless whole. According to the biological-animalist view, human animals (= human persons) are just another primate species—along with chimpanzees, orangutans, monkeys, and gorillas. The fact that human persons alone have inner lives (or any other psychological or moral properties) is not a particularly important fact about human persons. Proponents of the biological-animalist view have nothing to say about what distinguishes us from nonhuman primates. This is so, I suspect, because what distinguishes us from nonhuman primates is not biologically important.

On the biological-animalist view, what makes us the kind of beings that we are are our biological properties (like metabolism), and our continued existence depends only on the continued functioning of biological processes.[45] It is exclusively up to biologists to tell us what our natures are. A noted biological animalist, Eric Olson, says pointedly: "What it takes for us to persist through time is what I have called *biological continuity*: one survives just in case one's purely animal functions—metabolism, the capacity to breathe and circulate one's blood, and the like—continue."[46] Psychology is, as Olson says, "completely irrelevant to personal identity."[47]

Being a person and having the properties that are associated with being a person, on the biological-animalist view, are irrelevant to the kind of entity you fundamentally are. Person-making properties are temporary and contingent properties of human animals. Olson offhandedly refers to the properties in virtue of which a human animal is a person as "rationality, a capacity for self-consciousness, or what have you"; in Olson's view these are rather like properties of "being a philosopher, or a student, or a fancier of fast cars"—properties that are not part of one's nature.[48] According to biological animalism, what makes you you concerns the biological functions controlled by your lower brain stem.

If biological animalism is correct, then being a person is just an ontologically insignificant property of certain organisms. In that case, the question "When does a person begin?" would be ambiguous. Either it would mean: When does an organism—an entity that will acquire the property of being a person—begin? Or it could mean: When does an organism acquire the property of being a person? These questions have different answers: the time that a new organism begins is much earlier than the time that it acquires the property of being a person.

But we need not decide which way a biological animalist ought to construe the question "When does a person begin?" because there are reasons to reject the biological-animalist view independently of how it answers this question.

The main reason to reject the biological-animalist view is that it renders invisible our most important characteristics. The abilities of self-conscious, brooding, and introspective beings—from Augustine in the *Confessions* to analysands in psychoanalysis to former U.S. presidents writing their memoirs—are of a different order from those of tool-using, mate-seeking, dominance-establishing non-human primates—even though our use of tools, seeking of mates, and establishing dominance have their origins in our nonhuman ancestors. With respect to *the range of what we can do* (from planning our futures to wondering how we got ourselves into such a mess), and with respect to *the moral significance of what we can do* (from assessing our goals to confessing our sins), self-conscious beings are obviously unique—significantly different from non-self-conscious beings.

I agree with the biological animalists about our biological nature—as I said, I am a Darwinian—I just think that our biological nature does not exhaust our nature all things considered. For example, if Darwin is right, there are only two ultimate goals for human animals: survival and reproduction. But people have ultimate goals that cannot be assimilated to survival and reproduction. (Think of people willing to die in the service of an abstract idea like freedom.) Thus, I think that biological animalism does not do justice to the reality of human persons. So, let's turn to Thomistic animalism.

B. Thomistic Animalism

I use the term "Thomistic animalism" to describe a view that regards us as fundamentally animals, but does not construe human animals as biologists construe them. According to Thomistic animalism, any member of the biological species *Homo sapiens* is a person. But being a member of the *Homo sapiens* species is not like being a member of other species. According to Thomistic animalism, all and only members of the *Homo sapiens* species have immaterial spiritual souls that are not recognized by biologists.[49] Thus, according to Thomistic animalism, human persons are animals, but there are two kinds of animals: non-rational animals that do not have immaterial souls and rational animals that do have immaterial souls.

Norman M. Ford, author of two informative and provocative books on the beginning of persons,[50] is a major proponent of the view that I am calling "Thomistic animalism." Ford is concerned with what he usually calls "the human individual." As he put it, "I shall use all three ways of referring to the members of our biological species *Homo sapiens* as interchangeable and with the same meaning—human individual, human being and person."[51] This may sound like biological animalism, but it is crucially different. Unlike biological animalism, Thomistic animalism does not take biology to be the arbiter of the nature of animals, at least of human animals. Ford does not believe that "the human person can be satisfactorily explained in purely empirical terms." A human animal is not "just a living body that has the capacity to engage in rational self-conscious acts."[52] On the Thomistic-animalist view, a human animal is animated by an immaterial spiritual soul or a "human life-principle," which, after death, "is no longer present in the corpse."[53] Ford sees a "fundamental psychosomatic unity of soul and matter within the ontological unity of the human individual."[54] (Thus, I take Ford's view to be a form of substance dualism.)[55]

Although, on Ford's view, "person" officially is just another name for members of the *Homo sapiens* species, the "core of our personhood" is not a matter of biology: "Rape and perjury are immoral everywhere. This is so because morality is essentially related to the core of our personhood where human dignity and solidarity originate."[56] Thomistic animalism, then, takes us human persons to be fundamentally animals with important nonbiological properties that are unique to human persons. Moreover, Ford sometimes calls a spiritual soul "an immaterial life-principle."[57] If we need an immaterial life-principle to explain our being "living human individuals," why don't chimpanzees also need an immaterial life-principle to explain their being living nonhuman primates?

In any case, I think that Thomistic animalism is ultimately unsatisfactory for two principal reasons. First, Thomistic animalism tears apart the animal kingdom. Contrary to contemporary biological thought, Thomistic animalism makes membership in the species *Homo sapiens* very different from membership in any other species. It asserts that biology does not have the last word on *Homo sapiens*. Second, Thomistic animalism conceives of us human persons as having two parts: an immaterial soul and a material body. The constitution view offers an alternative that avoids both these difficulties while retaining moral and theological benefits of Thomistic animalism.[58]

On the constitution view, biology does have the last word on *Homo sapiens;* but biology does not have the last word on us human persons, all things considered. If we are constituted by human animals, but not identical to the human animals that constitute us, then we can give biology its full due—and with biologists, see the animal kingdom as a seamless whole—and still emphasize the very properties that Thomistic animalists insist on.

For example, unlike biologists, Ford locates the evolutionary difference between "a form of animal life" and human beings in a spiritual soul, evidence for which is that human beings have reflective self-awareness.[59] According to the constitution view, we can side with the biologists on the matter of the difference between human and nonhuman animals, and yet agree with Ford that reflective self-awareness does make us human persons unique. We just need to distinguish between human persons and human animals and refrain from using "human beings" or "human individuals" equivocally. We do not have to abandon standard biology in order to secure our uniqueness. Nor do we have to suppose that we have immaterial spiritual souls—or that any animal would need or have such a thing—in order to secure our uniqueness.

By conceiving of human persons as members of the species *Homo sapiens*, but essentially having nonbiological properties (immaterial souls), Thomistic animalism cannot make good sense of the respects in which we are like the rest of the animal kingdom and the respects in which we are not. By contrast, the constitution view clearly holds that we are part of the animal kingdom with respect to what constitutes us, but that our being essentially persons makes us unique in just the ways that Ford would like.

One consideration that is *not* among my reasons to reject Thomistic animalism is that it is presented as a Christian view.[60] Indeed, I think that theists who believe in (or even who want to leave open the possibility of) life after death have still another reason to reject Thomistic animalism: Animals essentially are organic; organic material essentially decays (it is corruptible). I do not see how an animal could possibly survive death. Ah, but the Thomistic animalist says, we are very special animals; we are animals-with-immaterial-souls, and an immaterial soul does not decay! In that case, if we are to survive death, we should be identified with the immaterial soul, not with animals at all. The constitution view, as I have argued elsewhere, is a better way to leave room for life after death than postulation of an immaterial soul.[61]

Thus, I believe that the constitution view is superior to both biological animalism and Thomistic animalism (as well as to substance dualism). Biological animalism does not recognize the ontological importance of the unique properties of human persons. Thomistic animalism, while recognizing the ontological importance of human persons, attributes the ontologically important properties to (putatively) immaterial features of members of the animal kingdom. By contrast, the constitution view both recognizes the ontological importance of the unique properties of human persons, and regards human persons as natural, material beings—without contravening any tenets of traditional theism or even of Christian doctrine. Now let's return to the matter of the coming into existence of a human person and its implications for thinking about abortion.

VII. Thinking about Abortion

This is an essay in metaphysics—specifically in the metaphysics of personal identity. It is not an essay on public policy, nor is it an essay on the legal issues concerning abortion in the United States. These matters, though important, are logically subsequent to the ones at issue here.[62] Nevertheless, the constitution view has one logical implication that is relevant to thinking about abortion. Thus, I want to add a coda to discuss this implication and reasons why it is useful in thinking about abortion.

According to the constitution view, as we have seen, a human organism exists before a human person comes into being: a human person comes into being when a human organism develops a rudimentary first-person perspective—at birth, or shortly before.[63] The obvious consequence of the constitution view for the issue of abortion is this: Any premise that implies that abortion before development of a rudimentary first-person perspective is the killing of an innocent person is false. If the constitution view is correct, then no sound anti-abortion argument can be based on such a premise.[64] This is all that follows from the constitution view. But it answers—in the negative—an important question: Does every human organism have the same ontological and moral status as you and me? This question is an important philosophical one for everyone—legislators, judges, as well as private individuals who have no official social roles—who thinks seriously about abortion.

Using "fetus" as short for "fetus before development of a rudimentary first-person perspective," the metaphysical implication of the constitution view is the following thesis—call it "(O)":

(O) A human fetus is an organism that does not constitute a person.

Thesis (O) has no direct implications for condoning or not condoning abortion. It certainly does not justify abortion. Indeed, one may endorse (O) and be just as opposed to procured abortions of any sort as someone who holds that every human embryo is a person. Thesis (O) is, however, significant for thinking about abortion, because it removes a whole category of arguments that short-circuit careful moral thought. The thesis that every fetus is a person implies that abortion is the killing of an innocent person. If the fetus is a person, abortion is morally impermissible regardless of the circumstances of the pregnant girl or woman. Morally speaking, the thesis that the fetus is a person renders the pregnant female invisible: it simply forecloses any consideration of the woman or girl per se who (for whatever reason) has an unwanted pregnancy. By contrast, (O) allows respect for pregnant females per se and not just as incubators. In thinking about abortion, it is morally important not to leave out respect for the pregnant girl or woman in her own right.[65] Thesis (O) opens up the field of discussion to include pregnant girls and women in their own right. There are three further reasons that (O) is helpful in thinking about abortion.

The first reason is that, by removing the premise that a fetus is a person, (O) clears the field of misleading arguments about, e.g., a "right to life." There can be no "right to life" until there is a person to be a subject of that right. It makes no sense to suppose that a nonexisting person has a right to be brought into existence. Moreover, "life" is used to refer both to biological life (taking in nutrition, locomotion, growing—biological characteristics that we share with other species) and to personal life (joys, hopes, plans for the future—nonbiological characteristics that appear in a biography). Human biological life derives value from making possible personal life. But to take human biological life—shorn of context and of considerations of quality—to be an absolute value in itself verges on idolatry. It puts allegiance to an abstract metaphysical view above the concrete needs of the actual people involved: it gives precedence to an abstraction—*life*—over the real lives of real people.

The second reason that (O) is helpful in thinking about abortion is this: Rejection of the thesis that the fetus is a person shifts the issue from a question about the morality of killing a person to a question about the morality of bringing into existence a person in various circumstances. The question of whether a person should be brought into existence is very different from the question of duties toward a person already in existence. This shift of questions—to whether a person should be brought into existence in various given circumstances— makes room for careful reflection that takes into account relevant considerations such as the health of the fetus, the health of the mother, the capacity of the mother (or others), financially and emotionally, to take on the responsibility of caring for an infant and bringing up a child, the quality of life that a child would likely have, the impact of a new child on the family, and the consequences for society of bringing a child into the world in the given circumstances. Discussions that assume that fetuses are persons simplemindedly screen off such morally relevant considerations from view.

Anyone who is considering an abortion is in a terrible situation. Everyone can agree that it would have been much better not to have become pregnant. But when the options are to have an abortion or to have a baby, there are circumstances in which the choice to have an abortion is the morally better choice. One such circumstance is a situation in which the fetus is anencephalic. Anencephaly is a fatal condition in which brain formation begins but goes awry, leaving a defective brain stem and malformed hemispheres. Anencephalic fetuses are never capable of long-term survival. Delivery of such a baby carries a high risk of hemorrhage and extreme trauma for the mother. Bringing such a baby into the world is not a wise use of health-care resources.

In such cases, I believe that abortion would be morally the right course of action. The anencephalic human organism will never have a rudimentary first-person perspective and will never come to constitute a person. Even Ford, who still counsels against abortion, agrees that such a fetus "will never be able to express rational activities." But Ford holds that a fetus with "anencephaly is a human individual with a rational nature on account of a divinely created immaterial soul or life-principle and who, due to a malformed cortex and brain damage, will never be able to express rational activities."[66]

The point is this: If (O) were false[67]—if abortion were morally impermissible on the grounds that a fetus is a person—then morally speaking, there could be no exceptions to the prohibition of abortion in the case of anencephaly, or in the case of rape or incest, or in the case of saving the pregnant woman's life. None of these considerations would be relevant to allowing abortion. (That most abortions have nothing to do with these extreme circumstances is irrelevant to the logical point.) Thus, another reason to welcome (O) is that (O)—unlike its denial—allows consideration of morally relevant circumstances in deciding about an abortion.

The third reason that (O) is helpful in thinking about abortion is that abortion is a complex issue, and (O), unlike the denial of (O), allows the complexity to be recognized. For example, who should make decisions about abortion? If (O) is denied, there is no moral room for decisions about abortion to be made by anyone. Given (O), the following line of thought is available (though not forced upon one):

It is reasonable that, in *any* decision, whoever will bear the burden for the effects of the decision should have control over making it. The ultimate bearer of responsibility for having a baby is primarily the pregnant girl or woman, and to a lesser extent her sexual partner, her doctor, and other caregivers whom she may call upon for help.[68] A new person does not come into existence until the fetus develops a rudimentary first-person perspective, perhaps at birth, perhaps shortly before birth at the earliest.[69] Since fetal development is a gradual process, the closer the fetus comes to developing a rudimentary first-person perspective, the more cautious someone considering abortion should be. So, as long as we can be sure that there is no rudimentary first-person perspective—up through, say, the second trimester of pregnancy—the decision to abort should be in the hands of the pregnant girl or woman and her allies.[70]

This line of thought leads to individual choice about matters of great personal importance and intimacy, but not to moral relativism. There is an analogy here with religion. We may tolerate individual religious choice, while not advocating religious relativism. One can be convinced that someone else is wrong on a vitally important matter, without feeling justified in interfering with her decision. Thesis (O)—the thesis that a fetus is not a person—allows (but does not require) individual moral judgment and tolerance for others' moral judgments about their own lives.

Thus, there are three important differences between the thesis that a fetus is not a person—(O)—and the denial of (O). First, (O) allows but does not require giving precedence to the concrete and particular (actual pregnant girls and women) over the abstract and general (the idea of life considered in isolation from anyone's actual experience of life). The thesis that a fetus is a person does the reverse. Second, (O) allows but does not require attending to the moral significance of the circumstances of a pregnancy. The thesis that a fetus is a person renders those circumstances morally irrelevant. Third, (O) allows but does not require individual moral judgment and tolerance for others' moral judgments about the most intimate details of their own lives.

To sum up this section: The constitution view, which is supported by arguments that have nothing to do with abortion,[71] implies that a fetus before development of a rudimentary first-person perspective is not a person. This section gives reasons to welcome this consequence. The overall reason to welcome it is that it opens the door to discussion of the considerations that I mentioned. If abortion were the killing of an innocent person, then none of the considerations that I mentioned—anencephaly, rape, incest, the pregnant person's suitability for parenthood, or the others—would even be relevant to the morality of abortion. There would be nothing to argue about. Putting aside the view that the fetus is a person is a necessary condition for discussion of the morality of abortion in various circumstances.

VIII. Conclusion

The constitution view of human persons is part of a comprehensive picture of the material world. It holds that human persons are constituted by bodies (i.e., organisms) without being identical to the constituting organisms. Such an account does justice both to our similarities to other animals and to our uniqueness. Moreover, I have argued that the constitution view is superior to biological animalism, Thomistic animalism, and other forms of substance dualism. According to the constitution view, a human person comes into existence when a human organism acquires a rudimentary first-person perspective. The onset of a first-person perspective marks the entry of a new entity in the world.

The constitution view has one important consequence for thinking about abortion. The consequence is that, for principled reasons that have nothing specifically to do with abortion, a fetus is not a person.[72] Just as a hunk of marble is in an ontologically distinct category from a statue, so is a fetus in an ontologically distinct category from a person. Thus, the constitution view gives one an *ontological* reason to deny that the fetus is a person. Anyone who takes it to be morally abhorrent to force a rape victim to bear the rapist's child has in addition a good *moral* reason to deny that the fetus is a person. Anyone who believes that there is even a possibility of morally relevant differences among pregnancies should welcome the thesis that follows from the constitution view: A fetus is not a person.

NOTES

Thanks to Gareth Matthews and Catherine E. Rudder for comments. I am also grateful to other contributors to this volume, especially Robert A. Wilson, Marya Schechtman, David Oderberg, Stephen Braude, and John Finnis.

1. Throughout this essay, I mean "we" to apply to the community of readers.

2. For example, see John Perry, "The Importance of Being Identical," in Amélie Oksenberg Rorty, ed., *The Identities of Persons* (Berkeley: University of California Press, 1976), 70.

3. For example, see Mark Johnston, "Human Beings," *Journal of Philosophy* 84 (1987): 64.

4. See Norman M. Ford, *The Prenatal Person: Ethics from Conception to Birth* (Malden, MA: Blackwell Publishing, 2002), 9, 15.

5. Ibid., 55. Moreover, everything in the natural world comes into existence gradually: solar systems, cherry blossoms, jellyfish, tractors and other artifacts. Thus, every natural entity has vague temporal boundaries, and hence is subject to vague existence;

but it does not follow that there is any vague identity. If *a*=*b* and *a* is vague, then *b* is vague in exactly the same respects. I discuss this further in my essay "Everyday Concepts as a Guide to Reality," *The Monist* (2006).

6. G. E. M. Anscombe, "Were You a Zygote?" in A. Phillips Griffiths, ed., *Philosophy and Practice* (Cambridge: Cambridge University Press, 1985), 111.

7. Ibid., 112.

8. This is a point that has been made by Roman Catholic writers. See, e.g., Norman M. Ford, *When Did I Begin? Conception of the Human Individual in History, Philosophy, and Science* (Cambridge: Cambridge University Press, 1988), 174–78. See also Anscombe, "Were You a Zygote?"

9. Many philosophers identify human organisms with human bodies. For example, Fred Feldman holds that human persons are (identical to) human organisms and that human organisms persist after death as corpses. See Fred Feldman, *Confrontations with the Reaper* (New York: Oxford University Press, 1992), 104–5. Although I do not identify persons and organisms, I do identify organisms and bodies.

10. Constitution is not a relation between parts and wholes. If *x* constitutes *y* at *t*, the difference between *x* and *y* is that *x* and *y* have different properties essentially and different persistence conditions. It is not a matter of *y*'s having a part that *x* lacks, or vice versa.

11. By "social sciences" I mean the disciplines of sociology, political science, history, and other disciplines that have groups of people in their domain. The domain of psychology includes conscious beings with beliefs, desires, and intentions. In the absence of anything immaterial, where is the domain of psychology located? The domain of psychology is located where the conscious beings with beliefs, desires, and intentions are located. Not every phenomenon in a material world has a definite spatial location—e.g., where was Smith's purchase of Shell Oil stock located?

12. I have discussed this at length in *Persons and Bodies: A Constitution View* (Cambridge: Cambridge University Press, 2000). See ch. 3.

13. Hector-Neri Castañeda developed this idea in several papers. See Castañeda, "He: A Study in the Logic of Self-Consciousness," *Ratio* 8 (1966): 130–57; and Castañeda, "Indicators and Quasi-Indicators," *American Philosophical Quarterly* 4 (1967): 85–100.

14. The term comes from Gareth B. Matthews, *Thought's Ego in Augustine and Descartes* (Ithaca, NY: Cornell University Press, 1992).

15. Gordon Gallup's experiments with chimpanzees suggest the possibility of a kind of intermediate stage between dogs (which have intentional states but no first-person perspectives) and human persons (who have first-person perspectives). In my opinion, Gallup's chimpanzees fall short of full-blown first-person perspectives (for details, see Baker, *Persons and Bodies*, 62–64). See Gordon Gallup, Jr., "Self-Recognition in Primates: A Comparative Approach to Bidirectional Properties of Consciousness," *American Psychologist* 32 (1977): 329–38.

16. The constitution view is an argument for this claim. The first-person perspective, along with the capacity to acquire a language, may be products of natural selection or may be specially endowed by God. But for whatever reason (either God's will or natural selection sans God), nonhuman primates have not developed robust first-person perspectives of the kind that we have.

17. I was motivated to distinguish between a robust and a rudimentary first-person perspective by my many critics, including Marc Slors, Anthonie Meijers, Monica Meijsing, Herman de Regt, and Ton Derksen.

18. Michael Lewis, "Myself and Me," in Sue Taylor Parker, Robert W. Mitchell, and Maria L. Boccia, eds., *Self-Awareness in Animals and Humans* (Cambridge: Cambridge University Press, 1994), 22.

19. So, rudimentary first-person perspectives have what Robert A. Wilson calls "action-traction." See Section V of his essay "Persons, Social Agency, and Constitution." *Social Philosophy and Policy* 22 (2) (2005): 49–69.

20. Gopnik is Professor of Psychology at the University of California at Berkeley, and Meltzoff is Codirector of the Institute for Learning and Brain Sciences at the University of Washington, where he is also Professor of Psychology.

21. Alison Gopnik and Andrew N. Meltzoff, "Minds, Bodies, and Persons: Young Children's Understanding of the Self and Others as Reflected in Imitation and Theory-of-Mind Research," in Parker, Mitchell, and Boccia, eds., *Self-Awareness in Animals and Humans*, 171.

22. Alison Gopnik, Andrew Meltzoff, and Patricia Kuhl, eds., *How Babies Think: The Science of Childhood* (London: Weidenfeld and Nicholson, 1999), 30.

23. See Ulric Neisser, "Criteria for an Ecological Self," in Philippe Rochat, ed., *The Self in Infancy: Theory and Research* (Amsterdam: North-Holland, Elsevier, 1995), 23. Neisser is a well-known cognitive psychologist at Cornell University.

24. See, for example, Jerome Kagan, *Unstable Ideas* (Cambridge, MA: Harvard University Press, 1989). Kagan is the Starch Professor of Psychology at Harvard.

25. See, for example, Cecilia Heyes and Anthony Dickinson, "The Intentionality of Animal Action," in Martin Davies and Glyn W. Humphreys, eds., *Consciousness: Psychological and Philosophical Essays* (Oxford: Blackwell, 1993), 105–20. Heyes is in the Department of Psychology at University College, London, and Dickinson is in the Department of Experimental Psychology at Cambridge University.

26. See Gallup, "Self-Recognition in Primates." Discussion of the mirror tests has become so widespread that the phenomenon of recognizing oneself in a mirror is routinely referred to simply by the initials MSR (mirror self-recognition) in psychological literature.

27. I do not expect the developmental psychologists to share my metaphysical view of constitution; I look to their work only to show at what stages during development certain features appear.

28. Daniel J. Povinelli, "The Unduplicated Self," in Rochat, ed., *The Self in Infancy*, 185. Povinelli is in the Cognitive Evolution Group at the University of Louisiana at Lafayette.

29. Jerome Kagan, "Is There a Self in Infancy?" in Michel Ferrari and Robert J. Sternberg, eds., *Self-Awareness: Its Nature and Development* (New York: The Guilford Press, 1998), 138.

30. Daniel J. Povinelli and Christopher G. Prince, "When Self Met Other," in Ferrari and Sternberg, eds., *Self-Awareness*, 88.

31. Povinelli, "The Unduplicated Self," 186. So it looks as if the scope of the self-concept that Gallup postulated to explain mirror behavior is really quite limited, contrary to Gallup's speculation.

32. Ulric Neisser, "Criteria for an Ecological Self," in Rochat, ed., *The Self in Infancy*, 18.

33. Philippe Rochat, "Early Objectification of the Self," in Rochat, ed., *The Self in Infancy*, 54. Rochat is in the Emory University Department of Psychology.

34. This latter detail is a needed technicality since, on the constitution view, *person* is a primary kind, and there may be nonhuman persons. "Human person" refers to a person constituted by a human organism.

35. Gareth Matthews suggested this argument.

36. Robert A. Wilson suggested (HP*).

37. "Regress argument" is a common philosophical term for the kind of argument sketched in the preceding paragraph.

38. I borrowed the example of the hammer from Robert Pasnau's excellent discussion of "has a capacity." See Robert Pasnau, *Thomas Aquinas on Human Nature: A Philosophical Study of Summa Theologiae 1a 75–89* (Cambridge: Cambridge University Press, 2002), 115.

39. There is (ontological) indeterminacy at the beginning of everything that comes into existence by means of a process. See my essay "Everyday Concepts as a Guide to Reality," *The Monist* (2006).

40. This is my interpretation of Dean Zimmerman's "The Constitution of Persons by Bodies: A Critique of Lynne Rudder Baker's Theory of Material Constitution," *Philosophical Topics* 30 (2002): 295–338.

41. Zimmerman asks how I differ from an emergent dualist (like William Hasker), who holds that a soul—a distinct substance, made of a unique kind of immaterial stuff—emerges from a body. Despite some affinities between my view and Hasker's, I think that it is implausible to suppose that there are immaterial substances in the natural world. Moreover: (1) On my view, the relation between a person and her body (as well as the relation between a person and the micro-elements that make her up) is an instance of a very general relation common to *all* macro-objects; whereas, according to Hasker, the relation between a person and her body is that a body is one part of a person, who also has a special immaterial part. (2) On my view, what emerges from material elements is never anything immaterial; on Hasker's view, the emergent self is an immaterial object. (3) I think that all the causal powers of a human person are constituted by causal powers at lower levels; whereas Hasker holds that the self has libertarian free will and can modify and direct the brain. See William Hasker, *The Emergent Self* (Ithaca, NY: Cornell University Press, 1999), 195.

42. Substance dualists countenance only one-way borrowing: the body borrows mental properties from the soul. Zimmerman supposes that the "emergent dualist will surely regard [my two-way borrowing] as simply a question of semantics" (Zimmerman, "The Constitution of Persons by Bodies," 316). He does not say why the substance dualist's one-way borrowing of mental properties from the soul by the body should be considered a matter of metaphysics, but borrowing in the other direction only a matter of semantics.

43. By "scientism" I mean the view that *all* correct explanations are scientific explanations. We must distinguish between scientific claims—claims made from *within* science—and claims made *about* science. One important claim about science (one that I reject) is that science is the arbiter of all knowable truth, that there is nothing to be known beyond what science delivers.

44. This is so, I believe, whether there is a Creator or not.

45. Eric T. Olson, *The Human Animal: Personal Identity without Psychology* (Oxford: Oxford University Press, 1997), 30.

46. Ibid., 16.

47. Eric T. Olson, "Was I Ever a Fetus?" *Philosophy and Phenomenological Research* 57 (1997): 97.

48. Olson, *The Human Animal*, 17.

49. See Ford, *When Did I Begin?* and *The Prenatal Person*.

50. The thesis that Ford elaborates and supports is (what is commonly taken to be) the official view of the Roman Catholic Church after the First Vatican Council, 1869–70. However, it is not the view of Thomas Aquinas, nor is it just an updated version of Aquinas's view. Aquinas, following Aristotle, thought that until the presence of a rational soul—

about twelve weeks into gestation—there was no human individual of any sort. See Robert Pasnau, *Thomas Aquinas on Human Nature*, 100–142. (An updated version of Aquinas's view, I believe, would place the beginning of a human person at the development of a brain that could support rational thought.) The Roman Catholic Church's official position is that human life must be protected from the time of conception. John Finnis pointed out to me that the doctrine is not that a fetus *is* a person, but that a fetus *must be treated as* a person. See, for example, Congregation for the Doctrine of the Faith, "Instruction on Respect for Human Life in Its Origin and on the Dignity of Procreation: Replies to Certain Questions of the Day," http://www.vatican.va/roman_curia/congrega tions/cfaith/documents/rc_con_cfaith_doc_19870222_respect-for-human-life_en.html (accessed April 4, 2004).

51. Ford, *When Did I Begin?* 67.

52. Ibid., 74.

53. Ibid., 16; Ford, *The Prenatal Person*, 13–16.

54. Ford, *When Did I Begin?* 74.

55. Although Thomistic animalists are substance dualists, I consider their view as a variety of animalism because they take their view from Thomas Aquinas, who followed Aristotle in holding that men (as he would say) are essentially animals.

56. Ford, *The Prenatal Person*, 17.

57. Ibid., 91.

58. See my "Material Persons and the Doctrine of Resurrection," *Faith and Philosophy* 18 (2001): 151–67; and my "Death and the Afterlife," in *The Oxford Handbook of Philosophy of Religion*, ed. William J. Wainwright (Oxford: Oxford University Press, 2004), 366–91.

59. Ford, *When Did I Begin?* 1. Moreover, Ford sometimes slips up and *contrasts* human persons and animals. See ibid., 75.

60. For what it's worth, I am a practicing Episcopalian, who accepts the Nicene Creed.

61. See my "Death and the Afterlife," in Wainwright, ed., *The Oxford Handbook of Philosophy of Religion*. I also believe that the constitution view can make better sense of the "two-natures" doctrine of Christ than can substance dualism. See my essay "Christians Should Reject Mind-Body Dualism," in Michael L. Peterson and Raymond J. VanArragon, eds., *Contemporary Debates in the Philosophy of Religion* (Maiden, MA: Blackwell Publishers, 2004), 327–37.

62. If I had written a different essay, U.S. Supreme Court cases—such as *Roe v. Wade* (1973) and *Casey v. Planned Parenthood* (1993)—would have been germane; but they are not germane to this metaphysical essay. Such legal considerations are at the wrong level of discourse for this essay.

63. In "Was I Ever a Fetus?", Eric T. Olson argued that on views like mine, I was never an early-term fetus. Distinguo! There is no x such that x was a fetus at t and I am identical to x. However, there is an x such that x was a fetus at t and I am now constituted by x. For my full reply to Olson's article, see my "What Am I?", *Philosophy and Phenomenological Research* 59 (1999): 151–59.

64. Moral theories like utilitarianism or Kantianism are of limited use in debates about abortion for two reasons: (1) The question of what beings qualify as being subject to moral theories is not answered by the theories themselves; and (2) in applying a moral theory to an actual case, all the "moral work" goes into describing the particulars of the case. In actual decisions about abortion, the particulars of the case carry the day.

65. Note that I am not using the fact that (O) allows respect for pregnant females per se, and not just as human incubators, as reason to accept (O), but rather as reason to

welcome (O) as a consequence of the constitution view. The reason to *accept* (O) is that it follows from the constitution view, which is a comprehensive view defended on grounds having nothing to do with fetuses.

66. Ford, *The Prenatal Person*, 95–96.

67. Thesis (O) is false if and only if either a fetus is not an organism, or a fetus is a person. I shall assume that those who deny (O) do not deny that a fetus is an organism, but rather hold that a fetus is a person.

68. Those who urge ill-prepared pregnant girls not to have abortions seem to melt away when the baby actually arrives; their concern for human life, as many have pointed out, seems to stop at birth.

69. Although a fetus may be sentient early on, it seems unlikely that it has a capacity to imitate or that it behaves in ways explainable only by attribution of beliefs, desires, and intentions until birth or shortly before birth. Thus, even in the absence of empirical research, I think it is safe to suppose that the requirements of a rudimentary first-person perspective are not met until birth or shortly before birth. I am not arguing from any attitude toward abortion of nearly full-term fetuses to a conclusion about the ontological status of the fetus. The thesis about the ontological status of the fetus—that a fetus before development of a rudimentary first-person perspective is not a person—follows from the constitution view, which was developed quite independently of these issues.

70. The reason that one may want to leave the state out of these decisions until there is a rudimentary first-person perspective is that laws limiting abortion are made by legislatures and upheld at times by courts filled with people who sincerely believe that women find fulfillment in being subordinate to men. A compassionate public policy would not leave the fate of women and girls who get pregnant in the hands of such people.

71. See my *Persons and Bodies*.

72. Nor, of course, is an embryo a person. Thus, any argument against embryonic stem cell research that presupposes that an embryo is a person is also unsound.

Part III / Persons at the End of Life

CHAPTER TWENTY-FOUR

The Biophilosophical Basis of Whole-Brain Death

James L. Bernat

> The boundaries which divide Life from Death are, at best, shadowy and vague. Who shall say where the one ends, and where the other begins?
>
> —EDGAR ALLEN POE, *THE PREMATURE BURIAL* (1844)

> The doctors came immediately one after the other: namely a Crow, an Owl, and a Talking-cricket.
>
> "I wish to know from you gentlemen," said the Fairy, turning to the three doctors who were assembled round Pinocchio's bed—"I wish to know from you gentlemen, if this unfortunate puppet is alive or dead! . . ."
>
> At this request the Crow, advancing first, felt Pinocchio's pulse; he then felt his nose, and then the little toe of his foot; and having done this carefully, he pronounced solemnly the following words:
>
> "To my belief the puppet is already quite dead; but if unfortunately he should not be dead, then it would be a sign that he is still alive!"
>
> "I regret," said the Owl, "to be obliged to contradict the Crow, my illustrious friend and colleague, but in my opinion the puppet is still alive; but if unfortunately he should not be alive, then it would be a sign that he is dead indeed!"
>
> "And you—have you nothing to say?" asked the Fairy of the Talking-cricket.
>
> "In my opinion the wisest thing a prudent doctor can do, when he does not know what he is talking about, is to be silent . . ."
>
> —CARLO COLLODI, *PINOCCHIO* (1881)

> Only a very bold man, I think, would attempt to define death.
>
> —HENRY K. BEECHER, *DEFINITIONS OF "LIFE" AND "DEATH" FOR*
> *MEDICAL SCIENCE AND PRACTICE* (1971)

I. Introduction

Notwithstanding these wise pronouncements, my project here is to characterize the biological phenomenon of death of the higher animal species, such as vertebrates. My claim is that the formulation of "whole-brain death" provides the most congruent map for our correct understanding of the concept of death. This essay builds upon the foundation my colleagues and I have laid since 1981 to characterize the concept of death and refine when this event occurs.[1] Although our society's well-accepted program of multiple organ procurement for transplantation requires the organ donor first to be dead, the concept of brain death is not merely a social contrivance to permit us to obtain the benefits of organ procurement.[2] Rather, the concept of whole-brain death stands independently as the most accurate biological representation of the demise of the human organism.

"Brain death" is the colloquial term for the determination of human death by showing the permanent cessation of the clinical functions of the brain, irrespective of the continued mechanically supported functioning of other bodily organs. Although the term "brain death" is hallowed by consensual usage that began in the 1960s, it is an unfortunate and misleading term because it implies erroneously that there are two types of death: brain death and ordinary death. In fact, death remains a unitary phenomenon, but one that may be determined in two ways: (1) by showing the irreversible cessation of breathing and circulation, or, (2) when breathing and circulation are mechanically supported, by showing the irreversible cessation of clinical brain functions.[3]

The concept of brain death has achieved a high degree of acceptance in Western society since the Harvard Medical School Ad Hoc Committee Report that first brought it to general public attention in 1968.[4] Since that time, brain-death determination has been codified into public law as a legal standard of death throughout the Westernized and developed world, as well as in a number of undeveloped countries.[5] In bioethics circles, brain death is viewed by many as an example of a previously controversial topic about which widespread consensus finally has been achieved, thus permitting the enactment of successful and well-accepted public policies.

Yet brain death has always had critics. Despite its general acceptance by most observant Christians and Jews as being consistent with Judeo-Christian religious beliefs and traditions,[6] some religious scholars have attacked brain death as fundamentally inconsistent with Christian or Jewish religious doctrines.[7] Some other scholars have argued for essential changes in the whole-brain death doctrine to embrace the "higher-brain formulation" that requires irreversible cessation of only cerebral hemispheric function and ignores the presence or absence of brain-stem functions.[8] Yet other scholars have pointed out purported inconsistencies in the definition and criterion of the accepted whole-brain death doctrine.[9] Recently, some scholars have called for abandoning brain death altogether because they claim that it is an unnecessary anachronism.[10]

Whereas previous critics attacked the edges of the doctrine of brain death, a new set of critics is attacking its very conceptual foundation. Most notably, the neurologist Alan Shewmon argues that any concept of death based upon brain function is wrong conceptually, because the brain enjoys no special status over other organs in the concept of death: the human organism is not dead until circulation stops irreversibly. He maintains that a defense of brain death based on viewing the brain as the organism's critical integrating and coordinating system is illogical, because many integrating and control functions are executed outside the brain.[11] Shewmon further points out that the existence of cases of brain-dead patients whose circulation and other organ functions have been successfully supported physiologically for months or longer negates the concept of brain death, because it is counterintuitive that a dead person could possibly exhibit circulation, growth, and parturition.[12] In a similar vein, the neurologist Robert Taylor argues that brain death represents a legal fiction that society has created to permit multiple organ procurement for transplantation—but that we all know that such patients really are not dead.[13]

A philosophical defense of whole-brain death has been offered by several scholars since the 1970s. Alexander Capron and Leon Kass were the first to point out that agreement on a concept of death must precede the design of tests for death or acceptance of a statute of death.[14] The neurologist Julius Korein observes that the brain is the critical system of the organism, whose permanent loss of functioning represents death.[15] In a series of papers over the 1980s and 1990s, with my Dartmouth colleagues Charles Culver and Bernard Gert, I argue that irreversible cessation of the clinical functions of the brain represents death because the brain is responsible for the functioning of the organism as a whole.[16] This defense of the whole-brain formulation of death was cited by the United States President's Commission for the Study of Ethical Problems in Medicine and Biomedical and Behavioral Research as the conceptual basis of brain death in their book *Defining Death*, in which they recommend the adoption by all states of the Uniform Determination of Death Act (UDDA).[17]

Previously, my colleagues and I proposed that an optimal analysis of death should be carried out in three sequential steps. The first task is to identify the definition of death by making explicit the indispensable characteristics of death that comprise our implicit, consensually agreed-upon concept of death. Next, we must seek a criterion of death that satisfies the definition by being both necessary and sufficient for death. Finally, we must devise a set of bedside tests of death to show that the criterion has been fulfilled. The tests should be chosen conservatively to exclude the possibility of false-positive determinations.[18]

The biophilosophical concepts on which the whole-brain formulation of death is based include emergent functions, the organism as a whole, and the irreplaceable critical system of the organism. In our previous articles, my colleagues and I had not developed these concepts fully. In light of attacks on the very conceptual foundation of whole-brain death, I now see the need to further develop these biophilosophical concepts. In this essay, I show that, with a more complete explication of these concepts, whole-brain death remains most congruent with our consensually agreed-upon concept of the death of the human organism.

II. The Paradigm of Death

Much of the disagreement in discussions of the definition and criterion of death derives from discord over what I call the "paradigm of death." "Paradigm," in this context, refers to a set of assumptions and conditions that frame the argument by making explicit the boundaries of the topic we are discussing, the class of phenomena to which it belongs, and the way in which it should be discussed. Failure to first agree on the paradigm of death leads to category noncongruence and thus to intractable disagreement. For example, failure to accept that death is fundamentally a biological phenomenon precludes concurrence on any unitary definition or criterion of death.

First, "death" is a nontechnical word that we all use correctly to refer to the cessation of an organism's life. Any attempt to precisely define it should capture this consensually agreed-upon and ordinary meaning. The philosophical task of defining death should not contrive to change this meaning by redefining death to suit a preconceived social or political agenda. Nor should the concept of death and the words we use to describe it be analyzed to such an advanced metaphysical level of abstractness that it is rendered devoid of its ordinary meaning.[19]

Second, as a matter of paradigm, I assert that death is a biological concept; thus, any definition of it must be compatible with biological observations and facts. Stating that death is a biological concept is not meant to denigrate the importance, richness, or beauty of cultural practices and religious rituals surrounding dying and death that are recorded throughout human history. Rather, it is only to state that because life fundamentally is a biological phenomenon, so must be its termination. A formulation of death should strive to be biologically coherent and to accurately and objectively represent the demise of the organism. Thus, I disagree with those scholars who hold that the definition of death is primarily a social matter that can be contrived.[20] I hold that although societies can establish laws and practices surrounding dying and death that may vary among cultures, the event of death is an objective, immutable, biological fact that can be studied, described, and modeled, but cannot be altered or contrived.[21]

Third, I restrict my purview here to the death of higher animal species, such as vertebrates. As a biological concept, death should be univocal across these species and not defined idiosyncratically for *Homo sapiens,* because, for example, we refer to the same concept when we say that a relative has died as we do when we say that our pet dog has died. Of course, humans are endowed with unique characteristics that distinguish them from lower species (including a soul, according to many religious doctrines), but the presence or absence of these features is not relevant to a biological concept of death. Even religious people who fervently believe that the human soul departs from the body at death can accept that death is a biological phenomenon. I choose to restrict my purview to higher animal species because, as I show later, the definition of death turns on the loss of the interrelatedness and unity of the complex organism. Such a concept may not be directly applicable to the death of the subunits of an organism, such as its cells, tissues, or organs; single-celled animals; or plants. For example, living "HeLa" cervical-cell culture lines continue to grow and divide in cell culture plates in experimental laboratories throughout the world, despite the death in 1951 of their eponymous progenitor Henrietta Lacks.

Fourth, because the concept of death is biological, it may be applied directly only to organisms: all living organisms must die and only living organisms can die. The term "death" often is used metaphorically, such as in the phrase "death of a culture." But nonmetaphorical direct usage must be restricted categorically to organisms. The expression "death of a person" usually refers to the death of the organism that was a person, but may also refer metaphorically to an organism's loss of personhood. "Personhood" is a psychosocial, spiritual, and legal concept, but not a biological concept. In the strict biological sense I employ here, the quality of personhood may be lost, but it cannot die except metaphorically speaking. Thus, in philosopher Jeff McMahan's proposal that there are two types of death—death of the organism and death of the person[22]—only the former comprises the topic of this strict biological discussion. The latter should more properly be called the loss of personhood.

Fifth, "alive" and "dead" comprise the only two fundamental underlying states of any organism. All organisms must be either alive or dead; none can be both or neither.[23] In this sense, alive and dead can be mapped as mutually exclusive and jointly exhaustive sets. In two recent articles, one by Amir Halevy and Baruch Brody, and the other by Linda Emanuel, it has been suggested that some organisms at some times may reside in ambiguous states that are neither dead nor alive but appear to have elements of both states, thus illustrating that the states of alive and dead are not jointly exhaustive.[24] Although such a view appears superficially plausible in the case of the life-status ambiguity of a brain-dead patient who has certain vital subsystems supported technologically while others are permanently absent, this view is not sound biologically. These authors have generated confusion because of their failure to distinguish between our ability to determine the exact underlying state of an organism and the nature of that underlying state. Thus, while it may be difficult for technical reasons in some cases to determine easily or confidently whether an organism is alive or dead at a given moment, this technical limitation does not necessarily imply that the organism resides in a hypothetical in-between state.

Sixth, death is an event and not a process. This fact results automatically from the preceding premise. The famous exchange of opinions between Robert Morison and Leon Kass in 1971 on this topic illustrates the two compelling sides of the argument.[25] Morison holds that death is a process because of the progressive and ineluctable loss of functions that occurs during dying. Kass counters that death is an event that represents the sudden transition from alive to dead. Both arguments are plausible. In some ways, death appears like a process, especially when it follows a gradual deterioration and loss of functions during a slow dying process. As Emanuel has pointed out, to an observer, it may appear arbitrary to stipulate any particular point along such an ineluctable dying process as the moment of death.[26] However, given that alive and dead are the only possible underlying states of an organism, the transition from the state of alive to the state of dead is necessarily sudden and instantaneous, at least in concept, because there is no intervening state. Of course, for technical reasons, we may be able to determine the time of the event of death only in retrospect and then only within a certain range of error. Dying is a process occurring when the organism is alive, and bodily disintegration is a process occurring once the organism is dead. Death is the event that separates the processes of dying and bodily disintegration and that marks the transition from the bodily state of alive to dead.[27]

Seventh, death is irreversible. It is impossible to return from the dead. Patients describing so-called near-death experiences have described memories of happenings they experienced when critically ill or incipiently dying, but not when dead. The very concept of death requires that it must be irreversible, by definition, because if one could return from such a state, one was not dead. I subscribe to philosopher David Cole's second definition of "irreversible," namely, that the loss of function cannot be reversed by anyone using present technology.[28] If future technologies become successful in permitting the reversal of loss of these seemingly irreversible functions, we will be forced to change our concepts of life and death to seek new signs of irreversibility.

III. The Structure and Functioning of a Higher Organism

The biophilosophical task of defining death begins with the tautology that the death of an organism is the cessation of the organism's life. Given this truism, we must first consider the concept of the life of an organism. Philosophers and biologists have known for ages that it is easier to describe the characteristics of life than to precisely define it.[29] For my purposes in defining death, it is necessary first to distinguish between the life of cells or other components of an organism and the life of the organism itself; I am concerned here with the latter.

In a provocative essay attempting to distinguish living from nonliving entities, the biologist Jacques Monod epitomizes the characteristics of all life forms: (1) "teleonomy," a coordination and correspondence of structure and function that suggests purpose; (2) "autonomous morphogenesis," the intrinsic self-reproduction of form; and (3) "reproductive invariance," the requirement that the source of information expressed in the structure of any biological form results entirely and only from a structurally identical form.[30] In a recent paper, physician Raphael Bonelli and his colleagues assert that all life forms have the following four characteristics: (1) dynamics, or signs of life, such as metabolism, growth, and locomotion; (2) integration, a process deriving from the mutual interaction of its component parts; (3) coordination, a regulatory process maintaining the constancy of the order of integration; and (4) immanency, the requirement that the preceding characteristics originate from and are intrinsic to the life form.[31]

An organism is a complex life form composed of individually living subunits, including cells, tissues, and organs. Each subunit is organized in a functional group, and is not merely a random aggregation of components. Thus, cells form functional subunits of tissues that in turn form functional subunits of organs. The interrelationships of the numerous hierarchies of functional subunits within an organism create an integrated, coordinated, functioning, and unified whole. This whole is the organism itself: the highest and most complex unit of life that subsumes all its living subsystems.

The hierarchies of functional units interrelate through "emergent functions." An emergent function is a property of a whole that is not possessed by any of its component parts.[32] Thus, a tissue has emergent functions not possessed by any of its component cells. An organ has emergent functions that are not possessed by any of its component tissues. And, most relevantly here, an organism has emergent functions that are not possessed by any of its component organ subunits.

An organism possesses an overall unity of operation encompassing and deriving from its emergent functions that has been called the "organism as a whole.[33] The organism as a whole is not merely the whole organism, that is, the sum of the organism's component parts. Thus, an otherwise healthy man who has both legs amputated may no longer be a whole organism, but he continues to function as an organism as a whole. The organism as a whole is greater than the sum of its component parts, owing to the presence of its emergent functions that reflect the coherent unity of the organism. The organism as a whole creates an overall unity that subsumes all the emergent functions of its organ and tissue subsystems.

Bonelli and his colleagues suggest four criteria by which the life of an organism can be distinguished from the life of its component parts: (1) completion, that the organism is not part of a greater whole but is intrinsically complete; (2) indivisibility, that no organism can be divided into two or more living organisms—thus, after any division in which the organism remains alive, the whole must reside in one of the parts; (3) self-reference, that the organism is the end in itself and does not derive its meaning from its component parts, all of which are unified by a founding principle within the organism itself; and (4) identity, that the living organism remains one and the same throughout life, despite incremental changes in its appearance and structure that may result in the loss or alteration of its parts, and that may eventually result in the complete replacement of all its component atoms.[34]

All living organisms possess mechanisms by which they obtain, select, process, compare, store, and utilize information from their internal milieu and their environment to produce goal-oriented output in the form of biological behavior that favor the continued life and health of the organism. The portion of the organism's internal structure dedicated to information-processing that directs such goal-oriented output is called a "control system."[35] Control systems are the emergent functions of organisms that are essential to the operation of the organism as a whole.

An organism's control systems vary in their importance in their contribution to the health and continued life of the organism. The most important control system is the "critical system" of the organism. The critical system is the irreplaceable, indispensable, complex, structural-functional control system that maintains the health and life of the organism, without which the organism no longer can function as a whole.[36] The vital importance of this system for the continued health of the organism is the functional equivalent in the organism of the cellular concept "autopoesis," or self-repair, one of the determining features of life.[37] No organism can survive the loss of its critical system. With the loss of the critical system, the organism loses its life-characterizing processes, especially its anti-entropic capacity, and entropy (disorder) inevitably increases. The inexorable increase in entropy is conceptually tied to the irreversibility of the process.[38]

IV. Death of the Organism

Death of the organism is the irreversible loss of the capacity of the organism to function as a whole that results from the permanent loss of its critical system. This concept may be stated formally: Death is defined as the permanent cessation of the critical functions of the organism as a whole. In higher animal species, the criterion of death that satisfies this definition by being both necessary and sufficient for death is the permanent cessation of the clinical functions of the brain. The brain is the critical system of the organism without which the organism cannot function as a whole.

The term "clinical functions" refers to the set of functions of the brain that can be determined by bedside clinical examination without having to employ sophisticated laboratory techniques. The bedside measurement of the brain's clinical functions requires performing the standard clinical tests for brain death—namely, the determination of complete unresponsiveness, apnea (absent breathing), and absent cranial nerve-innervated reflexes—and ascertaining a structural cause producing an irreversible loss of the brain's clinical functions.[39] When all the clinical brain functions have ceased irreversibly, the organism is dead. This is the meaning of the colloquial term "brain death."

The brain is the irreplaceable critical system of the organism. It can neither be transplanted nor can any of its exquisite emergent functions, such as conscious awareness, be simulated by a machine or artifice. If the science fiction of brain transplantation or artificial brain synthesis ever were to become possible in the future (which I strongly doubt), such a technology would require us to completely redefine human life and personal identity.

The other organs of the body maintain the health and proper operation of the critical system. Thus, the heart pumps blood to perfuse the brain, the lungs provide intake of oxygen and output of carbon dioxide for optimal neuronal metabolic demands, the intestine provides nutrition and hydration essential for neuronal function, and the liver and kidneys detoxify ingested material and excrete metabolic waste products necessary for neuronal metabolism. These subsidiary organs provide metabolic conditions to optimize functioning and maintain the health of the critical system.

Global interruption of oxygen, glucose, or blood flow to brain neurons for as brief an interval as ten seconds results in the loss of consciousness. This loss of an essential emergent function may be only temporary if the oxygen, glucose, or blood flow is rapidly restored thereafter. But interruption of these vital substrates and functions for longer than ten minutes can result in the destruction of the organism's critical system and therefore cause death.

Prior to the late 1950s, all patients who had suffered the irreversible cessation of clinical brain functions immediately and permanently lost breathing and circulation and were declared dead. Contemporary technology now permits the mechanical replacement of respiration and, hence, continued support for heartbeat and circulation, despite the loss of the critical system. A brain-dead patient also may retain liver and kidney functions and enteric absorption of foods and fluids provided by a feeding gastrostomy tube. The persistence of these subsidiary organ functions is a direct consequence of technology, because none would be possible without mechanical ventilation. The continued operation of these organs exemplifies how some of an organism's subsystems can be kept functioning with technological assistance, despite the loss of the critical system.

But what is the significance of these functioning subsystems with regard to the organism as a whole once the critical system has been destroyed? The significance of their continued functioning is analogous to that of an isolated, perfused kidney maintained outside the body or to the continued growth and division of cells in a laboratory cell culture. They are merely artificially supported organ and tissue subsystems whose overall control, interrelatedness, and unity is forever gone because of the loss of the critical system. Bonelli and his colleagues explain in greater operational detail why, in brain death, the organism as a whole has ceased functioning; it is because the complete loss of brain functions results in the loss of the organism's immanence, integration, coordination, identity, completion, and final totality.[40]

What are the precise quantity and location of brain functions comprising the critical system of the organism that must be lost for the organism to be dead? Brain-death proponents differ on this important question. The most widely accepted formulation upon which public laws have been drafted around the world is the whole-brain formulation. This formulation requires the loss of clinical functions from all principal components of the brain, including the cerebral hemispheres, thalamus, hypothalamus, and brain stem. The whole-brain formulation holds that the functions of the organism as a whole—hence, those of the critical system—are distributed throughout diverse regions of the brain. For example, conscious awareness requires the cerebral hemispheres, thalamus, hypothalamus, and brain stem; breathing and blood pressure regulation require the brain stem; and the executive control system that processes information to integrate and regulate homeostasis is located in the hypothalamus.

Not every brain neuron is necessary, however, for the operation of the critical system of the organism and the functioning of the organism as a whole. For example, the neurons of the brain stem that comprise the critical system are those in a central core encompassing the ascending reticular activating system and its projections to the thalamus and cerebral hemispheres. Only these brain-stem neurons are consequential to the critical system, because they are essential to generating wakefulness, which is a necessary precondition for conscious awareness.

A few scholars have claimed that because brain-dead patients may retain some measurably functioning brain neurons, the whole-brain formulation of death has been disproved.[41] They cite the presence of electroencephalographic (EEG) activity that has been recorded in some unequivocally brain-dead patients as evidence that not all functions of the whole brain have ceased.[42] However, the presence of isolated nests of functioning neurons that do not contribute to the operation of the critical system of the organism or to the functioning of the organism as a whole remain consistent with the whole-brain formulation. Despite the unnecessarily categorical language of the UDDA, the whole-brain formulation does not require the cessation of the functioning of every neuron, but only those which contribute to the critical system subserving the organism as a whole.[43]

Proponents of the higher-brain formulation of death hold that permanent cessation of only cerebral hemispheric and thalamic functions is sufficient for death.[44] Thus, a commonsense interpretation of their formulation would consider patients in persistent vegetative states and infants with anencephaly to be dead. However, the higher-brain formulation fails as a concept of death for several reasons.[45] Most importantly, the higher-brain formulation does not strive to make explicit the traditional, implicit concept of death. By declaring patients dead who are regarded as alive in every society and culture, it contrives a redefinition of death. But most relevant to our considerations here, it is a nonbiological concept, because it does not seek to identify the critical system of the organism or consider the functioning of the organism as a whole.

In the United Kingdom, largely as a result of the influence of the neurologist Christopher Pallis,[46] the concept of brain-stem death has become popularized and codified into law.[47] The brain-stem formulation holds that the permanent absence of brain-stem function alone is sufficient for death. Proponents of the brain-stem formulation argue that because nearly all brain inputs and outputs pass through the brain stem, and because the brain stem is the center for breathing, blood pressure control, and wakefulness, that its permanent cessation of functioning is death. Pallis additionally points out that most of the accepted tests for whole-brain death are tests of brain-stem functions.

The brain-stem formulation has two weaknesses. First, by not requiring cessation of thalamic and cerebral hemispheric activity, it provides for the improbable but still possible occurrence of a primary-brain-stem stroke or other lesion that produces a profound locked-in syndrome, that is, a state of preserved conscious awareness, but with paralysis so profound that evidence of the preserved awareness may be difficult to ascertain. Such a macabre scenario is at least imaginable in which a patient who remains aware has been incorrectly determined to be dead because of apnea, absent cranial nerve reflexes, and unresponsiveness. Of course, such a state would require *some* degree of continued functioning of the ascending reticular activating system of the brain stem, the thalami, and the cerebral hemispheres. Second, the brain-stem formulation eliminates the use of confirmatory tests of brain death, such as those measuring intracranial blood flow and EEG. Both intracranial blood flow and EEG may persist in "brain-stem death" when it is produced by a primary-brain-stem catastrophe that does not also produce markedly raised intracranial pressure.[48]

In addition to being a philosophically coherent formulation, whole-brain death works well in practice because the tests showing absence of brain-stem functions confirm that all the clinical functions of the brain have ceased. In the usual case of massive brain trauma, intracranial hemorrhage, or hypoxic-ischemic (lack of oxygen and circulation) neuronal injury suffered during cardiopulmonary arrest, swelling of the diffusely damaged brain causes intracranial pressure to rise, and this usually exceeds mean arterial blood pressure and sometimes exceeds systolic blood pressure. At this point, intracranial circulation ceases and essentially all neurons that were not killed by the primary traumatic, cerebrovascular, or hypoxic-ischemic injury are killed by the secondary ischemic injury. The marked rise in intracranial pressure produces the clinical syndrome of bilateral transtentorial herniation (damaging shifts of brain within intracranial compartments) that compresses and infarcts (destroys cells by lack of blood flow) the brain stem.[49]

The whole-brain-death tests that show the absence of brain-stem function in the setting of bilateral transtentorial herniation serve as a valid confirmation that all neurons contributing to the functioning of the critical system have been destroyed. By contrast, in a primary-brain-stem catastrophe, such as a massive brain-stem hemorrhage, the brain stem may have been destroyed without also killing the neurons of the thalamus, hypothalamus, and cerebral hemispheres. Thus, the presence of clinical signs of brain-stem failure from a primary brain stem or cerebellar lesion does not have the same confirmatory significance of global neuronal dysfunction as the same signs do in the case of a cerebral lesion with transtentorial herniation. In the case of a primary-brain-stem or cerebellar lesion, under a whole-brain formulation, confirmatory tests would be necessary to determine that death has occurred and especially to eliminate the possibility of a false-positive death determination where a profound locked-in syndrome has been produced.

V. The Time of Death

An issue of both practical and theoretical importance is the identification of the time of death.[50] Physicians Joanne Lynn and Ronald Cranford point out that there are four possible choices for stating the time of death: T_1, when the critical function is lost; T_2, when the critical function is observed to be lost; T_3, when the critical function is irreversibly lost; and T_4, when the critical function is demonstrated to be irreversibly lost.[51]

Given the requirement that death must be irreversible, the T_1 and T_2 times can be excluded. From a purely theoretical perspective, T_3 represents the most logical time of death. However, it is intrinsic to the physical examination for death that physicians must determine it at the bedside. Death may have occurred earlier, but physicians must perform tests to prove this before declaring a patient dead. Therefore, for practical reasons, it is most common for physicians to state the time of death as T_4. The T_4 time for death declaration is consistent with physicians' practices throughout the world and throughout history. Thus, using brain tests or circulatory tests, the event of death is determined primarily in retrospect.

VI. The Future of Death

Since 1950, we have witnessed the development of remarkable life-sustaining technologies that were unimaginable previously. The development of those technologies is the principal reason that we are now faced with the task of analyzing the concept of death. Prior to the second half of the twentieth century, death was a unitary phenomenon: with the failure of certain bodily systems critical to life, all the remaining vital systems inevitably and quickly also ceased irreversibly. In those times, we did not have to consider whether an organism that had lost certain vital systems while retaining others was alive or dead, because such cases were impossible. But now that we have the technological capacity to support ventilation, and hence circulation, we have been forced to address the biophilosophical meaning of death and are compelled to identify the indispensable characteristic defining death. I hold that the defining characteristic of death is the permanent cessation of the critical functions of the organism as a whole, confirmed by demonstrating the permanent cessation of functioning of the critical system of the organism.

The achievements in the medical field since 1950 raise the question of what impact future technological developments will have on the concept and determination of death. Since the early 1980s, intensive care unit (ICU) technology has advanced to such an extent that some brain-dead patients can have their heartbeat, circulation, and other organ subsystems physiologically maintained for months. Prior to the development of this ICU technology, it was impossible for physicians to maintain a brain-dead patient's heartbeat and circulation for more than a week. Now, because of advances in ICU technology, more instances of prolonged maintenance have been reported. Shewmon recently reported a series of mostly young brain-dead patients whose heartbeat and circulation were able to be maintained for months, and, in one incredible case, for years.[52]

I can foresee future technological advances that will enable us to support or mimic the vital functions of breathing, heartbeat, and circulation, and those of the kidney, liver, and pancreas. I can also imagine the development of high-technology computerized monitoring and control systems in the ICU that will reproduce some of the roles of the hypothalamus in ensuring homeostasis.

However, despite the advances in artificial-intelligence technology and theory, I cannot imagine any machine that will ever reproduce conscious awareness. The design of the critical system of the organism represents an unparalleled level of complexity far surpassing that of any other organ. Indeed, some scientifically knowledgeable philosophers have argued that the neural organization of consciousness is so utterly complex that not only will our technology never be able to reproduce it, we never will be able even to understand it.[53]

Future technological advances should be able to help us to more accurately ascertain and localize the precise set of neurons that is responsible for the critical functions of the organism as a whole and that are necessary and sufficient for the operation of the critical system. In this way, it will permit the doctrine of whole-brain death to mature and become more fully refined as the precise nature of the critical system is identified. But future technological advances will not alter the concept of death, because they will never be able to replace the indispensable critical system of the organism. Thus, while future technologies may make death determination more rapid and accurate, they will not alter the concept that death is the permanent loss of the critical system of the organism.

VII. Conclusion

Although historically the concept of brain death evolved to facilitate organ transplantation, I have shown that the biophilosophical formulation of whole-brain death stands alone as the most congruent map by which to understand the biological phenomenon of death. Moreover, whole-brain death enjoys a broad intuitive appeal even among people who have not rigorously scrutinized its conceptual basis. The combination of its intuitive appeal and its biophilosophical coherence has resulted in a high degree of public consensus sufficient to enact more or less uniform laws permitting whole-brain death determination throughout the world.

The remaining areas of controversy center around religious disagreements with the concept of brain death, the extent to which the practice of brain-death determination remains useful in our society, and whether organisms are truly dead or only incipiently dying once their brains have irreversibly ceased functioning. Given the increasing acceptance of brain death throughout the world, however, there is no reason to believe that these areas of persisting controversy will interfere with the established public consensus on the determination of human death.

NOTES

1. See, especially, James L. Bernat, Charles M. Culver, and Bernard Gert, "On the Definition and Criterion of Death," *Annals of Internal Medicine* 94, no. 3 (1981): 389–94; James L. Bernat, Charles M. Culver, and Bernard Gert, "Defining Death in Theory and Practice," *Hastings Center Report* 12, no. 1 (1982): 5–9; James L. Bernat, "How Much of the Brain Must Die in Brain Death?" *Journal of Clinical Ethics* 3, no. 1 (1992): 21–26; and James L. Bernat, "A Defense of the Whole-Brain Concept of Death," *Hastings Center Report* 28, no. 2 (1998): 14–23.

2. The concept of brain death evolved and was first put into practice because of the need for heart-beating cadaver donors for vital-organ transplantation and to permit the cessation of life-sustaining therapy on hopelessly brain-damaged patients. Only later did scholars adequately defend why the brain-dead patient was truly dead. The parallel historical evolution of brain death and organ procurement is described in Martin S. Pernick, "Brain Death in a Cultural Context: The Reconstruction of Death, 1967–1981," in Stuart J. Youngner, Robert M. Arnold, and Renie Schapiro, eds., *The Definition of Death: Contemporary Controversies* (Baltimore, MD: Johns Hopkins University Press, 1999), 3–33.

3. Previously, I showed that the time at which cessation of breathing and circulation causes death is when the brain has become destroyed as a result of lack of oxygen and blood flow. Thus, the unitary criterion of death is the irreversible loss of all clinical brain functions. Physicians may determine when death occurs by using tests showing the irreversible cessation of breathing and circulation when mechanical ventilation is not employed or anticipated, but they must use tests showing the irreversible cessation of clinical brain functions when ventilation (and, hence, circulation) are mechanically supported. See the further discussion of this point, including clinical examples, in Bernat, Culver, and Gert, "On the Definition and Criterion of Death."

4. Ad Hoc Committee of the Harvard Medical School to Examine the Definition of Brain Death, "A Definition of Irreversible Coma: Report of the Ad Hoc Committee of the Harvard Medical School to Examine the Definition of Brain Death," *Journal of the American Medical Association* 205, no. 5 (1968): 337–40. Henry K. Beecher, whose admonition I quoted at the beginning of this essay, chaired the committee that drafted this report. The social context in which this report was written has been analyzed in Mita Giacomini, "A Change of Heart and a Change of Mind? Technology and the Redefinition of Death in 1968," *Social Science and Medicine* 44, no. 10 (1997): 1465–82.

5. A recent study of brain-death legislation around the world reveals brain-death laws in sixty-seven of seventy-eight surveyed countries. See Eelco F. M. Wijdicks, "Brain Death Worldwide," *Neurology* 58, no. 1 (2002): 20–25.

6. Even in the early era of brain-death discussions, religious leaders and other scholars argued that brain death was compatible with the teachings and traditions of Christianity and Judaism. See Frank J. Veith et al., "Brain Death I. A Status Report of Medical and Ethical Considerations," *Journal of the American Medical Association* 238, no. 15 (1977): 1651–55. More recent statements also support this view. Pope John Paul II pronounced the compatibility of the practices of brain-death determination and organ transplantation with Roman Catholic teachings in his address to the eighteenth International Congress of the Transplantation Society in Rome on August 29, 2000, available on-line at http://www.vatican.va/holy_father/john_paul_ii/speeches/2000/jul-sep/documents/hf_jp=ii_spe_20000829_transplants_en.html. For a Talmudic argument that the concept of brain death is compatible with Orthodox Judaism, see Fred Rosner and Moses D. Tendler, "Defi-

nition of Death in Judaism," *Journal of Halacha and Contemporary Society* 17 (1989): 14–31. Most Islamic authorities accept brain death as consistent with Islamic teachings. See, for example, Basim A. Yaqub and Saleh M. Al-Deeb, "Brain Death: Current Status in Saudi Arabia," *Saudi Medical Journal* 17, no. 1 (1996): 5–10. I recently reviewed the current ethical and religious issues in brain death in James L. Bernat, *Ethical Issues in Neurology*, 2d ed. (Boston: Butterworth-Heinemann, 2002), 257–60.

7. For an example of Roman Catholic opposition to brain death, see Paul A. Byrne, Sean O'Reilly, and Paul M. Quay, "Brain Death—An Opposing Viewpoint," *Journal of the American Medical Association* 242, no. 18 (1979): 1985–90; and Josef Seifert, "Is Brain Death Actually Death? A Critique of Redefinition of Man's Death in Terms of 'Brain Death'," *The Monist* 76, no. 2 (1993): 175–202. For an example of Orthodox Jewish opposition, see J. David Bleich, "Establishing Criteria of Death," in Fred Rosner and J. David Bleich, eds., *Jewish Bioethics* (New York: Sanhedrin Press, 1979), 277–95.

8. For examples of the higher-brain formulation of death argument, see Robert M. Veatch, "The Whole-Brain-Oriented Concept of Death: An Outmoded Philosophical Formulation," *Journal of Thanatology* 3, no. 1 (1975): 13–30; and Stuart J. Youngner and Edward T. Bartlett, "Human Death and High Technology: The Failure of the Whole-Brain Formulations," *Annals of Internal Medicine* 99, no. 2 (1983): 252–58.

9. These purported inconsistencies are summarized in Amir Halevy and Baruch Brody, "Brain Death: Reconciling Definitions, Criteria, and Tests," *Annals of Internal Medicine* 119, no. 6 (1993): 519–25.

10. See Robert D. Truog, "Is It Time to Abandon Brain Death?" *Hastings Center Report* 27, no. 1 (1997): 29–37. Truog states that brain death is anachronistic because it evolved at a time when, because of legal sanctions, physicians were extremely reluctant to discontinue life-sustaining therapy until the patient was dead. Now that legal doctrines permit discontinuing life-sustaining therapy, brain death no longer is a necessary concept. He argues further that brain-death determination is now practiced solely because it is a prerequisite for multiple organ procurement. Truog suggests that we unlink organ procurement from brain death, dispense altogether with brain-death determination, and permit multiple organ procurement with informed consent when the patient is beyond harm because of incipient dying.

11. D. Alan Shewmon, "'Brainstem Death,' 'Brain Death,' and Death: A Critical Reevaluation of the Purported Equivalence," *Issues in Law and Medicine* 14, no. 2 (1998): 125–45.

12. D. Alan Shewmon, "Chronic 'Brain Death': Meta-Analysis and Conceptual Consequences," *Neurology* 51, no. 6 (1998): 1538–45. Shewmon's current criticisms of brain death are particularly fascinating because, prior to 1994, he was one of the strongest proponents of brain death. For his personal account of how and why he diametrically transformed his views, see D. Alan Shewmon, "Recovery from 'Brain Death': A Neurologist's Apologia," *Linacre Quarterly* 64, no. 1 (1997): 30–96.

13. Robert M. Taylor, "Re-examining the Definition and Criterion of Death," *Seminars in Neurology* 17, no. 3 (1997): 265–70. Taylor compares the legal fiction of brain death to that of "legal blindness." We all know that patients who are declared legally blind are not necessarily completely blind, but, as a society, we have decided that their visual loss is sufficiently profound to grant them the benefits reserved for those who are completely blind. He argues that, analogously, we all know that the brain dead are not truly dead, but are close enough to being dead for society to permit multiple organ procurement from them.

14. Alexander M. Capron and Leon R. Kass, "A Statutory Definition of the Standards for Determining Human Death: An Appraisal and a Proposal," *University of Pennsylvania Law Review* 121, no. 1 (1972): 87–118.

15. See the full account of the critical-system argument in Julius Korein, "The Problem of Brain Death: Development and History," *Annals of the New York Academy of Sciences* 315 (1978): 19–38; Julius Korein, "Brain States: Death, Vegetation, and Life," in James E. Cottrell and Herman Turndorf, eds., *Anesthesia and Neurosurgery*, 2d ed. (St. Louis, MO: C. V. Mosby Co., 1986), 293–351; and Julius Korein, "Ontogenesis of the Brain in the Human Organism: Definitions of Life and Death of the Human Being and Person," in Rem B. Edwards, ed., *Advances in Bioethics* (Greenwich, CT: JAI Press, 1997), 2:1–74.

16. See the discussion of this point in the articles listed in note 1, especially Bernat et al., "On the Definition and Criterion of Death"; and Bernat, "A Defense of the Whole-Brain Concept of Death."

17. President's Commission for the Study of Ethical Problems in Medicine and Biomedical and Behavioral Research, *Defining Death: A Report on the Medical, Legal and Ethical Issues in the Determination of Death* (Washington, DC: U.S. Government Printing Office, 1981), 31–43.

18. The philosophical basis for these three levels of analysis are rigorously explicated in Bernat et al., "On the Definition and Criterion of Death," 390–92.

19. Linda Emanuel is guilty of pursuing the concept of death to an unhelpfully metaphysical level when she writes that "there is no state of death. . . . [T]o say 'she is dead' is meaningless because 'she' is not compatible with 'dead'." See Linda L. Emanuel, "Reexamining Death: The Asymptotic Model and a Bounded Zone Definition," *Hastings Center Report* 25, no. 4 (1995): 27.

20. For example, see Robert M. Veatch, "The Conscience Clause: How Much Individual Choice in Defining Death Can Our Society Tolerate?" in Youngner et al., eds., *The Definition of Death*, 137–60; and Dan W. Brock, "The Role of the Public in Public Policy on the Definition of Death," in Youngner et al., eds., *The Definition of Death*, 293–307.

21. Important examples of public laws codifying communally accepted practices about death that are founded on a society's accepted concept of death include the statute of death and the practice of organ procurement from dead persons. Nearly all states in the United States have enacted determination-of-death statutes specifically recognizing brain death. Although these social issues are not intrinsic to the definition and criterion of death, they are relevant to how well the concept of death is accepted and implemented by society. I have discussed the relationship that these practical and social issues have to the soundness of an underlying concept of death in Bernat, "A Defense of the Whole-Brain Concept of Death."

22. Jeff McMahan, "The Metaphysics of Brain Death," *Bioethics* 9, no. 2 (1995): 91–126. Although many people, myself included, would not wish our organisms to survive if we permanently lost the qualities of our personhood, it is important to separate death from loss of personhood. For example, patients surviving in a persistent vegetative state (PVS) arguably may have lost their personhood at the time they suffered their profound brain damage, but may remain alive for several years thereafter. The best-known PVS patients were Karen Ann Quinlan and Nancy Beth Cruzan, two young women whose tragic illnesses were memorialized in highly publicized, precedent-setting American judicial decisions concerning termination of life-sustaining treatment. John Lizza has further confused the topic with his distinctions between different types of personhood and his claim

that it is only persons and not organisms who literally die. See John P. Lizza, "Defining Death for Persons and Human Organisms," *Theoretical Medicine and Bioethics* 20, no. 5 (1999): 439–53.

23. See the defense of this assertion in Fred Feldman, *Confrontations with the Reaper: A Philosophical Study of the Nature and Value of Death* (New York: Oxford University Press, 1992), 111.

24. Halevy and Brody, "Brain Death"; Baruch Brody, "How Much of the Brain Must Be Dead," in Youngner et al., eds., *The Definition of Death*, 71–82; Emanuel, "Reexamining Death."

25. Robert S. Morison, "Death: Process or Event?" *Science* 173, no. 998 (1971): 694–98; Leon Kass, "Death as an Event: A Commentary on Robert Morison," *Science* 173, no. 998 (1971): 698–702.

26. Emanuel, "Reexamining Death," 29–31.

27. See Bernat et al., "On the Definition and Criterion of Death." The conceptual view of death as an instantaneous event that separates the underlying states of alive and dead also is defended in Feldman, *Confrontations with the Reaper*, 108–10.

28. David J. Cole, "The Reversibility of Death," *Journal of Medical Ethics* 18, no. 1 (1992): 26–30.

29. For example, see the discussion on this topic in Lynn Margulis and Dorion Sagan, *What Is Life?* (New York: Simon and Schuster, 1995); and Francis Crick, *Life Itself: Its Origin and Nature* (New York: Simon and Schuster, 1981).

30. Jacques Monod, *Chance and Necessity: An Essay on the Natural Philosophy of Modern Biology* (New York: Alfred A. Knopf, 1971), 3–22.

31. Raphael Bonelli, Enrique H. Prat, and Johannes Bonelli, "Philosophical Considerations on Brain Death and the Concept of the Organism as a Whole," *Psychiatria Danubina* 21, no. 1 (2009): 3–8. This essay of theirs, cited with permission, is a refinement of the authors' earlier work; see Johannes Bonelli et al., "Brain Death: Understanding the Organism as a Whole," *Medicina e Morale* 3 (1999): 497–515.

32. Martin Manner and Mario Bunge, *Foundations of Biophilosophy* (Berlin: Springer-Verlag, 1997), 29–30.

33. Jacques Loeb, *The Organism as a Whole* (New York: G. P. Putnam's Sons, 1916). I and my coauthors also rely on this concept in Bernat et al., "On the Definition and Criterion of Death," 390–92.

34. Bonelli et al., "Philosophical Considerations."

35. Korein, "The Problem of Brain Death," 24–26.

36. Ibid., 26–28.

37. Margulis and Sagan, *What Is Life?*, 61–64.

38. See the discussion on the relationship between entropy and control systems in D. R. Brooks et al., "Entropy and Information in Evolving Biological Systems," *Biology and Philosophy* 4 (1989): 407–32; and Ilya Prigogine, *From Being to Becoming: Time and Complexity in the Physical Sciences* (San Francisco: W. H. Freeman and Co., 1980), 176.

39. For a summary of the accepted bedside and laboratory tests for brain death, see Medical Consultants to the President's Commission for the Study of Ethical Problems in Medicine and Biomedical and Behavioral Research, "Guidelines for the Determination of Death: Report of the Medical Consultants on the Diagnosis of Death to the President's Commission for the Study of Ethical Problems in Medicine and Biomedical and Behavioral Research," *Neurology* 32, no. 4 (1982): 395–99; and Eelco F. M. Wijdicks, "Determining

Brain Death in Adults," *Neurology* 45, no. 5 (1995): 1003–11. For the most current account of tests, see Eelco F. M. Wijdicks, "The Diagnosis of Brain Death," *New England Journal of Medicine* 344, no. 16 (2001): 1215–21.

40. Bonelli et al., "Philosophical Considerations."

41. For example, see the defense of this point in Robert M. Veatch, "The Impending Collapse of the Whole-Brain Definition of Death," *Hastings Center Report* 23, no. 4 (1993): 18–24.

42. Madeline M. Grigg et al., "Electroencephalographic Activity after Brain Death," *Archives of Neurology* 44, no. 9 (1987): 948–54.

43. Because, in its relevant portion, the UDDA states that "an individual who has sustained . . . irreversible cessation of all functions of the entire brain, including the brain stem, is dead," some commentators have claimed that any measurable brain function negates the presence of whole-brain death. See Veatch, "The Impending Collapse." But it is clear from the President's Commission discussion accompanying the UDDA that they intend the term "functions" in the UDDA to mean only what I have referred to as "clinical functions" that are measurable by bedside physical examination and not "physiological activities," such as the functioning of an isolated group of cells, whose measurement requires laboratory determination. Thus, to interpret the UDDA's stated requirement for "cessation of all functions of the brain" to also encompass cessation of laboratory-measured physiological activity is simply an incorrect reading of the statute. Despite its categorical language, the UDDA does *not* require the cessation of all neuronal functions in the brain, but only the brain's clinical functions. See the clear explanation of this point in President's Commission, *Defining Death*, 32–36, 75–76.

44. Arguments supporting the higher-brain formulation of death include Robert M. Veatch, "Brain Death and Slippery Slopes," *Journal of Clinical Ethics* 3, no. 3 (1992): 181–87; Richard M. Zaner, ed., *Death: Beyond Whole-Brain Criteria* (Dordrecht, The Netherlands: Kluwer Academic Publishers, 1988); and Karen G. Gervais, *Redefining Death* (New Haven, CT: Yale University Press, 1986).

45. See David Lamb, *Death, Brain Death, and Ethics* (Albany: State University of New York Press, 1985), 41–50. I have most recently reviewed the shortcomings of the whole-brain formulation as a concept of death in James L. Bernat, "Philosophical and Ethical Aspects of Brain Death," in Eelco F. M. Wijdicks, ed., *Brain Death* (Philadelphia, PA: Lippincott, Williams and Wilkins, 2001), 171–88.

46. Christopher Pallis, *ABC of Brainstem Death*, 2d ed. (London: British Medical Journal Publishers, 1996); and Christopher Pallis, "Further Thoughts on Brainstem Death," *Anaesthesia and Intensive Care* 23, no. 1 (1995): 20–23.

47. Working Group Convened by the Royal College of Physicians and Endorsed by the Conference of Medical Royal Colleges and Their Faculties in the United Kingdom, "Criteria for the Diagnosis of Brain Stem Death," *Journal of the Royal College of Physicians of London* 29, no. 5 (1995): 381–82.

48. For clinical and pathological examples, see J. Ogata et al., "Primary Brainstem Death: A Clinico-Pathological Study," *Journal of Neurology, Neurosurgery, and Psychiatry* 51, no. 5 (1988): 646–50; and Michael Kosteljanetz et al., "Clinical Brain Death with Preserved Cerebral Arterial Circulation," *Acta Neurologica Scandinavica* 78, no. 5 (1988): 418–21.

49. These intracranial processes are described in Fred Plum and Jerome B. Posner, *The Diagnosis of Stupor and Coma*, 3d ed. (Philadelphia, PA: F. A. Davis Co., 1980), 87–101.

50. See the discussion of this topic in Stuart J. Youngner, Robert M. Arnold, and Michael A. DeVita, "When Is 'Dead'?" *Hastings Center Report* 29, no. 6 (1999): 14–21.

51. Joanne Lynn and Ronald E. Cranford, "The Persisting Perplexities in the Determination of Death," in Youngner et al., eds., *The Definition of Death*, 101–14.

52. Shewmon, "Chronic 'Brain Death'." These were highly unusual cases. In nearly every brain-death determination, all treatments are stopped. In these unusual cases, the motivations for continuing treatment despite brain death included religious beliefs, the failure of family members to accept the diagnosis, and to continue pregnancy in order to permit delivery.

53. Colin McGinn, "Can We Solve the Mind-Body Problem?" in Ned Block, Owen Flanagan, and Güven Güzeldere, eds., *The Nature of Consciousness: Philosophical Debates* (Cambridge, MA: MIT Press, 1997), 529–42. McGinn explains that the profound neurobiological complexity of consciousness may be *forever* beyond human understanding because of our biological cognitive limitations, in much the same way that the complexities of nuclear physics are forever beyond the understanding of a chimpanzee because of the biological limitations of its cognitive capacity.

CHAPTER TWENTY-FIVE

The Definition of Death in Jewish Law

Fred Rosner, M.D.

Rapid advances in biomedical technology and therapeutic procedures have generated new moral dilemmas and accentuated old ones in the practice of medicine. The vast recent strides made in medical science and technology have created options that only a few decades ago would have been considered to be in the realm of science fiction. New discoveries and techniques in organ transplantation, assisted reproduction, and gene therapy, to cite but a few, have created a keen awareness of the ethical issues that arise from humans' enhanced ability to control their destiny.

Together with these advances has come a shift of emphasis in the physician-patient relationship from beneficence and paternalism to the primacy of patient autonomy and self-determination. Economic factors and considerations also play a greater role in individual and societal medical decision making. Religion has always been and continues to be an important determinant of ethical decision making. This chapter presents general principles of Jewish medical ethics, the structure of Jewish law, differences between secular and Jewish ethics, and the definition of death in Jewish law.

The General Principles of Jewish Medical Ethics

Judaism is guided by the concept of the supreme sanctity of human life and of
the dignity of man created in the image of God. The preservation of human life
in Judaism is a divine commandment. Jewish law requires physicians to do everything in their power to prolong life, but prohibits the use of measures that
prolong the act of dying. The value attached to human life in Judaism is far
greater than that in Christian tradition or in Anglo-Saxon common law. To save
a life, all Jewish religious laws are automatically suspended, with the only exceptions being idolatry, murder, and forbidden sexual relations, such as incest.
In Jewish law and moral teaching, the value of human life is infinite and beyond
measure, so that any part of life—even if only an hour or a second—is of precisely the same worth as 70 years of it.[1-4]

In Jewish tradition a physician is given specific divine license to practice
medicine. According to Maimonides and other codifiers of Jewish law, it is an
obligation upon physicians to use their medical skills to heal the sick. Physicians in Judaism are prohibited from withholding their healing skills and are
not allowed to refuse to heal unless their own life would be seriously endangered thereby.

Judaism is a right-to-life religion. This obligation to save lives is both individual and communal. Certainly a physician, who has knowledge and expertise
far greater than that of a layperson, is obligated to use his or her medical skills
to heal the sick and thereby prolong and preserve life. It is erroneous to suppose
that having recourse to medicine shows lack of trust and confidence in God, the
Healer. The Bible takes it for granted that medical therapy is used and actually
demands it. In addition, in Judaism a patient is obligated to seek healing from
human physicians and not rely on faith healing. The Talmud states that no wise
person should reside in a city that does not have a physician. Maimonides rules
that it is obligatory upon humans to accustom themselves to a regimen that
preserves their body's health and heals and fortifies it when it is ailing.

The extreme concerns in Judaism about the preservation of health and the
prolongation of life require that a woman's pregnancy be terminated if it endan-
gers her life, that a woman use contraception if a pregnancy would threaten her
life, that an organ transplant be performed if it can save or prolong the life of a
patient dying of organ failure, and that a postmortem examination be performed
if the results of the autopsy may provide immediate life-saving information to
rescue another dying patient. Judaism sanctions animal experimentation to find

the cure for human illnesses, provided there is no pain and suffering to the animal, since Judaism prohibits cruelty to animals. Judaism also allows patients to accept experimental medical or surgical treatments, provided no standard therapy is available and the experimental therapy is administered by the most experienced physicians, whose intent is to help the patient and not just to satisfy their academic curiosity.

The infinite value of human life in Judaism prohibits euthanasia or mercy killing in any form. Handicapped newborns, the mentally retarded, the psychotic, and patients dying of any illness or cause have the same right to life as you and I, and nothing may be done to hasten their death. On the other hand, there are times when specific medical or surgical therapy is no longer indicated, appropriate, or desirable for a terminal, irreversibly ill patient. There is no time, however, when general supportive care, including food and water, can be withheld or withdrawn, thereby hastening the patient's death.

The Structure of Jewish Law

The Pentateuch, or Five Books of Moses, is known as the Torah and is the fundamental source of all Jewish religious law. The Torah is sometimes referred to as the written or biblical law, as opposed to the oral law, which represents the unwritten traditions that interpreted, applied, and supplemented the written Torah.

The widely accepted reduction to writing of the legal matter of the oral law is known as the Talmud, which consists of 63 tractates of opinions and teachings of many rabbis who analyzed, interpreted, dissected, and commented on the written or biblical law. The first part of the authoritative Babylonian Talmud was redacted and written by Rabbi Judah the Prince in the second century. The Talmud was completed by Rabbi Ashi in the fifth century. The major commentary on both the Bible and the Talmud is that of Rabbi Shlomo ben Yitzchak (1040–1105), known as Rashi.

The heads of the rabbinic academies in Babylon during the sixth through ninth centuries were called *Gaonim*. They were the first to produce systematic codes of Jewish law by summarizing the conclusions of the lengthy talmudic discussions. At the beginning of the second millennium, the center of Jewish learning shifted to North Africa, where famous talmudic commentators such as Rabbenu Chananel flourished. Rabbi Isaac of Fez, known as Alfasi (1013–1103), wrote a famous work that is a talmudic commentary and code of Jewish law at the same time.

During the eleventh to thirteenth centuries, a group of French and German rabbis known collectively as Tosafot wrote important commentaries and annotations which, in addition to that of Rashi, appear alongside the text in printed editions of the Talmud. The most illustrious Jew of the Middle Ages is the Spaniard Moses Maimonides (1138–1204), rabbi, philosopher, physician, astronomer, ethicist, and much more. His most famous work, *The Mishneh Torah*, is a monumental compilation and systematization of all biblical, talmudic, and Gaonic law. It remains to this day a classic and authoritative 14-volume Jewish legal code.

Over the next two centuries, additional commentaries on and digests of talmudic debate were composed by famous Jewish scholars such as Rabbi Moses ben Nachman (1195–1270), known as Nachmanides, Rabbi Menachem HaMeiri (1249–1315), Rabbi Solomon ben Adret (1215–1310), known as Rashba, and Rabbi Asher ben Yechiel (1250–1327), known as Rosh. The next two landmark codes were those of Rabbi Jacob ben Asher (1269–1343), known as Tur, and Rabbi Joseph Karo (1488–1575), whose work is known as *Shulchan Aruch*. Numerous commentaries by later rabbinic authorities and decisors made the *Shulchan Aruch* the accepted standard work of Jewish law, which it remains today, alongside Maimonides' *Mishneh Torah*.

The major rabbinic literature of the past four centuries consists of responsa, which are formal replies to legal queries addressed to rabbinic scholars of all generations. These responsa deal with social, political, and economic as well as legal problems and issues of their times. Hundreds of volumes of responsa have been authored by many rabbis over many centuries. This "case law" literature is part of the Jewish legal mainstream and serves as precedent authority for subsequent responsa.

Secular Ethics versus Jewish Ethics

Whereas much of the modern secular ethical system is based on rights, Judaism is an ethical system based on duties and responsibilities. "Indeed, there is no word for rights in the very language of the Hebrew Bible and of the classic sources of Jewish law. In the moral vocabulary of the Jewish discipline of life we speak of human duties, not of human rights, of obligations, not entitlement. The Decalogue is a list of Ten Commandments, not a bill of Human Rights."[5]

In Judaism, beneficence and altruism are promoted over mere nonmaleficence. The physician-patient relationship is viewed as a covenant, in contrast to the notion of a relationship between freely contracting individuals.[6]

In current secular ethics, the principle of absolute autonomy for the patient takes precedence over all the other values, including beneficence and even life itself. This approach has been criticized by prominent Catholic bioethicists,[7] and it is not consonant with Jewish ethical thinking.

> Judaism restricts the notion of autonomy to actions that are morally indifferent. Where conflicting values arise, each individual is bound to act in accordance with a high standard of normal moral conduct . . . Therefore, in medical situations that involve ethical conflicts, the solution is based on the appropriate Jewish law that governs both the physician and the patient. This approach can be termed a *moral-religious paternalism* as opposed to the Hippocratic *individual-personal paternalism* of the physician.[6]

Thus, secular ethics attributes a relative value to life, whereas Judaism ascribes a supreme value to life. Therefore, in Judaism, an autonomous decision to destroy life is unacceptable, suicide is morally and legally forbidden, refusal of life-saving treatment is not respected, and active euthanasia is strictly prohibited.

Euthanasia is opposed without qualification in Jewish law, which condemns as sheer murder any active or deliberate hastening of death, whether the physician acts with or without the patient's consent. Some rabbinic views do not require the physician to resort to "heroic" methods, but sanction the omission of machines and artificial life-support systems that serve only to draw out the dying patient's agony, provided, however, that basic care, such as food and good nursing, is provided. Judaism requires the physician to do everything in his or her power to prolong life, but prohibits the use of measures that prolong the act of dying. Judaism also distinguishes between withholding (sometimes allowed) and withdrawing (never allowed) a certain treatment, whereas the secular and Catholic ethical systems do not make such a distinction.

Judaism is thus concerned with covenantal obligations and individual responsibilities, which is very different from secular ethics, which is based on individual rights, such as autonomy, liberty, and privacy. With this background on basic principles of Jewish medical ethics, the structure of Jewish law, and some of the differences between secular and Jewish ethics, one can better understand the remainder of this essay on the definition of death in Jewish law.

The Definition of Death in Jewish Law

Jewish tradition views death as inevitable and just. Judaism differentiates between the body and the soul, acknowledging resurrection for the body,[8] and immortality for the soul. The traditional view is that death occurs upon the separation of the soul from the body. Since this phenomenon does not lend itself to direct empirical observation, the classical secular definition of death has been the absence or cessation of breathing and heartbeat.

The era of organ transplantation, coupled with rapid advances of biomedical technology, led to a reevaluation of the traditional definition of death and the emergence of the concept of brain death, or whole-brain death including brainstem death. In fact, the suggestion has been made that anencephaly be equated with "brain absent" (i.e., lacking cerebral hemispheres) and be accepted as another definition of death to enable anencephalic neonates to serve as organ donors.[9] A logical extension of such thinking is to declare patients in irreversible coma or in a persistent vegetative state to be dead in order to harvest their organs. Should society stretch, bend, or abandon the dead-donor rule?[10] The American Medical Association recently withdrew its suggestion that the dead-donor rule might be broken to allow organs to be removed from anencephalics prior to death.

Judaism certainly rejects such suggestions of redefining death, since patients with spontaneous respiration and heartbeat are considered fully alive in all respects. Does Judaism, however, accept the concept of whole-brain death, whereby the patient has no spontaneous respiration but a heart that continues to beat? Cerebral death is certainly not acceptable in Judaism as a definition of death because unconsciousness does not remove the humanhood or personhood from a patient. But if the whole brain, including the brainstem, which controls vital bodily functions such as respiration, is permanently and irreversibly nonfunctional, does Judaism consider such a situation as equivalent to death? Must the patient also have asystole in Jewish law before being considered dead? One prominent Jewish bioethicist writes that:

> much of the debate concerning the definition of death misses the mark. A definition of death cannot be derived from medical facts or scientific investigation alone. The physician can only describe the physiological state which he observes; whether the patient meeting that description is alive or dead, whether the human organism in that physiological state is to be treated as a living person or as a corpse, is an

ethical and legal question. The determination of the time of death, insofar as it is more than a mere exercise in semantics, is essentially a theological and moral problem, not a medical or scientific one.[11]

There is at present an intense debate among rabbinic authorities as to whether Jewish law recognizes whole-brain death as a definition of death. In Judaism, the classic and primary source indicating that death coincides with irreversible cessation of respiration is a passage in the Babylonian Talmud, tractate Yoma, which enumerates circumstances under which one may or must desecrate the Sabbath in order to save a human life.[12] "Every danger to human life suspends the [laws of the] Sabbath. If debris [of a collapsing building] falls on someone and it is doubtful whether he is there or whether he is not there, or if it is doubtful whether he is alive or whether he is dead . . . one must probe the heap of the debris for his sake [even on the Sabbath]. If one finds him alive, one should remove the debris but if he is dead, one leaves him there" until after the Sabbath. The Talmud then explains as follows: "How far does one search [to ascertain whether he is dead or alive]? Until [one reaches] his nose. Some say: Up to his heart . . . Life manifests itself primarily through the nose as it is written: *In whose nostrils was the breath of the spirit of life*" (Gen. 7:22).

Rashi states that, if no air emanates from his nostrils, he is certainly dead. Rashi further explains that some authorities suggest the heart be examined for signs of life, but the respiration test is considered of greatest import. The two major Codes of Jewish law universally accepted throughout Judaism, the *Mishneh Torah* of Moses Maimonides and the *Shulchan Aruch* of Joseph Karo, both rule that, if one cannot detect signs of respiration at the nose, the patient is certainly dead.[13,14] Neither Maimonides nor Karo requires examination of the heart. Cessation of respiration seems to be the determining physical sign for the ascertainment of death. Thus, Jewish law seems to accept the concept that whole-brain death with resultant absent spontaneous respiration is equivalent to death, irrespective of the presence or absence of a beating heart. Respirator dependency in a patient with polio or amyotrophic lateral sclerosis is obviously not equated with death, since these patients clearly have brain function including brainstem function but require mechanical assistance to breathe. Death in Judaism requires permanent and irreversible cessation of respiration.

Some rabbis, however, state that the lack of respiration was thought to be indicative of prior cessation of cardiac activity. Medieval rabbis and physicians thought that warm air from the heart is expelled through the nose and cold air, which cools the heart, enters through the nose. It was thus believed that respiration without cardiac activity is impossible.[11] Furthermore, in his commentary on the pivotal talmudic passage cited above, Rashi states that "at times life is not evident at the heart but is evident at the nose." This statement, according to some writers, indicates that, if life is not evident at the nose but is evident at the heart, cardiac activity would itself be sufficient to indicate that the person is still alive.[12] These writers therefore require cessation of both cardiac and respiratory functions to confirm that a person is dead.

These two rabbinic views accepting or rejecting whole-brain death as a valid Jewish legal definition of death are thus based on different interpretations of the talmudic commentary of Rashi and on subsequent medieval and modern rabbinic interpretations of the pivotal talmudic passage and other classic Jewish sources. These diametrically opposing views, which have resulted in considerable debate and controversy in Orthodox Jewish circles over the past two decades, are not based on secular moral principles or on social policy. Rather, these views are rooted in fine points of Jewish law, which the rabbinic authorities of each generation are empowered to interpret.

To support the view that whole-brain death is equated with death in Judaism, the concept of physiological decapitation was introduced.[15] In Judaism, if a human being or animal is decapitated, they are immediately counted as dead, irrespective of cardiac or other bodily movement. The death throes of a decapitated person are not considered residual life any more than the twitching of a lizard's amputated tail. These death throes or twitchings are only reflex activities demonstrating that cellular life continues for a while after the death of the whole organism, human or animal. The decapitated state itself is recognized in Jewish law as equivalent to death. Complete destruction of the brain is said to be the equivalent of physiological decapitation and therefore a valid definition of death. Loss of the ability to breathe spontaneously is a crucial criterion for determining whether complete destruction of the brain has occurred. Thus, if sophisticated neurological examination and testing of a patient indicate irreversible total loss of the function of the whole brain, including brainstem function, the patient is as if decapitated and therefore dead, even if the heart is still beating. Judaism also recognizes the fact that, even after the organism has been pronounced dead, individual cells may continue to function for some time thereafter in various parts of the body. The movement of a severed tail of a lizard is said to be purely reflex or autonomous in nature and does not indicate that the tail is alive. A series of rabbinic responsa on organ transplants and the definition of death by the late Rabbi Moshe Feinstein strongly support this concept of physiological decapitation.

Additional rabbinic sources support the thesis of physiological decapitation. Based on a talmudic discussion in tractate Chullin, Karo's authoritative Code of Jewish Law describes individuals "who are considered dead even though they are still alive."[16] These include those whose neck has been broken. These people are considered dead in that they impart ritual defilement and render their wives widows even though they may still have spastic or convulsive movements and even have heartbeats. The reason is that the connection between the brain and the body has been severed by the severance of the spinal cord or by the severance of the blood supply to the brain. It thus seems that the death of the whole brain is the legal definition of death in Jewish law. This definition has been adopted by the Israeli Chief Rabbinate and by many but not all orthodox rabbis and orthodox Jewish physicians.[17]

Those who reject the physiological decapitation concept point to Rashi's comment in the pivotal talmudic passage in tractate Yoma, where Rashi says that the absence of respiration is conclusive "if the patient appears dead in that there is no movement of his limbs." Other medieval and more recent rabbinic authorities echo Rashi's statement. Rabbi Tzvi Ashkanazi (1660–1718), known as *Chacham Tzvi*, concludes that "there can be no respiration unless there is life in the heart, for respiration is from the heart and for its benefit."[18] Rabbi Moses Sofer (1762–1839), known as *Chatam Sofer*, states that absent respiration is equated with death only if the patient "lies as an inanimate stone and there is no pulse whatsoever."[19] Modern interpreters of Rashi's statement that the patient "appears dead in that there is no movement of his limbs," when looking at a brain-dead individual on a respirator, see a pink person. They do not see a person with the ashen blue-gray pallor classically associated with death. The person looks more like a sleeping individual.

Those who support the thesis of physiological decapitation dismiss the statement of *Chacham Tzvi* because he did not have our present knowledge of the circulatory system and, in his scheme of things, the heart was a "respiratory" organ, involved in the warming and cooling of the air. Furthermore, during the time of *Chatam Sofer*, the interval between whole-brain death and cessation of cardiac activity was a matter of minutes, since ventilators were not available to maintain blood oxygenation in the absence of an independent ability to breathe.

The controversy is ongoing. The disagreement, however, is not purely a theoretical discussion of fine points in talmudic law. Practical results and ramifications flow from the two opposing views. Those who reject the physiological decapitation hypothesis, which equates total irreversible destruction of the brain including the brainstem with death, are faced with the following problems. First, secular society, which accepts brain death, will not pay for a patient's care after death. Hence, who will pay for that care between the declaration of brain death and cessation of cardiac activity? Second, is not a brain-dead patient in an intensive care unit unnecessarily denying that bed to another living patient who needs intensive care? Is that not an inappropriate use of a scarce resource (i.e., an ICU bed)? Furthermore, how can most organ transplantations be performed if one has to wait for cardiac standstill before organ harvesting from the donor? Most organs, if not continuously perfused, cannot be successfully transplanted into needy recipients.

Those who require irreversible cardiac and respiratory arrest to pronounce a patient dead not only reject the physiological decapitation thesis, but also do not accept the thesis that cessation of spontaneous respiration is equated with death and that spontaneous respiration and life itself are one and the same. There is considerable evidence in classic Jewish sources indicating that irreversible lack of respiration and death are synonymous. The soul departs through the nostrils at death, just as it is the nostrils into which the Lord blows the soul of life at birth (Gen. 2:6). Other sources, however, indicate that life may at times continue even after respiration has ceased, suggesting "that absence of respiration is at best a sign that death may be presumed to have occurred but is not, in itself, one and the same as death."[11]

Summary and Conclusion

Judaism is guided by the principle that life is sacred, is of supreme value, and is a gift from God. Physicians and patients are obligated to heal and seek healing, respectively. The prolongation of life, where medically possible, is required, but the prolongation of dying is wrong. Physicians and patients are governed by the norms of Jewish law even if such rules and regulations occasionally conflict with the moral attitudes of a secular society.

The definition of death in Jewish law is critically important in this era of organ transplantation, since the saving of lives is an absolute Jewish mandate to individuals and to Jewish society in general. There is at present an intense debate among rabbinic authorities as to whether Jewish law (*halacha*) recognizes death of the whole brain, including the brainstem, as a definition of death. The classic definition of death in Judaism, as found in the Talmud and Codes of Jewish Law, is the irreversible absence of respiration in a person who appears dead (i.e., shows no movements and is unresponsive to all stimuli). Jewish writings provide considerable evidence for the thesis that the brain and the brainstem control all bodily functions, including breathing and heartbeat. It therefore follows that irreversible total cessation of all brain function, including that of the brainstem, is equated with death. This situation is said to be the figurative equivalent of physiological decapitation, whereby the decapitated person is certainly dead, even if the heart transiently continues to beat.

The other rabbinic view rejects the analogy of decapitation and requires cardiac standstill in addition to cessation of respiration before death can be pronounced. Proponents of both views honestly and deeply feel the correctness of their interpretation of the classic Jewish sources. How can one respect this religious diversity within the Jewish rabbinic community in a formally secular society? New York State law requires medical examiners to take into consideration the religious, cultural, and ethnic sensitivities of families before deciding on the performance of an autopsy. The separation of church and state in the constitution of the United States ensures that no physician is obligated to perform an act contrary to his or her religious convictions. No Catholic physician is obligated to perform an abortion. Similarly, no Jewish physician is obligated to remove the life-support systems from a brain-dead patient if the physician believes that the patient is still alive by virtue of a beating heart. Thus, objections to brain death within the orthodox Jewish community can inform a secular moral perspective such as the one underlying American jurisprudence or "mainstream" bioethics.

NOTES

1. Jakobovits, I., *Jewish Medical Ethics*. New York: Bloch, 1959.

2. Rosner, F., and Bleich, J. D., *Jewish Bioethics*. New York: Sanhedrin Press, 1979.

3. Feldman, D. M., and Rosner, F., *Compendium on Medical Ethics*. 6th ed. New York: Federation of Jewish Philanthropies.

4. Rosner, F., *Modern Medicine and Jewish Ethics*. 2d ed. Hoboken, NJ: Ktav & Yeshiva University Press, 1991.

5. Jakobovits, I., *The Timely and the Timeless: Jews, Judaism and Society in a Storm Tossed Decade*. New York: Bloch, 1989, 128.

6. Steinberg, A., Medical ethics: Secular and Jewish approaches. In Rosner, F. (ed). *Medicine and Jewish Law*. Northvale, NY: Aronson, 1990, 19–39.

7. Pellegrino, E., and Thomasma, D. C. *For the Patient's Good*. New York: Oxford University Press, 1988.

8. Rosner, F. (transl)., *Moses Maimonides' Treatise on Resurrection*. New York: Ktav, 1982.

9. Council on Ethical and Judicial Affairs, American Medical Association, The use of anencephalic neonates as organ donors. *JAMA* 1995;273:1614–18.

10. Arnold, R. M., and Youngner, S. J., The dead donor rule: Should we stretch it, bend it, or abandon it? *Kennedy Inst Ethics J* 1993;2:263–78.

11. Bleich, J. D., Establishing criteria of death. In *Contemporary Halakhic Problems*. New York: Ktav & Yeshiva University Press, 1977, 372–93.

12. Rosner, F., and Tendler, M. D. Definition of death in Judaism. *J Halacha Contemp Soc* 1989;17 (spring):14–31.

13. Maimonides, M., *Mishneh Torah*, Laws of the Sabbath 2:19.

14. Karo, J., *Shulchan Aruch, Orach Chayim* 329:4.

15. Tendler, M. D., Cessation of brain function: Ethical implications in terminal care and organ transplants. *Ann NY Acad Sci* 1978;315:394–497.

16. Karo, J., *Shulchan Aruch, Yoreh Deah* 370:1.

17. Jakobovits, Y., Brain death and heart transplants: The Israeli Chief Rabbinate's directives. *Tradition* 1989;24:1–14.

18. Ashkenazy, T., Responsa *Chacham Tzvi* 77.

19. Sofer, M., Responsa *Chatam Sofer, Yoreh Deah* 338.

An Unfounded Diagnosis

Revisiting the Medical and Metaphysical
Justifications of "Brain Death"

David A. Jones

There is an impressive consensus in favor of accepting brain death as death, despite a number of philosophical criticisms of the concept (Bernat 2005). Indeed, organ retrieval from brain-dead patients has come to be accepted throughout the world, and brain death is generally seen as providing more reliable criteria for death than cardiopulmonary criteria. Nevertheless, while this practical consensus has grown, there is no agreed rationale for the practice (McCullagh, 1993, pp. 7–103; Youngner, Landefeld, Coulton, Juknialis, and Leary, 1989; Tomlinson, 1990).

The problem of identifying the rationale for brain death is well illustrated by a 1989 survey of health care professionals. In this study, 195 doctors, nurses, and decision makers were asked about their understanding of brain death (Youngner et al., 1989, pp. 2208–9). Sixty-three percent correctly identified the legal definition of death. Only 35 percent correctly applied the whole brain criterion to the legal status of patients when given different scenarios. They were then asked for their own personal opinions concerning two patients: one brain dead, the other in persistent vegetative state (PVS).[1] Whereas the great majority (95 percent) identified the brain-dead patient as dead, the reasons they gave were split three ways. Only 28 percent appealed to whole-brain destruction or complete loss of bodily integration, which could be called the official justification for brain death. A further 38 percent gave a reply that referred to the fact that the brain-dead patient had irreversibly lost consciousness or *higher* brain function. More startling still, 34 percent gave a reply that seemed to imply that the patient was really *still alive* but should be treated *as though* he or she were dead. Given some of the reasons why they thought that the brain-dead patient was dead, it is not surprising that 38 percent of these respondents also thought the patient in PVS was dead as well. Although this study was conducted almost twenty years ago, studies in the last five years have shown similar results (White, 2003; Siminoff, Burant, and Youngner, 2004).

The precise figures given here are not important. They would no doubt be different were the group taken from a different cross section of the population or from a different country. What is revealing about these results is that they show that there are *significant differences of belief* about what justifies brain death underlying the present practical consensus, and these differences show up both among health care professionals and among the wider public. When identifying brain death with death, people commonly appeal to one of three distinct rationales. These may be termed the medical, the metaphysical, and the moral justifications. This paper focuses on a critique of the medical and metaphysical justifications.[2]

The Medical Justification of "Brain Death"

The medical rationale is based on the idea that brain death has not changed the definition of death in any deep sense but has given us a better, more clinically sensitive, set of criteria for diagnosing death. According to this view, the concept of death is the same as it has always been; only the medical tests have changed.

The body is an integrated organism, a system of interrelated systems and organs. When an organ is described as alive, what is meant is not that it is itself a living whole, but that it remains viable and functionally intact and that many of its cells are alive. When a body is described as alive, this is because it is an integrated living organism. The body is not to be identified with any one organ, not even with the brain. I am not just a brain in a suit but I am a living organism, an organized whole.

One prominent account of brain death identifies the brain as the organ that integrates and organizes the rest of the body. The nervous system and, less directly, the endocrine system are controlled from the brain. The brain is the organ of organization. If the brain dies, it is argued, the body is no longer a single living organism. It seems to be maintained artificially for a brief time, but in reality the balance and integration have already gone. There is no spontaneous functioning. The body may appear to be alive, but, it is argued, this appearance is deceptive. It is the brain that makes the body function as a whole, so when the brain dies, the body has died, and all that is left is a collection of separate subsystems artificially maintained that give the appearance, but not the reality, of life (President's Commission, 1981, p. 35; Grisez and Boyle, 1979).

If this account is accepted, then a number of things are immediately clear. First, it is clear why brain-dead patients, *of necessity*, deteriorate rapidly even with assistance. Final systemic collapse cannot be far away. This is because the bodies do not have their own center of integration but are kept in a fragile balance from outside. It is also apparent why these patients are utterly different from people in PVS or other mentally impaired individuals. A patient in PVS can live for many years with only nursing assistance. A brain-dead body is always on the point of collapse.

In the United Kingdom, there has been a further attempt to identify brain death with *brainstem death* (Conference of Medical Royal Colleges 1976). It is argued that once the brainstem is destroyed, the brain can no longer function, conscious thought is impossible, and the body is no longer integrated. However, while the functioning of the brainstem seems to be necessary for the functioning of the higher brain (and so of consciousness), the destruction of the brainstem does not leave the upper brain destroyed; thus the organic basis to support thought is still intact. Further, some patients with lesions in the brainstem have briefly regained consciousness after stimulation of the brain above the lesion (Hassler 1977 quoted by Shewmon 1989, p. 36). A conscious man is obviously not dead, whatever the state of his brainstem!

What is required for death is the destruction of the organic basis of the living body, not the simple absence of present functioning of the brain (Byrne, O'Reilly, and Quay, 1979, pp. 1987–89). Most legal definitions of death outside the United Kingdom prefer "whole brain" definitions of brain death. However, what the United Kingdom criteria has in common with most other legal criteria for death is that they include, explicitly or implicitly, reference to the brainstem. In this way, they demonstrate a concern with the *integrated functioning* of the brain and not only with consciousness. They show that the concept of death being used is not fundamentally different from the traditional concept of death: "irreversible loss of function of the whole organism" (Lamb, 1994, p. 1031; also, e.g., Iglesias, 1991, and Bernat, 1992). The *concept* of death has not changed, only the *criteria*.

This account of brain death has proved attractive to doctors, philosophers, and legislators, because it maintains the traditional *concept* of death while assimilating modern advances in science and medicine. It allows the benefits of organ transplantation from brain-dead donors without putting at risk patients in PVS or other vulnerable groups. It seems to distinguish clearly the dead from the dying. Thus, this account has become the standard justification for identifying brain death as death in many legal, medical, and ethical bodies (Capron and Kass, 1972; Conference of Medical Royal Colleges, 1979; Grisez, 1979; President's Commission, 1981; Chagas, 1986; Capron, 1987; White, Angstwurm, and Carrasco de Paula, 1989; Pallis, 1990; Iglesias, 1991; Tonti-Filippini, 1991; Bernat, 1992; Capron, 1993; Lynn, 1993; Lamb, 1994; Pentz, 1994; Conference of Medical Royal Colleges 1995; Steinberg, 1996). If governmental or medical bodies provide a rationale for accepting brain death, they typically prefer the medical justification.

Somatic Survival with Brain Death

The medical justification involves two empirical claims: (1) that the well-defined clinical syndrome conventionally called "brain death" does in fact mean that the whole of the brain has lost all its function irreversibly and (2) that the body (as a whole) dies with the brain. However, there is mounting evidence against both of these claims. In the United Kingdom and several other countries, brain death is diagnosed without observing the electrical activity of the brain (measured by the electroencephalogram, EEG). When such patients have been investigated, it is found that a number of them still show signs of electrical activity. Nevertheless, these patients conform well to other brain-death criteria and seem to have no better hope of recovery. Similarly, the results of autopsy on brain-dead patients show that often areas of intact tissue remain. The brain has not been physically destroyed. Such findings clearly demonstrate that the clinical syndrome called "brain death" does not in fact involve the destruction of the entire brain.

To preserve the organs of a brain-dead body, various forms of hormone treatment have been suggested and tried. A particular concern is to prevent the patient from developing an excess urinary output known as diabetes insipidus. However, a proportion of brain-dead patients do not develop diabetes insipidus, even without hormone treatment. This means that in these patients there is residual pituitary function, and hence brain function, because the hypothalamus of the brain regulates the pituitary gland. Thus, some brain function may be intact after a clinical diagnosis of brain death.

For brain death to be diagnosed, the body must be unresponsive in a variety of ways, including, importantly, the inability to breathe spontaneously. However, in many brain-dead patients, the body is not completely unresponsive. There remain various reflexes of the esophagus and other reflex reactions. Most startling is the way in which such bodies commonly react to incision during organ harvesting. The heartbeat quickens and the blood pressure rises rapidly. The reaction is so extreme that at least in some hospitals in England and Australia (to the author's knowledge), organ-harvesting operations are routinely carried out with the brain-dead patient under *general anesthetic!* The fact that other hospitals paralyze the patient without using general anesthetic does not suffice to quiet one's anxieties; rather, the opposite happens. The body is clearly a responsive system.

Finally, although the medical justification rests on the claim that brain death is intrinsically unstable because there is no inner principle of balance, stability, dynamism, or spontaneity, some brain-dead patients have been maintained for a number of weeks. This has happened, for example, when doctors have endeavored to maintain the bodies of brain-dead pregnant mothers in the hope that their children can be delivered alive. These cases are unusual, but even in ordinary cases of brain death, it has been discovered that the time these patients can be sustained can be doubled by certain hormone treatments.

How are we to describe what is going on here? What is it that is "sustained" or "maintained" or "prolonged" or "survives"? The most natural and least contrived way to describe these cases is to say that the life of the body is sustained and is maintained by artificial supports. In the medical literature, these cases are sometimes described as *somatic survival* with brain death (Parisi, Kim, Collins, and Hilfinger, 1982). Clearly, the life of these bodies is sustained by artificial means (ventilation and perhaps other forms of treatment), but that is also true of other very sick patients who are unquestionably alive. Somatic survival is survival.[3]

Responses to Criticism

Defenders of the medical justification cope with this empirical counterevidence in several ways. First, many examples of bodily responsiveness (as the rise in blood pressure in reaction to the organ-harvesting operation) are dismissed as *spinal reflexes.* They do not show that the brainstem (and thus the brain) is functional. Brain death exists despite these responses. The evidence of electrical and other activity of the brain is sometimes acknowledged, but a distinction is made between the death of the brain as a whole (or the functional death of the brain) on the one hand and the death of the entire brain on the other. It is acknowledged that individual neurons may continue to fire, but it is asserted that these isolated pockets of activity have no significance, for the *brain-as-a-whole* no longer exists as a functioning organ (Bernat, 1992, pp. 24–25). This distinction is an application to the brain of a principle already well understood concerning the body: the body as a whole can die, though the entire body (every cell and organ) is not yet dead. This distinction is obviously essential to the whole idea of transplanting live organs from dead patients.

Another common response to the acknowledged presence of EEG activity (and indeed to other signs of life in brain-dead patients) is to point to the poor prognosis of such patients. According to Pallis (1990),

> Even over the last 20 years there have been far more misdiagnoses of death based on cardiovascular criteria than there have been in relation to brain death. The record here is reassuring. Patients fulfilling clinical criteria of brain stem death (and in whom ventilation was continued) have all developed asystole. And none have ever regained consciousness before that. (Pallis, 1990, p. 12; also Lamb, 1991)

One further response to the more extraordinary cases is to say that these examples are, for the most part, exceptional cases of *misdiagnosis*, which should not alter our confidence in the concept of brain death or in the general reliability of clinical practice. This is especially so with reference to accounts of prolonged somatic survival. It is known that most brain-dead patients suffer cardiac arrest within hours or a few days; therefore, exceptional examples can be put down to misdiagnosis.

There are more cautious commentators who think that misdiagnosis is widespread and thus want more stringent clinical tests before brain death is declared (Evans, 1989; Byrne and Nilges, 1993; Kaukinen, 1995). These criticisms have practical implications, but they do not necessarily invalidate the concept of brain death as the moment of death ascertainable by clinical tests (Iglesias, 1991). Nor is it reasonable to expect 100 percent accuracy from these tests, for absolute certainty is no part of medicine. It is surely a good thing if brain-death criteria mark a significant advance on previous means of diagnosing death. Diagnosis of death has never been infallible, but is it better now than it has been in the past.

Response to These Responses

The problem with many of these responses is that they do not address the central concern. It is generally admitted that brain-dead patients have a poor prognosis, but "bad prognosis as such cannot be a criterion for a diagnosis of brain death" (Kaukinen, Mäkelä, Häkkinen, and Martikainen, 1995, p. 78). This also undermines the soothing reassurances of reliable diagnosis given by Pallis and others. Upon examination, the evidence supporting diagnosis turns out to be the poor outcome of these patients (still appealed to in Conference of Medical Royal Colleges 1995, pp. 381–382). Yet, at the risk of repetition, showing inevitably poor prognosis is a long way from showing that the patient is already dead.

Furthermore, examples of somatic survival after brain death cannot be dismissed as misdiagnosis. In presenting a rare example of extended survival with brain death, Shewmon (1997b) described a child who had sustained massive brain damage due to meningitis. The child showed a flat EEG and no spontaneous respiration and fulfilled all the clinical criteria for brain death. Further tests confirmed this extraordinary diagnosis: evoked potentials showed no cortical or brain stem responses; magnetic resonance angiogram showed no intracranial blood flow. At Shewmon's presentation, it was illuminating to see the reaction to this evidence by a physician who accepted the received medical justification of brain death. He stated calmly that this case must be one of misdiagnosis. This was even after a slide had been shown of the MRI scan showing "the entire brain, including the brain stem, had been replaced by ghost-like tissues and disorganised proteinaceous fluids" (Shewmon, 1997b). The child was evidently brain dead, though his body survived fourteen years (and still did at the time of that discussion).

This case is the most extreme, but it is only one of many well-documented cases of prolonged somatic survival with brain death (Jones, 1995, p. 268). The question of prolonged somatic survival in brain-dead pregnant women has become so well known as to attract considerable comment (*Journal of Clinical Ethics*, 1993, 4, no. 4, devoted an entire issue to the ethical aspects of keeping the bodies of such women alive). These cases are exceptional, but they are not cases of misdiagnosis. They are important for this reason: that they show there is *no necessary connection* between brain death and the death of the body. If this is the case when the body survives for a prolonged period, it is also in the usual case of a much briefer somatic survival. The brain dies but the body itself has not yet died, even if it will die soon.

Somatic Death

So deeply entrenched is the dogma that the brainstem mediates integrative function that one is inclined to say, "If the brainstem does not do this, what organ does it? And if bodily death is not brain death, what is it?—for it cannot be the death of every cell or organ."

The integration of the body seems to be a function of the organism as a whole, rather than a function of any one organ, even the brain. The brain stem stabilizes, regulates, and modulates an already existing integrated organism (Shewmon, 2001). This preexisting integration includes the maintenance of temperature, blood pressure, respiration, circulation, the assimilation of nutrients and elimination of waste, the many aspects of metabolism, resistance to infection, and responses to stress such as that dramatic response to the incision that makes it necessary to administer general anesthetic to the donor during organ retrieval. Assisted ventilation does not replace the lungs (which still function to exchange gases) but merely replaces the movement of the diaphragm. Respiration as a metabolic process and an activity of the body as a whole is not artificially maintained or replaced. Nor is the heartbeat maintained artificially, but it continues spontaneously so long as the supply of oxygen is not cut off. In fact, the body of a brain-dead patient may well receive less support than some other patients who are clearly still alive. *A fortiori*, the bodies of brain-dead patients are still alive.

The death of the body is not identical to the death of any one organ. The body can continue to exist even if its heart should stop, so long as some replacement can be found (as is clearly shown by heart transplants and lung bypass machines). However, the maintenance of spontaneous heartbeat is one sign of continued life of the body in which the heart still beats. The body does not die until it undergoes systemic collapse when it cannot regain its vital balance. The ability of the body to maintain itself as a whole and resist spiraling entropy depends on general features of the vital systems (this is what is meant by bodily integration). Once this integration is lost, destruction occurs. No one should be declared dead unless there is destruction of the vital systems of the body.

The medical justification of brain death relies on the argument that the various forms of medical support "mask" the death of the patient (President's Commission, 1981, pp. 35–36; Tomlinson, 1984, p. 381). Yet medical support (such as assisted ventilation, kidney dialysis, or implantation of a pacemaker) does not mask death so much as prevent death. The body is not artificially alive. It is alive in the ordinary sense, but its life is supported by technology. Even with this support, the body dies eventually. When a body is really dead (in the old-fashioned sense of irreversibly lacking heartbeat, respiration, and integrated metabolism), then pumping air into it cannot disguise the fact. The balance cannot be restored from outside.

This account of somatic survival with brain death effectively undermines the medical justification for identifying brain death with death (Jonas, 1974; Becker, 1975; Green and Wikler, 1980; Byrne, O'Reilly, Quay, and Salsich, 1982/83; Tomlinson, 1984; Wreen, 1987; Seifert, 1993; Youngner, 1992; Wikler, 1993; Singer, 1995a, 1995b; McMahon, 1995; Truog, 1997; Shewmon, 1997a, 2001). Whereas the practice of organ harvesting from beating-heart cadavers has been accepted, it has not been established that the bodies of these patients are in fact dead. Many operating theater staff find organ harvesting traumatic precisely because it seems to involve the death of a warm and well-maintained body with a beating heart (Youngner, Allen, and Bartlett, 1985; Rothstein, 1995). These reactions are not to be dismissed as misplaced emotions, but rather they are the recognition of the fact of the life of these bodies, often in the face of an official denial of that fact. The medical justification relies on a story that is no longer plausible and, in fact, never was to a great number of people. *The bodies of brain-dead patients are not dead.*

The Metaphysical Justification of "Brain Death"

Metaphysical justifications of brain death as death distinguish *the death of the person from the death of the biological organism.* Those who justify brain death in this way would extend the concept to cover other patients who were clearly alive but who had lost consciousness, as in the case of patients in PVS. These theorists talk about higher brain death (Veatch, 1993) or neocortical death (Puccetti, 1988), because it is theorized that severe brain damage in the higher parts of the brain, as occurs in PVS, is enough to render conscious thought impossible. There are some problems with the diagnosis of PVS and with deciding how much brain damage makes conscious thought impossible (Capron, 1987; Shewmon, 1989), but it seems obvious that at least those clinically diagnosed as whole-brain dead must have irreversibly lost consciousness. It is precisely these cases the Harvard report had in mind when it defined death as irreversible coma (Beecher, 1968).

There are a number of different forms of the metaphysical justification of brain death as the death of the person. These vary according to the underlying metaphysical account of the person being set forth. There are consequently more or less refined forms of this justification. The following list is not exhaustive but covers the main forms of the argument in use in the contemporary discussion.

Cartesian Dualism

A position popular among the general public that is also accepted by a minority of philosophers holds that the human person consists of two things: a mind (also identified with "the soul" or "the spirit") and a body. Its most famous philosophical advocate was René Descartes. The mind is the thinking thing *res cogitans;* in contrast, the body is a kind of machine. The means of the interaction of mind and body is obscure, but it certainly happens via the brain or some part of the brain that collects sensory information and controls the rest of the body (including the voluntary muscles). The brain is, thus, the interface between mind and body, the place where the two interact. If the brain is irreversibly destroyed, then the mind or soul is cut loose from the body. The person, as a composite of soul and body, has died. So long as it could be empirically verified that the organic basis of conscious thought has been destroyed, then one could confidently declare the person dead, even though the body lives on. This is often the picture behind comments such as "My son died three years ago, this is just an empty shell," used to describe a patient in PVS.

Although this view remains influential in the popular imagination and does have some philosophic following, in this century it has been undermined by a thoroughgoing philosophical critique. The idea that the person is a "ghost inside a machine" creates many problems in epistemology. How can one know that there is an "external world"? How can one know that other bodies have minds "inside" them? If we can never experience things as someone else does, how can we know that they have experiences at all? While these questions may seem fatuous to someone unfamiliar with them (surely we *know* that other people and things exist), philosophers have failed to give good rational arguments to show how we could in principle know these things. While there were many proposed solutions, none ever gained widespread acceptance. If these questions are less debated now, it is not because a solution was ever found, but because philosophers grew tired of the fruitless quest.

The problem with these questions is that they assume a view of the person that is false. When they dissociated "internal" (mind) from "external" (body) in principle, they found it was not possible to join them up again. The only solution to this problem is not to dissociate the two in the first place but to acknowledge the holism of the human person. What we see is outside of us. This is a real relation. We do not see internal images (though seeing may involve internal images); we see objects in the world. The grammar (the concepts) of looking or seeming are parasitic on the practice of seeing. Perception does not concern some inner and private world but is a real relation to external perceptible things. Even pain is to be understood in reference to possible damage and to natural behavior and not simply to some inner private object called "my pain." This was well exposed by Wittgenstein almost fifty years ago:

> If I say of myself that it is only from my own case that I can know what the word "pain" means—must I not say the same of other people too? And how can I generalize the *one* case so irresponsibly?
>
> Now someone tells me that he knows what pain is only from his own case!—Suppose everyone had a box with something in it: we call it a "beetle." No one can look into anyone else's box, and everyone says he knows what a beetle is only by looking at *his* beetle.—Here it would be quite possible for everyone to have something different in his box. One might even imagine such a thing constantly changing.—But suppose the word "beetle" had a use in these people's language?—If so it would not be used as the name of a thing. The thing in the box has no place in the language-game at all; not even as a *something:* for the box might even be empty.—No, one can "divide through" by the thing in the box; it cancels out, whatever it is. (Wittgenstein, 1953, p. 293)

That is to say: If we construe the grammar of the expression of sensation on the model of "object and designation," the object drops out of consideration as irrelevant.

These considerations not only are about language but also expose the problems with the underlying concept of the person. We cannot properly understand perception and language if we think of the person as an immaterial mind interacting with a body. The person has to be construed as a whole being living in the world.

Lockean Persons

The dominant analysis of the human person in the present English-speaking philosophical community takes its influence less from Descartes than from John Locke. Already in the seventeenth century Hobbes had offered a materialist alternative to Cartesian dualism. Locke steered a middle path between Descartes and Hobbes, maintaining a subjective starting point for the person but without committing himself to the causal relations of the mental and the physical. Whatever the basis of consciousness might be, some living things have it and some do not. This was his starting point. Given that some creatures are certainly conscious, what concerns these self-conscious creatures is the continuity of their personality (memories, commitments, attitudes). It is thus that psychological continuity constitutes the person as a person (at *this* point there is a convergence with Descartes). So, if the possibility of any psychological life is cut off (by irreversible brain damage), then there is no "person." A body might continue to live on, but because this body is no longer the bearer of any psychological attributes, it cannot be a person. *A fortiori,* it cannot be the same person it was before, thus the person must have died.[4]

This account has the advantage of holding that the death of the person follows logically and immediately from the irreversible loss of consciousness. The death of the person is nothing else but the loss of those conscious attributes. There is no need to speculate about the nature or causes of consciousness. So long as we are confident that conscious thought is no longer possible, then *de facto* we have shown that "the person" is dead. However, this advantage carries with it a defect. The unwillingness to identify the person with a substance (material or immaterial) generates many paradoxes. If personal identity comprises the identity of conscious attributes (rather than anything "underlying"), then it seems it can be lost by degrees. A phrase such as "He is not the person he used to be" could be taken literally. Over time, persons would gradually cease to be themselves and become other persons (this conclusion is explicitly embraced by Parfit, 1986). There is no possibility of counting persons through time for, though there is continuity, there is never strict identity, but rather continuous change. You never meet the same person twice, but then you never are the same person twice either!

This account of the person is highly contrived. It could mean that, if somehow a number of persons in the future had my memories and character, there would be *no matter of fact* as to which one was in fact me. If they all actually possessed my memories and character, they would all have an equal claim to be continuous with me and I should be as concerned for them as myself. Parfit has an extensive analysis of being concerned for oneself and hopes to show by his analysis that long-term selfishness is irrational (though, of course, crude and immediate selfishness would become more rational). Such considerations, however high-minded, are beside the point. Someone may have more concern for another than for himself or herself (say a mother for her child), but she does not think that she is the same person as her child! She may prefer that she die and her daughter live, but she does not believe that she will live in (or as) the daughter. I hope that when I die, God will raise me from the dead. This wish is emphatically not a wish that God should raise someone very like me (with my memories and character). The identity of persons is not a relation of similarity (as if twins by becoming similar enough could become the same person), nor is it even a relation of continuity, for every time someone falls asleep consciousness is interrupted and character and attitudes can certainly undergo dramatic and disruptive change within the biography of the same person.

Locke treats the word *person* to denote an extra quality added to being a human being, rather as the word *magnet* denotes an extra quality that a piece of metal might gain and then lose. "A piece of iron gets magnetised and so *becomes* a magnet; later it may get demagnetised and *stops* being a magnet though it is still the same piece of iron" (Anscombe, 2005, p. 268). Faced with this account, what are we to say? One common response is to point out how arbitrary this view of the person is. Once *person* is uncoupled from the readily identifiable human being and made to rely on variable qualities, such as intelligence, memory, or awareness, then there can be no nonarbitrary way to say who passes the test of personhood and who fails. Those with stricter marking criteria (so to speak) will fail all infants until they can speak, adults with severe dementia, and even those with learning disabilities and will also fail those in a coma whom we have decided not to revive. Those with more lenient criteria will pass all who have a glimmer of consciousness or any possibility of achieving this. Following this argument to its logical conclusion, a rigorous criterion of personhood should exclude all children from personhood until they were fully autonomous persons and able to take legal responsibility for their actions, at around sixteen or so (that is, until they became competent adults or what is known in English law as "Gillick competent" minors). Before this point they might be deemed "prepersons."

This incorrigible arbitrariness undermines the credibility of a Lockean account of the human person. In place of this arbitrary insubstantial account of personhood, a number of other philosophers have argued that we need to retrieve the ancient sense of ourselves as substantial beings of a particular kind, as rational animals. As Wiggins says, "By *person* we mean a *certain sort of animal,* and for purposes of both politics and morality that is the best thing for us to mean" (Wiggins, 1980, p. 187; see also Anscombe, 2005, p. 268).

Aristotelian Substances

The most sophisticated metaphysical accounts of brain death as death are those that renounce any form of dualism. They are based on the metaphysics of Aristotle (Matthews, 1979) or of Thomas Aquinas (Shewmon, 1985). These authors hold that we are indeed animals of a particular kind and, like other animals, are conceived, born, and die. The significance of human death may be different, but the biological conditions for human death are the same as those for other animals. Human death is the death of a biological organism.

According to the Thomist/Aristotelian view, death is the passing away of one substance (the living animal) and the coming to be of another, or others (the corpse). This is counterintuitive for some modern commentators, e.g., McMahon (1995):

> one might hold that the living organism and the corpse are not one and the same thing. The corpse is not a phase in the history of a body that was once alive; rather, it is a different substance altogether, one that pops into existence upon the death of the organism. I assume, however, that this is even less plausible than the idea that we *may* continue to exist after death as corpses. (McMahon, 1995, p. 99)

If one substitutes "comes to be" for the satirical phrase "pops into existence," this is a fair and accurate account of the Thomist/Aristotelian position. Why is it thought to be so implausible? The reason depends on the understanding of *material stuff* appealed to. We are presumably supposed to agree with the remark that "a corpse is a phase in the history of a body." Because what exists is the body, the presence or absence of life is only accidental to its identity. This becomes more explicit later when he says, "When the entire brain dies, that is certainly sufficient for the ceasing to exist of the mind, but not,'in the normal case, of the ceasing to exist of the brain. A dead, nonfunctional brain is still a brain" (McMahon, 1995, p. 103).

This is precisely what an Aristotelian would deny. What is it that makes the brain a brain? Is it its chemical composition? If we liquefy a dead brain, would it still be a brain? Clearly not. What makes the brain the brain is not only that it contains certain chemical or physical stuff; but also that it has a particular form, shape, and structure. The brain makes sense only as the organ of an animal, and this accounts for its structure and function. What happens when it dies? At a basic level, it ceases to have the functional structure (the metabolizing dynamic form) that it had. It may still have the outward appearance of a brain but the similarity ends there. The remains of a once living object are, at a biological (and hence metaphysical) level, a different sort of thing than a living being. Indeed, the remains are generally an accidental juxtaposition of many things, including chemical compounds and larger structures, which are no longer held together by being a part of a living unity, but now only by inertia (what has not yet fallen apart). If it is admitted that what makes a brain a brain has to do with its *shape* or *structure,* then one should say that "shape" and "structure" should not here be interpreted in a superficial and static way but should refer to the structured life of a living, functioning whole.

The death of an animal is then the passing away of one form (the form of the living animal) and the coming to be of other forms that were once included (implicitly) within the form of the living animal. So, for instance, the life of cells and organs that once took their place within a larger substantial whole (that is, as a part of a whole animal) now become the substantial forms for separate remains. The skin cells or the kidney could be removed and live separately with a life that is no longer the life of the whole animal. Other structures like bones, or chemicals like water and glucose, become stuff that exists in its own right, no longer essentially a part of a living whole. The death of an animal always leaves some form or forms that were once implicit in it. The question arises: Could the living animal die and leave "remains" that were still a living whole but were no longer the same living animal? Could there be a substantial change where the animal died but what remained still had some life as a whole of its own?

Shewmon has developed his own views considerably (Shewmon, 1985, 1989, 1997a, 2001). In 1985 he imagined removing an intact living brain from a human being and keeping it alive in a vat. Assuming the rest of the body continued to live, like the body of a brain-dead patient, we face the question: Which body is the patient, the brain (without the rest of its body), or the rest of the body (without its brain)? The answer seems clear. The brain is the same person and the brainless body is a sort of living human remains. The rest of the body has a life that came from a human person but that is no longer human life, for human life is essentially the life of a *rational* animal. The life of a brainless body is like the life of an individual organ that continues to live for a while outside the body (a heart or a kidney).

This manner of reasoning would have the same practical consequences as the other metaphysical justifications of brain death: It would identify the death of the person with the destruction of that part that makes human consciousness possible. After this, the body would still be alive, but it would not be the same human animal any more; rather, it would be the living remains that came to be when the rational animal passed away (Shewmon, 1985).

This account takes the human being seriously as a certain sort of animal. It does not identify the person with one organ (the brain), nor with an immaterial part (the mind), nor with a set of powers and attributes (the personality). The person is a whole living rational animal. However, an essential part of that animal is its brain, the vehicle of its rational powers. Without this organ, what remains is not really a human being any more. Matthews (1979) thinks the same is true of a decerebrated cat. A cat without a brain is not a cat (as a dead cat is not a cat). It is in truth a different sort of thing.

Shewmon's argument, however, is not compelling, because it gratuitously assumes that in every case (even in these contrived cases), the *number* of persons involved must remain constant. Yet consider a case where a brain is divided in two and each half brain survives (as *seems* physiologically possible, at least for the upper brain). What if half the brain were removed and the other half left with the body? We would be confused as to the identity of each. We would say either that one of the two halves was a newly created person, or that both halves were newly created persons, and *neither* one was identical to the person who underwent the operation. This is similar to Shewmon's case where the whole brain is taken out of a living body. We might say that the brain took with it the old person and a new, profoundly mentally impaired person had come into being, or perhaps that the person had split in two, and neither was identical to the person who underwent the operation. We can resolve this case without being obliged to postulate a humanoid animal, a living human being that is not a human person.

Now consider the case in which half of the brain of a patient is destroyed *in situ*. Perhaps there are clinical states that come close to this. Would we have any doubts at all that this is the same person who underwent the operation? None at all. Note that it may be *either half* of the brain that is destroyed without affecting the example. There is no single *bit* of the brain, nor the brain as a whole, nor of any other organ that is the carrier of identity; rather, it is the living organism as a whole that endures through time. Note then that *separation* of the body into two raises questions of identity that pose no problem when what is involved is not division but destruction. It is the presence of an *alternative candidate* (with an equal or better claim to continuity with the person) that causes us to have doubts about someone's identity. Brain death involves no splitting of the person, no problems of identity due to alternative candidates, but simply the destruction of an organ. In the case of brain death, there is no doubt as to the *identity* of the person. We know both *who* that person is and that that person is *alive*, though mentally impaired.

The general philosophical literature continues to debate issues of personal identity considering, among other things, the implications for personal identity of brain transplant operations. There have been attempts to use these considerations to resolve the status of brain-dead individuals (Green and Wikler, 1980; Shewmon, 1985; McMahon, 1995). Yet this whole approach has been well criticized because, *even if this approach is right about personal identity,* questions of identity do not, in themselves, resolve questions of life or death.

To justify brain death, we need to know when an individual is dead—that is, what constitutes the conditions and meaning of death that explain and validate brain-death criteria, not whether an individual is the same individual who existed before. In short, we need to know something about the conditions that are necessary for an individual's being alive as opposed to dead, not whether an individual is still a particular individual or person (Agich and Jones, 1986, p. 268).

Actualism

The most significant elements of human life involve our consciousness and rational powers. These include all our voluntary actions, eating, talking, and playing football no less than our acts of pure and private contemplation. However, it is obvious that we do not exercise these powers all the time, as sleep, drugs, or injury may prevent us from using them. Shewmon (in 1985) accepted the personhood of the early embryo because, though he or she does not do any *actual* thinking, he or she has the capacity to grow a brain, to develop his or her rational powers, and this is something inherent in his or her nature. It follows from this that one doesn't have to actually exercise a power in order to possess it radically, as a capacity of one's nature. In this regard, our rational powers should not be treated differently from our other powers. To be sure, they are more important to us, more interesting, more characteristic of our essence, but they are all equally powers of a substance, the living human person. Like all powers they have to develop and mature, they can be exercised or neglected, they are not in use all of the time, and they may be impeded by injury or illness.

If a man loses his sight, we do not say this makes him a different person. Taking this metaphor too literally is what causes problems for the Lockean approach to personal identity. It is logically possible that one person (with sight) ceases to be, and another (blind) comes to be in his place, but we do not have sufficient reason to suppose any such thing really occurs. The person is still the same being; he has lost only a capacity. In like manner, it is indeed a subtle form of *actualism* to think that we must possess a functioning brain to be the same rational animal (a point made by Seifert, 1993, against Shewmon, 1985, and later conceded by Shewmon, 1997a). The brain function may be destroyed, but the capacity is still an intrinsic part of our nature. We do not become members of another species by severe brain damage. We are not literally "vegetables" ("He would never want to be a vegetable" is quoted with approval by Gillett, 1986; this is bad metaphysics as well as bad manners). We remain human beings and, as such, subjects of rational powers even if injury or illness persistently prevent us from exercising them.

It has been claimed (Lizza, 1993, p. 355) that there is a consensus of classical and modern philosophical thought upholding reason as a constitutive part of human nature and, therefore, "some potential for cognitive function is necessary for personhood." However, this follows only if "some potential" relates to the very fact of the person's being alive and human (and therefore possessed of a human nature). If "some potential for cognitive function" means a present ability, then immaturity or injury is not being taken seriously. A newborn infant has no present ability to speak, but few philosophers have thought of newborn infants as nonhuman or nonpersons. Rationality is part of human nature, as are our five senses, our ability to laugh and cry and walk, and many other things. These characteristics develop in us and may be lost (in the sense that we can no longer exercise them) without our ceasing to be human. This is true of every power of an animal, including our most extraordinary rational powers. They may be impeded, but they are lost radically only when the animal dies and the living being, in which all these powers inhered, is no more.

The dividing line between life and death comes not when this or that ability is lost but only when the organism can no longer be maintained as a unity. Death is marked by a transition from unity to multiplicity, even if some of the parts then retain a life of their own, for a time. It is the point at which an individual no longer functions as an integrated biological unit.

This holist account of the life and death of the human being is, in fact, the traditional Judeo-Christian one (Pentz, 1994). The dogmatic teaching of the Catholic Church is that the rational soul is *per se* "the form of the body" (Council of Vienne, 1311). What is wrong then with saying that the soul acts on the body via the brain? This assumes that the body already exists before the soul acts on it. In fact, it is the soul that constitutes the body as a living body. The soul is the form of the body, not an invisible motor moving it.

Thomas Aquinas gives the classical statement of the soul as the form of the body (*Summa Theologiae*, Ia, Q 75, Q 76). He asks the question whether the whole soul is in each part of the body. To this he replies that it is, but it does not have the same relation to each part and does not have the same relation to any of the parts as it does to the whole: "Its relation to the whole is not the same as its relation to the parts; for it relates to the whole primarily and essentially, as to its proper object; but it relates to the parts secondarily, inasmuch as they are ordered to the whole" (*Summa Theologiae*, Ia, Q 76, art. 8). In this way it is true to say that the brain is a vehicle for the soul, or that the soul is present in the brain, in as much as the brain is an organ of the whole. Yet if the whole can survive without this organ, then *de facto* the soul is still present in that whole and in the parts, inasmuch as they are parts of the whole. So long as the organism as a whole is still alive, he or she is the same animal, the same human being, the same person. So, *the person is not dead until his or her body dies.*

Conclusion

The very persistence of the term *brain death* is evidence of the conceptual confusion surrounding its use. People do not refer to patients as *heart dead* or *circulation dead,* for if someone is dead, he or she is dead, *simpliciter.* That medical workers, lawyers, and the public persist in making the verbal distinction between "death" and "brain death" shows that the identification of brain death with death is far from agreed. Brain death seems to represent a different sort of death than ordinary death, a hint of the tension between different justifications of the concept. Even those who work in the area are confused about how to justify the identification of brain death with death (Youngner et al., 1989; Tomlinson, 1990).

Having carefully distinguished the medical and metaphysical issues, I have argued that the bodies of brain-dead patients are not dead and the person is not dead until his or her body dies. If these theses are accepted, then there needs to be an immediate reexamination of the permissible limits of organ procurement. Organ harvesting is permissible on live donors only when it does no serious harm to any function. Only if it can be established beyond doubt that the patient is dead may vital organs be removed. Preparations of the body for organ harvesting may be made, with the patient's permission, if they do no harm to the patient, but one must be wary of treating one patient for the sake of another (Jones 2000). The living patient must always remain the primary object of treatment.

NOTES

This article contains selected material from a longer article, David Albert Jones, O.P., "Metaphysical Misgivings about 'Brain Death,'" in M. Potts, P. Byrne, and R. G. Nilges (eds.), *Beyond Brain Death: The Case against Brain-Based Criteria for Human Death* (pp. 121–138), Dordrecht: Kluwer Academic Publishers, 2000, reprinted with the kind permission of Springer Science and Business Media.
    1. Brain death is a distinct clinical syndrome from PVS and has a different prognosis (Jennet, 1972). Someone in PVS may survive for months or years, whereas someone in brain death will suffer total systemic collapse within hours or days. The person in PVS can breathe spontaneously and has a functioning brainstem. The person with brain death cannot

breathe spontaneously and does not have a functioning brainstem. In all those countries that have accepted brain related criteria for death, the person with brain death is classified as dead, whereas the person with PVS is classified as alive, albeit living in a severely debilitated state. In addition to these two states or syndromes there are other unresponsive or minimally responsive clinical states that are now distinguished (Laureys, 2004).

2. For a critical discussion of the moral justification for accepting brain death as death, see my earlier work (Jones, 2000), from which most of the material for this article is drawn.

3. When this paper was part of a longer paper published in 2000, it relied on medical evidence gathered by Evans and Hill, 1989; Shewmon, 1989; McCullagh, 1993, pp. 7–56; Jones, 1995; Kaukinen et al., 1995; Shewmon, 1997a. The last ten years have not undermined but have rather reinforced this evidence as similar phenomena have been reported many times (e.g., Bohatyrewicz et al., 2007; Döşemeci, Cengiz, Yilmaz, and Ramazanoglu, 2004; Joffe and Antony, 2007; Linos, Fraser, Freeman, and Foot, 2007; Sethi et al., 2008).

4. A usefully clear example is provided by John Harris: "most current accounts of the criteria for personhood follow John Locke in identifying self-consciousness coupled with fairly rudimentary intelligence as the most important features . . . [the human individual] will gradually move from being a potential or a pre-person into an actual person when she becomes capable of valuing her own existence. And if, eventually, she permanently loses this capacity, she will have ceased to be a person" (Harris, 1995, pp. 8–9).

REFERENCES

Agich, G., and Jones, R. P. 1986. Personal identity and brain death: A critical response. *Philosophy and Public Affairs* 15: 267–274.

Anscombe, G. E. M. 2005. *Human Life, Action and Ethics*. M. Geach and L. Gormally (eds.). Exeter, UK: Imprint Academic.

Aquinas, T. 1947. *Summa Theologiae*. London: Blackfriars.

Becker, L. 1975. Human being: The boundaries of the concept. *Philosophy and Public Affairs* 4: 334–359.

Beecher, H. K. 1968. A definition of irreversible coma. Report of the ad hoc committee of the Harvard Medical School to examine the definition brain death. *JAMA* 205: 337–340.

Bernat, J. L. 1992. How much of the brain must die in brain death? *Journal of Clinical Ethics* 3(1): 21–26.

Bernat, J. L. 2005. The concept and practice of brain death. *Progress in Brain Research* 150: 369–379.

Bohatyrewicz, R., Walecka, A., Bohatyrewicz, A., Zukowski, M., Kepinski, S., Marzec-Lewenstein, E., et al., 2007. Unusual movements, "spontaneous" breathing, and unclear cerebral vessels sonography in a brain-dead patient: A case report. *Transplantation Proceedings* 39(9): 2707–2708.

Byrne, P. 2008. "Brain death": Enemy of life and truth. *Renew America*, 25 June.

Byrne, P. A., O'Reilly, S., and Quay, P. M. 1979. Brain death: An opposing viewpoint. *JAMA* 242: 1985–1990.

Byrne, P. A., and Nilges, R. G. 1993. The brain stem in brain death: A critical review. *Issues in Law and Medicine* 9(1): 3–21.

Byrne, P. A., O'Reilly, S., Quay, P. M., and Salsich, P. 1982/83. Brain death: The patient, the physician, and society. *Gonzaga Law Review* 18, no. 3, 429–516.

Capron, A. M. 1987. Anencephalic donors: Separate the dead from the living. *Hastings Center Report* 17(1): 5–9.

Capron, A. M. 1993. The tell-tale heart: Public policy and the utilization of non-heart-beating donors. *Kennedy Institute of Ethics Journal* 3: 251–262.

Capron, A., and Kass, L. 1972. A statutory definition of the standards for determining human death: An appraisal and a proposal. *University of Pennsylvania Law Review* 121(1): 87–88, 102–118.

Chagas, C. (ed). 1986. *The Artificial Prolongation of Life and the Determination of the Exact Moment of Death*. Vatican City: Pontifical Academy of Sciences.

Conference of Medical Royal Colleges and their Faculties in the United Kingdom, 1995. Criteria for the diagnosis of brain stem death. *Journal of the Royal College of Physicians, London* 29: 381–382.

Conference of Medical Royal Colleges and Their Faculties in the United Kingdom, 1976. Diagnosis of brain death. *British Medical Journal* 2: 1187–1188.

Conference of Medical Royal Colleges and Their Faculties in the United Kingdom, 1979. Diagnosis of death. *British Medical Journal* 1: 332.

Döşemeci, L., Cengiz, M., Yilmaz, M., and Ramazanoglu, A. 2004. Frequency of spinal reflex movements in brain-dead patients. *Transplantation Proceedings* 36(1): 17–19.

Evans, D. W., and Hill, D. J. 1989. The brain stems of organ donors are not dead. *Catholic Medical Quarterly* 40(3): 113–120.

Gillett, G. R. 1986. Why let people die? *Journal of Medical Ethics* 12: 83–86.

Green, M. B., and Wikler, D. 1980. Brain death and personal identity. *Philosophy and Public Affairs* 9: 103–133.

Grisez, G., and Boyle, J. M. 1979. *Life and Death with Liberty and Justice. A Contribution to the Euthanasia Debate*. Notre Dame, IN: University of Notre Dame Press.

Hardacre, H. 1994. Response of Buddhism and Shinto to the issue of brain death and organ transplantation. *Cambridge Quarterly for Healthcare Ethics* 3: 585–601.

Harris, J. 1995. Euthanasia and the value of life. In John Keown (ed.), *Euthanasia Examined*. Cambridge: Cambridge University Press.

Hassler, R. 1977. Basal ganglia systems regulating mental activity. *International Journal of Neurology* 12: 53–72.

Iglesias, T. 1991. Death and the beginning of life. *Ethics and Medicine* 7(2): 8–17.

Jennett, B., and Plum, F. 1972. Persistent vegetative state after brain damage: A syndrome in search of a name. *The Lancet* 1 (April 1): 734–37.

Joffe, A. R., and Anton, N. R. 2007. Some questions about brain death: A case report. *Pediatric Neurology* 37(4): 289–291.

Jonas, H. 1974. Against the stream. In H. Jonas, *Philosophical Essays: From Ancient Creed to Technological Man*. Englewood Cliffs, NJ: Prentice-Hall.

Jones, D. A. 1995. Nagging doubts about brain death. *Catholic Medical Quarterly* 47(3): 263–273.

Jones, D. A. 2000. Metaphysical misgivings about brain death. In M. Potts, P. Byrne, and R. G. Nilges (eds.), *Beyond Brain Death: The Case Against Brain Based Criteria for Human Death*. Dordrecht, The Netherlands: Kluwer Academic Publishers.

Kaukinen, S., Mäkelä, K., Häkkinen, V. K., and Martikainen, K. 1995. Significance of electrical activity in brain-stem death. *Intensive Care Medicine* 21: 76–78.

Lamb, D. 1991. Death in Denmark. *Journal of Medical Ethics* 17: 100–101.

Lamb, D. 1994. What is death? In R. Gillon (ed.), *Principles of Health Care Ethics*. New York: John Wiley & Sons.

Laureys, S., Owen, A. M., and Schiff, N. D. 2004. Brain function in coma, vegetative state, and related disorders. *The Lancet Neurology* 3(9): 537–546.

Linos, K., Fraser, J., Freeman, W., and Foot, C. 2007. Care of the brain-dead organ donor. *Current Anaesthesia and Critical Care* 18(5–6): 284–294.

Lizza, J. P. 1993. Persons and death: What's metaphysically wrong with our current statutory definition of death? *Journal of Medicine and Philosophy* 18: 351–374.

Lynn, J. 1993. Are the patients who become organ donors under the Pittsburgh Protocol for "non-heart-beating donors" really dead? *Kennedy Institute of Ethics Journal* 3: 167–178.

Matthews, G. B. 1979. Life and death as the arrival and departure of the psyche. *American Philosophical Quarterly* 16: 151–156.

McCullagh, P. 1993. *Brain Dead, Brain Absent, Brain Donors*. New York: John Wiley & Sons.

McMahon, J. 1995. The metaphysics of brain death. *Bioethics* 9: 91–126.

Pallis, C. 1990. Return to Elsinore. *Journal of Medical Ethics* 16: 10–13.

Parfit, D. 1986. *Reasons and Persons*. Oxford: Oxford University Press.

Parisi, J. E., Kim, R. C., Collins, G. H., and Hilfinger, M. F. 1982. Brain death with prolonged somatic survival. *New England Journal of Medicine* 306: 14–16.

Pentz, R. D. 1994. Veatch and brain death: A plea for the soul. *Journal of Clinical Ethics* 5: 132–135.

President's Commission for the Study of Ethical Problems in Medicine and Biomedical and Behavioral Research. 1981. *Defining Death: Medical, Legal and Ethical Issues in the Determination of Death*. Washington, DC: U.S. Government Printing Office.

Puccetti, R. 1988. Does anyone survive neocortical death? In R. Zaner (ed.), *Death: Beyond Whole Brain Criteria*. Dordrecht, The Netherlands: Kluwer Academic Publishers.

Rothstein, J. 1995. Attending to transitions: A medical student's encounter with transplantation. *Making the Rounds in Health, Faith and Ethics* 1(4): 1–5.

Seifert, J. 1993. Is "brain death" actually death? *The Monist* 76: 173–202.

Sethi, N. K., Sethi, P., Torgovnick, J., Arsura, E., Schaul, N., and Labar, D. 2008. EMG artifact in brain death electroencephalogram, is it a cry of "medullary death"? *Clinical Neurology and Neurosurgery* 110(7): 729–731.

Shewmon, D. A. 1985. The metaphysics of brain death, persistent vegetative state and dementia. *The Thomist* 49(1): 24–80.

Shewmon, D. A. 1989. "Brain death": A valid theme with invalid variation, blurred by semantic ambiguity. In R. White, H. Angstwurm, and I. Carrasco de Paula (eds.), *Working Group on the Determination of Brain Death and Its Relationship to Human Death*. Vatican City: Pontifical Academy of Sciences.

Shewmon, D. A. 1997a. Recovery from "brain death": A neurologist's apologia. *Linacre Quarterly* 64: 30–96.

Shewmon, D. A. 1997b. Address given at the International Conference of the Linacre Centre for Healthcare Ethics, Cambridge.

Shewmon, D. A. 2001. The brain and somatic integration: Insights into the standard biological rationale for equating "brain death" with death. *Journal of Medicine and Philosophy* 26(5): 457–478.

Siminoff, L., Burant, C., and Youngner, S. J. 2004. Death and organ procurement: Public beliefs and attitudes. *Social Science and Medicine* 59(11): 2325–2334.

Singer, P. 1995a. Is the sanctity of life terminally ill? *Bioethics* 9: 327–343.

Singer, P. 1995b. *Rethinking Life and Death.* Oxford: Oxford University Press.

Steinberg, A. 1996. Definition of death. *Nephrology Dialysis Transplantation* 11: 961–963.

Linacre Centre for Health Care Ethics. 1994. Submission to the Select Committee of the House of Lords on Medical Ethics. In *Euthanasia: Clinical Practice and the Law.* London: Linacre Centre.

Tomlinson, T. 1984. The conservative use of the beam dead criterion: a critique. *Journal of Medicine and Philosophy* 9: 377–394.

Tomlinson, T. 1990. Misunderstanding death on a respirator. *Bioethics* 4: 253–264.

Tonti-Filippini, N. 1991. Determining when dead has occurred. *Linacre Quarterly* 58(1): 25–49.

Truog, R. D. 1997. Is it time to abandon brain death? *Hastings Center Report* 27(1): 29–37.

Veatch, R. M. 1993. The impending collapse of the whole-brain definition of death. *Hastings Center Report* 23(4): 18–24.

White, R., Angstwurm, H., and Carrasco de Paula, I. (eds.). 1989. *Working Group on the Determination of Brain Death and Its Relationship to Human Death.* Vatican City: Pontifical Academy of Sciences.

White, G. 2003. Intensive care nurses' perceptions of brain death. *Australian Critical Care* 16(1): 7–14.

Wiggins, D. 1980. *Sameness and Substance.* Oxford: Basil Blackwell.

Wikler, D. 1993. Brain death: A durable consensus? *Bioethics* 7: 239–246.

Wittgenstein, L. 1953. *Philosophical Investigations.* G. E. M. Anscombe (trans.). Oxford: Basil Blackwell.

Wreen, M. 1987. The definition of death. *Public Affairs Quarterly* 1(4): 87–99.

Youngner, S. J. 1992. Defining death: A superficial and fragile consensus. *Archives of Neurology* 49: 570–572.

Youngner, S. J., Allen, M., Bartlett, E. T., et al. 1985. Psychosocial and ethical implications of organ retrieval. *New England Journal of Medicine* 313: 321–324.

Youngner, S. J., Landefeld, C. S., Coulton, C. J., Juknialis, B. W., and Leary, M. 1989. "Brain death" and organ retrieval: A cross-sectional survey of knowledge and concepts among health professionals. *JAMA* 261(15): 2205–2210.

CHAPTER TWENTY-SEVEN

St. Thomas on the Beginning and Ending of Human Life

William A. Wallace

St. Thomas is well known for his teaching that the beginning of human life is a gradual process, that the human soul is not infused into the incipient organism at fertilization but rather is prepared for by a succession of forms that dispose the matter for the reception of a rational soul. Less well known is his speculation that the reverse process may occur at the ending of human life, namely, that the human soul may depart from the body before all signs of life have disappeared from it. There are sensible signs that processes like these might occur, for example, in the stages of "quickening" mothers feel when pregnant and in the gradual loss of faculties experienced by moribund individuals in the period before their death. Yet, until fairly recently, there was little medical information available that would lend support to such thinking. Thus it is commonly taught that human life in the most proper sense begins at fertilization, when the rational soul is infused into the body, and terminates at death, when the human soul departs from the body.

In this essay I sketch a few developments in medical science that encourage us to look again at St. Thomas's teaching on the beginning and ending of human life, not to make the point that his doctrines are perennially valid, but rather to stimulate our development of a natural philosophy along Aristotelian-Thomistic lines that is adequate to deal with problems now arising in embryology and neuroscience. Unfortunately, in recent times the philosophy of nature has languished within Thomism and has largely been replaced by a philosophy of science that is incapable of dealing with distinctively human problems, particularly those relating to the soul and its relation to the body. Natural philosophy is an integral part of the Thomistic synthesis and it would be a serious mistake to let it now fall by the wayside. Its neglect can only place in peril the more fashionable metaphysical themes that continue to attract attention in the present day.

St. Thomas's Teaching

With regard to human generation, Aquinas followed Aristotle in holding that the conception of a male child was not completed until the fortieth day after intercourse, whereas that of the female child lasted until the ninetieth day. The only instance of immediate conception he cites is that of Jesus Christ, on the basis that Christ's conception, unlike that of other humans, should not have to await the complete formation of his natural flesh. On this account Christ was conceived instantly by the divine power of the Holy Spirit, and thus in miraculous fashion (*In 3 Sent.*, d.3, q.5, a.2). For all others conception is a gradual process. Animation, of course, is immediate in the sense that a soul of some type is present as soon as the male's semen fertilizes the material provided by the female, but this is not a human soul at the outset. In its earliest stage it is a nutritive soul (*anima vegetativa*), which regulates the early growth of the embryo; when development is sufficient to support sensation, the nutritive soul is replaced by a sense soul (*anima sensitiva*); and this in turn is ultimately replaced by the human soul (*ST 1a*, q.118, a.1, ad 4). In this teaching Aquinas is simply following Aristotle's account in *On the Generation of Animals* (729a–744b). Aristotle recognizes that it is difficult to determine precisely when the rational soul comes to be present in the embryo and simply states that it comes from outside and is divine (*G.A.* 736b). St. Thomas picks up on this teaching and explicitly holds that the intellective soul (*anima intellectiva*) is created by God and infused into the embryo at the completion of the human's coming-to-be, and that this soul once present performs all the functions of previous forms in the incipient organism (*ST 1a*, q.118, a.2, ad 2). So, for him, this complete conception of the male child does not occur until after forty days, and that of the female until after ninety days, as just mentioned.[1]

An interesting feature of Aristotle's teaching on the earlier stages of animal generation is the role he assigns to the nutritive soul and the sense soul in the developmental process. In the case of the former, he assumes that the semen and the unfertilized embryo, while still separated from each other, already possess a nutritive soul, although they do so only potentially. Such an embryo thus lives the life of a plant, first with the mother drawing nourishment to it and then with the embryo beginning to nourish itself as a whole; when this second stage occurs the nutritive soul loses its potential status and comes to be present actually (*G.A.*, 736b). Similarly, at the onset of animal life the sense soul is present only potentially. For it to become actually present sense organs have to develop in the organism, and particularly the sense of touch, so that the embryo can experience sensation. Since there can be various degrees of sensation, moreover, and in the higher animals all of the sense organs have to be developed before a specific animal is produced, Aristotle held that the developing animal embryo first becomes an animal in general and then one of a particular type. The transition process can then occupy a considerable period of time. That serves to explain why the sensitive soul in the developing human, the animal with the most refined sense powers, requires at least forty days to reach complete actuality.

St. Thomas apparently subscribed to this aspect of Aristotle's teaching and in so doing introduced the concept of a transient entity, an *ens in via,* into the discussion. The text in which he does so occurs in *SCG 2,* c.89, where Aquinas is discussing the intermediate souls or substantial forms that function in the generation of higher animals and humans. The successive replacement of forms in these cases takes place by a series of natural generations and corruptions, and thus, when leading up to the human soul, the form which is most perfect (*forma perfectissima*), there will be found many intermediate forms and generations. These intermediates, St. Thomas writes, are not complete in species but are on the way (*in via*) to a determinate species, and thus they are not generated with a permanent status but only transiently, so that, through them, the ultimate species may be arrived at.[2]

Although St. Thomas is frequently cited for his advocacy of "delayed hominization," as it is now commonly called, little attention has been paid to the obverse of that process, what might be termed "early dehominization," where the human soul departs from the body at some period of time before all bodily functions have ceased. Aquinas gives indication that he endorsed this view of the ending of human life, although he does not seem to have developed his thought on that subject. The text in which he does so is his exposition of Proposition

1 of the *Liber de causis,* where he compares what happens in the generation of a human being with what happens at corruption. He writes: "For it is obvious that in the generation of an individual human being one finds in the material subject first existence, then the living thing and after that a human; for it is an animal before it is a man, as is said in the second book of *On the Generation of Animals.* And again, in the process of corruption, first [the individual] loses the use of reason and remains alive and breathing, then it loses life and remains a being, because it does not corrupt into nothingness."[3] Although this statement occurs in a commentary where St. Thomas is exposing the thought of the author of *De causis,* it seems that here he is speaking in his own voice. He clearly understands Aristotle's teaching on delayed hominization, and applies the reverse process, without objection, to suggest at least the possibility of early dehominization.

Hominization

All of this discussion, it goes without saying, took place in a thought context where nothing was known about cells or of the existence of ova and spermatazoa, where the microscope was more than three hundred years off, and molecular biology yet another three hundred years or so after that. Only within the past few decades, however, have substantial advances been made in embryology, and so now we stand at the apex of a development taking place over many centuries that awaits translation into the philosophical language of Aristotle and Aquinas. One way of effecting this translation is to focus on the concept of nature, first as instantiated in human nature, and then in the various natural kinds found in the world of nature—animals, plants, minerals, and the elements from which all of these are constituted. Aristotle defined nature as a principle within bodies that initiates their characteristic activities and reactivities, and identified it with the basic matter of which they are composed, but more properly with the form that energizes that matter and stabilizes these bodies as substances (*Physics,* 193ab). This latter was called substantial form within the Aristotelian tradition, but for purposes here it is better referred to as natural form, because it is by it that a thing's nature is known. Natural forms are immediately intelligible: if we know what a cat is, or what an oak is, or what sulphur is, and are able to define these, it is because we have grasped their natures and have come to know them through their natural forms.[4]

The natures of objects of ordinary experience seem relatively unproblematic, but natures prove difficult to grasp when we move into the realm of the very small. Atoms and molecules went undetected for centuries, and the vast number of subatomic particles that have recently been detected defy attempts at clear understanding. One may speak of the nature of water or iron, but does it make sense to attribute a nature to an electron, or a neutron, or a proton? Although these are entities to which we assign physical existence, they do not seem to be intelligible as wholes or subsistent entities, but rather as parts that enter into the composition of other things. Moreover, most subatomic particles are either charged or radioactive: if the first, they can be quickly attracted to, and absorbed into, the being of another entity; if the second, while being what they are they are already breaking down into something else. Having granted them physical existence, one would be hesitant to exclude them entirely from the world of nature, but at the same time it would not seem necessary to attribute to them stable natures such as are found in the macroscopic objects of ordinary experience. To the extent that they have natures, these are perhaps best thought of as transient natures, the type found in transient entities or *entia vialia,* beings only "on the way" or becoming, not existing or subsisting in their own right.

Pursuant to this line of reasoning, the findings of modern science would indicate that transient natures play a more important part in the universe than hitherto expected, certainly far beyond the role attributed them by St. Thomas. According to the "Big Bang" theory of its origin, evidences of which are still discernible at the edges of our expanding universe, subatomic particles were the first entities to appear and have continued to play a key role in the evolution of stars and galaxies. Immediately after creation there was an extremely brief period of elementary particle activity at very high energies; then came a longer period for the formation of chemical elements and compounds, from which stars and planets were formed some five billion years ago; then periods of biogenesis during which were produced, at least on the planet Earth, the plants and animals inhabiting its surface; and finally the period of hominization, the culmination of biogenesis, when *homo sapiens* was created by God and the human race made its first appearance.

To translate this sequence into the language of natures, and also to incorporate both creation and evolution within it, we propose to indicate a natural form by the letters NF, then add to it subscripts to designate different types of natures—"t" for transient, "i" for inorganic, "p" for plant, "a" for animal, and "h" for human, and to represent a creative act with a double-shafted arrow and an evolutionary process with a single-shafted arrow. The sequence described above then may be written as follows:

$$0 \gg NF_t > NF_i > NF_p > NF_a \gg NF_h \qquad (1)$$

The idea is that from nothing (*ex nihilo*), indicated by the zero (0) at the far left, God created the primordial matter that exploded into a universe of elementary particles, here designated as entities with transient natures (NF_t). From these, over time and still under the causal action of the First Agent, the chemical substances we know as elements and compounds were educed from the potency of protomatter, all of these possessing stable inorganic natures (NF_i). Then, by a steady process of evolution under the divine causality, when proper conditions were realized first plant natures (NF_p) and then animal natures (NF_a) emerged into being, as selected regions of the universe came to be populated with the higher forms of flora and fauna. Finally, at the last stage, when all was ready for the most perfect form to appear, a new creative initiative on God's part was required. This is shown by the second arrow with a double shaft, here indicating the direct creation of the human soul (NF_h). The natural processes of evolution may be sufficient to bring organisms to a level just below that of thought and volition, but of themselves they cannot progress to the final stage. God himself must complete the process, producing *ex nihilo* the human soul, tailored to match the ultimate disposition of matter as this has been prepared, over billion of years, for its reception. And this creative act, according to Catholic teaching, would be repeated each time throughout the centuries that a new human person came into existence, with its matter being likewise disposed, through the procreative action of the human parents, to receive an individual, incommunicable, and immortal soul.

According to this model, transient natures were involved in the formation of the universe, cosmogenesis, as it is currently understood. It remains now to see how such natures may be involved in the generation of organisms. One way of doing this is to update St. Thomas's medieval view of plant generation and express it in a notation similar to that used in formula (1). For this we continue to designate a plant nature by NF_p, but now add additional subscripts to indicate the parent plant and its offspring as well as the intermediate nature that effects the transition between the two. The new subscripts are the following: "pP" refers to the parent plant, "pO" to the offspring, numerically different from the parent but pertaining to the same species, and "pT" to the transient plant-like nature of the seed during its development. Then we have:

$$NF_{pP} > NF_{pT} > NF_{pO} \tag{2}$$

The agency involved in the first transition, from NF_{pP} to NF_{pT}, is a natural agency associated with the powers of a plant nature. Chemical materials are absorbed by the parent organism through its powers of nutrition, growth, and reproduction to form the genetic materials contained in the seed. Then, after separation from the parent, a form of life persists in the seed. This begins its own internal development through the incipient plant-like form, NF_{pT}, which St. Thomas referred to as an "active force" (*vis activa*) that gives it a plant nature "according to first act" (*secundum actum primum*) though it is not yet a form in the full sense (*ST 1a*, q.118, a.1, ad 3 & ad 4). This suffices to draw nourishment to the incipient organism and direct its growth until its quantitative parts are sufficiently articulated to sustain a stable, individual plant nature of the species. At that point a new plant form, NF_{pO}, is educed from the potentiality of matter, and a new individual of the species has been produced.[5]

The generation of a human individual is obviously more complex, but for St. Thomas it proceeds along analogous lines. Here again we would update his medieval account by importing into it information from modern embrylogical research, the details of which cannot be explained in this brief account.[6] We employ the same notation as heretofore, using subscripts similar to those in formula (2), with the subscript "hP" now referring to the human parent at the beginning of the process and the subscript "hO" to the human offspring at the end. In this case two transient natures are required, one plant-like, represented by the subscript "pT," the other animal-like, represented by the subscript "aT." The formula for human generation may then be written as follows:

$$2NF_{hP} > nNF_{pT} > mNF_{aT} \gg 1NF_{hO} \tag{3}$$

This formula is similar to (2) but is definitely more complex. As before, the subscript "hP" refers to the human parents at the beginning of the process and the subscript "hO" to the human offspring at the end. Since human generation is bisexual, the process starts with two mature human souls or natures (indicated by the "2" preceding the NF_{hP}), one female and the other male, and it terminates in one human offspring (indicated by the "1" preceding the NF_{hO}), since we are not now considering the production of twins. The double-shaft on the last arrow shows that the soul of the offspring is created directly by God, although the organic materials suitable for the soul's reception have been procreated by the parents.

The intermediate stages are symbolized by the two intermediate terms representing two transient natures, one plant-like, designated by subscript "pT," the other animal-like, represented by subscript "aT." But note here that a small "n" and a small "m" have been prefixed to the two symbols so as to number these types of genetic material. In the normal case and in our modern understanding, the process starts with two seeds (n=2), an egg and a sperm cell, although there might be more than one sperm if multiple births were being discussed. They combine to form a unicellular zygote, but that cell quickly divides and sub-divides to form a complex cell mass that grows and nourishes in a way analo-gous to plant life—hence the subscript "pT." In later stages of development this embryonic human develops organs of sensation and movement and so mani-fests the characteristics of animal life—hence the subscript "aT." Note again the "m" before the term NF_{aT}. Recent embryological studies have shown that the number "m" is not necessarily the same as the number "n," whatever that might be, nor is it necessarily the "1" that precedes the individual human offspring, $1NF_{hO}$. The initial cell mass is apparently made up of pluripotential cells that are not predetermined as to the number of organisms it will eventually produce. Twinning can take place during its development and, what is even more un-usual, recombination can take place where splitting had previously occurred. Thus it is not always the case that n=2 and m=2, as one might expect. What starts out as apparently one organism might end up as two or more, and what starts out as two or more might end up as one.

When can one be sure that twinning or recombination will no longer occur and that the developing embryo has become irreversibly individual? Empirical evidence suggests that this occurs at the beginning of the third week after fer-tilization, when the "primitive streak" first appears in the embryo. Through this streak the cells of the embryo first become organized "into one whole multicel-lular individual living human being, possessing for the first time a body axis and bilateral symmetry" (Ford, p. 172). The appearance of one primitive streak thus signals that only one embryo proper (and thus a human individual) has been formed and begun to exist. At this time the embryo "becomes one living body, informed or actuated by a human form, life-principle or soul that arises through the creative power of God" (ibid.).

This extraordinary finding provides strong confirmation of St. Thomas's view that transient natures continue to inform the incipient human organism for some time after the initial formation of the zygote. If God had created the human soul and infused it into the zygote at fertilization, then a stable individual of human nature would already have been formed. And, were another individual to be formed subsequent to that time, this would be an instance of asexual genera-tion—a type of generation found in lower forms but not proper to humans. The phenomena of twinning and recombination therefore give unexpected support to St. Thomas's teaching that unstable natures, that is, transient natures, continue to inform the developing organism until such time as the proper dispositions are at hand for the irreversible formation of an individual human being. Only at that moment does God create a new soul, a substantial form that has a transcendental order to the matter so prepared for it, and infuse this intellectual soul into such matter, with the result that a new human person finally comes into being.

Dehominization

St. Thomas's suggestion that the human soul might depart from the body at some time previous to the cessation of various life signs, such as heartbeat in his day and brain death in our own, has not received as much consideration as his views on hominization. Two recent developments, however, bear on the account of dehominization he gives in his commentary on the *Liber de causis* and encourage us to give a closer look at the ending of human life. The first is a proposal from a neurophysiologist, Dr. Alan Shewmon, who has been studying brain death, persistent vegetative state, and dementia and speculating about the relevance of Thomistic concepts to their solution.[7] The other is an analysis of human death and dying provided by Mieczysaw A. Krpiec, O.P., a philosopher who, along with Karol Wojtya (Pope John Paul II), pioneered the movement known as Lublin Thomism and from its phenomenological perspective has been doing research in anthropology.[8]

Shewmon takes his point of departure from hypothetical brain-vat experiments wherein a human body is reduced to a brain alone, floating in a warm solution and connected to various machines that replace its normal body functions. This type of thought experiment is used by Shewmon to inquire into the minimum part of the human body that is capable of supporting the human essence. The conclusion he comes to is that the brain is the critical structure for sustaining the human soul and mediating consciousness. If it were removed from the body by a skillful neurosurgeon, the organism's condition would be that of a brainless vegetative substance, the same as that of a person who has suffered total brain death. If still connected to life support systems, moreover, even though the cerebral cortex had been removed, as long as the brainstem was left intact the body need not die but could still be maintained in a vegetative state. On the other hand, if such systems were disconnected from the floating brain, the brain would die and with it the person, because the spiritual soul would leave the body at brain death.[9]

The case of dementia is more difficult to analyze, for it requires determining not only when irreversible damage had been done to the cerebral cortex but also pinpointing the specific part of the cortex that is necessary for the functioning of the human intellect and will. This part, which Shewmon sees as also essential for the functioning of the cogitative sense (*vis cogitativa*), he locates in the "tertiary association area" of the cortex. When this part is destroyed the human person dies and the rational soul departs, leaving only a humanoid animal body behind.[10]

Shewmon does not make explicit use of the concept of transient natures in his analysis of dehominization, but he does invoke a Thomistic concept that is closely related to it, namely, that of virtual presence. In his view, as in St. Thomas's, the spiritual soul contains virtually all the powers of animal and vegetative souls, and thus these souls may be said to be virtually present in the person. Should the right material dispositions be present, these souls can become actualized. For example, structural damage to critical parts of the brain may be so severe that it forces a substantial change and results in the death of the person. Then the human soul leaves the body and a new soul is educed from the potency of matter: in severe instances of dementia this will be a sense soul, in instances of irreversible persistent vegetative states, a nutritive soul alone.

Shewmon's analysis may now be summed up in formula (4), which turns out to be almost the obverse of our previous formulas:

$$NF_h > NF_{aT} > NF_{pT} > NF_i \tag{4}$$

Human cogitation is so dependent on the brain that, if the areas of the brain that are used by the cogitative sense for its operations are impaired or removed, they will cease to be informed by the human soul, which will be replaced by an animal soul virtually contained within the human. Expressed in the language of natures, in such a case human nature, NF_h, degenerates into a transient animal-like nature, NF_{aT}, and the individual shows the symptoms of dementia. If further deterioration takes place, such that the cerebral cortex no longer functions and only the brainstem remains intact, the transient animal-like nature gives way to a transient plant-like nature, NF_{pT}, and the individual passes into the persistent vegetative state. And finally, when life signs cease altogether, not even this transient nature can be sustained in the organism and the body corrupts completely into inorganic matter, NF_i, the "dust of the earth" from which it originally came.

Possibly because of his use of the "brain-vat" scenario, Shewmon may be viewed as writing science fiction and his thought dismissed as far-fetched speculation.

This need not be the case, however, particularly when his ideas are taken up in the philosophical context provided by Father Krpiec. In discussing the death of a human person Krpiec makes a distinction between physical death, the cessation of life signs when the soul is thought to leave the body, which he calls "physical death," and death "understood actively," that is, death as a real experience of the human spirit.[11] The latter experience occurs at the moment when the person becomes capable of making a final decision about life, a moment that represents the culmination of all the changeable acts performed during the entire span of bodily existence. Active death, Krpiec argues, is a transtemporal experience that takes place in the realm of the spirit and beyond the point at which the individual can return to the temporal and changeable condition of earthly life.[12] Thus, it does not coincide with the co-activity of the body. The implication is that the human soul at the moment of active death has already departed from the body and subsists as an individual substance.

If one grants the absence of brain activity in the personal experience of death, one may draw a further corollary. According to St. Thomas's theory of knowledge, all human knowing in the state of union with the body occurs by reflection on phantasms (*ST 1a*, q.84, a.7), which are produced by the cogitative power through the intermediary of various brain states. As long as the soul operates with phantasms, it can make changes through its higher powers of intellect and will, and it does not reach the point of ultimate decision. Conversely, at the moment in time when phantasmal activity ceases, these changes are no longer possible and the individual's rational life is over. If the intellect and will function later, they do so as separated substances and not as operative powers of a natural body. In other words, the person's truly human and changeable existence is ended, and the human soul, precisely as human, ceases to have any proper function it can exercise in the body.

If this analysis is correct, and the body continues to manifest vital activities, it probably does so as a humanoid organism. The body is specifically human, and thus should be classified under the human species, but it no longer possesses a stable human nature and will gradually decline and decay. Its life functions in this state can be seen as those of a transient nature, human in origin but sensory and vegetative in actual operation. There is therefore a succession of substantial forms in the humanoid organism, and the overall dying process can aptly be referred to as one of dehominization.

This surprising conclusion based on the work of Shewmon and Krpiec reinforces our earlier reasoning about transient natures based on the work of Ford, Pastrana, and others. When the two strains of thought relating to hominization and dehominization are put together, they constitute a strong counter-argument to those who would maintain that Thomism is dead, that it is a fossilized, archaic body of teaching, of antiquarian interest only, of no possible application in our miracle age of science and technology. Quite the opposite is true, and particularly in fields of knowledge relating to a Thomistic philosophy of nature and of science. Problems of greatest importance for human life are now awaiting solution: what to do at the beginning of life—contraception, "choice," *in vitro* fertilization, frozen embryos, surrogate motherhood, abortion directly or indirectly procured; what to do at the end of life—dementia, persistent vegetative state, "when to pull the plugs," a question increasingly being asked in hospitals. St. Thomas obviously has much to contribute to the solution of such problems. But there is another side of the coin. The philosophy of nature and of science has been much neglected in the recent Thomistic tradition. This is a difficult field of study, one in which much work needs to be done, particularly in applying hylomorphic concepts to natural processes at the micro-level, for example, carrying the discussion of the "dispositions of matter" beyond the point it had reached in the thirteenth century. Problems relating to natures and transient natures have been broached in this essay, as have those relating to individuation and cogitation, but no claim can be made that the answers given are definitive.[13] New empirical data are constantly being made available, and unfortunately they are much more readily accessed than is a philosophical tradition that has been developing over seven centuries. Yet there is still much to be harvested in that tradition. Perhaps the stimulus provided by new discoveries in the physical and biological sciences will serve as a catalyst to our uncovering more of the riches that are there contained.

NOTES

1. St. Thomas goes into further detail on the process of human generation in four places: *In 2 Sent.*, d.18, q.2, aa.1,3; *Summa contra gentiles 2*, cc. 86–89; *De potentia*, q.3, aa.9–12; and *ST 1a*, q.118. All of these texts are analyzed by Michael A. Taylor in his "Human Generation in the Thought of Thomas Aquinas: A Case Study on the Role of Biological Fact in Theological Science" (S.T.D. diss., The Catholic University of America, 1981). A more extensive analysis that relates Thomas's teaching to studies in modern embryology is Norman M. Ford, *When did I begin? Conception of the human individual in history, philosophy and science* (Cambridge: Cambridge University Press, 1989), pp. 19–64.

2. The Latin here reads as follows: "Nec est inconveniens si aliquid intermediorum generatur et statim postmodum interrumpitur: quia intermedia non habent speciem completam, sed sunt in via ad speciem; et ideo non generantur ut permaneant, sed ut

per ea ad ultimum generatum perveniatur." In a following paragraph Aquinas spells out in more detail what he means by these intermediates: "Quanto igitur aliqua forma est nobilior et magis distans a forma elementi, tanto oportet esse plures formas intermedias, quibus gradatim ad formam ultimam veniatur, et per consequens plures generationes medias. Et ideo in generatione animalis et hominis in quibus est forma perfectissima, sunt plurimae formae et generationes intermediae, et per consequens corruptiones, quia generation unius est corruptio alterius. Anima igitur vegetabilis, quae primo inest, cum embryo vivit vita plantae, corrumpitur, et succedit anima perfectior, quae est nutritiva et sensitiva simul, et tunc embryo vivit vita animalis; hac autem corrupta, succedit animal rationalis ab extrinseco immisa, licet praecedentes fuerint virtute seminis."

3. "Manifestum est autem in generatione unius particularis hominis quod in materiali subiecto primo invenitur esse, deinde invenitur vivum, postmodum autem est homo; prius enim ipse est animal quam homo, ut dicitur in secundo *De generatione animalium*. Rursumque in via corruptionis primo amittit usum rationis et remanet vivum et spirans, secundo amittit <vitam> et remanet ipsum ens, quia non corrumpitur in nihilum"— *Super librum De causis expositio*, ed. H. D. Saffrey (Fribourg: Société Philosophique; Louvain: Editions E. Nauwelaerts, 1954), p. 6.

4. For a fuller explanation of these difficult concepts, see W. A. Wallace, "The Intelligibility of Nature: A Neo-Aristotelian View," *The Review of Metaphysics*, 38 (1984), pp. 33–56, and "Nature as Animating: The Soul in the Human Sciences," *The Thomist*, 49 (1985), pp. 612–648.

5. For details, see Taylor, "Human Generation," pp. 273–326, for the passages in the *Summa* in which this process is described. Apparently St. Thomas explained the process somewhat differently in each of the four places in which he discusses it, depending on the biological authority he was using at the time. Probably the fullest treatment is that in *De potentia,* analyzed by Taylor on pp. 223–266, where Thomas makes more use of medical terminology deriving from Avicenna than in the other places. One text that is particularly helpful is *De potentia,* q.3, a.12, which reads as follows: "Secundum quod Philosophus probat in XV *De animalibus,* semen non deciditur ab eo quod fuit actu pars, sed quod fuit superfluum ultimae digestionis; quod nondum erat ultima assimilatione assimilatum. Nulla autem corporis pars est actu per animam perfecta, nisi sit ultima assimilatione assimilata; unde semen ante decisionem nondum erat perfectum per animam, ita quod anima esset forma eius; erat tamen ibi aliqua virtus, secundum quam iam per actionem animae erat alteratum et deductum ad dispositionem propinquam ultimae assimilationi; unde et postquam decisum est, non est ibi anima, sed aliqua virtus animae" (Marietti ed., p. 77).

6. The essentials are provided by Norman Ford, *When did I begin?*, pp. 65–182, but see also Gabriel Pastrana, O.P., "Personhood and the Beginning of Human Life," *The Thomist*, 41 (1977), pp. 247–294; A. P. Smith, O.P., "Transient Natures at the Edges of Human Life: A Thomistic Exploration," *The Thomist*, 54 (1990), pp. 191–227; and W. A. Wallace, O.P., "Nature and Human Nature as the Norm in Medical Ethics," *Catholic Perspectives on Medical Morals*, ed. E. D. Pellegrino et al., Dordrecht: Kluwer, 1989, pp. 25–53.

7. See his "The Metaphysics of Brain Death, Persistent Vegetative State, and Dementia," *The Thomist*, 49 (1985), pp. 24–80; also his "Ethics and Brain Death: A Response," *The New Scholasticism*, 61 (1987), pp. 321–344.

8. See his *I-Man: An Outline of Philosophical Anthropology*, translated by Marie Lescoe et al. and abridged by F. J. Lescoe and R. B. Duncan (New Britain, Conn.: Mariel Publications, 1985), pp. 166–186.

9. Shewmon writes, "It should therefore be equally evident that, in the natural context, a person will die (and his spiritual soul will leave the body) the moment his brain dies, irrespective of whether the rest of the body maintains some vegetative integrity of not."—"The Metaphysics of Brain Death," p. 47; see also pp. 44–48.

10. Ibid., pp. 52–60.

11. In his *I-Man: An Outline of Philosophical Anthropology*, pp. 177–178.

12. Ibid., p. 179.

13. For a fuller exposition, see W. A. Wallace, "Aquinas's Legacy on Individuation, Cogitation, and Hominization," *Thomas Aquinas and His Legacy*, ed. D. M. Gallagher (Washington, D.C.: The Catholic University of America Press, 1994), pp. 173–193, which carries forward his investigations in "Nature, Human Nature, and the Norm in Medical Ethics." See also his *The Modeling of Nature: Philosophy of Science Based on a Philosophy of Nature in Synthesis*, (Washington, D.C.: The Catholic University of America Press, 1997).

CHAPTER TWENTY-EIGHT

The Impending Collapse of the Whole-Brain Definition of Death

Robert M. Veatch

For many years there has been lingering doubt, at least among theorists, that the currently fashionable "whole-brain-oriented" definition of death has things exactly right. I myself have long resisted the term "brain death" and will use it only in quotation marks to indicate the still common, if ambiguous, usage. The term is ambiguous because it fails to distinguish between the biological claim that the brain is dead and the social/legal/moral claim that the individual as a whole is dead because the brain is dead. An even greater problem with the term arises from the lingering doubt that individuals with dead brains are really dead. Hence, even physicians are sometimes heard to say that the patient "suffered brain death" one day and "died" the following day. It is better to say that he "died" on the first day, the day the brain was determined to be dead, and that the cadaver's other bodily functions ceased the following day. For these reasons I insist on speaking of persons with dead brains as individuals who are dead, not merely persons who are "brain dead."

The presently accepted standard definition, the Uniform Determination of Death Act, specifies that an individual is dead who has sustained "irreversible cessation of all functions of the entire brain, including the brain stem."[1] It also provides an alternative definition specifying that an individual is also dead who has sustained "irreversible cessation of circulatory and respiratory functions." The President's Commission for the Study of Ethical Problems in Medicine and Biomedical and Behavioral Research made clear, however, that circulatory and respiratory function loss are important only as indirect indicators that the brain has been permanently destroyed (p. 74).

Doubts about the Whole-Brain-Oriented Definition

It is increasingly apparent, however, that this consensus is coming apart. As long ago as the early 1970s some of us doubted that literally the entire brain had to be dead for the individual as a whole to be dead.[2]

From the early years it was known, at least among neurologists and theorists who read the literature, that individual, isolated brain cells could be perfused and continue to live even though integrated supercellular brain function had been destroyed. When the uniform definition of death said *all functions of the entire brain* must be dead, there was a gentleman's agreement that cellular level functions did not count. The President's Commission recognized this, positing that "cellular activity alone is irrelevant" (p. 75). This willingness to write off cellular level functions is more controversial than it may appear. After all, the law does not grant a dispensation to ignore cellular level functions, no matter how plausible that may be. Keep in mind that critics of soon-to-be-developed higher brain definitions of death would need to emphasize that the model statute called for loss of *all* functions.

By 1977 an analogous problem arose regarding electrical activity. The report of a multicenter study funded by the National Institutes of Neurological Diseases and Stroke found that all of the functions it considered important could be lost irreversibly while very small (2 microvolt) electrical potentials could still be obtained on EEG. These were not artifact but real electrical activity from brain cells. Nevertheless, the committee concluded that there could be "electrocerebral silence" and therefore the brain could be considered "dead" even though these small electrical charges could be recorded.[3]

It is possible that the members of the committee believed that these were the result of nothing more than cellular level functions, so that the same reasoning that permitted the President's Commission to write off little functions as unimportant would apply. However, no evidence was presented that these electrical potentials were arising exclusively from cellular level functions. It could well be that the reasoning in this report expanded the existing view that cellular functions did not count to the view that some minor supercellular functions could be ignored as long as they were small.

More recently the neurologist James Bernat, a defender of the whole-brain-oriented definition of death, has acknowledged that:

> the bedside clinical examination is not sufficiently sensitive to exclude the possibility that small nests of brain cells may have survived . . . and that their continued functioning, although not contributing significantly to the functioning of the organism as a whole, can be measured by laboratory techniques. Because these isolated nests of neurons no longer contribute to the functioning of the organism as a whole, their continued functioning is now irrelevant to the dead organism.[4]

The idea that functions of "isolated nests of neurons" can remain when an individual is declared dead based on whole-brain-oriented criteria certainly stretches the plain words of the law that requires, without qualification, that *all functions of the entire brain* must be gone. That exceptions can be granted by individual private citizens based on their personal judgments about which functions are "contributing significantly" certainly challenges the integrity of the idea that the whole brain must be dead for the individual as a whole to be dead.

There is still another problem for those who favor what can now be called the "whole-brain definition of death." It is not altogether clear that the "death of the brain" is to be equated with the "irreversible loss of function." At least one paper appears to hold out not only for loss of function but also for destruction of anatomical structure.[5] Thus we are left with a severely nuanced and qualified whole-brain-oriented definition of death. For it to hold as applied in the 1990s, one must assume that function rather than structure is irreversibly destroyed and that not only can certain cellular-level functions and microvolt-level electrical functions be ignored as "insignificant," but also certain "nests of cells" and associated supercellular-level functions can as well.

By the time the whole-brain-oriented definition of death is so qualified, it can hardly be referring to the death of the whole brain any longer. What is particularly troublesome is that private citizens—neurologists, philosophers, theologians, and public commentators—seem to be determining just which brain functions are insignificant.

The Higher-Brain-Oriented Alternative

The problem is exacerbated when one reviews the early "brain death" literature. Writers trying to make the case for a brain-based definition of death over a heart-based one invariably pointed out that certain functions were irreversibly lost when the brain was gone. Then, implicitly or explicitly, they made the moral/philosophical/religious claim that individuals who have irreversibly lost these key functions should be treated as dead.

While this function-based defense of a brain-oriented definition of death served the day well, some of us realized that the critical functions cited were not randomly distributed throughout the brain. For instance, Henry Beecher, the chair of the Harvard Ad Hoc Committee, identified the following functions as critical: "the individual's personality, his conscious life, his uniqueness, his capacity for remembering, judging, reasoning, acting, enjoying, worrying, and so on."[6]

Of course, all these functions are known to require the cerebrum. If these are the important functions, the obvious question is why any lower brain functions would signal the presence of a living individual. This gave rise to what is now best called the *higher-brain-oriented definition of death:* that one is dead when there is irreversible loss of all "higher" brain functions.[7] At first this was referred to as a cerebral or a cortical definition of death, but it seems clear that just as some brain stem functions may be deemed insignificant, likewise, some functions in the cerebrum may be as well. Moreover, it is not clear that the functions of the kind Beecher listed are always necessarily localized in the cerebrum or the cerebral cortex. At least in theory someday we may be able to build an artificial neurological organ that could replace some functions of the cerebrum. Someone who was thinking, feeling, reasoning, and carrying on a conversation through the use of an artificial brain would surely be recognized as alive even if the cerebrum that it had replaced was long since completely dead. I have preferred the purposely ambiguous term "higher brain function," as a way to make clear that the key philosophical issue is which of the many brain functions are really important.

Although that way of putting the question may offend the defenders of the more traditional whole-brain definition of death, once they have made the move of excluding the cellular, electrical, and supercellular functions they consider "insignificant," they are hardly in a position to complain about the project of sorting functions into important and unimportant ones.

Criticisms of the Higher Brain Formulations

Several defenders of the whole-brain-oriented concept have claimed that defining death in terms of loss of certain significant brain functions involves a change in the concept of death. This, however, rests on the implausible claim of Alex

Capron, the executive director of the President's Commission, that the move from a heart-oriented to a whole-brain-oriented definition of death is not a change in concept at all, but merely the recognition of new diagnostic measures for the traditional concept of death (p. 41). It is very doubtful, however, that the move to a whole-brain-oriented concept of death is any less of a fundamental change in concept than movement to a higher-brain-oriented one. From the beginning of the debate many people with beating hearts and dead brains would have been alive under the traditional concept of death focusing on fluid flow, but are clearly dead based on a then-newer whole-brain-oriented concept. Most understood this as a significant change in concept. In any case, even if there is a greater change in moving to a definition of death that identifies certain functions of the brain as significant, the mere fact that it is a conceptual change should not count against it. Surely, the critical question is which concept is right, not which concept squares with traditional views.

A second major charge against the higher-brain-oriented formulations has been that we are unable to measure precisely the irreversible loss of these higher functions based on current neurophysiological techniques (p. 40). By contrast it has been assumed that the irreversible loss of all functions of the entire brain is measurable based on current techniques.

Although lay people generally do not realize it, the measurement of death based on any concept can never be 100 percent accurate. The greatest error rates have certainly been with the heart-oriented concepts of death. Many patients have been falsely determined to have irreversibly lost heart functions. In earlier days we simply did not have the capacity to measure precisely. Even today there may be no reason to determine precisely whether the heart could be restarted in the case of a terminally ill, elderly patient who is ready to die.

There is even newly found ambiguity in the notion of irreversibility.[8] We are moving rapidly toward the day when organs for transplant will be obtained from non-heart-beating cadavers who have been determined to be dead based on heart function loss. It will be important for death to be pronounced as quickly as possible after the heart function has been found irreversibly lost. It is not clear, however, whether death should be pronounced when the heart has permanently stopped (say, following a decision based on an advance directive to withdraw a ventilator), but could be started again. In the minutes when it could be started, but will not be because the patient has refused resuscitation, can we say that the individual is dead?

Likewise, it is increasingly clear that we must acknowledge some, admittedly very small, risk of error in measuring the irreversible loss of all functions of the entire brain. Alan Shewmon has argued that the determination of the death of the entire brain cannot be made with as great a certainty as some neurologists would claim.[9] Some neurologists have persisted in claiming that brains are dead (or have irreversibly lost all function) even though electrical function still remains.[10] Clearly, brains with electrical function must have some living tissues; claims these brains are dead must rest on the assumption that remaining functions are insignificant.

None of this should imply that the death of the brain cannot be measured with great accuracy. But it is wrong to assume that similar or greater levels of accuracy cannot be obtained in measuring the irreversible loss of key higher functions, including consciousness. The literature on the persistent vegetative state repeatedly claims that we can know with great accuracy that consciousness is irreversibly lost.[11] The AMA's Councils on Scientific Affairs and Ethical and Judicial Affairs have concluded that the diagnosis can be made with an error rate of less than one in a thousand.[12] In fact the President's Commission itself said that "the Commission was assured that physicians with experience in this area can reliably determine that some patients' loss of consciousness is permanent."[13]

Even if we could not presently measure accurately the loss of key higher functions such as consciousness, that would have a bearing only on the clinical implementation of the higher-brain-oriented definition, not the validity of the concept itself. Defenders of the higher brain formulation might continue to use the now old-fashioned measures of loss of all function, but only because of the assurance that if all functions are lost, the higher functions certainly are. Such a conservative policy would leave open the question of whether we could some day measure the loss of higher functions accurately enough to use the measures clinically.

Still another criticism is the claim that any higher brain formulation would rely on a concept of personhood or personal identity that is philosophically controversial (pp. 38–39). Personhood theories are notoriously controversial. It is simply wrong, however, to claim that any higher-brain-oriented concept of death is based on either personhood or personal identity theories. I, for one, have acknowledged the possibility that there are living human beings who do not satisfy the various concepts of personhood. As long as the law is only discussing whether someone is a living individual, the debate over personhood is irrelevant.

Perhaps the most serious charge against the higher-brain-oriented formulations is that they are susceptible to the so-called slippery slope argument.[14] Once one yields on the insistence that all functions of the entire brain must be irreversibly gone before an individual is considered dead, there seems to be no stopping the slide of eliminating functions considered insignificant. The argument posits that once totally and permanently unconscious individuals who have some other brain functions (such as brain stem reflexes) remaining are considered dead, someone will propose that those with only marginal consciousness similarly lack significant function and soon all manner of functionally compromised humans will be defined as dead. Since being labelled dead is normally an indicator that certain moral and legal rights cease, such a slide toward considering increasing numbers of marginally functional humans as dead would be morally horrific.

But is the slippery slope argument plausible? In its most significant form, such an argument involves a claim that the same principle underlying one apparently tolerable judgment also entails other, clearly unacceptable judgments. For example, imagine we were trying to determine whether the elderly could be excluded from access to certain health care services based on the utilitarian principle of choosing the course that produced the maximum aggregate good for society. The slippery slope argument might be used to show that the same principle entails implications presumed clearly unacceptable, such as excluding health care from the socially unproductive. To the extent that one is certain that the empirical assumptions are correct (for example, that the utilitarian principle does entail excluding care from the unproductive) and one is confident that such an outcome would be morally unacceptable, then one might attempt to use slippery slope arguments to challenge the proposal to withhold health care from the elderly. The same principle used to support one policy also entails other policies that are clearly unacceptable.

The slippery slope argument is valid insofar as it shows that the principle used to support one policy under consideration entails clearly unacceptable implications when applied to different situations. In principle, there is no difference between the small, potentially tolerable move and the more dramatic, unacceptable move. However, as applied to the definition of death debate, the slippery slope argument can actually be used to show that the whole-brain-oriented definition of death is less defensible than the higher-brain-oriented one.

As we have seen, the whole-brain-oriented definition of death rests on the claim that irreversible loss of all functions of the entire brain is necessary and sufficient for an individual to be dead. That, in effect, means drawing a sharp line between the top of the spinal cord and the base of the brain (i.e., the bottom of the brain stem). But is there any principled reason why one would draw a line at that point?

In the early years of the definition of death debate, the claim was made that an individual was dead when the central nervous system no longer retained the capacity for integration. It was soon discovered, however, that this could be taken to imply that one was "alive" as long as some spinal cord function remained. That was counterintuitive (and also made it more difficult to obtain organs for transplant). Hence, very early on it was agreed that simple reflexes of the spinal cord did not count as an indicator of life. Presumably the principle was that reflex arcs that do not integrate significant bodily functions are to be ignored.

But why then do brain stem reflexes mediated through the base of the brain stem count? By the same principle, if spinal reflexes can be ignored, it would seem that some brain stem reflexes might be as well. An effort to show that brain stem reflexes are more integrative of bodily function is doomed to fail. At most there are gradual, imperceptible gradations in complexity between the reflexes of the first cervical vertebra and those of the base of the brain stem. Some spinal reflexes that trigger extension of the foot while the contralateral arm is withdrawn certainly cover larger distances.

Whatever principle could be used to exclude the spinal reflexes surely can exclude some brain stem reflexes as well. We have seen that the defenders of the whole-brain-oriented position admit as much when they start excluding cellular level functions and electrical functions. Certainly, those who exclude "nests of cells" in the brain as insignificant have abandoned the whole brain position and are already sliding along the slippery slope.

By contrast the defenders of the higher-brain-oriented definition of death can articulate a principle that avoids such slipperiness. Suppose, for example, they rely on classical Judeo-Christian notions that the human is essentially the integration of the mind and body and that the existence of one without the other is not sufficient to constitute a living human being. Such a principle provides a bright line that would clearly distinguish the total and irreversible loss of consciousness from serious but not total mental impairments.

Likewise, the integration of mind and body provides a firm basis for telling which functions of nests of brain cells count as significant. It avoids the hopeless task of trying to show why brain stem reflexes count more than spinal ones or trying to show exactly how many cells must be in a nest before it is significant. There is no subjective assessment of different bodily functions, no quibble about how much integration there must be for the organism to function as a whole. The principle is simple. It relies on qualitative considerations: when, and only when,   .
there is the capacity for organic (bodily) and mental function present together in

a single human entity is there a living human being. That, I would suggest, is the philosophical basis for the higher-brain-oriented definition of death. It avoids the slippery slope on which the defenders of the whole-brain-oriented position have found themselves; it, and only it, provides a principled reason for avoiding the slippery slope.

Conscience Clauses

There is one final development that signals the demise of the whole-brain-oriented definition of death as the single basis for declaring death. It should be clear by now that the definition of death debate is actually a debate over the moral status of human beings. It is a debate over when humans should be treated as full members of the human community. When humans are living, full moral and legal human rights accrue. Saying people are alive is simply shorthand for saying that they are bearers of such rights. That is why the definition of death debate is so important. It is also why, in principle, there is no scientific way in which the debate can be resolved. The determination of who is alive—who has full moral standing as a member of the human community—is fundamentally a moral, philosophical, or religious determination, not a scientific one.

In a pluralistic society, we are not likely to reach agreement on such moral questions, which is why no one definition of death has carried the day thus far. When one realizes that there are many variants on each of the three major definitions of death, each of which has some group of adherents, it seems unlikely that any one position is likely to gain even a majority any time soon. For example, defense of the higher-brain-oriented position stands or falls on the claim that the essence of the human being is the integration of a mind and a body, a position reflecting religious and philosophical assumptions that are not beyond dispute. (Other defenders of the higher brain position, for example, are more Manichaean, holding that only the mind is important; they apparently are committed to a view that a human memory transferred to a computer with a capacity to continue mental function would still have all the essential ingredients of humanness and that the same living human being continues to live on the computer hard drive.) These are disputes not likely to be resolved soon.

As a society we have a method for dealing with fundamental disputes in religion and philosophy. We tolerate diversity and affirm the right of conscience to hold minority beliefs as long as actions based on those beliefs do not cause insurmountable problems for the rest of society. That is precisely what in 1976 I proposed doing in the dispute over the definition of death.[15] I proposed a definition of death with a conscience clause that would permit individuals to choose their own definition of death based on their religious and philosophical convictions. I did not say at the time, but should have, that the choices would have to be restricted to those that avoid violating the rights of others and avoid creating insurmountable social problems for the rest of society. For example, I assume that people would not be able to pick a definition that required society to treat them as dead even though they retained cardiac, respiratory, mental, and neurological integrating functions. Likewise, I assume that people would not be permitted to pick a definition that would insist that they be treated as alive when all these functions were absent. There are minimal public health considerations that would set limits on the choices available, but certainly the three major options would be tolerable: heart-, whole-brain-, and higher-brain-oriented definitions.

The state of New Jersey has gone part of the way recently by adopting a law with a conscience clause that would permit religious objectors to designate in advance that a heart-oriented definition should be used in pronouncing their deaths.[16] Since it is now widely accepted that anyone can write an advance directive mandating withdrawal of life support once one is permanently unconscious, any persons who favor a higher-brain-oriented definition of death already have the legal right to make choices that end up with them dead in anyone's sense of the term very shortly after they had lost higher brain functions. Permitting them to designate that they be called dead when they are permanently unconscious changes very little.

There is a litany of worries over conscience clauses that defenders of the whole-brain-oriented definitions cite. They worry about life insurance paying off at different times, depending on which definition is chosen, and about homicide charges being dependent on such choices, but these are already with us when people are permitted to use advance directives to control the timing of their deaths. They worry about health insurance costs, but for those who choose a higher-brain-oriented formulation the only implication is lower costs. For those who choose a heart-oriented definition potentially higher health insurance costs could result, but that position is held only by a small minority, and it is technically so difficult to maintain a beating heart in someone whose brain is dead that the costs will probably not be significant. If they were, the problem could be addressed by clarifying that standard health insurance would not cover the medical costs for maintaining someone who is "alive with a dead brain." None of these problems has arisen in New Jersey, and none is likely to arise. In short, there is no reason to suspect that the use of a conscience clause will result in social chaos—only in greater respect for minority religious and philosophical views that would otherwise be suppressed by the tyranny of the majority. For convenience it would probably be prudent to adopt a single "default definition" favored by a majority; it would make little difference which definition is used as long as the minority who had strong preference for an alternative had the right to designate in advance its choice of another definition. As with surrogate decisionmaking for terminal care and the procurement of cadaver organs, I think it would be reasonable for the next of kin to have the right of surrogate decisionmaking in the case of minors or mentally incompetent individuals who had not expressed a preference while competent.

Crafting New Public Law

Changing current law to conform to these suggestions will be complex and should be done with deliberate speed, but it should be done. Two changes would be needed in the current definition of death: (1) incorporating the higher brain function notion and (2) incorporating some form of the conscience clause.

Present law makes persons dead when they have lost all functions of the entire brain. It is uniformly agreed that the law should incorporate only this basic concept of death, not the precise criteria or tests needed to determine that the whole brain is dead. That is left up to the consensus of neurological experts.

All that would be needed to shift to a higher brain formulation is a change in the wording of the law to replace "all functions of the entire brain" with some relevant, more limited alternative. There are at least three options: references to higher brain functions, cerebral functions, or consciousness. While we could simply change the wording to read that an individual is dead when there is irreversible cessation of all higher brain functions, that poses a serious problem. We are now suffering from the problems created by the vagueness of the referring to "all functions of the entire brain." Even though referring to "all higher brain functions" would be conceptually correct, it would be even more ambiguous. It would lack needed specificity.

This specificity could be achieved by referring to irreversible loss of cerebral functions, but we have already suggested two problems with that wording. Just as we now know there are some isolated functions of the whole brain that should be discounted, so there are probably some isolated cerebral functions that most would not want to count either. For example, if, hypothetically, an isolated "nest" of cerebral motor neurons were perfused so that if stimulated the body could twitch, that would be a cerebral function, but not a significant one for determining life any more than a brain stem reflex is. Second, in theory some really significant functions such as consciousness might some day be maintainable even without a cerebrum—if, for example, a computer could function as an artificial center for consciousness. The term "cerebral function" adds specificity but is not satisfactory.

The language that seems best if integration of mind and body is what is critical is "irreversible cessation of the capacity for consciousness." That is, after all, what the defenders of the higher brain formulations really have in mind. (If someone were to claim that some other "higher" function is critical, that alternative could simply be plugged in.) As is the case now, the specifics of the criteria and tests for measuring irreversible loss of capacity for consciousness would be left up to the consensus of neurological expertise, even though measuring irreversible loss of capacity for a brain function such as consciousness involves fundamentally nonscientific value judgments. If the community of neurological expertise claims that irreversible loss of consciousness cannot be measured, so be it. We will at least have clarified the concept and set the stage for the day when it can be measured with sufficient accuracy. We have noted, however, that neurologists presently claim they can in fact measure irreversible loss of consciousness accurately.

A second significant change in the definition of death would be required to incorporate the conscience clause. It would permit individuals, while competent, to execute documents choosing alternative definitions of death that are, within reason, not threatening to significant interests of others. While the New Jersey law permits only the alternative of a heart-oriented definition, my proposal, assuming irreversible loss of consciousness were the default definition, would permit choosing either heart-oriented or whole-brain-oriented definitions as alternatives.

The New Jersey law presently permits only competent adults to execute such conscience clauses. This, of course, excludes the possibility of parents choosing alternative definitions for their children. I had long ago proposed that, just as legal surrogates have the right to make medical treatment decisions for their wards provided the decisions are within reason, so they should be permitted to choose alternative definitions of death provided the individual had never expressed a preference. This would, for example, permit Orthodox Jewish parents to require that the state continue to treat their child as alive even though he or she had suffered irreversible loss of consciousness or of total brain function. (Whether the state also requires insurers to continue paying for support of these individuals deemed living is a separate policy issue.) While the New Jersey law tolerates only variation with an explicitly religious basis, I would favor variation based on any conscientiously formulated position.

As a short-cut the law could state that patients who had clearly irreversibly lost consciousness because heart and lung function had stopped could continue to be pronounced dead based on criteria measuring heart and lung function. That this was simply an alternative means for measuring permanent loss of consciousness would have to be set out more clearly than in the present Uniform Determination of Death Act. I see no reason to continue including the alternative measurement in the legal definition. I would simply allow it to fall under the criteria to be articulated by the consensus of experts. This leads to a proposal for a new definition of death, which would read as follows:

> An individual who has sustained irreversible loss of consciousness is dead. A determination of death must be made in accordance with accepted medical standards.
>
> However, no individual shall be considered dead based on irreversible loss of consciousness if he or she, while competent, has explicitly asked to be pronounced dead based on irreversible cessation of all functions of the entire brain or based on irreversible cessation of circulatory and respiratory functions.
>
> Unless an individual has, while competent, selected one of these definitions of death, the legal guardian or next of kin (in that order) may do so. The definition selected by the individual, legal guardian or next of kin shall serve as the definition of death for all legal purposes.

If one favored only the shift to consciousness as a definition of death without the conscience clause, only paragraph one would be necessary. One could also craft a similar definition using the whole-brain-oriented definition of death as the default definition. Some have proposed an additional paragraph prohibiting a physician with a conflict of interest (such as an interest in the organs of the deceased) from pronouncing death. I am not convinced that paragraph is needed, however.

A Principled Reason for Drawing the Line

It has been puzzling why what at first seemed like a rather minor debate over when a human was dead should have persisted as long as it has. Many thought the definition of death debate was a technical argument that would be resolved in favor of the more fashionable, scientific, and progressive brain-oriented definition as soon as the old romantics attached to the heart died off. It is now clear that something much more complex and more fundamental is at stake. We have been fighting over the question of who has moral standing as a full member of the human moral community, a matter that forces on us some of the most basic questions of human existence: the relation of mind and body, the rights of religious and philosophical minorities, and the meaning of life itself.

I am not certain whether some version of the higher-brain-oriented definition of death will be adopted in any legal jurisdiction anytime soon, but I am convinced that the now old-fashioned whole-brain-oriented definition of death is becoming less and less plausible as we realize that no one really believes that literally all functions of the entire brain must be irreversibly lost for an individual to be dead. Unless there is some public consensus expressed in state or federal law conveying agreement upon exactly which brain functions are insignificant, we will all be vulnerable to a slippery slope in which private practitioners choose for themselves exactly where from the top of the cerebrum to caudal end of the spinal cord to draw the line. There is no principled reason to draw it exactly between the base of the brain and the top of the spine. Better that we have a principled reason for drawing it. To me, the principle is that for human life to be present—that is, for the human to be treated as a member in full standing of the human moral community—there must be integrated functioning of mind and body. That means some version of a higher-brain-oriented formulation.

NOTES

1. President's Commission for the Study of Ethical Problems in Medicine and Biomedical and Behavioral Research, *Defining Death: Medical, Legal and Ethical Issues in the Definition of Death* (Washington, D.C.: U.S. Government Printing Office, 1981), p. 2. Page numbers for subsequent citations are in the text.

2. Robert M. Veatch, "The Whole-Brain-Oriented Concept of Death: An Outmoded Philosophical Formulation," *Journal of Thanatology* 3 (1975): 13–30.

3. Earl A. Walker et al., "An Appraisal of the Criteria of Cerebral Death: A Summary Statement," *JAMA* 237 (1977): 982–86, at 983.

4. James L. Bernat, "How Much of the Brain Must Die on Brain Death?" *The Journal of Clinical Ethics*, 3, no. 1 (1992): 21–26, at 25.

5. Paul A. Byrne, Sean O'Reilly, and Paul M. Quay, "Brain Death: An Opposing Viewpoint," *JAMA* 242 (1979): 1985–90.

6. Cited in Robert M. Veatch, *Death, Dying, and the Biological Revolution* (New Haven: Yale University Press, 1976), p. 38.

7. Robert M. Veatch, "Whole-Brain, Neocortical, and Higher Brain Related Concepts," in *Death: Beyond Whole-Brain Criteria*, ed. Richard M. Zaner (Dordrecht, Holland: D. Reidel Publishing Company, 1988), pp. 171–86.

8. David J. Cole, "The Reversibility of Death," *Journal of Medical Ethics* 18 (1992): 26–30.

9. Alan D. Shewmon, "Caution in the Definition and Diagnosis of Infant Brain Death," in *Medical Ethics: A Guide for Health Professionals*, ed. John F. Monagle and David C. Thomasma (Rockville, Md.: Aspen Publishers, 1988), pp. 38–57.

10. Stephen Ashwal and Sanford Schneider, "Failure of Electroencephalography to Diagnose Brain Death in Comatose Patients," *Annals of Neurology* 6 (1979): 512–17.

11. Ronald B. Cranford and Harmon L. Smith, "Some Critical Distinctions between Brain Death and the Persistent Vegetative State," *Ethics in Science and Medicine* 6 (Winter 1979): 199–209; Phiroze L. Hansotia, "Persistent Vegetative State," *Archives of Neurology* 42 (1985): 1048–52.

12. Council on Scientific Affairs and Council on Ethical and Judicial Affairs, "Persistent Vegetative State and the Decision to Withdraw or Withhold Life Support," *JAMA* 263 (1990): 426–30, at 428.

13. President's Commission for the Study of Ethical Problems in Medicine and Biomedical and Behavioral Research, *Deciding to Forego Life-Sustaining Treatment: Ethical, Medical, and Legal Issues in Treatment Decisions* (Washington, D.C.: U.S. Government Printing Office, 1983), p. 177.

14. Bernat, "How Much of the Brain Must Die on Brain Death?" pp. 21–26.

15. Veatch, *Death, Dying, and the Biological Revolution*, pp. 72–76.

16. New Jersey Declaration of Death Act, N.J.S.A. 26: 6A–5.

CHAPTER TWENTY-NINE

Against the Stream

Comments on the Definition and Redefinition of Death

Hans Jonas

The by now famous "Report of the *Ad Hoc* Committee of the Harvard Medical School to Examine the Definition of Brain Death" advocates the adoption of "irreversible coma as a new definition of death."[1] The report leaves no doubt of the practical reasons "why there is need for a definition," naming these two: relief of patient, kin, and medical resources from the burdens of indefinitely prolonged coma; and removal of controversy on obtaining organs for transplantation. On both counts, the new definition is designed to give the physician the right to terminate the treatment of a condition which not only cannot be improved by such treatment, but whose mere prolongation by it is utterly meaningless to the patient himself. The last consideration, of course, is ultimately the only valid rationale for termination (and for termination only!) and must support all the others. It does so with regard to the reasons mentioned under the first head, for the relief of the patient means automatically also that of his family, doctor, nurses, apparatus, hospital space, and so on. But the other reason—freedom for organ use—has possible implications that are not equally covered by the primary rationale, which is the patient himself. For with this primary rationale (the senselessness of mere vegetative function) the Report has strictly speaking defined not death, the ultimate state, itself, but a criterion for permitting it to take place unopposed—e.g., by turning off the respirator. The Report, however, purports by that criterion to have defined death itself, declaring it on its evidence as already given, not merely no longer to be opposed. But if "the patient is declared dead on the basis of these criteria," i.e., if the comatose individual is not a patient at all but a corpse, then the road to other uses of the definition, urged by the second reason, has been opened in principle and will be taken in practice, unless it is blocked in good time by a special barrier. What follows is meant to reinforce what I called "my feeble attempt" to help erect such a barrier on theoretical grounds.

My original comments of 1968 on the then newly proposed "redefinition of death"[2] were marginal to the discussion of "experimentation on human subjects," which has to do with the living and not the dead. They have since, however, drawn fire from within the medical profession, and precisely in connection with the second of the reasons given by the Harvard Committee why a new definition is wanted, namely, the *transplant* interest, which my kind critics felt threatened by my layman's qualms and lack of understanding. Can I take this as corroborating my initial suspicion that this *interest*, in spite of its notably muted expression in the Committee Report, was and is the major motivation behind the definitional effort? I am confirmed in this suspicion when I hear Dr. Henry K. Beecher, author of the Committee's Report (and its Chairman), ask elsewhere: "Can society afford to discard the tissues and organs of the hopelessly unconscious patient when they could be used to restore the otherwise hopelessly ill, but still salvageable individual?"[3] In any case, the tenor and passion of the discussion which my initial polemic provoked from my medical friends left no doubt where the surgeon's interest in the definition lies. I contend that, pure as this interest, viz., to save other lives, is in itself, its intrusion into the *theoretical* attempt to define death makes the attempt impure; and the Harvard Committee should never have allowed itself to adulterate the purity of its scientific case by baiting it with the prospect of this *extraneous*—though extremely appealing—gain. But purity of theory is not my concern here. My concern is with certain practical consequences which under the urgings of that extraneous interest can be drawn from the definition and would enjoy its full sanction, once it has been officially accepted. Doctors would be less than human if certain formidable advantages of such possible consequences would not influence their judgment as to the theoretical adequacy of a definition that yields them—just as I freely admit that my shudder at one aspect of those consequences, and at the danger of others equally sanctioned by that definition, keeps my theoretical skepticism in a state of extreme alertness.

Since the private exchanges referred to (which were conducted in the most amicable spirit of shared concern) somewhat sharpened my theoretical case and in addition brought out some of the apprehensions that haunt me in this matter—and which, I think, should be in everyone's mind before final approval of the new definition takes matters out of our hands—I base the remainder of this paper on a statement titled "Against the Stream" which I circulated among the members of the informal group in question.[4]

I had to answer three charges made à propos of the pertinent part of my *Daedalus* essay: that my reasoning regarding "cadaver donors" counteracts sincere life-saving efforts of physicians; that I counter precise scientific facts with vague philosophical considerations; and that I overlook the difference between death of "the organism as a whole" and death of "the whole organism," with the related difference between spontaneous and externally induced respiratory and other movements.

I plead, of course, guilty to the first charge for the case where the cadaver status of the donor is in question, which is precisely what my argument is about. The use of the term "cadaver donor" here simply begs the question, to which only the third charge (see below) addresses itself.

As to the charge of vagueness, it might just be possible that it vaguely reflects the fact that mine is an argument—a precise argument, I believe—*about* vagueness, viz., the vagueness of a condition. Giving intrinsic vagueness its due is not being vague. Aristotle observed that it is the mark of a well-educated man not to insist on greater precision in knowledge than the subject admits, e.g., the same in politics as in mathematics. Reality of certain kinds—of which the life-death spectrum is perhaps one—may be imprecise in itself, or the knowledge obtainable of it may be. To acknowledge such a state of affairs is more adequate to it than a precise definition, which does violence to it. I am challenging the undue precision of a definition and of its practical application to an imprecise field.

The third point—which was made by Dr. Otto Guttentag—is highly relevant and I will deal with it step by step.

a. The difference between "organism as a whole" and "whole organism" which he has in mind is perhaps brought out more clearly if for "whole organism" we write "every and all parts of the organism." If this is the meaning, then I have been speaking throughout of "death of the organism as a whole," not of "death of the whole organism"; and any ambiguity in my formulations can be easily removed. Local subsystems—single cells or tissues—may well continue to function locally, i.e., to display biochemical activity for themselves (e.g., growth of hair and nails) for some time after death, without this affecting the definition of death by the larger criteria of the whole. But respiration and circulation do not fall into this class, since the effect of their functioning, though performed by subsystems, extends through the total system and insures the functional preservation of its other parts. Why else prolong them artificially in prospective "cadaveric" organ donors (e.g., "maintain renal circulation of cadaver kidneys in situ") except to keep those other parts "in good shape"—viz., alive—for eventual transplantation? The comprehensive system thus sustained is even capable of continued overall metabolism when intravenously fed, and then, presumably, of diverse other (e.g. glandular) functions as well—in fact, I suppose, of pretty much everything not involving neural control. There are stories of comatose patients lingering on for months with those aids; the metaphor of the "human vegetable" recurring in the debate (strangely enough, sometimes in support of redefining death—as if "vegetable" were not an instance of life!) say as much. In short, what is here kept going by various artifices must—with the caution due in this twilight zone—be equated with "the organism as a whole" named in the classical definition of death—much more so, at least, than with any mere, separable part of it.

b. Nor, to my knowledge, does that older definition specify that the functioning whose "irreversible cessation" constitutes death must be spontaneous and does not count for life when artificially induced and sustained (the implications for therapy would be devastating). Indeed, "irreversible" cessation can have a twofold reference: to the function itself or only to the spontaneity of it. A cessation can be irreversible with respect to spontaneity but still reversible with respect to the activity as such—in which case the reversing external agency must continuously substitute for the lost spontaneity. This is the case of the respiratory movements and heart contractions in the comatose. The distinction is not irrelevant, because if we could do for the disabled brain—let's say, the lower nerve centers only—what we can do for the heart and lungs, viz., *make* it work by the continuous input of some external agency (electrical, chemical, or whatever), we would surely do so and not be finicky about the resulting function lacking spontaneity: the functioning as such would matter. Respirator and stimulator could then be turned off, because the nerve center presiding over heart contractions (etc.) has again taken over and returned *them* to being "spontaneous"—just as systems presided over by circulation had enjoyed spontaneity of function when the circulation was only nonspontaneously active. The case is wholly hypothetical, but I doubt that a doctor would feel at liberty to pronounce the patient dead on the ground of the nonspontaneity at the cerebral source, when it can be *made* to function by an auxiliary device.

The purpose of the foregoing thought-experiment was to cast some doubt (a layman's, to be sure) on the seeming simplicity of the spontaneity criterion. With the stratification and interlocking of functions, it seems to me, organic spontaneity is distributed over many levels and loci—any superordinated level enabling its subordinates to be naturally spontaneous, be its own action natural or artificial.

c. The point with irreversible coma as defined by the Harvard group, of course, is precisely that it is a condition which precludes reactivation of any part of the brain in *every* sense. We then have an "organism as a whole" minus the brain, maintained in some partial state of life so long as the respirator and other artifices are at work. And here the question is not: has the patient died? but: how should he—still a patient—be dealt with? Now *this* question must be settled, surely not by a definition of death, but by a definition of man and of what life is human. That is to say, the question cannot be answered by decreeing that death has already occurred and the body is therefore in the domain of things; rather it is by holding, e.g., that it is humanly not justified—let alone, de-manded—to artificially prolong the life of a brainless body. This is the answer I myself would advocate. On that philosophical ground, which few will contest, the physician can, indeed should, turn off the respirator and let the "definition of death" take care of itself by what then inevitably happens. (The later utiliza-tion of the corpse is a different matter I am not dealing with here, though it too resists the comfortable patness of merely utilitarian answers.) The decision to be made, I repeat, is an axiological one and not already made by clinical fact. It begins when the diagnosis of the condition has spoken: it is not diagnostic it-self. Thus, as I have pointed out before, no redefinition of death is needed; only, perhaps, a redefinition of the physician's presumed duty to prolong life under all circumstances.

d. But, it might be asked, is not a definition of death made into law the sim-pler and more precise way than a definition of medical ethics (which is difficult to legislate) for sanctioning the same practical conclusion, while avoiding the twilight of value judgment and possible legal ambiguity? It would be, if it really sanctioned the same conclusion, and no more. But it sanctions indefinitely more: it opens the gate to a whole range of other possible conclusions, the extent of which cannot even be foreseen, but some of which are disquietingly close at hand. The point is, if the comatose patient is by definition dead, he is a patient no more but a corpse, with which can be done whatever law or custom or the deceased's will or next of kin permit and sundry interests urge doing with a corpse. This includes—why not?—the protracting of the in-between state, for which we must find a new name ("simulated life"?) since that of "life" has been preempted by the new definition of death, and extracting from it all the profit we can. There are many. So far the "redefiners" speak of no more than keeping the respirator going until the transplant organ is to be removed, then turning it off, then beginning to cut into the "cadaver," this being the end of it—which sounds innocent enough. But why must it be the end? Why turn the respirator off? Once we are assured that we are dealing with a cadaver, there are no logical reasons against (and strong pragmatic reasons for) going on with the artificial "animation" and keeping the "deceased's" body on call, as a bank for life-fresh organs, possibly also as a plant for manufacturing hormones or other biochemical compounds in demand. I have no doubts that methods exist or can be perfected which allow the natural powers for the healing of surgical wounds by new tissue growth to stay "alive" in such a body. Tempting also is the idea of a self-replenishing blood bank. And that is not all. Let us not forget research. Why shouldn't the most wonderful surgical and grafting experiments be conducted on the complaisant subject-nonsubject, with no limits set to daring? Why not immunological explorations, infection with diseases old and new, trying out of drugs? We have the active cooperation of a functional organism declared to be dead: we have, that is, the advantages of the living donor without the disadvantages imposed by his rights and interests (for a corpse has none). What a boon for medical instruction, for anatomical and physiological demonstration and practicing on so much better material than the inert cadavers otherwise serving in the dissection room! What a chance for the apprentice to learn *in vivo*, as it were, how to amputate a leg, without his mistakes mattering! And so on, into the wide open field. After all, what is advocated is "the full utilization of modern means to maximize the value of cadaver organs." Well, this is it.

Come, come, the members of the profession will say, nobody is thinking of this kind of thing. Perhaps not; but I have just shown that one *can* think of them. And the point is that the proposed definition of death has removed any reasons not to think of them and, once thought of, not to do them when found desirable (and the next of kin are agreeable). We must remember that what the Harvard group offered was not a definition of irreversible coma as a rationale for breaking off sustaining action, but a definition of death by the criterion of irreversible coma as a rationale for conceptually transposing the patient's body to the class of dead things, *regardless* of whether sustaining action is kept up or broken off. It would be hypocritical to deny that the redefinition amounts to an antedating of the accomplished fact of death (compared to conventional signs that may outlast it); that it was motivated not by exclusive concern with the patient but with certain extraneous interests in mind (organ donorship mostly named so far); and that the actual use of the general license it grants is implicity anticipated. But no matter what particular use is or is not anticipated at the moment, or even anathematized—it would be naive to think that a line can be drawn anywhere for such uses when strong enough interest urge them, seeing that the definition (which is absolute, not graded) negates the very principle for drawing a line. (Given the ingenuity of medical science, in which I have great faith, I am convinced that the "simulated life" can eventually be made to comprise practically every extraneural activity of the human body; and I would not even bet on its never comprising *some* artificially activated neural functions as well: which would be awkward for the argument of nonsensitivity, but still under the roof of that of nonspontaneity.)

e. Now my point is a very simple one. It is this. We do not know with certainty the borderline between life and death, and a definition cannot substitute for knowledge. Moreover, we have sufficient grounds for suspecting that the artificially supported condition of the comatose patient may still be one of life, however reduced—i.e., for doubting that, even with the brain function gone, he is completely dead. In this state of marginal ignorance and doubt the only course to take is to lean over backward toward the side of possible life. It follows that interventions as I described should be regarded on a par with vivisection and on no account be performed on a human body in that equivocal or threshold condition. And the definition that allows them, by stamping as unequivocal what at best is equivocal, must be rejected. But mere rejection in discourse is not enough. Given the pressure of the—very real and very worthy—medical interests, it can be predicted that the permission it implies in theory will be irresistible in practice, once the definition is installed in official authority. Its becoming so installed must therefore be resisted at all cost. It is the only thing that still can be resisted; by the time the practical conclusions beckon, it will be too late. It is a clear case of *principiis obsta*.

The foregoing argumentation was strictly on the plane of common sense and ordinary logic. Let me add, somewhat conjecturally, two philosophical observations.

I see lurking behind the proposed definition of death, apart from its obvious pragmatic motivation, a curious revenant of the old soul-body dualism. Its new apparition is the dualism of brain and body. In a certain analogy to the former it holds that the true human person rests in (or is represented by) the brain, of which the rest of the body is a mere subservient tool. Thus, when the brain dies, it is as when the soul departed: what is left are "mortal remains." Now nobody will deny that the cerebral aspect is decisive for the human quality of the life of the organism that is man's. The position I advanced acknowledges just this by recommending that with the irrecoverable total loss of brain function one should not hold up the naturally ensuing death of the rest of the organism. But it is no less an exaggeration of the cerebral aspect as it was of the conscious soul, to deny the extracerebral body its essential share in the identity of the person. The body is as uniquely the body of this brain and no other, as the brain is uniquely the brain of this body and no other. What is under the brain's central control, the bodily total, is as individual, as much "myself," as singular to my identity (fingerprints!), as noninterchangeable, as the controlling (and recipro- cally controlled) brain itself. My identity is the identity of the whole organism, even if the higher functions of personhood are seated in the brain. How else could a man love a woman and not merely her brains? How else could we lose ourselves in the aspect of a face? Be touched by the delicacy of a frame? It's this person's, and no one else's. Therefore, the body of the comatose, so long as— even with the help of art—it still breathes, pulses, and functions otherwise, must still be considered a residual continuance of the subject that loved and was loved, and as such is still entitled to some of the sacrosanctity accorded to such a subject by the laws of God and men. That sacrosanctity decrees that it must not be used as a mere means.

My second observation concerns the morality of our time, to which our "re- definers" pay homage with the best of intentions, which have their own subtle sophistry. I mean the prevailing attitude toward death, whose faintheartedness they indulge in a curious blend with the tough-mindedness of the scientist. The Catholic Church had the guts to say: under these circumstances let the patient die—speaking of the patient alone and not of outside interests (society's, medi- cine's, etc.). The cowardice of modern secular society which shrinks from death as an unmitigated evil needs the assurance (or fiction) that he is already dead when the decision is to be made. The responsibility of a value-laden decision is replaced by the mechanics of a value-free routine. Insofar as the redefiners of death—by saying "he is already dead"—seek to allay the scruples about turning the respirator off, they cater to this modern cowardice which has forgotten that death has its own fitness and dignity, and that a man has a right to be let die. Insofar as by saying so they seek to provide an even better conscience about keeping the respirator on and freely utilizing the body thus arrested on the threshold of life and death, they serve the ruling pragmatism of our time which will let no ancient fear and trembling interfere with the relentless expanding of the realm of sheer thinghood and unrestricted utility. The "splendor and misery" of our age dwells in that irresistible tide.

NOTES

Written in 1970, this essay is a postscript to Essay 5 in H. Jonas, *Philosophical Essays: From Ancient Creed to Technological Man* (Englewood Cliffs, NJ: Prentice-Hall, 1974).

1. See Essay 5, note 11.
2. Editor's Note: See Essay 5, pp. 129–31.
3. See Essay 5, p. 114.
4. Of its members I name the renal surgeon Dr. Samuel Kountz, specializing in kidney transplantation, and Drs. Harrison Sadler and Otto Guttentag, all of the Medical Center of the University of California in San Francisco.

CHAPTER THIRTY

Brain Death and Personal Identity

Michael B. Green and Daniel Wikler

The legal and medical definition of death has recently changed in many states from cessation of heart and lung function to so-called brain death. Patients who have suffered irreversible loss of brain function but continue to breathe would have been accounted alive under previous medical practice and legal statute. They are now pronounced dead. Though the changes are sanctioned by leading medical and legal authorities, they have proceeded in a climate of some confusion, a symptom of which was a recent ruling by a Florida judge: "This lady is dead and has been dead and she is being kept alive artificially."[1] In part this confusion is merely the result of misunderstanding on the part of judges and the public of what those authorities proposing redefinition have in mind, but it also mirrors the conceptual disarray in the brain-death literature.[2] Though a large number of physicians, jurists, and philosophers now hold that brain death is death, there is little agreement about the justification for the redefinition or about the nature of the task of "redefinition" itself.

The principal arguments for classifying brain-dead patients as dead can be sorted into two groups. Those of the first type, which we will call the biological arguments, hold that redefinition is required by new developments in biomedical science. The second sort of argument proposes the redefinition as a solution to a moral problem, that of indefinitely and pointlessly maintaining the irreversibly comatose, and hence justified on moral grounds. Each kind of argument has an initial persuasiveness, but this is lost when the arguments are set out and examined in detail. We will argue, in Sections I and II, respectively, that neither of these kinds of arguments supports the thesis that brain-dead patients are dead.

In so arguing, we undermine the principal theoretical sources of support for the new definition of death. Our ultimate intention is, however, to support the brain-death definition. To justify it, we provide, in Section III, what we regard as the first satisfactory rationale for regarding brain death as death. Our argument is ontological rather than biological or moral, having to do with the conditions of existence of persons.[3] We sketch what we believe to be the best theory of personal identity and draw a corollary on brain death which supports the view that persons cease to exist at that moment.

Our conclusion, then, is that brain-dead patients are indeed dead, though not for the reasons that they are now thought of as dead. Whether the brain dead should be considered dead *under the law* is, we argue in Section IV, another issue entirely; we think they should, but provide an argument for the legal redefinition which is wholly independent of our philosophical claim.

I. The Biological Arguments

Brain death—the irreversible cessation of brain function—involves two catastrophic changes in functioning. One is coma, the permanent loss of consciousness and awareness of the world. The other is the loss of the brain's ability to regulate certain autonomic body processes, such as respiration, which contribute to maintenance of internal homeostasis. These losses involve cessation of functioning of different parts of the brain (here for convenience to be called "upper" and "lower," respectively—the details do not matter) and each can occur without the other.[4] The early, influential Harvard Report used the title "A Definition of Irreversible Coma," but consisted of instructions on diagnosing cessation of both upper and lower brain functioning, and left the reader unclear as to which event was meant to mark the patient's death.[5] The subsequent medical literature is not unanimous on this point, but the established view now seems to be that brain death is to be understood as cessation of all brain functioning.[6]

This point is widely misunderstood. In the celebrated case of Karen Quinlan, for example, none of the parties to the dispute over termination of care advanced the claim that she was dead or brain dead, even though she was thought to be in a "persistent vegetative state," that is, shorn of mental capacities.[7] It was thus unfortunate that the case was publicized as a test case for the new definition. Ms. Quinlan was (and is, as of this writing) alive according to the dominant medical brain death conception, since her lower brain continued to regulate her breathing and other life processes. Death is marked, on this view, by death of the *whole* brain. Permanent loss of consciousness has no bearing on the matter if the lower brain continues to do its work. Why have most medical authorities thought that loss of this capacity, as occurs in whole brain death, should be counted as death? As we shall argue in Section II, most of the support for redefinition derives from moral considerations. Nevertheless, two arguments have appeared which attempt to uphold the redefinition on medical grounds. The first claims that despite appearances, this is nothing more than an application of the traditional definition of death, one which has heretofore been almost universally accepted. The second sees whole brain death as a departure from tradition, but one justified on scientific grounds. We shall present and counter these in turn.

Brain Death as the Traditional Standard

Has brain death been our traditional definition of death? According to *Black's Law Dictionary*, death is "the ceasing to exist; defined . . . as a total stoppage of the circulation of the blood, and a cessation of the animal and vital functions consequent thereon, such as respiration, pulsation, etc." Since a brain-dead patient, with machine assistance, can exhibit all of these vital signs, it would seem that a pronouncement of death on such a patient would be a clear deviation from the old standard. Yet some of those arguing for the redefinition of death deny this.[8] Their argument first makes a distinction between the state of death and the signs or clinical indicators by which the presence of that state is detected. Thus, a switch from a set of cardiovascular indicators to the set of brain-death indicators need not mean that one tests for different states before declaring brain death.[9] Indeed, according to their argument, the traditional heart-lung test has been a test for brain death all along.

The claim that the traditional heart-lung test has always been used to detect brain death is to be secured by the following sub-argument. The presence of heartbeat and breathing in the healthy individual is a sign, not only of heart and lung function, but also of a certain underlying *capacity*, in particular the capacity for spontaneous respiration and heartbeat. Call this Capacity S. The state of death is assumed, on this account, to be the loss of this capacity. The presence of heartbeat and breathing is a good indicator of the presence of S under ordinary circumstances. When heartbeat and breathing are occurring as the result of machine maintenance of life-functions, however, the test yields a false positive. The advent of these artificial aids has made development of a more accurate test mandatory. And (the argument continues) this is what the direct tests for brain function are. Capacity S is lodged in the lower brain; use of the EEG and similar indicators of brain death give us a direct reading on the presence of S regardless of clinical context. Hence brain death represents only a technological refinement of the traditional indicators of death, and no change in the definition of death at all.

The troubles with this argument are twofold. First, Capacity S—the capacity for spontaneous heartbeat and respiration—is *not* lodged in the lower brain. If it were, a functional lower brain would guarantee the presence of S. But it does not. If "spontaneous" means unassisted by machine, S is a capacity of the body as a whole. Hence brain death is not the same as loss of Capacity S. Second, loss of Capacity S was not the state tested for by the traditional tests for death. Persons requiring pacemakers because of heart injury, or respirators due to spinal injury, also lack this capacity. But they are surely not to be counted as dead for that reason by the concept of death embodied in the traditional definition. Machine dependence *in general* has no bearing on one's status as alive or dead.[10] But Capacity S involves nothing more than general machine independence: the ability to breathe and to circulate blood without artificial support. But since the absence of S has never been the state of death, it hardly matters that brain death is an unfailing indicator of it. Hence it is no argument for adoption of a brain-death definition that the new clinical indicators of brain death are simply refinements of the traditional cardiovascular indicators for the state of death.

Brain Death as a New Standard

What is lodged in the lower brain is not Capacity S but *neural* capacity for spontaneous respiration and heartbeat. The second argument seeks to provide justification for attaching special importance to this source of machine independence. Two grounds have, in fact, been independently advanced. The first is that brain death is, as a matter of medical fact, soon followed by death of the living system as a whole. The second sees brain death itself as the death of that system.[11] Neither ground is sufficient.

The first is easily dispatched. As Becker observed, "though the loss of one vital function (say loss of the capacity to eliminate wastes) may inevitably *bring about* death, it does not constitute death by itself."[12] Brain death portends bodily death, but does not constitute it. The interval during which a brain-dead patient can be maintained by artificial life-supports is at present quite limited, a fact which Lamb cites in support of a brain-death definition of death; but surely it could be extended, perhaps indefinitely.[13] It is difficult to see why the brevity of the interval should have any bearing on the definition of death. There are a host of medical conditions which, given the current power of medicine, also inevitably lead to death of the system as a whole, just as renal failure did only a few years ago. There was and is no temptation to regard the onset of these conditions as the occasion of death, and, failing further argument, this judgment extends naturally to the brain.[14]

The other ground for attaching special importance to death of the (lower) brain, its alleged central role in the functioning body system, purports to offer a way of distinguishing brain death from other misfortunes which may eventually be fatal. The contention here is that the brain is more than merely one vital organ among others; in some important sense it is the body system. Lamb states:

> Since the brain stem, not the heart, is recognized as the specific area which regulates all vital processes, it follows that after brain stem death the heart and other organs can never function again naturally. . . . The recognition that the brain stem, not the heart, is the central vital agency suggests a recent "paradigm shift" within the medical profession.[15]

Lamb then proceeds to document the shift to a definition of death based on brain death—even in patients with hearts still beating—on the part of several eminent medical specialists.

Lamb's argument deserves careful attention, not least because the almost universal acceptance of the death of the lower brain as a definition of death in the medical community might seem to invoke the authority of expert opinion. We shall question this authority.

The argument involves *inter alia* two steps, both of which we find questionable. First, that a paradigm shift has occurred among scientists; and second, that this gives the rest of us reason to identify death with brain death.

The problem with the first step lies in what is promised by the term "paradigm shift." If this is more than mere phrase-mongering, we will want evidence that there has been some sort of theoretical crisis in medical science which preceded the alleged shift. We must see medical science in theoretical crisis, analogous to other critical junctures in the history of science, replete with rival comprehensive theories which appear to be incommensurable. But there are none here. As Lamb himself states, the essential scientific facts were all quite well known before anyone gave any thought to changing the definition of death:

> There was, and still is, no doubt concerning the causal relationship between cerebral death and a cessation of the heartbeat. However, it was then (i.e., before the new definition became popular) maintained that death came only with the latter.[16]

Scientists command autonomy in setting some definitions, whether in the course of paradigm shifts or in ordinary science. If, as has happened in the history of science, a chemist wants to change the definition of "acid" to suit theoretical needs, it is up to him and his peers to decide the issue. The revised definition of acid is correct if it augments predictive and explanatory power, and this is a matter in which only the scientist is expert; the rest of us accept the redefinition on faith. The change in the definition of death, however, does not seem to be the sort of response to scientific needs that commands our allegiance. Many of the specialists supporting the change are not scientists at all in the narrow sense of being theory-builders, as they would have to be if we are to be bound to follow their example. They are, rather, medical practitioners. And even those scientists who support this change might not be doing so in their role as theory-builders, since they may simply be responding to the practitioner's statement of need for a definition which facilitates the acquisition of fresh organs and of more room in the intensive care units. To accept Lamb's argument we would need to see new scientific laws formulated or other evidence of the new definition's theoretical, as opposed to moral or practical, utility. Without such evidence, recent wholesale change of opinion within the medical community tells us nothing more than that many physicians have chosen to pronounce brain-dead patients dead.

The reader may feel that even if Lamb's appeal to authority fails to establish the centrality of the brain in the body's system of life-functions, that role is intuitively clear. Certainly the brain's work is different from that of any other vital organ. It is the organizer, the integrator; the other organs form the workforce regulated by its commands. And, as Becker points out, the body's life is surely a matter of *systemic* functioning: the continued interaction of a hierarchy of biological and chemical subsystems.[17] What we need is a criterion for determining death of the system; and what better candidate than loss of the command center which maintains systemic integration?

A more careful assessment of the lower brain's role, however, does not support the conclusion that brain death constitutes the cessation of systemic functioning. The fact that the lower brain is the element in the system which keeps other elements acting as a system does not make its continued functioning essential. It is still one among many organs, and, like other organs, could conceivably be replaced by an artificial aid which performed its function. The respirators and other life-supports which maintain body functioning after lower brain death collectively constitute a sort of artificial lower brain, and development of a more perfect mechanical substitute is merely a technological problem. When the lower brain's job is performed by these substitutes, the body's life-system continues to function as a system. The nonessential character of brain death may be brought out by some mechanical analogies: the heating system in a home can continue to function even after its thermostat fails, so long as the furnace is turned on and off manually (or by a substitute machine); an airplane continues to fly even after the autopilot fails if human pilots are able to take control. The source of control is not important; what matters is whether the job is done. The artificial life-supports now in use perform the brain's work rather poorly, as shown by the rapidity with which death of the body usually follows brain death; but not so poorly that the artificially maintained system is no system at all.[18]

Thus permanent cessation of lower brain functioning, which is the event known as brain death in the medical literature on the subject, does not mark the moment of death. Indeed, it does not even bear on the question of whether the patient is alive or dead, for any of the reasons found in the medical literature. Just how these arguments miss their mark so badly will be discussed later in this essay.

II. The Moral Arguments

It is morally right to discontinue care of a brain-dead patient. Does this show that brain-dead patients are dead? The answer depends on what one takes the activity of defining death to be. One often cited paper states that

> when we speak of human death . . . we are making a statement with policy implications. We are saying that it is now appropriate to behave towards the individual in a different way. . . . It is appropriate to begin burial ritual and for the deceased's friends and family to begin the mourning process. . . . If the individual is a holder

of public office, say, the President of the United States, the Vice President would assume the office of the President. Thus, human death is a social and moral concept quite beyond the biological. . . . The only reason the definition of death receives any attention at all in the realm of public policy is that the term summarizes and legitimates what might be called "death behavior," a radically different set of social relationships and actions.[19]

This passage suggests that to redefine death is to call for new patterns of "death behavior." If declaring a patient dead upon final cessation of breathing amounted to calling for burial and mourning at that time, then to pronounce death upon brain death would be to prescribe these practices at the earlier time. Presumably, then, on this view, the way to decide when death occurs is to determine when "death behavior" should begin.

"Death behavior" at the bedside might include mourning, turning off life-support equipment, and removing vital organs for transplantation. Ordinarily there will be little point to delay these acts past the time of brain death, at least not for the patient's sake. Roland Puccetti writes:

If someone suggested to me that my body might survive death of the neocortex for several months or years, provided it were fed and cleaned properly, etc., that would have no greater appeal to me than preservation of my appendix in a bottle of formaldehyde. For in the sense in which life has value for human beings, I would have been dead all that time.[20]

Taken to mean that life would be no more valuable to the patient than death, there can be no nonreligious objection to this assessment. The brain-dead patient has no capacity for happiness, has no interests, and arguably has no rights. Further attempts to maintain the patient's functional integrity would do him no good and are not morally required of us. The question to be answered, however, is whether the moral proposition that maintenance of the brain dead preserves nothing of value and may be ceased when convenient shows that the brain dead are dead. Many of the medical articles on brain death seem to suggest that it does. There is little real argument of any kind for regarding the brain dead as dead, but the authors regularly mention the pointlessness of maintaining those in irreversible coma and the difficulties for the transplant surgeon caused by waiting for breathing to stop. These concerns clearly motivate the redefinition— again, no new *scientific* data appeared to support the shift—and, in the absence of other argument, seem to appear to the medical authors to justify the redefinition as well.[21] This view of redefinition is explicitly stated by one philosopher:

The only way of choosing (between competing definitions of death) is to decide whether or not we attach any value to the preservation of someone irreversibly comatose. Do we value "life" even if unconscious, or do we value life only as a vehicle for consciousness?[22]

This account of the task of defining death, however, has unacceptable, even absurd, consequences. If our society came to value sports so much that the cripple's sedentary existence was thought to have no value, we would hardly find it congenial to reclassify the lame as dead. In any case, the value of life often drops well before brain death; years before, in some cases of senility. Indeed, many of us would prefer death over continued existence at the level of some profoundly retarded, institutionalized human beings. For all that, there is no temptation to say that these human beings are dead. When they do die, the change is obvious. A reclassification of healthy, profoundly retarded humans as dead would amount to ontological gerrymandering.

Thus the account of defining death which is assumed by the moral arguments is a faulty one, and a source of its error is the way in which the speech act of pronunciation of death is construed. It is certainly true that a person who pronounces a patient dead usually acts differently and expects others to do likewise. But it does not follow that to pronounce a patient dead *is* to state an intention to act differently and to call upon others to follow suit. The conclusion does not follow, even if the sole motives of the person pronouncing death are the statement of intent and the prescription to others. The argument conflates three aspects of speech acts: what is said, the effects of saying it, and the motives for saying it. Two speakers can presumably agree on whether a patient has died even if they endorse different sorts of mourning practices; indeed, even if one of them thinks the practices should begin before death, or only after a decent interval. And, of course, the speaker's intent in pronouncing death may be just to inform his listeners about the condition of the deceased, with no intention of prescribing any practice.

The reason that pronouncing death *seems* to be prescribing termination of care, and the reason that citing the moral advantages of medical abandonment *seems* to be a way of arguing for a redefinition of death as brain death, is that certain moral premises are simply assumed without question or argument: one is that there is no point to giving medical care to the dead and the other is that life should always be preserved. If these positions are abandoned, the pressure to change the definition of death is immediately relieved. We have only to realize that the moment of pulling the plug need not be the moment of death to see that defining death is a different job from deciding when it is best to remove the life-support systems. The heart-lung definition of death did not, and could not, itself, have required pointless maintenance of the brain dead. That severe prescription emerges only when we add the premise that the living must not be abandoned. What the moral arguments show, then, is not that the brain dead are dead but that the brain dead need not be cared for. The moral argument addresses a moral issue which is, unfortunately, confused by many with the task of defining death. Our argument in Section III supports the redefinition, not by demonstrating that the brain dead have a worthless existence, but by showing that they have no existence at all.

III. An Ontological Argument

To state that an ailing patient, Jones, is still alive, is in fact to make two claims; the second of which is usually taken for granted. One is that the patient is alive. The other is that the patient is (remains) *Jones*.[23] It is natural to assume that the living patient, who entered the hospital as Jones, must still be Jones (who else could it be?).[24] But we will show that this is mistaken. If we do establish that the patient, even if alive, is not Jones, and if no one else is Jones, then we will have established that Jones does not exist. And this, of course, establishes that Jones is dead. *Jones'* death thus occurs *either* at the time that the patient dies, if the patient has remained Jones; *or* at the time the patient ceased to be Jones, whichever comes first. If, as we contend, the patient ceased to be Jones at the time of brain death, then Jones' brain death is Jones' death.[25] Thus, if the loss of capacity for mental activity which occurs at brain death constitutes death, it is not for moral reasons, nor for biological reasons, but for *ontological* reasons.[26]

We need, then, to show that the patient ceases to be Jones when brain death strips the body of its psychological traits. We accomplish this by drawing a corollary about brain death from what we believe to be the correct theory of personal identity.[27] In what follows, we sketch the theory briefly, emphasizing the role which the theory attributes to the brain function. Then we state the corollary and use it to show that the criteria of personal identity thus derived do not permit identity to survive the kinds of changes which brain death involves. The result justifies a definition of death as brain death.[28]

Accounts of Personal Identity

It will seem to some—particularly to philosophers familiar with the literature on personal identity—that there exists a very short argument proving that brain-dead patients are not identical to the persons who once were associated with their bodies. Bernard Gert states:

> . . . if a body does not have any psychological features, then it is not a person, and hence the question of personal identity cannot even arise.[29]

This argument, however, must be recognized as an enthymeme, a full statement of which involves the acknowledgment of two quite substantial metaphysical assumptions. The first of these is an account of what is essential for an individual to belong to a certain kind; in the present case, the claim is that an entity is a person only if it has psychological properties. The second assumption is that it is essential for the continued existence of an individual that it remain a member of the kind to which it belongs. Otherwise, although having the capacity for psychological states might be essential to being a person, it could simply be the case that being a person, like being a musician, was a property that a given individual could acquire or lose in the course of a lifetime without ceasing to be the same individual. Each of these assumptions is notoriously controversial. There is nothing approaching a definitive account of the essence of personhood. And apparent counterexamples to the second assumption abound in nature: a bit of radioactive uranium, for example, may decay and become lead without ceasing to exist.[30] Indeed, on some accounts of what a person is, even persons come into the world as non-persons and, retaining their identity, enter that category upon suitable psychological development. Thus at least one boundary of that kind is permeable.

The approach we take here permits us to remain agnostic on the issue of kind-essentialism and on whether membership in a kind is essential to retention of identity. We offer instead an argument which establishes a claim about the essential properties of a given *individual*. The claim is that the continued possession of certain psychological properties by means of a certain causal process is an essential requirement for any given entity to be identical with the individual who is Jones. Thus, we can afford to remain uncommitted on whether persons are essentially beings with psychological properties and on whether Jones is essentially a person. We demonstrate instead that Jones, whatever kind of entity he is, is essentially an entity with psychological properties. Thus, when brain death strips the patient's body of all its psychological traits, Jones ceases to exist.

What is required to show that Jones is an individual who essentially possesses certain psychological capacities is an adequate account of personal identity. The literature on this topic generally assumes that certain individuals are identifiable as persons and then gives an account of the criteria according to which a person existing at one time is to be identified with one existing at a later time. For convenience of exposition, we will continue to talk as though the individuals we pick out are persons, but this will not affect the force of our argument. We need only claim that in normal cases we are able to identify the individual Jones (whether or not he is a person) in order to show that this individual's identity is essentially connected with the possession of certain psychological properties.

Two sorts of personal identity criteria have been proposed. One concerns continuity and connectedness of personality, memory, and other mental phenomena; the other stresses spatio-temporal continuity of the physical body. On the "mentalist" view, two "person-stages" are stages of the same person, just in case the latter is a continuation of the earlier personality and can remember what the earlier one has done.[31] The body-continuity view makes no such requirement; having the same body is sufficient and necessary.

The mentalist's basic argument is the apparent conceivability of body-switching. We can, the mentalist asserts, readily imagine persons coming to inhabit other person's bodies, or switching bodies between them. It certainly seems possible to imagine oneself waking up in another's body. We might have a hard time convincing others who we were, but we feel that we should know it in an instant. The fact that our body might be unfamiliar would be beside the point from the subjective point of view. When we narrate these examples as we usually do, it is plain that we are using a mentalist criterion of personal identity. To the extent that the descriptions of events in these examples are intuitively correct, argues the mentalist, we have established the soundness of the mentalist criterion.

The body-continuity theorists, however, have an effective counter to this argument. What is disputed is not whether these examples can be imagined, but how they ought to be interpreted. Let us suppose that a person *did* wake up feeling that he was Jones, but had a new body, or that two persons seemed able to remember events which had happened in the lives of the persons who had heretofore had the other's body. This does not show that a transfer of bodies has occurred. The subjective phenomenon might be delusive. Many persons have thought they were Napoleon or some other person; they may even have known enough about the other's life and personality to mimic the other person convincingly. If Jones and Smith woke up, each claiming to be the other, this folie à deux would simply be the situation which the mentalist mistakenly calls a body-switch. The difficulty for the mentalist is that an additional criterion of personal identity must be found, one which would establish that the memories are not delusional. But the surest criterion for genuine memory is that the re-membered event be one which happened in the rememberer's own history. The circularity is apparent.

Can the mentalist show that the putative identity changes in the body-transfer examples are not merely identity-preserving changes of psychological qualities? Not unless the examples are narrated in greater detail; everything that happens in the example mentioned above is consistent with a body-theorist's interpretation. But the mentalist can elaborate the story in a way that rules out this possibility and thus demonstrates the conceptual possibility of a person being serially identical with distinct bodies.

This consists of making clear *why* the narrated changes occur. The body theo-rist's counter-construal is silent on this point, but one's imagination can supply a range of possible causes. Jones might have been subjected to brainwashing by someone who wanted him to feel and act like Smith. Or Jones might have endured a psychotic episode in which the character of his friend, Smith, provided the organizing motif for his delusions. Or the delusions might coincidentally have formed a coherent personality and imagined life-history which duplicated that of Smith, a total stranger.

Other explanations could be dreamed up, but we need not extend this list. What is important for our purposes is the fact that the body-theorist's counter-construal appears plausible *only because* the alleged body-transfer narrative per-mits us to assume the applicability of one or another of these explanations. But suppose a body-switch narrative could be told in sufficient detail to preclude the typical body-theorist interpretations. If all these possible explanations of the qualitative changes were ruled out, we would have no reason to suppose that mere qualitative change had occurred. Then, unless the body-theorist is pre-pared to offer, in addition to a reconstrual of identity change as qualitative change, some new and powerful *explanation* for the latter, his argument will fail to convince. We would look for some other account.

The likely alternative, of course, would be that of the mentalist: these changes occurred because the persons switched bodies. This account, too, can be con-vincing only upon the assumption that an adequate explanation of events is offered, that is, an explanation of how (what we want to call) Jones' assumption of Smith's body occurred. And the explanation or explanations which would be acceptable here will characteristically be different from those which would have been accepted as accounting for personality changes. In fact, the explanations can be enumerated. If one believes in a Cartesian soul, the body-transfer must involve some sort of incorporeal unhitching from Jones' body and subsequent rehitching onto Smith's. The mentalist, however, is not tied to Cartesian dualism. Even if he grants that all mental events are physical events, there is a way that an event in Smith's life could come to be remembered by a person with Jones' body. Since memory is (presumably) stored in the brain, and since recall is (presumably) an activity of the brain, the switching of bodies between Smith and Jones could be brought about by transplanting Smith's brain into Jones' body and vice versa.[32]

To put the point in general terms: body-transfer will have occurred if and only if the sort of explanation of the continuity of a person's psychological properties is the same as that which explains this continuity in ordinary life histories (that is, those involving no body transfer). Personal identity presupposes a characteristic causal tie between person-stages (what the cause is, exactly, depends on what, empirically, causes psychological continuity). Indeed, this causal tie *is* the criterion of personal identity.[33]

Persons can switch bodies, then, if the causal connections between the psychological events in the respective bodies are the same as those which normally obtain among the psychological events which occur in the history of a normal human body. We know these causes to operate primarily within the neural system; specifically the brain. Thus it is that brain-transplantation would also constitute transfer of a person from one body to another. *Personal* identity, then, seems to be congruent with *brain* identity. This proves to be a happy result in consideration of several of the familiar cases. Consider, for example, a decapitated person whose head and body are each sustained by high-technology medicine.[34] If the head can communicate with us, and shows psychological connectedness and continuity with the erstwhile person, there can be little doubt that it *is* that person and the body is not.

But the equation of personal and brain identity needs to be qualified. Suppose that during a brain-transplantation experiment, the brain is inadvertently subjected to a process which removes all memory traces from it; indeed, "unwires" the brain so completely that the owner's entire complement of mental traits and capacities is permanently erased.[35] We feel no urge to regard the individual resulting from placing the unwired brain in a "new" body as the person previously associated with the brain. Brain identity alone is insufficient for personal identity. The reason for this follows immediately from the account given above: the ordinary causal processes which link events in a personal history involve more than spatio-temporal continuity of brain tissue. They also require continuity of certain brain *processes*, carried out through microstructural and microfunctional registrations in the brain tissue. Two body-stages which fail to be linked by continuity of these processes will fail to be stages of the same person, even if identity of the brain is preserved.[36]

Identity and Brain Death

Our argument that personal identity does not survive brain death requires but one further observation. We have throughout this discussion spoken of body transfers, cases in which a person's identity "leaves" one body and "arrives" at another. We have undertaken to state the conditions under which the entire transfer occurs. We have a fortiori stated the conditions under which each component of the transfer occurs; in particular, under which the ceasing to be associated with one body occurs. When a brain and its ongoing ordinary physiological processes are removed from one body to another, personal identity follows. But it is not necessary that the functioning brain reach its destination for identity to have vacated the donor body. If the brain fails to find a new home and is destroyed, the person's history comes to an end; the continued life functioning of the person's former body is as irrelevant to the issue as it would be had the brain been lodged in the intended new body and the resulting person continued to live.

We submit that, in quite ordinary clinical circumstances, a brain-dead body has similarly been stripped of the identity of the formerly associated person; and this holds true even if that body continues to live. It is not necessary that the brain actually be removed for personal identity to quit the body. The reason that brain removal cancels personal identity in the donor body, after all, is that the resulting body cannot thereafter have the kind of causal relation to earlier person-body stages which is required for the personal identity to hold. Brain death has the same result. Indeed, it is unimaginable that the identity question could be much affected by the physical removal of a permanently malfunctioning (and possibly liquified) brain from a living brain-dead body. Brain death and brain removal have much the same result; the dead brain serves only to add bulk to the body if left intact. If, as has been established above, removal of the conscious, functioning brain leaves us with a body not identical to the person formerly associated with it, surely removal of a dead brain leaves just the same thing; and no more remains when the brain dies in place.

Personal identity can, in theory, survive an operation in which the brain is removed from the body; it will lodge either in the brain (if suitably maintained) or in a new host body. If the brain dies, whether in its customary body or elsewhere, so does the person whose brain it is. The continuation of life in the body is immaterial in deciding this question.[37] That body is no more Jones than would be the continuation of the life of each of his cells in Petri dishes, or of each of his organs in the proper solution, after an ordinary death; it is merely better integrated tissue and organ functioning. We have, then, an argument for regarding a person's brain death as that person's death tout court which avoids both covert moral prescriptions and spurious appeals to the authority of biomedical science. The death of persons, unlike that of bodies, regularly consists in their ceasing to exist.

We have now only to relate our ontological argument to the brain-death controversy. We have argued, following other personal identity theorists, that a given person ceases to exist with the destruction of whatever processes there are which normally underlie that person's psychological continuity and connectedness. We know these processes are essentially neurological, so that irreversible cessation of upper-brain functioning constitutes the death of that person. Whole-brain death is also death for persons, but only because whole-brain death is partly comprised of upper-brain death. Tests for either will be tests for death.

Of course, our view does not imply that a person dies with his last moment of consciousness. What matters is the preservation of the substrate, not the psychological states which it produces. Hence a person who suffers brain death during sleep dies at the time of brain death, not the time of onset of sleep. Similarly, a person in a persistent coma might be alive if enough of the brain remained structurally and functionally intact.

Further, it does not follow from our argument that all humans lacking the substrate of consciousness are dead. Anencephalic infants are lacking at birth the cortical material necessary for the development of cognitive functioning and, arguably, consciousness. Still, due to possession of a functioning brain stem, they may have spontaneous breathing and heartbeat, and a good suck. Accounts which simply identified life with upper brain function would have to classify these infants as dead, which they obviously are not. We, on the other hand, need only point out that the identity criteria for the anencephalic, never-to-be conscious infant do not involve causal substrates for higher level psychological continuity. The conditions for life and existence will be those of human bodies rather than those of persons.

Finally, we emphasize that our argument, requiring no moral premises, is not sufficient to yield moral conclusions. We show that the brain dead are dead, but it does not follow that brain death is the appropriate moment to turn off ventilators or to remove organs. These acts, and other "death behavior" might be in order at some earlier time, as circumstances dictate. The relationship between defining and pronouncing death, and discontinuing care will receive further discussion in our section on the legal definition of death.

IV. The Legal Definition of Death

We have argued for the definition of death as brain death, and hence have no major quarrel with the current trend toward that definition in statutory and case law.[38] But neither, in our opinion, should those who reject our arguments and who cleave to the traditional heart-lung definition. The reasons we will give for this are moral ones. Our position calls for some explaining, especially in view of our insistence (in Section II) that moral considerations should be resolutely ignored in formulating a definition of death.

To Becker, allowing moral considerations to determine a definition of death is a cowardly evasion:

> Rigging the definition of death . . . while tempting, is an avoidance of the real issue. The real issue is whether, and if so when, it is moral to give up trying to prolong the patient's life . . . It seems best to face this problem directly—by defining when it is permissible to give up life-saving efforts—and not to evade the problem by introducing an ad hoc definition of death.[39]

But Becker offers no argument to support this last claim. Perhaps he felt he could assume agreement on the importance of being true to the facts. If so, his confidence is misplaced. However imperative truth is in theoretical work, the cardinal virtues of our social institutions are justice and utility. These will, we feel, attach to a policy that *does* evade the problem (assuming, for the sake of argument, that it is a problem) worrying Becker.

Becker feels, as do we, that discontinuation of medical care of brain-dead patients is morally acceptable, even mandatory. By Becker's definition of death, such action amounts to giving up life-saving efforts. If this sort of medical action were to be endorsed by statute or other governmental sanction, it might take the form of releasing physicians from the legal obligation to preserve the life of the irreversibly comatose.[40] The standard argument against this sort of policy is that it threatens a slide down a slippery slope: today we endorse the withdrawal of care from the comatose; perhaps tomorrow from the senile, the moderately retarded, the nonproductive. The likelihood of such a slide is probably impossible to measure with any confidence, but it surely is not negligible. Some persons now being retained in institutions for the mentally retarded, after all, have a cognitive life not much different from Karen Quinlan's. And the historical precedent (admittedly under vastly different sociopolitical conditions) has already been set.[41]

Whatever danger exists of a drift toward unjustified euthanasia would be significantly lessened if the statute licensing termination of care of brain-dead patients were one which classified them as dead rather than alive; one which, given a heart-lung definition of death, evaded the euthanasia issue. For the public, whether justifiably or not, seems willing to regard brain-dead patients as dead. A brain-death statute thus has the virtue of leaving official public policy on euthanasia, presently quite restrictive, apparently unchanged. This legal step would portend a threat to the senile and retarded only if the public came to think of them as *dead*, an eventuality which is most unlikely. The danger of the slippery slope is, then, blocked by setting a precedent which would be nearly invulnerable to distortion. Since almost all parties to the euthanasia dispute agree that the best (minimum) policy would be one which authorized withdrawal of care of the permanently comatose but no one else, licensing "letting die" by brain-death statute would be an ideal step.

Are there any serious moral objections to such an evasion? The fact that the policy would (in the view of those endorsing the heart-lung definition of death) embody a falsehood may count against it. But public policy should be granted some autonomy in these matters. The question of whether (to take an historical example) tomatoes should be classified as a vegetable or a fruit for tax purposes ought to be decided by political and economic considerations, not by biological ones.[42] It is true that an evasion in brain-death legislation would serve to dampen rather than stimulate public debate on these matters. But given the dangers alleged to be inherent in such debate, this may count against an "honest" statute.[43]

Those who (mistakenly, in our view) do not agree that brain death *is* death, then, may still have reason to support brain-death legislation authorizing withdrawal of life supports from brain-dead patients. Such support will be automatically coming from those convinced, as we are, that brain dead patients are dead (though, as we argue here, such a conclusion is not always sufficient to dictate public policy). The philosophical arguments determine the truth of the definition but not the morality of propounding it.

V. Death as Brain Death

We have argued that the death of a person's brain is that person's death. Since we believe that the argument we provide constitutes the only grounds for accepting the theoretical definition of death as brain death, it is important to reemphasize the differences between our argument and those which have been most widely accepted.

We have distinguished a number of *biological* arguments for defining death as brain death. They can all be faulted for their focus on the brain stem since (by our argument) it is loss of upper brain function which marks the person's death. Death of the brain stem is no more constitutive of death *simpliciter* than death of the kidneys or of other vital organs. The arguments we have criticized in Section I rest either on unwarranted identification of the brain stem with the body's biosystem as a whole or on erroneous appeals to the authority of medico-legal tradition or current medical opinion. On our view, the central question about death—which state of a person's body constitutes death—is answered in large part by means of a *metaphysical* argument. The only purely "biological" question is how this state can be clinically identified, and it is on this issue—not the former—that we must defer to medical expertise.

The *moral* argument proceeds from the intuition that the existence of the brain-dead patient is without any value to itself or others. Those using this argument construe the definition of death as a prescription of certain actions. The argument is successful in supporting the conclusion that care should be withdrawn from the brain dead. It can even be used to support a statute calling these patients dead. But it in no way shows that the brain dead *are* dead; this issue is never engaged.

Our argument, by contrast, is free of moral premises. The notion of "person" enters in, not because of any moral view concerning what sorts of entities have rights, but because the most likely account of personal identity serves to show that after brain death the person who entered the hospital has literally ceased to exist. Our claim that the person has died, of course, follows immediately from this. The account of personal identity uses as "data" determinations of the identities of persons and bodies in certain circumstances, but involves no testing of moral intuitions. And the moral issues concerning the patient's care are left open.

There is one more point our argument clarifies. It comes as no surprise that the continued capacity for a mental life is what makes our life valuable. Without it, life would not be worth living. But the connection between our having a capacity for a mental life and that life being of value to us is even tighter than many have supposed. For the position we hold here is not simply that a mindless future life would be of no value to us, but that such a life, whatever else might be true of it, could not be ours.

Finally, we have shown that whatever one's stance on the theoretical issues mentioned above, there may be sound moral reasons to support the current trend in public policy which extends the definition of death to include the brain dead. For those who think that brain-dead patients are still alive, this is a moral evasion. But if we wish to keep our official policy on euthanasia strict to avoid any slippery-slope difficulties, it is an ideal evasion. It is extremely implausible that the public, which believes that the brain dead are dead, could ever come to believe that the profoundly retarded or the grossly senile are dead; even though the mental life of some of these may not be much greater than that of brain-dead patients. This would prevent an extension and abuse of the statute which might follow upon (what those not persuaded by our previous arguments would consider) a more straightforward account assessing the "quality of life," one which would involve prescriptions of the form "killing (or 'letting die') is impermissible except when. . . ." And we have noted that public policy is entitled to such autonomy. Brain dead patients are in fact dead but that is not the reason to have their bodies die.

We have tried, then, to deal with the delicate topics of brain death, death, and personal identity, keeping in mind that the spheres of morality, ontology, science, and public policy, while related, are quite distinct. Our solution to the problem, we believe, gives each sphere its due without arrogating the domain of the others.

NOTES

Daniel Wikler gratefully acknowledges suggestions from those who commented on an ancestor of this essay read at the University of Wisconsin, Georgetown University, and Oberlin College, and from Norman Fost, David Mayo, and Elliott Sober, and thanks the Joseph P. Kennedy, Jr. Foundation for financial support. The present work is a descendant of a union of that paper and a paper by Michael B. Green, who expresses his appreciation for the support of the Minnesota Center for Philosophy of Science and of its Director, Grover Maxwell. Dr. Green also thanks William Winslade, Co-Director of the UCLA Program in Medicine, Law & Human Values, for providing the opportunity to investigate the topic of this essay.

1. *New York Times*, 5 December 1976.

2. Though the literature on brain death is large, it has been remarkably free of argument. The medical literature, especially, gives the reader the impression that no argument is needed. (This sentiment is discussed in part I and II below.) The arguments which we seek to refute are our reconstruction of what we believe to be the assumptions of the leading writers on the subject. Our references to that literature will be accordingly sparse. Two appropriately argumentative papers, with which we take special care to note parts of agreement and contrast, appeared in *Philosophy & Public Affairs:* Lawrence Becker's

"Human Being: The Boundaries of the Concept," vol. 4, no. 4 (Summer 1975): 334–359, and David Lamb's "Diagnosing Death," vol. 7, no. 2 (Winter 1978): 144–153.

3. The notion that brain death marks the "death of the person" is common in writing on brain death, but usually receives little explicit explication or support, deriving instead either from an intuitive essentialism (see Robert Veatch, *Death, Dying and the Biological Revolution: Our Last Quest for Responsibility,* New Haven: Yale University Press, 1976) or moral considerations (see below, Section II). We distinguish these approaches below; see fn. 28.

4. We will use the terms "upper" and "lower" to designate the parts of the brain which sponsor cognitive and regulative functions, respectively. These are not terms of the physiologist's art; it is possible that this neat division of brain parts is false to the facts and that some sections of the brain are involved in both kinds of activity, but we do not see how the present discussion would be thereby undermined.

5. *Journal of the American Medical Association* 205 (1968): 337–340.

6. The physiological facts are elegantly summarized in Peter McL. Black, "Brain Death," *New England Journal of Medicine* 299 (17 August 1978): 338–344; and (24 August 1978): 393–401.

7. New Jersey Supreme Court: In the Matter of Karen Quinlan, an alleged incompetent. 79 NJ 10, 355 A2and 647 (1976). Our analysis of the matter will vindicate common intuition that Karen Quinlan was already dead while what was once her body continued to live.

8. This version of the argument is implicit in much of the brain-death literature, but it has not been spelled out in the form given here. Arguments resembling (inexactly) the one given here may be found in Clarence Crafoord, "Cerebral Death and the Transplant Era," *Diseases of the Chest* 55, no. 2 (February 1969): 141–145; and Robert Schwager, "Medicine and Irreversible Coma," in Tom Beauchamp and Seymour Perlin, eds., *Ethical Issues in Death and Dying* (Englewood Cliffs, 1977).

9. For certain practical reasons, some statutes have written brain death into the legal definition of death alongside, rather than in place of, the traditional heart-lung definition. See Alexander M. Capron and Leon R. Kass, "A Statutory Definition of the Standards for Determining Human Death: An Appraisal and a Proposal," *University of Pennsylvania Law Review* 121, no. 1 (November 1972): 87–118.

10. A point well argued in Becker, "Human Being." See p. 355.

11. As Black notes in "Brain Death," these two grounds have given rise to two other kinds of validation studies for brain-death indicators. Those interested in the role of brain death in causing so-called somatic death (death of the rest of the body) have been concerned to demonstrate that somatic death is inevitable once the appropriate indications of brain death appear. Those emphasizing the central place of the brain in the body system are concerned to learn just when the brain disintegrates; what happens to the rest of the body, and when, is treated as immaterial.

12. Becker, "Human Being," p. 353.

13. See Lamb, "Diagnosing Death," p. 174; Black, "Brain Death."

14. There is a series of classic eighteenth-century experiments by LeGallois on rabbit fetuses and pups which makes this point forcibly. LaGallois noted that if these organisms were decapitated above the pneumogastric nerve, the body of the organism remained alive for a period of time equal to that required for suffocation to occur in an organism at that developmental level. For very young rabbits, this was a period of several hours! Thus, the proximal cause of death in each case was asphyxiation, not the decapitation

which produced it. The moral is obvious. If there is nothing peculiar in maintaining that these decapitated bodies, though waning, were still alive, there is nothing peculiar about maintaining the same position vis-à-vis brain-dead organisms so long as we are constrained to consider biological considerations alone. For an account of the LeGallois experiments, see Solomon Diamond, *The Roots of Psychology* (New York: Basic Books, 1974), pp. 41–44.

15. Lamb, "Diagnosing Death," pp. 146–147.

16. Ibid., p. 147.

17. Becker, "Human Being," p. 353.

18. In denying the relevance of lower brain death in determining death of the body, we follow Becker; we have been concerned here to defend him against Lamb. Were it not for our views on the identity of the brain-dead patient, we would also endorse his positive view that "a human organism is dead when, for whatever reason, the system of those reciprocally dependent processes which assimilate oxygen, metabolize food, eliminate wastes, and keep the organism in relative homeostasis are arrested in a way which the organism itself cannot reverse" ("Human Being," p. 353). Except for the final clause concerning spontaneous reversal, the fundamental idea is sound: bodily death consists of functional disintegration. This definition is appropriately vague; it cannot be used to specify an instant of bodily death in most cases, but it serves to rule out a host of illegitimate candidates.

19. Robert M. Veatch, "The Whole-Brain Oriented Concept of Death: An Out-Moded Philosophical Formulation," *Journal of Thanatology* 3 (1975): 13–30. Our continuation of the argument is not meant to represent Veatch's view since our development of this argument is not entirely consonant with his. We endorse Veatch's conclusions and our arguments are complementary to his (though see below, fn. 28). See his *Death, Dying and the Biological Revolution,* chaps. 1–2.

20. Roland Puccetti, "The Conquest of Death," *The Monist* 59 (1976): 252.

21. If the chief medical impetus for recognizing brain death as death was a moral one, why would the medical criteria for brain death focus on death of the *whole* brain rather than on death of the upper brain alone? The patient whose upper brain is lost has, after all, a life just as low in quality as that of the patient whose whole brain is gone. Medical articles are mostly silent on this issue. An exception is *The Lancet's* editorial on the occasion of a statement on brain death by the Conference of Royal Colleges and Faculties of the United Kingdom. Their remark that "How long life support should be provided for such survivors of brain damage is a harrowing question, but vegetative patients are not brain dead and the questions of ethics and of the use of resources are different" (13 November 1976, p. 1065) reaffirms the focus on lower rather than higher, brain death, but does not explain the reasons for this focus. The tests for whole brain death were more reliable than those for upper brain death alone, but recent articles disavow this as the reason. Our conversations with medical specialists give us the impression that physicians, so used to attempting to restore the body to functional integrity, cannot bring themselves to pronounce death upon a breathing body which maintains itself with only nutritional and custodial care. Our diagnosis, then, is that moral concern to let the patients lapse, constrained by tradition, caused the physicians to adopt an otherwise unmotivated attitude of respect for the lower brain, identifying its continued functioning with life itself.

22. Jonathan Glover, *Causing Death and Saving Lives* (Middlesex, 1977), p. 45.

23. The term "patient" is used neutrally to designate the entity in the hospital bed. For a discussion of the relation of existence and identity, see Roderick Chisholm, "Coming

into Being and Passing Away," in Stuart F. Spicker and H. Tristram Englehardt, eds., *Philosophical Medical Ethics: Its Nature and Significance* (Dordrecht, Holland, 1977), especially p. 171.

24. That brain-dead patients can nevertheless be alive is argued in Section I, above.

25. It is worth emphasizing that we are not speaking of two distinct events, loss of identity and death, which occur in the life of every individual. Once Jones is no longer the living entity we call "the patient," Jones is gone and dead. That his body lives or dies is immaterial. As Becker himself notes ("Human Being," p. 354), the continued life of organs and other entities which were once a part of a living person does not constitute continued life of that person. What matters is whether these tissues *are* that person. Indeed, Jones would be dead, even if his living body were to become another person— assuming, as we shall show, that such talk makes sense. This shows that the issue is not whether the patient is *a* person after brain death. It is whether the patient is *that* person, Jones.

26. Gareth Matthews offers an ontological argument for brain death in his "Life and Death as the Arrival and Departure of the Psyche," *American Philosophical Quarterly* 16, no. 2 (April 1979): 151–157. Matthews' argument, which proceeds from a neo-Aristotelian notion of *psyche* distinct from current conceptions of "person," identifies death of an organism with the loss of the capacity for self-regulation in the way distinctive of its kind. We find his proposal unsuccessful; a comprehensive examination of Matthews' position would not fall within the scope of this article.

27. The theory is essentially the view developed by John Perry in a series of articles; see his contributions to his edited volume *Personal Identity* (Berkeley and Los Angeles: University of California Press, 1975) and to Amelie Rorty, ed., *The Identities of Persons* (Berkeley and Los Angeles: University of California Press, 1976); and his review of Bernard Williams' *Problems of the Self* in *Journal of Philosophy* 73, no. 13 (15 July 1976): 416–438. Bernard Gert's "Personal Identity and the Body," *Dialogue*, September 1971, pp. 458–478, from which we also learned much, is in important respects similar. A similar theory is embodied in Jewish law, according to Rabbi Azriel Rosenfeld, who has noted its importance for the brain-death controversy; see his "The Heart, the Head, and the Halakhah," *New York State Journal of Medicine* (15 October 1970): 2615–2619.

28. The notion that the brain-dead patient has "ceased to exist as a person" (see fn. 3, above) has both a moral and an ontological interpretation. The moral claim is simply that the patient's life now lacks the features that make life more valuable for people than death. Our ontological claim is that the person who entered the hospital, he whose body is now brain dead, no longer exists (though his body or some of its parts may both exist and live). Robert Veatch, in his *Death, Dying and the Biological Revolution* holds that "to define the death of a human being, we must recognize the characteristics that are essential to humanness. . . . We use the term *death* to mean the loss of what is essentially significant to an entity—in the case of man, the loss of humanness" (p. 26). "To ask what is essentially significant to a human being is a philosophical question—a question of ethical and other values. Many elements make human beings unique—their opposing thumbs, their possession of rational souls . . . and so on. Any concept of death will depend directly upon how one evaluates these qualities" (pp. 29–30). This seems to be a hybrid: moral considerations dictating our ontological conclusion. Veatch conducts his search for what is "essentially human" and "essential to man's nature" by contrasting various "traditions" ("the empiricalist philosophical tradition seems to be represented in the emphasis on consciousness. . . . At least in the Western tradition, man is seen as an

essentially social animal," p. 41), by drawing upon his own and others' intuitions on man's essence, and by citing perceived moral dangers of adopting the views he opposes.

It would be hard to argue for or against this view except by citing one's own intuitions on "man's nature," if any. We avoid the evident difficulties of this approach by constructing a step-by-step argument using the intuitive "data" on personal identity drawn on by Locke and his successors. Though our argument, like Veatch's, appeals in the end to intuitions, it appeals to conceptual intuitions, not moral ones, on which there is considerable consensus, and which are used to test a concept (personal identity) which is considerably better defined than Veatch's "human existence." Our individual-essentialism is, relative to Veatch's (and others') kind-essentialism, better methodology if not better metaphysics.

29. Gert, "Personal Identity and the Body," pp. 475–476.

30. Berent Enç, "Natural Kinds and Linnaean Essentialism," *Canadian Journal of Philosophy* 5, no. 1 (1 September 1975): 83–102. See also Marjorie Price, "Identity through Time," *Journal of Philosophy* 74, no. 4 (April 1977): 201–217.

31. A person-stage is a person in a given time interval. A person *simpliciter* is a series of person-stages. The problem of personal identity, thus conceived, is to state the criteria determining which person-stages are stages of the same entity.

32. That a materialist view of mind and person can coexist with our view that persons cease to exist before their bodies do is denied by Saul Kripke ("Naming and Necessity," in G. Harman and D. Davidson, eds., *Semantics of Natural Languages,* Dordrecht, 1972, p. 334 and fn. 73). Kripke, after attacking a crude materialist view, admits that a sophisticated materialist cum mentalist would identify the person with a body *whose brain enjoyed the proper physical organization.* Kripke claims that even this latter approach falls prey to modal difficulties, but he does not attempt to show this, and we have not been persuaded of any incompatability of materialism with our position by the objections he does offer (for a fuller treatment of Kripke's views; see Fred Feldman, "Kripke on the Identity Theory," *Journal of Philosophy* 71, no. 24 [October 1974]: 666 ff.). The outcome of this debate is not relevant to our present purposes, however. Although we have spoken of memory as though it is a brain process, thus suggesting support of a mind-brain identity thesis, all we require is that mental life be nomologically dependent on brain-functioning and that the capacity for consciousness should follow the undamaged brain wherever it might go. This we take modem neuroscience to have established beyond controversy.

33. Body-continuity theorists aim their fire at examples which, like Locke's, leave the causes unspecified. The brain-transplantation variants escape their attention (a point made by Perry in his review of B. Williams, *Problems of the Self,* and by Gert, "Personal Identity and the Body") and the various arguments used against the Lockean cases score no points against them.

34. Or, substitute brain for head, assuming that the brain can be hooked up to sensory devices and provided with some means of self-expression. An early treatise on medical jurisprudence, *Manual of Medical Jurisprudence and State Medicine* by M. Ray (London, 1836, ad ed.), p. 499, stated that "individuals who are apparently destroyed in a sudden manner, by certain wounds, diseases or even decapitation, are not really dead, but are only in conditions incompatible with the persistence of life." On our own view, the body may well be *alive*—so may the head—but only one is the person who was once whole.

Becker, "Human Being," p. 358, says: "Bizarre questions may be raised, of course. Is a human brain separated from its body and kept 'functioning' a human being? . . . I admit to being at a loss for a reply to such cases, let alone an answer." Again, Becker has addressed the wrong question: we want to know not (only) if the brain is *a* human being, but *which* human being, where the "human being" means "person." Becker would presumably find our question unanswerable as well; we simply regard the case as more easily conceivable than Becker professes to do. On the conceivability of isolated brains having psychological states, see Bernard Gert, "Can a Brain have a Pain," *Philosophy and Phenomenological Research* 27, no. 3 (March 1967): 432–436, and references cited therein. For a case in which such a state may already have existed in an isolated brain, see fn. 19 in Puccetti, "The Conquest of Death."

35. This sort of imagery is, of course, fatuous. We can foresee no reason why a variant which is truer to the facts should not provide the same conclusion, however. Perry refers to this process as a "brain zap" in his review of B. Williams, *Problems of the Self.*

36. Contrast this case from Gert's "Personal Identity and the Body": Jones is hypnotized and made to think, feel, and otherwise resemble Smith in all mental respects. Then the brain is transplanted into Smith's body. The resulting individual is Jones, even though it is psychologically similar to Smith and has Smith's body. The reason is that, in this case, the causal relations between body-stages (hypnosis as well as transplantation) are personal-identity preserving. (In fact, this case involves considerable philosophical license: if hypnosis or other psychological procedures could produce the vast changes alleged here, our concept of personal identity would be considerably different from what it is.)

37. The same would be true if a new person's brain, carrying that person's brain structure and processes, were transplanted into the body. The result would be a living person, but not the person, now dead, whose body it formerly was.

38. Two unresolved problems of detail pose problems for those writing brain-death statutes. One is how to specify medical criteria of brain death in a way that assures a minimum of false positives. The second is the harmonious accommodation of the quite different criteria which will be used by physicians and coroners called upon to pronounce death in settings as diverse as intensive care units, accident sites, and cornfields. Neither of these has significant theoretical interest.

39. Becker, "Human Being," pp. 356–357.

40. Since doctors are rarely, if ever, prosecuted for decisions to cease medical support of the permanently comatose, such a statute might not be needed.

41. Leo Alexander, "Medical Science Under Dictatorship," *New England Journal of Medicine* 241, no. 2 (14 July 1949): 39–47.

42. Though once the rules are set, those adversely affected may try to use a biological argument to reverse the ruling and to advance their interests. See Charles M. Rick, "The Tomato," *Scientific American* 239 (2 August 1978): 76–86.

43. There are two positions which are immune to our argument on public policy. We shall state these without any discussion, though both raise important issues deserving greater consideration. First, those who both disagree with our conclusions and believe that it would be a good thing to have a debate leading to a policy of limited euthanasia would not want to take the muted course we advocate. Second, there are those who will be concerned about an important difference between the "tomato" case and the topic of this paper. The justification for the evasive public policy in the present case rests on the assumption that those making policy have made a correct *moral judgment* on a very important topic and that this decision justifies the evasive legislation. There is no comparable

moral decision in the tomato case, just prudential considerations, so that no "evasion" arises, merely pragmatic redefinition. Thus, the tactic advocated here, even if it is supported in this case by a correct moral judgment, is implicitly authorizing lawmakers to employ evasive or conceptually mistaken legislation when, in their best judgment, moral considerations lead them to conclude it would be justified. The path advised here may be an instance of a kind of policy making which, even if justified in this individual case taken in isolation, should probably not be encouraged.

CHAPTER THIRTY-ONE

On the Definition of Death

John P. Lizza

When a neurological criterion for determining death was formally introduced in the recommendation of the 1968 Ad Hoc Committee of the Harvard Medical School, the conceptual basis for accepting the criterion was unclear.[1] As Martin Pernick notes, the committee shifted back and forth between endorsing the loss of consciousness, as opposed to the loss of bodily integration, as the conceptual foundation for the new criterion that the committee eventually proposed.[2] Indeed, the committee's characterization of the criterion as "irreversible coma" reflected this ambiguity, as the term had been used in the past to describe the condition of individuals in deep coma or persistent vegetative state.[3] In fact, although the committee proposed a new criterion for determining death, it had little to say about the definition or concept of death for which the criterion was proposed.

One of the first attempts to clearly articulate the conceptual foundation for the neurological criterion appeared in the work of James Bernat, Charles Culver, and Bernard Gert, when they proposed "the permanent cessation of functioning of the organism as a whole" as a definition of death.[4] One reason they gave for rejecting the irreversible loss of consciousness as the conceptual basis for the neurological criterion was that it would entail classifying as dead those individuals who had irreversibly lost consciousness but retained brainstem function (e.g., individuals in permanent vegetative state). Because Bernat, Culver, and Gert thought that such individuals could not be classified as dead, they invoked the loss of organic integration as the basis for the neurological criterion. They then maintained that, because individuals in permanent vegetative state retain the integrative functions of the brainstem, they were still integrated organisms and therefore still alive. The influential President's Commission for the Study of Ethical Problems in Medicine and Biomedical and Behavioral Research took a similar position in 1981.[5]

Bernat, Culver, and Gert's definition of death was soon challenged. Stuart Youngner and Edward Bartlett showed that the rationale behind the biological *definition* of death as the loss of integration of the organism as a whole does not support the whole-brain *criterion* of death that the President's Commission and others endorse.[6] Instead, it supports only the adoption of a more limited brainstem criterion, because the brainstem, not neocortical structures, is supposedly responsible for integrating the organism in a life-sustaining way. In addition, because "the permanent cessation of the functioning of the organism as a whole" is supposed to capture the idea that any organism dies when it loses its internal, organic integration, it is unclear why it is necessary that higher-brain functions must cease, because those functions are not essential to the integration of the organism as a whole. Higher-brain functions would appear to be as necessary to the functioning of the organism as a whole as, say, fingernail growth. Indeed, precisely because the proponents of the above definition do not regard higher-brain functions as necessary for the integration of the organism as a whole, they do not regard individuals in permanent vegetative state as dead.

The problem with the definition, however, as Youngner and Bartlett pointed out, is that it has the absurd implication that certain kinds of patients, whom we think are alive, would be "dead." Consider, for example, patients with locked-in syndrome, who have a fairly specific and limited lesion in the ventral pons, causing disconnection of the upper motor neurons in the brain from lower motor neurons in the spinal cord. The portions of their brains responsible for consciousness and cognition, however, remain intact. It is easy to imagine such a patient's having additional lesions in those portions of the brain that play a role in the regulation of heartbeat, respiration, blood pressure, and hormonal balance. Because individuals who have lost all brain functions have been sustained for months and even longer, it is also not hard to imagine sustaining such a locked-in patient. The problem, however, is that even though the patient retains consciousness, acceptance of spontaneous brainstem functions as necessary for organic integration would entail that this patient has irreversibly lost organic integration and therefore is dead.

A second major challenge to Bernat, Culver, and Gert's definition of death has come from those who argue that the human organism as a whole may remain alive despite the loss of all brain function. Cases of postmortem pregnancy and the extraordinary case reported by D. Alan Shewmon in which a male with no brain function was sustained for more than twenty years challenge the claim that brain function is necessary for organic integration.[7] Also, the view that individuals who have lost all brain function but receive artificial life support are not integrated organisms but merely collections of organic parts has been effectively critiqued by many scholars, including Becker,[8] Truog,[9] Halevy and Brody,[10] Grant,[11] Seifert,[12] Byrne et al.,[13] Taylor,[14] Veatch,[15] Gervais,[16] Wikler,[17] and Shewmon.[18] Indeed, at the Third International Symposium on Coma and Death in 2000, Dr. Shewmon delivered on his claim to "drive the nails into the coffin" of the idea that organic integration requires brain function.[19] At bottom, individuals who have lost all brain function but continue to function in such biologically integrated ways for such lengthy time frames are integrated organisms of some sort and cannot be classified as corpses or dead organisms.

If these challenges to the currently accepted definition of death have merit, then we are faced with a choice: We must either retain the definition of death as the loss of organic integration and give up the current whole-brain, neurological criterion or come up with an alternative definition of death that is consistent with accepting a neurological criterion. I propose that we do the latter and shall argue that the irreversible loss of organic integration is an incorrect conceptual basis for accepting a neurological criterion of death. The correct basis appeals to the essential significance of consciousness in the lives of people. I think that, all along, the real reason that we have been willing to accept "brain death" as death is not because we were sure that it entailed the loss of integration of the organism as a whole, but because we were sure that it constituted the irreversible loss of consciousness and every other mental capacity and function. Because so many of us believe that the potential for consciousness is essential (necessary) to the kind of being that we are, we are willing to accept its loss as the end of our lives. In my view, death can be defined as the irreversible loss of psychophysical integration, where *psycho* refers to a capacity or potential for conscious experience of the world. The irreversible loss of consciousness can thus serve as a criterion for the determination of death.

If an organism is alive in cases such as "postmortem" pregnancy, the question arises: What is alive? It does not automatically follow that the person is alive, as claimed by those who wish to maintain that death is the loss of organic integration but reject the neurological criterion for death. Advocates of a consciousness-related formulation of death do not consider such a being to be a living person. In their view, a person cannot persist through the loss of all brain function or even the loss of just those brain functions required for consciousness and other mental functions. Thus, if an advocate of the consciousness-related formulation of death wishes to maintain that the person dies even though some being is alive in these cases, what remains alive must be a different sort of being. It must either be a human being, as distinct from a person, or a being of another sort (e.g., a "humanoid" or "biological artifact"). By "humanoid" or "biological artifact," I mean a living being that has human characteristics but falls short of being human, a form of life created by medical technology. Indeed, this may be the most sensible thing to say about such a living being. Whereas a person is normally transformed into a corpse at death, technology has intervened in this natural process and made it possible for a person to die in new ways. Instead of a person's death being followed by remains in the form of an inanimate corpse, it is now possible for a person's remains to take the form of an artificially sustained, living organism devoid of the capacity for consciousness and any other mental function.

This distinction between the person and the human organism and the idea that a person may die even though the biological organism that in part constituted it may remain alive may cause some consternation. Aren't persons organisms? How can a person's death be different from that of a human organism? Do persons literally die? Or is death a concept that applies only to organisms? The answers to these questions are not so simple. In the history of philosophy and religion, many views reject the strict identification of the human being or person with a biological organism or human body. Dualism and nonreductive materialism are two examples. In addition, views of the person such as those of Aquinas, Meilaender, Strawson, Lowe, Wiggins, and Baker are consistent with predicating "death" literally to persons.[20] Thus, how one understands the relation between the person and human organism may affect what one is willing to accept as the definition and criteria for death.

A substantive concept of persons provides the correct conceptual grounding for a consciousness-related formulation of death. However, the arguments in favor of this formulation have been clouded, in part because some of its main proponents, such as Robert Veatch, Michael Green, and Daniel Wikler, have relied on a problematic qualitative or functionalist concept of person, instead of a more defensible substantive concept.[21] Veatch, for example, is careful to construct his definition of death in terms of the death of the human being, not the person. He also distances himself from the argument of Green and Wikler, because he believes their view defines death in terms of the loss of personal identity, which he believes is problematic. All along, Veatch assumes that *person* is a qualitative or functional specification of the human being, rather than, itself, a substantive concept. His concern is thus that the functionalist theory of personhood may entail that a person no longer exists in cases of dementia in which all traces of rationality and many other cognitive abilities are lost. Veatch believes, however, that a death has not occurred in such cases. In addition, Veatch is specifically critical of Green and Wikler's argument, because their view defines death in terms of the loss of personal identity. Veatch believes that we can conceive of cases in which personal identity in the Lockean sense may be lost, but a death has not occurred. According to Veatch, Green and Wikler's theory would commit them to drawing the absurd conclusion that someone who has lost psychological continuity—for example, by suffering complete amnesia—has necessarily died. However, Veatch asks us to suppose that this human being who has suffered complete amnesia subsequently develops a new set of beliefs, memories, and other psychological characteristics that we associate with personhood. According to Veatch, even though we might regard such a being as a new person, it is counterintuitive to say, as he believes Green and Wikler must say, that a death occurred in such a case.

Veatch believes that human beings, not persons, are the kind of thing that dies. However, Veatch accepts what he says is the traditional Judeo-Christian concept of a *human being* as an essential union of mind and body.[22] Because such a union may still exist even though someone suffers complete amnesia, the human being would still exist. A death has not occurred. However, because an irreversible loss of consciousness, as in permanent vegetative state, would entail the destruction of the essential union of mind and body, Veatch believes that the traditional Judeo-Christian concept of the human being warrants accepting a consciousness-related criterion of death. He regards individuals in permanent vegetative state as dead. Because these individuals have crossed the bright line between dementia (diminished mental capacity) and amentia (no mental capacity), their essential union of mind and body has been destroyed.

Karen Gervais also criticized Green and Wikler's view on grounds similar to those of Veatch.[23] She argues that as long as the biological substrate for consciousness remains intact, despite the complete loss of memories, a death has not occurred. However, Gervais believes that the same *person* continues to exist. At this point, she is invoking a substantive concept of personhood and rejecting the functionalist view that she attributes to Green and Wikler and assumed by Veatch. In contrast to Veatch, Gervais treats persons as the kind of thing that can literally die. I believe that she is correct in this, and that Veatch erred in failing to recognize a substantive concept of person. She also reinterprets Veatch's argument in a way that essentially equates her substantive concept of person with Veatch's substantive concept of human being. What is common to Gervais and Veatch is that they both accept the idea that what dies is a substantive entity that is essentially mind and body. Gervais calls such a being a "person," whereas Veatch refers to it as a "human being." Gervais, like Veatch, also accepts a consciousness-related formulation of death that would treat individuals in permanent vegetative state as dead. Veatch's error thus lies in his assumption that there is no alternative to the qualitative or functionalist view of the person and personal identity. Insofar as Gervais invokes a substantive concept of person, she puts the argument for a consciousness-related formulation of death on more coherent, conceptual grounds.

P. F. Strawson's definition of a person as an individual to which we can necessarily apply both predicates that ascribe psychological characteristics (P-predicates) and predicates that ascribe corporeal characteristics (M-predicates) is an example of the use of "person" in this substantive sense. In Strawson's view, and even assuming with Bernat, Culver, and Gert that death is a biological or corporeal concept, it is neither a category mistake nor a metaphor to predicate death to persons. Wiggins and Lowe's substantive views of the person, as well as Baker's constitutive view, can also provide the conceptual grounding for a consciousness-related formulation of death. Because all of these views understand a person as a living substantive being with minimally the capacity for consciousness, the irreversible loss of this capacity would mean the end of a person's life.[24]

Bernat, Culver, and Gert challenge this view. Bernat asserts, "As a biological concept, death should be univocal across these (higher animal) species and not defined idiosyncratically for *Homo sapiens,* because, for example, we refer to the same concept when we say that a relative has died as we do when we say that our pet dog has died."[25] He argues that acceptance of the irreversible loss of consciousness as a criterion of death for persons or human beings violates the requirement that death must mean the same thing for all higher animal species and offends against the common usage and understanding that death must be the same for these types of organisms.

Bernat's position is puzzling. First, he offers no general explanation of when the definition of death varies across species and when it is does not. For example, why is it acceptable to have a definition of death for vertebrates that does not apply to invertebrates, but unacceptable to have a definition of death for human beings or persons that does not apply to other higher animal species? How exactly does the kind of thing that dies influence the definition of death for that kind of thing? While Bernat at least recognizes variation in the definition of death across species, he never examines the details of what impact the kind of thing that dies has on the definition of death.

Second, even if the definition of death for a human being, pet dog, and members of other higher animal species is the same, this may be because all of these organisms have some form of consciousness or sentience. Indeed, consciousness or sentience may be an essential property of these kinds of being, such that its irreversible loss would entail the death or ceasing to exist of these types of organism. This opens up a number of options for a consciousness-related theorist. For example, consciousness-related theorists could maintain that the irreversible loss of consciousness and sentience in a dog would entail the loss of integration of the organism *as a whole* and hence would mean its death. In this view, an artificially sustained dog in permanent vegetative state may not be a dog at all. Instead, it may be the remains of a dog, a different kind of biological organism, or, perhaps more descriptively, a kind of biological artifact.

Alternatively, a consciousness-related theorist could rely on a distinction between persons and organisms (e.g., that persons are constituted by but not identical to or reducible to living organisms). In this view, the death of the person is understood as different from the death of the organism. This distinction provides consciousness-related theorists with further options, depending on what they consider to be the necessary and sufficient conditions of personhood. For example, if the capacity or potential for consciousness and sentience is necessary and sufficient for being a person but is not a necessary condition for being an organism, then the definition of the death of the person would be different than that of the organism. This particular account of personhood might classify dogs as persons, because they exhibit consciousness and sentience. In this case, the definition of death of a human being *qua* person would be the same as that of the dog *qua* person. Moreover, the definition of death of the human being *qua* organism might be the same as that of the dog *qua* organism. However, if more than consciousness and sentience is required for personhood—e.g., the capacity for language, rationality, or moral responsibility—then the dog would be excluded from the class of persons. The death of the human person would then be different from the death of these other kinds of being.

Bernard Gert also appears to acknowledge that the definition of death depends on the kind of thing that dies.[26] In the light of experiments in which monkeys were kept alive for some time after their heads were severed from their bodies,[27] Gert now believes that it is necessary to include the irreversible loss of consciousness in the definition of death. He writes, "When a monkey's severed head responds to sounds and sights, claiming that it is dead alters the ordinary understanding of death far more than claiming that the monkey is still alive."[28] To accommodate this ordinary understanding of death, Gert, now joined by Charles Culver and K. Danner Clouser, amends the earlier biological definition of death that he, Bernat, and Culver had proposed. In place of the former definition of death as "the permanent cessation of the functioning of the organism as a whole," Gert, Culver, and Clouser now offer the following: "death is the permanent cessation of all observable natural functioning of the organism as a whole, and the permanent absence of consciousness in the organism as a whole, and in any part of the organism."[29] The amendment is needed to accommodate the fact that the monkeys were alive, even though they had ceased to function as organic wholes. Gert earlier explained that it is necessary to include the clauses about the absence of consciousness in the definition of death, because "the importance of consciousness to a conscious organism has no counterpart in nonconscious animals or plants."[30]

In this amended definition of death that Gert, Culver, and Clouser believe applies to all organisms, (1) permanent cessation of all observable natural functioning of the organism as a whole and (2) irreversible loss or absence of consciousness are jointly necessary and sufficient for death. However, neither is individually sufficient for death. Thus, these authors continue to reject the higher-brain formulation of death because, as Gert expressed in earlier work, "Taking permanent loss of consciousness as sufficient for the death of a human being makes the death of a human being something *completely distinct* from the death of lower organisms."[31] In addition, Gert thinks that such a definition "does not state what we ordinarily mean when we speak of death."[32] In support of this claim, he states, "We ordinarily regard permanently comatose patients in persistent vegetative states who are sufficiently brain damaged that they have irreversibly lost consciousness as still alive."[33]

Gert, Culver, and Clouser take the presence of consciousness in the severed head of the monkey as sufficient for the continued life of the monkey. In their recent consideration of a variation on the case in which the monkey's decapitated body is also artificially sustained, they hold that the monkey continues to exist as the artificially sustained severed head, not the artificially sustained apian body. They explain,

> In our previous account, we recognized the importance of consciousness, claiming that "consciousness and cognition are sufficient to show the functioning of the organism as a whole in higher animals but they are not necessary." If we had taken science fiction more seriously, we might have anticipated the recent research that has demonstrated that consciousness of a part of the organism is possible independent of the functioning of the organism as a whole. In these science fiction stories, it is quite clear that the organism as a whole has ceased to function, although a part of the organism remains conscious. We now realize that when consciousness is maintained in a part of the organism, even though that part, namely the head or the brain, has been separated from the rest of the organism, the organism has not died.
>
> We erred in not recognizing consciousness as sufficient for life, independent of the functioning of the organism as a whole.[34]

However, at this point, Gert, Culver, and Clouser fail to consider, as Shewmon and others have pointed out, that the brain is not necessary for there to be an integrated organism. And if the brain is not necessary, neither is the head. The artificially sustained decapitated apian body is a living organism of some kind, as it continues to function in an integrated way, albeit through artificial life support. In fact, it would probably require less artificial support than the severed head. If the dependence on artificial support is not a reason for thinking that the severed head is dead, it is not a reason for thinking that the decapitated body is dead. The difficulty is that most biologists and ordinary people would probably identify the artificially sustained decapitated body as the continuation of the life of an organism. Indeed, those who reject the loss of all brain function as a criterion of death maintain that the human organism with no brain function may persist through artificial support. If the head of such an artificially sustained whole-brain dead human being were severed, it is unclear why this would make any difference in how they regard the nature of the artificially sustained brainless body. Thus, there is probably more biological reason for identifying the artificially sustained whole-brain dead or (hypothetically) artificially sustained decapitated body as a human organism, rather than the severed head.

At this point, Gert, Culver, and Clouser might argue that, because the functioning of the whole-brain dead body is not "natural" but artificially sustained, the individual is dead. Indeed, according to their latest definition of death, lower-order organisms that are never conscious are dead when they lose "all observable *natural* functioning of the organism as a whole" (emphasis added).[35] Thus, assuming that frogs are never conscious, the definition would entail that a frog on permanent artificial life support, especially if the support involves multiple organs, is dead, because it has lost "all observable natural functioning as a whole." However, this is strongly counterintuitive, especially if the frog could catch prey, exchange oxygen for gaseous wastes, take in nourishment and eliminate waste, and so on. Entropy would clearly not have set in. Would any biologist say that the frog is dead? Would ordinary people say that the frog is "dead"?

Gert, Culver, and Clouser's aim to provide a trans-species definition of death that captures the ordinary meaning of death thus fails. Because there are plenty of organisms that function as a whole without a brain and because the artificially sustained decapitated human body could be one of them, the "ordinary" sense of what it means for an organism to die would not apply to the artificially sustained decapitated human body. We would not consider other organic beings (e.g., animals lower on the phylogenic scale or plants) to have died, because they were dependent on artificial life support. Similarly, if we assume with Gert, Culver, and Clouser that there is a trans-species biological meaning of death, we should not consider the artificially sustained decapitated human body to be dead, simply because it requires artificial support.

Gert, Culver, and Clouser also equivocate on what they call the severed head. Is it a "part of an organism" or an "organism"? Or do they think that this part of the organism (the artificially sustained severed head) is enough for it to still be a human organism? Again, the artificially sustained decapitated body would more likely count as a type of organism than the severed head, because there is so much more natural structure and integrated functioning among subsystems to sustain life in the case of the decapitated body than there is in the case of the severed head. Indeed, it is unclear whether it is correct to call the artificially sustained severed head an "organism" at all. Instead, it would seem to be more a form of life created by technology—a cyborg with organic parts, rather than an organism. However, it is then not at all clear that, even if the ordinary understanding of human life and death were strictly biological, such a sense of life and death would apply to artificially sustained severed heads, because such cyborgs are not biological organisms in the usual sense. Indeed, because Gert, Culver, and Clouser hold that consciousness is sufficient for human life "independent of the functioning of the organism as a whole," the form of life that constitutes or supports a human consciousness need not necessarily be the life of an organism. Therefore, the death of the human person need not be tied to the death of an organism. If a human being or person can be alive independent of the organism as a whole, then it is the human being's consciousness that is definitive of a human life. However, if consciousness is definitive of human life, then its irreversible loss is definitive of human death.

In sum, Gert, Culver, and Clouser's revision in the definition of death in response to consideration of the hypothetical case of the artificially sustained severed head tries to do justice to the intuition that the person would still be alive. However, in doing so, they ignore the implication of the criticism of the whole-brain neurological criterion, i.e., that the human organism would continue to exist in the form of the artificially sustained decapitated body, not in the form of the severed head. Because we cannot be in two places at once and because they correctly identify the continuation of the person with the severed head, the continuation of the integration of the organism as a whole (what supposedly we share with all forms of organic life) becomes irrelevant to understanding what it means for us to be alive. Consciousness, rather than integration as a whole organism, appears definitive of our existence. However, if consciousness is essential to our existence, then its irreversible loss, as in cases of permanent vegetative state and whole-brain death, would be sufficient for our death.

It should be noted that the significance of consciousness in our lives is not derived from strictly biological considerations of what it means for us to be integrated organisms like other biological organisms. Instead, its significance comes from the *value* that we place on consciousness in our understanding of the kind of being that we are. In short, the possibility of the bifurcation of our existence into an artificially sustained severed head and an artificially sustained organic body shows that the death of the person or human being is different from the death of other kinds of being.

Does taking the permanent loss of consciousness as sufficient for the death of a human being make the death of a human being something *completely distinct* from the death of lower organisms, as Gert claims? The answer depends on what we mean by "completely distinct" and "lower organism." As noted above, Bernat recognizes that the definition of death for higher-order organisms (presumably those that can be said to be conscious) is different from the definition of death for lower-order organisms. This is so, precisely because of the role that consciousness plays in the lives of these beings. If the definition of death for higher-order organisms were not different from that of lower-order organisms, then there would be no need for Bernat, Gert, and Culver to amend their original definition of death. The irreversible loss of the integration of the organism as a whole would have been sufficient.

However, when it comes to human beings or persons, our nature *is* different from that of other kinds of beings. While we do have a biological nature, that biological nature can be sustained in unprecedented ways. As an artificially sustained severed head, it would be the continuation of our consciousness as a kind of cyborg, rather than a natural human organism, along with the fact that we would continue to recognize, relate to, and value the individual as the same person, that ground our belief that death has not occurred. Absent the identification of this being as a locus of value in a network of conscious, social relations, there would be no reason to consider the person to still be alive. In this hypothetical case, the biological considerations of the integration of an organism as a whole would play little, if any, role in our understanding of what it means for us to continue to be alive. While the artificially sustained severed head would retain some type of psychophysical integration, it would not be the type of natural psychophysical integration or "integration of the organism as a whole" found in ordinary forms of life. Thus, the death of the person could be understood as the loss of "psychophysical integration," but there would now be new ways in which the integration could be maintained. Accordingly, there would be new ways in which the psychophysical integration could irreversibly cease. Insofar as these possibilities represent new ways for people to live and die, the life and death of persons would be distinct from the life and death of other organisms.

The underlying problem with Bernat, Culver, and Gert's view is their framing of the issue of how to define death within a "biological paradigm." According to them, death is a biological concept that may be applied directly and literally only to organisms. Any other use of "death," such as the death of a person, is a metaphorical use of the term or, at best, elliptical for saying that the organism that was the person has died. The paradigm can be summarized as the belief that death is fundamentally or strictly a biological phenomenon. Although they claim that they are trying to capture the ordinary common sense understanding of death, the definition and criteria of death are understood to be within the province of biologists or physicians to define.

The alternative to this "medical" or "biological" paradigm of death is to think that, because human nature is not simply biological, human death is a metaphysical, ethical, and cultural phenomenon *in as equally a fundamental sense* as it is a biological phenomenon. The definition and criteria of death are therefore as much matters involving metaphysical reflection, moral choice, and cultural acceptance, as they are biological facts to be discovered. For these reasons, we should not expect there to be a unitary definition or criterion of death applicable to all organisms or even just higher-order organisms. However, this is an implication that I believe enriches us and not one that should be obfuscated and avoided by pretending that the definition and criteria of death for persons or human organisms are strictly biological or medical matters. It promotes an understanding of our nature as beings that are open-ended rather than timelessly fixed, as having an active role in creating and determining the bounds of our being rather than being passive recipients of physical forces. Moreover, it's true.

Bernat asserts that because life is fundamentally a biological phenomenon, defining death is fundamentally biological.[36] The problem with this claim is that it is incomplete. We are not interested in when life as such ceases but when the life of certain kinds of beings ceases. The theoretical underpinning of this claim is the Aristotelian idea, reiterated and developed most notably in the work of the contemporary philosopher David Wiggins, that "Everything that exists is a *this such*."[37] This "Thesis of the Sortal Dependency of Individuation" entails (paraphrasing Wiggins) that any judgment that a thing that is alive is the same thing that dies has no chance of being true unless two preconditions are satisfied: (a) that there exists some known or unknown answer to the question "same *what?*" and (b) this answer affords some principle by which the entities of this particular kind—some kind containing things that are such as to live and die—may be traced through space and time and reidentified as one and the same. The corollary to this principle is: "Everything that ceases to exist ceases to exist as a *this such*." Thus, if death is a form of ceasing to exist, we can only maintain that the death of the human being or person is fundamentally or strictly biological, if we accept that the human being or person, what dies or ceases to exist, is fundamentally or strictly identical to a biological being.[38] If there are moral, metaphysical, and cultural aspects of human beings or persons that are essential to their nature, then the death of these entities, their ceasing to exist, cannot be understood in purely biological terms.[39] Thus, the death of the human being or person is no less a metaphysical, moral, and cultural phenomenon than it is a biological one.

Another way of putting my critique of the medical or biological paradigm of death is to say that any strictly biological definition of death assumes some materially reductionistic view about humanity or personhood. Those reductionistic views, however, conflict with what many philosophers and lay people believe about humans or persons. Thus, because any strict biological definition of death assumes some reductionistic view, those who reject the reductionistic views ought to reject the idea that defining death is a strictly biological matter. In short, the currently accepted biological definition of death as "the permanent cessation of the functioning of the organism as a whole" and even the amended biological definition that Gert, Culver, and Clouser have proposed have taken the soul out of defining death, literally for some, figuratively for others. It sterilizes the debate over the definition of death from its ontological and ethical complexities. Worse, it commits the all-too-common error in bioethics of mistakenly assuming that what is fundamentally a metaphysical and ethical issue can be resolved by medicine or biology.

Bernat, Gert, Culver, and Clouser would likely protest at this point that to reject the biological paradigm of death and accept the irreversible loss of conscious as a criterion for death would be to radically change the ordinary meaning of death. However, I believe the opposite. Because human death has always signified a transformation from our being a person or human being into the remains of one, to ignore how our psychological, moral, and cultural nature defines the kind of being that we are and to focus exclusively on our biological nature to define our coming into being and passing away distorts the ordinary meaning of human life and death.

Technology has intervened in the natural life-history of human beings in unprecedented ways. Just as we can now live in ways that were previously impossible, we can now die in new ways that are made possible by medical technology. The new medical realities present us with the challenge of how we ought to project the terms *life* and *death*. Some of the assumptions about the meaning of death that may have governed our use of the term in the past may thus need to be given up in light of the new cases. It may be more important to preserve other assumptions about the psychological, moral, and cultural meaning of human life and death at the expense of giving up some of the biological assumptions about the meaning of these terms. What is clear, however, is that this issue of how we ought to project "life" and "death" to the new cases is not one that can be settled by consideration of the meaning of terms, as if meaning were something timelessly fixed. While words cannot mean just anything, the debate about how to project the terms must be understood within a framework of interests, values, and history of use within which words have their meaning.

In his *Cruzan* dissent, Justice Stevens wrote: "for patients . . . who have no consciousness and no chance of recovery, there is a serious question as to whether the mere persistence of their bodies is 'life' as that word is commonly understood, or as it is used both in the Constitution and the Declaration of Independence."[40] Stevens was asking about the meaning of life and death within the context of the U.S. Constitution and the framework of the moral and legal rights of living persons recognized in that constitution. His question was not framed in strictly biological terms. When we ask for a definition and criterion for death that can be used in practical cases, it would be a mistake to frame this issue in strictly biological terms, because it is not in terms of persons or human beings as strictly biological beings that we are interested in an answer to the question. We are interested in the life and death of persons as understood as psychological, moral, and cultural beings, as well as biological beings. Indeed, if we frame the question in strictly biological terms, we rule out the psychological, moral, and cultural dimension of persons from the start and thereby distort the purpose of why we seek to answer the question in the first place. Moreover, as I have argued above, pushing a strictly biological account of life and death leads to strongly counterintuitive results when it comes to what we say about various actual and hypothetical cases. Most of us would not wish to identify ourselves with artificially sustained, brainless integrated human organisms, even though the strictly biological account of life and death leads to that absurd conclusion. If we resist this conclusion, we are resisting it because we think of our nature as something more than biological.[41]

NOTES

1. Ad Hoc Committee of the Harvard Medical School to Examine the Definition of Brain Death, A definition of irreversible coma, *Journal of the American Medical Association* 1968, 205: 337–340.

2. Pernick, M. S., Brain death in a cultural context, in Youngner, S. J., Arnold, R. M., and Schapiro, R., eds., *The Definition of Death: Contemporary Controversies* (Baltimore: Johns Hopkins University Press, 1999), 12.

3. Joynt, R. J., A new look at death, *Journal of the American Medical Association* 1984, 252: 682.

4. Bernat, J., Culver, C., and Gert, B., On the criterion and definition of death, *Annals of Internal Medicine* 1981, 94: 389–394.

5. President's Commission for the Study of Ethical Problems in Medicine and Biomedical and Behavioral Research, *Defining Death: Medical, Ethical, and Legal Issues in the Determination of Death* (Washington, DC: U.S. Government Printing Office, 1981).

6. Youngner, S., and Bartlett, E., Human death and high technology: The failure of the whole-brain formulations, *Annals of Internal Medicine* 1983, 99: 252–258.

7. Field, D. R., Gates, E. A., Creasy, R. K., Jonsen, A. R., and Laros, R. K., Maternal brain death during pregnancy, *Journal of the American Medical Association* 1988, 260(6): 816–822; Bernstein, I. M., Watson, M., Simmons, G. M., Catalano, M., Davis, G., and Collins, R., Maternal brain death and prolonged fetal survival, *Obstetrics and Gynecology* 1989, 74(3): 434–437; Anstötz, A., Should a brain-dead pregnant woman carry her child to full

term? The case of the "Erlanger baby," *Bioethics* 1993, 7(4): 340–350; Shewmon, D. A., Chronic "brain death": Meta-analysis and conceptual consequences, *Neurology* 1998, 51: 1538–1545; Shewmon, D. A., Letters and replies. *Neurology* 1999, 53: 1369–1372.

8. Becker, L. C., Human being: The boundaries of the concept, *Philosophy and Public Affairs* 1975, 4: 335–359.

9. Truog, R. D., Is it time to abandon brain death?, *Hastings Center Report* 1997, 27(1): 29–37.

10. Halevy, A., and Brody, B., Brain death: Reconciling definitions, criteria, and tests, *Annals of Internal Medicine* 1993, 119: 519–525; Brody, B., How much of the brain must be dead?, in Youngner, S. J., Arnold, R. M., and Schapiro, R., eds., *The Definition of Death: Contemporary Controversies* (Baltimore: Johns Hopkins University Press, 1999), 71–82.

11. Grant, A. C., Human brain death in perspective: Comments on the spinal dog and decapitated frog, presented at the Third International Symposium on Coma and Death, Havana, February 22–25, 2000, and published in Machado, C., and Shewmon, D. A., eds., *Brain Death and Disorders of Consciousness* (New York: Kluwer, 2004).

12. Seifert, J., Is "brain death" actually death?, *The Monist* 1993, 76(2): 175–202.

13. Byrne, P. A., O'Reilly, S., Quay, P., and Salsich, Jr., P. W., Brain death: The patient, the physician, and society, in Potts, M., Byrne, P. A., and Nilges, R. G., eds., *Beyond Brain Death: The Case Against Brain Based Criteria for Human Death* (Dordrecht: Kluwer, 2000), 21–89.

14. Taylor, R. M., Re-examining the definition and criterion of death, *Seminars in Neurology* 1997, 17: 265–279.

15. Veatch, R. M., Brain death and slippery slopes, *Journal of Clinical Ethics* 1992, 3(3): 181–187; Veatch, R. M., Maternal brain death: An ethicist's thoughts, *Journal of the American Medical Association* 1982, 248: 1102–1103.

16. Gervais, K. G., *Redefining Death* (New Haven: Yale University Press, 1986), 146–147.

17. Wikler, D., Who defines death? Medical, legal and philosophical perspectives, in Machado, C., ed., *Brain Death: Proceedings of the Second International Conference on Brain Death* (Amsterdam: Elsevier, 1995), 13–22.

18. Shewmon, D. A., "Brainstem death," "brain death," and death: A critical reevaluation of the purported evidence, *Issues in Law and Medicine* 1998, 14: 125–145; Shewmon, D. A., Recovery from "brain death": A neurologist's apologia, *Linacre Quarterly* 1997, 64(1): 30–96.

19. Shewmon, D. A., The "critical organ" for the "organism as a whole": Lessons from the lowly spinal cord, presented at the Third International Symposium on Coma and Death, Havana, February 22–25, 2000, and published in Machado and Shewmon, *Brain Death and Disorders of Consciousness*.

20. See the selections from Aquinas, Meilaender, Strawson, Lowe, and Baker in this anthology (Chapters 4, 5, 9, 10, and 11) and Chapter 6 of Wiggins, D., *Sameness and Substance* (Cambridge: Harvard University Press, 1980).

21. Green, M., and Wikler, D., Brain death and personal identity, *Philosophy and Public Affairs* 1980, 9: 105–133; Veatch, R. M., The impending collapse of the whole-brain definition of death, *Hastings Center Report* 1993, 23(4): 18–24. There are a number of difficulties with various versions of the qualitative or functionalist view of persons: (1) that to avoid circularity, it must presuppose a substantive view of persons (see Butler, J., appendix to *The Analogy of Religion, Natural and Revealed to the Constitution and Nature*. London: Knapton, 1736; Lowe, E. J., Real selves: Persons as a substantial kind, in Cockburn, D., ed., *Human Beings*. New York: Cambridge, 1991 [reprinted as Chapter 10 in this volume]); (2) that it fails to adequately account for moral responsibility (see Molyneux, W., Letter of Molyneux to Locke, 23 Dec. 1693, in *The Works of John Locke* VIII. London 1794, 329;

Chapter 6 of Reid, T., *Essays on the Intellectual Powers of Man*. London, 1785; and Korsgaard, C., Personal identity and the unity of agency: A Kantian response to Parfit, *Philosophy and Public Affairs* 1989, 18(2): 101–132); (3) that it fails to explain intuitions about thought experiments regarding personal identity (see Lockwood, M., When does a life begin?, and The Warnock report: A philosophical appraisal, both in Lockwood, M., ed., *Moral Dilemmas in Modern Medicine*. Oxford: Oxford University Press, 1985; Wiggins, D., *Sameness and Substance*. Cambridge: Harvard University Press, 1980; Unger, P., *Identity, Consciousness and Value*. New York: Oxford, 1990; and McMahan, J., *The Ethics of Killing: Problems at the Margins of Life*. New York: Oxford, 2002); and (4) that it cannot account for the essential cultural and relational nature of persons (see Chapter 7 of Lizza, J., *Persons, Humanity, and the Definition of Death*. Baltimore: Johns Hopkins University Press, 2006).

22. Veatch, R. M., The impending collapse.

23. Gervais, *Redefining Death*, 126.

24. For a more extended argument and development of this view, see Lizza, J. P., *Persons, Humanity, and the Definition of Death* (Baltimore: Johns Hopkins University Press, 2006).

25. Bernat, J. M., The biophilosophical basis of whole-brain death, *Social Philosophy and Policy* 2002, 19(2): 330 (as Chapter 24 in this anthology).

26. Gert, B., A complete definition of death, In Machado, C., ed., *Brain Death* (Amsterdam: Elsevier, 1995). See also Chapter 11 of Gert, B., Culver, C. M., and Clouser, K. D., *Bioethics: A Systematic Approach* (New York: Oxford, 2006).

27. White, R. J., Wolin, L. R., Masopust, L., Taslitz, N., and Verdura, J., Cephalic exchange transplantation in the monkey, *Surgery* 1971, 70: 135–139.

28. Gert, B., A complete definition of death, 26.

29. Gert, Culver, and Clouser, *Bioethics*, 290.

30. Gert, A complete definition of death, 28.

31. Ibid. (emphasis added).

32. Ibid., 29.

33. Ibid.

34. Gert, Culver, and Clouser, *Bioethics*, 293–294.

35. Gert, Culver, and Clouser, *Bioethics*, 290.

36. Bernat, J., Reply to J. Lizza's letter to the editor, *Hastings Center Report* 1999, 28: 3.

37. Wiggins, *Sameness and Substance*, 15.

38. If death is not a type of ceasing to exist, then it is unclear what *would* count as a type of ceasing to exist. However, for a challenge to the claim that a person's death does not entail the person's ceasing to exist, see Chapter 6 of Feldman, F., *Confrontations with the Reaper* (New York: Oxford, 1992).

39. By "essential," I follow Aristotle's understanding of an essential property as a property that is necessary for something to exist as the kind of thing that it is. Its loss would therefore entail the ceasing to exist of that kind of thing (Aristotle, *Metaphysics* VII). This view does not entail that every aspect or characteristic of a person has to be understood in more than purely biological terms. Persons undergo a host of biological activity that can be explained and predicted in purely biological terms. My claim is that the issue of when the life of a human being or person ends, like when it begins, cannot be understood in purely biological terms. This is because "person" and "human being" are not merely biological beings.

40. *Nancy Beth Cruzan, by her Parents and Co-Guardians, Lester L. Cruzan et ux. v. Director, Missouri Department of Health et al.*, 497 US 261, 1990.

41. I would like to thank Springer publications and the Johns Hopkins University Press for permission to incorporate some passages from the following works into this article: Lizza, J. P., The conceptual basis of brain death revisited: Loss of organic integration or loss of consciousness?, in Machado and Shewmon, *Brain Death*; and Lizza, J. P., *Persons, Humanity, and the Definition of Death* (Baltimore: Johns Hopkins University Press, 2006).

CHAPTER THIRTY-TWO

Selection from *Controversies in the Determination of Death: A White Paper*

The Philosophical Debate

The President's Council on Bioethics

Why do we describe the central question of this inquiry as a *philosophical* question? We do so, in part, because this question cannot be settled by appealing exclusively to clinical or pathophysiological facts. Those facts were our focus in the previous chapters in which we sought to clarify important features of "total brain failure," a condition diagnosed in a well-defined subset of comatose, ventilator-dependent patients. As a condition, it is the terminus of a course of pathophysiological events, the effects of which account for certain clinically observable signs (all manifestations of an incapacitated brainstem) and for confirmatory results obtained through selected imaging tests. A patient diagnosed with this condition will never recover brain-dependent functions, including the capacity to breathe and the capacity to exhibit even minimal signs of conscious life. If the patient is sustained with life-supporting technologies, this condition need not lead immediately to somatic disintegration or failure of other organ systems. These facts are all crucial to answering the question, *Is a human being with total brain failure dead?* But determining the significance of these facts presents challenges for philosophical analysis and interpretation.

In this chapter, we set forth and explore two positions on this philosophical question. One position rejects the widely accepted consensus that the current neurological standard is an ethically valid one for determining death. The other position defends the consensus, taking the challenges posed in recent years as opportunities to strengthen the philosophical rationale for the neurological standard.

At the outset, it is important to note what is common to these two opposing positions. *First, both reject the idea that death should be treated merely as a legal construct or as a matter of social agreement.* Instead, both embrace the idea that a standard for determining death must be defensible on biological as well as philosophical grounds. That is to say, both positions respect the *biological reality* of death. At some point, after all, certainty that a body is no longer a living whole is attainable. The impressive technological advances of the last several decades have done nothing to alter the reality of death, even if they have complicated the task of judging whether and when death has occurred in particular circumstances. In light of such complications, however, both positions share the conclusion that a human being who is not known to be dead should be considered alive.

Second, neither position advocates loosening the standards for determining death on the basis of currently known clinical and pathophysiological facts. There is a well-developed third philosophical position that is often considered alongside the two that are the main focus of this chapter. This third position maintains that there can be two deaths—the death of the *person*, a being distinguished by the capacities for thought, reason, and feeling, and the death of the *body* or the *organism*. From the perspective of this third philosophical position, an individual who suffers a brain injury that leaves him incapacitated with regard to certain specifically human powers is rightly regarded as "dead as a person." The still living body that remains after this death is not a human being in the full sense. Philosopher John Lizza discusses the living organism left behind after the "person" has died in the following way:

> Advocates of a consciousness-related formulation of death do not consider such a being to be a living person. In their view, a person cannot persist through the loss of all brain function or even the loss of just those brain functions required for consciousness and other mental functions. . . . [W]hat remains alive must be a different sort of being . . . a form of life created by medical technology. . . . Whereas a person is normally transformed into a corpse at his or her death, technology has intervened in this natural process and has made it possible . . . for a person's remains to take the form of an artificially sustained, living organism devoid of the capacity for consciousness and any other mental function.[1]

Thus, advocates of this third position effectively maintain that in certain cases there can be two deaths rather than one. In such cases, they argue, a body that has ceased to be a person (having "died" the first death) can be treated as deceased—at least in certain ways. For example, according to some advocates of this position, it would be permissible to remove the organs of such individuals while their hearts continue to beat. The patients most often cited as potential heart-beating organ donors, based on this concept of death, are PVS patients and anencephalic newborns (babies born with very little, if any, brain matter other than the brainstem). Organ retrieval in such cases might entail the administration of sedatives to the allegedly "person-less" patient because some signs of continued "biological life" (such as the open eyes and spontaneous breathing of the PVS patient) would be distracting and disturbing to the surgeons who procure the patient's organs.

Serious difficulties afflict the claim that something that can be called "death" has occurred even as the body remains alive. One such difficulty is that there is no way to know that the "specifically human powers" are irreversibly gone from a body that has suffered any injury shy of total brain failure. In Chapter Three [of *Controversies in the Determination of Death*], we cited neurologist Steven Laureys's observation that it is impossible to ascertain scientifically the inward state of an individual—and features of this inward state (e.g., thinking and feeling) are always cited as marks of a distinctively *human* or *personal* life. It is very important here to recall the marked differences in appearance between the individual with total brain failure and the individual with another "consciousness-compromising" condition. The latter displays several ambiguous signs—moving, waking up, and groaning, among others—while the former remains still and closed off from the world in clinically ascertainable ways.[2]

A related problem with this "two deaths" position is that it expands the concept of death beyond the core meaning it has had throughout human history. Human beings are members of the larger family of living beings, and it is a fundamental truth about living beings that every individual—be it plant or animal—eventually dies. Recent advances in technology offer no warrant for jettisoning the age-old idea that it is not as persons that we die, but rather as members of the family of living beings and as animals in particular. The terminus of the transformation that occurs when a human being is deprived by injury of certain mental capacities, heartbreaking as it is, is not *death*. We should note, again, that some technological interventions administered to the living might be deemed *futile*—that is, ineffective at reversing or ameliorating the course of disease or injury—and that an ethically valid decision might be made to withdraw or withhold such interventions. There is no need, however, to call an individual *already dead* in order to justify refraining from such futile interventions.

In summary, the two positions that we present in this chapter share the conviction that death is a single phenomenon marking the end of the life of a biological organism. Death is the definitive end of life and is something more complete and final than the mere loss of "personhood."

I. Position One: There Is No Sound Biological Justification for Today's Neurological Standard

The neurological standard for death based on total brain failure relies fundamentally on the idea that the phenomenon of death can be *hidden*. The metaphor employed by the President's Commission and cited in Chapter One [of *Controversies in the Determination of Death*] expresses this idea: When a ventilator supports the body's vital functions, this technological intervention obscures our view of the phenomenon. What seem to be signs of continued life in an injured body are, in fact, misleading artifacts of the technological intervention and obstacles to ascertaining the truth. To consult brain-based functions, then, is to look through a "second window" in order to see the actual condition of the body.

The critical thrust of Position One can be summarized in this way: There is no reliable "second window" on the phenomenon of death. If its presence is not made known by the signs that have always accompanied it—by breathing lungs and a beating heart—then there is no way to state with confidence that death has occurred. Only when all would agree that the body is ready for burial can that body, with confidence, be described as dead. If blood is still circulating and nutrients and oxygen are still serving to power the work of diverse cells, tissues, and organ systems, then the body in which these processes are ongoing cannot be deemed a corpse.

Soon after the Harvard committee argued that patients who meet the criteria for "irreversible coma" are already dead, some philosophers and other observers of the committee's work advanced an opposing view. The counterarguments presented then by one such philosopher, Hans Jonas, are still useful in framing the objections raised today against the neurological standard. In his 1974 essay, "Against the Stream," Jonas dissented from the Harvard committee's equation of "irreversible coma" and death and counseled, instead, a conservative course of action:

We do not know with certainty the borderline between life and death, and a definition cannot substitute for knowledge. Moreover, we have sufficient grounds for
suspecting that the artificially supported condition of the comatose patient may
still be one of life, however reduced—i.e., for doubting that, even with the brain
function gone, he is completely dead. In this state of marginal ignorance and doubt
the only course to take is to lean over backward toward the side of possible life.[3]

With these words, Jonas underscored a point that is pivotal to Position One:
There can be uncertainty as to where the line between life and death falls even
if we are certain that death is a biologically real event. In patients with total
brain failure, the transition from living body to corpse is in some measure a
mystery, one that may be beyond the powers of science and medicine to penetrate and determine with the finality that is possible when most human beings die.

Have advances in the scientific and clinical understanding of the spectrum
of neurological injury shown that Jonas's stance of principled (and therefore
cautious) uncertainty was incorrect? Today we have a more fine-grained set of
categories of, as he put it, "artificially supported . . . comatose patients"—some
of whom meet the criteria for total brain failure and others who have hope of
recovering limited or full mental function. Only the first group is considered to
be dead by today's "brain death" defenders. Even with respect to this group,
however, there is still reason to wonder if our knowledge of their condition is
adequate for labeling them as dead. If there are "sufficient grounds," as Jonas
put it, for suspecting that their condition may still be one of life, then a stance
of principled and hence cautious uncertainty is still the morally right one to
take.

This line of inquiry brings us to Shewmon's criticisms summarized earlier in
Chapter Three [of *Controversies in the Determination of Death*] of the accepted
pathophysiological and clinical picture of patients with "brain death" (total
brain failure). Do Shewmon's criticisms constitute the "sufficient grounds" to
which Jonas appeals? To answer this question, these criticisms and the evidence
supporting them must first be considered in greater depth.

In 1998, the journal *Neurology* published an article by Shewmon entitled,
"Chronic 'Brain Death': Meta-Analysis and Conceptual Consequences." In that
article, Shewmon cites evidence for the claim that neither bodily disintegration
nor cessation of heartbeat *necessarily* and *imminently* ensues after brain death.[4]
Shewmon's evidence is drawn from more than one hundred documented cases
that demonstrate survival past one week's time, with one case of survival for

more than fourteen years.[5] Furthermore, he demonstrates that such factors as age, etiology, and underlying somatic integrity variably affect the survival probability of "brain dead" patients. Observing that asystole (the absence of cardiac contractions colloquially known as "flatline") does not necessarily follow from "brain death," Shewmon concludes that it is the overall integrity of the body (the "underlying somatic plasticity") *rather than the condition of the brain* that exerts the strongest influence on survival. These facts seem to contradict the dominant view that the loss of brain function, in and of itself, leads the body to "fall apart" and eventually to cease circulating blood.

Critics of this meta-analysis have challenged the data on which Shewmon based his conclusions, claiming that many of the patients in the cases that he compiles might not have been properly diagnosed with whole brain death (in our usage, total brain failure). They also point out the rarity with which such cases are encountered, compared with the frequency of rapid descent to asystole for patients accurately diagnosed.[6] To point out the rarity of prolonged survival, however, is to admit that the phenomenon does, in some cases, occur. Whether it might occur more often is difficult to judge because patients with total brain failure are rarely treated with aggressive, life-sustaining interventions for an extended time.

If it is possible—albeit rare—for a body without a functioning brain to "hold itself together" for an indefinite period of time, then how can the condition of total brain failure be equated with biological death? Or, to put the question in Jonas's terms, does this fact not give "sufficient grounds" for suspecting that such patients might still be alive, although severely injured? The case for uncertainty about the line between life and death is further strengthened by considering the somatic processes that clearly continue in the body of a patient with total brain failure.

In a paper published in the *Journal of Medicine and Philosophy* in 2001, Shewmon details the integrated functions that continue in a body in the condition of "brain death." Table 2 reproduces a list of somatically integrative functions that are, in Shewmon's words, "*not* mediated by the brain and possessed by at least some [brain dead] bodies."[7]

Readers not well-versed in human physiology might find this list hard to follow. Its significance, however, can be simply stated: It enumerates many clearly identifiable and observable physiological mechanisms. These mechanisms account for the continued health of vital organs in the bodies of patients diagnosed with total brain failure and go a long way toward explaining the lengthy survival of such patients in rare cases. In such cases, globally coordinated work

Table 2 Physiological Evidence of "Somatic Integration"

- Homeostasis of a countless variety of mutually interacting chemicals, macromolecules and physiological parameters, through the functions especially of liver, kidneys, cardiovascular and endocrine systems, but also of other organs and tissues (e.g., intestines, bone and skin in calcium metabolism; cardiac atrial natriuretic factor affecting the renal secretion of renin, which regulates blood pressure by acting on vascular smooth muscle; etc.);
- Elimination, detoxification and recycling of cellular wastes throughout the body;
- Energy balance, involving interactions among liver, endocrine systems, muscle and fat;
- Maintenance of body temperature (albeit at a lower than normal level and with the help of blankets);
- Wound healing, capacity for which is diffuse throughout the body and which involves organism-level, teleological interaction among blood cells, capillary endothelium, soft tissues, bone marrow, vasoactive peptides, clotting and clot lysing factors (maintained by the liver, vascular endothelium and circulating leucocytes in a delicate balance of synthesis and degradation), etc.;
- Fighting of infections and foreign bodies through interactions among the immune system, lymphatics, bone marrow, and microvasculature;
- Development of a febrile response to infection;
- Cardiovascular and hormonal stress responses to unaesthetized incision for organ retrieval;
- Successful gestation of a fetus in a [brain dead] pregnant woman;
- Sexual maturation of a [brain dead] child;
- Proportional growth of a [brain dead] child.

Souce: D. A. Shewmon, "The Brain and Somatic Integration: Insights into the Standard Biological Rationale for Equating 'Brain Death' with Death," *J Med and Phil* 26, no.5 (2001): 457–78.

continues to be performed by multiple systems, all directed toward the sustained functioning of the body as a whole. If being alive as a biological organism requires being a whole that is more than the mere sum of its parts, then it would be difficult to deny that the body of a patient with total brain failure can still be alive, at least in some cases.

None of this contradicts the claim that total brain failure is a unique and profound kind of *incapacitation*—and one that may very well warrant or even morally *require* the withdrawal of life-sustaining interventions. According to some defenders of the concept of medical futility, there is no obligation to begin or to continue treatment when that treatment cannot achieve any good or when it inflicts disproportionate burdens on the patient who receives it or on his or her family. Writing many years before the somatic state and the prognostic possibilities of total brain failure were well-characterized, Jonas emphasized the need to accept that sustaining life and prolonging dying is not always in the patient's interest:

> The question [of interventions to sustain the patient] cannot be answered by decreeing that death has already occurred and the body is therefore in the domain of things; rather it is by holding, e.g., that it is humanly not justified—let alone demanded—to artificially prolong the life of a brainless body . . . the physician can, indeed should, turn off the respirator and let the "definition of death" take care of itself by what then inevitably happens.[8]

To summarize, Position One does *not* insist that medicine or science can know that all or even some patients with total brain failure are still living. Rather, Position One makes two assertions in light of what we now know about the clinical presentation and the pathophysiology of total brain failure. The first is that there are "sufficient grounds" for doubt as to whether the patient with this condition has died. The second is that in the face of such persistent uncertainty, the only ethically valid course is to consider and treat such a patient as a still living human being. Finally, such respectful consideration and treatment does not preclude the ethical withdrawal or withholding of life-sustaining interventions, based on the judgment that such interventions are futile.

II. Position Two: There Is a Sound Biological Justification for Today's Neurological Standard

Position One is the voice of "principled and hence cautious uncertainty." We should not claim to know facts about life and death that are beyond the limits of our powers to discern, especially when the consequence might be to place a human being beyond the essential and obligatory protections afforded to the living. The recent critical appraisals of total brain failure ("whole brain death") offered by Shewmon and others only underscore the limits to our ability to discern the line between life and death.

Position Two is also motivated by strong moral convictions about what is at stake in the debate: The bodies of deceased patients should not be ventilated and maintained as if they were still living human beings. The respect owed to the newly dead demands that such interventions be withdrawn. Their families should be spared unnecessary anguish over purported "options" for treatment. Maintaining the body for a short time to facilitate organ transplantation is a reasonable act of deference to the need for organs and to the opportunity for generosity on the part of the donor as well as the family. Notwithstanding this need and opportunity, the true moral challenge that faces us is to decide in each case whether the patient is living or has died. To help us meet that challenge, the clinical and pathophysiological facts that call the neurological standard into question should be re-examined and re-evaluated. On the basis of such a reexamination and reevaluation, Position Two seeks to develop a better rationale for continuing to use the neurological standard to determine whether a human being has died.

A. The Work of the Organism as a Whole

Early defenders of the neurological standard of "whole brain death" relied on the plausible intuition that in order to be a living organism any animal, whether human or non-human, must be a *whole*. Ongoing biological activity in various cells or tissues is not in itself sufficient to mark the presence of a living organism. After all, some biological activity in cells and tissues remains for a time even in a body that all would agree is a corpse. Such activity signifies that disparate *parts* of the once-living organism remain, but not the organism *as a whole*. Therefore, if we try to specify the moment at which the "wholeness" of the body is lost, that moment must come before biological activity in all of its different cells or tissues has ceased. As Alexander Capron, former executive director of the President's Commission, has repeatedly emphasized, the fact that this moment is *chosen* does not mean that it is *arbitrary*; the choice is not arbitrary if it is made in accordance with the most reasonable interpretation of the biological facts that could be provided.[9]

The neurological standard's early defenders were not wrong to seek such a principle of wholeness. They may have been mistaken, however, in focusing on the *loss of somatic integration* as the critical sign that the organism is no longer a whole. They interpreted—plausibly but perhaps incorrectly—"an organism as a whole" to mean "an organism whose parts are working together in an integrated way." But, as we have seen, even in a patient with total brain failure, some of the body's parts continue to work together in an integrated way for some time—for example, to fight infection, heal wounds, and maintain temperature. If these kinds of integration were sufficient to identify the presence of a living "organism as a whole," total brain failure could not serve as a criterion for organismic death, and the neurological standard enshrined in law would not be philosophically well-grounded.

There may be, however, a more compelling account of *wholeness* that would support the intuition that after total brain failure the body is no longer an organismic whole and hence no longer alive. That account, which we develop here with Position Two, offers a superior defense of "total brain failure" as the standard for declaring death. With that account, death remains a condition of the organism as a whole and does not, therefore, merely signal the irreversible loss of so-called higher mental functions. But reliance on the concept of "integration" is abandoned and with it the false assumption that the brain is the "integrator" of vital functions. Determining whether an organism remains a *whole* depends on recognizing the persistence or cessation of the fundamental vital *work* of a living organism—the work of self-preservation, achieved through the organism's need-driven commerce with the surrounding world. When there is good reason to believe that an injury has irreversibly destroyed an organism's ability to perform its fundamental vital work, then the conclusion that the organism as a whole has died is warranted. Advocates of Position Two argue that this is the case for patients with total brain failure. To understand this argument, we must explore at some length this idea of an organism's "fundamental work."

All organisms have a *needy* mode of being. Unlike inanimate objects, which continue to exist through inertia and without effort, every organism persists only thanks to its own exertions. To preserve themselves, organisms *must*—and *can* and *do*—engage in commerce with the surrounding world. Their constant need for oxygenated air and nutrients is matched by their ability to satisfy that need, by engaging in certain activities, reaching out into the surrounding environment to secure the required sustenance. This is the definitive work of the organism *as an organism*. It is what an organism "does" and what distinguishes every organism from non-living things.[10] And it is what distinguishes a *living* organism from the dead body that it becomes when it dies.

The work of the organism, expressed in its commerce with the surrounding world, depends on three fundamental capacities:

1. Openness to the world, that is, receptivity to stimuli and signals from the surrounding environment.
2. The ability to act upon the world to obtain selectively what it needs.
3. The basic felt need that drives the organism to act as it must, to obtain what it needs and what its openness reveals to be available.

Appreciating these capacities as mutually supporting aspects of the organism's vital work will help us understand why an individual with total brain failure should be declared dead, even when ventilator-supported "breathing" masks the presence of death.

To preserve itself, an organism must be open to the world. Such openness is manifested in different ways and at many levels. In higher animals, including man, it is evident most obviously in consciousness or felt awareness, even in its very rudimentary forms. When a PVS patient tracks light with his or her eyes, recoils in response to pain, swallows liquid placed in the mouth, or goes to sleep and wakes up, such behaviors—although they may not indicate *self*-consciousness—testify to the organism's essential, vital openness to its surrounding world. An organism that behaves in such a way cannot be dead.

Self-preserving commerce with the world, however, involves more than just openness or receptivity. It also requires the ability to *act* on one's own behalf—to take in food and water and, even more basically, to breathe. Spontaneous breathing is an indispensable action of the higher animals that makes metabolism—and all other vital activity—possible. Experiencing a felt inner need to acquire oxygen (and to expel carbon dioxide) and perceiving the presence of oxygen in its environment, a living body is moved to act on the world (by contracting its diaphragm so that air will move into its lungs). An organism that breathes spontaneously cannot be dead.

Just as spontaneous breathing in itself reveals an organism's openness to and ability to act upon the world, it also reveals a third capacity critical to the organism's fundamental, self-preserving work: What animates the motor act of spontaneous breathing, in open commerce with the surrounding air, is the inner experience of need, manifesting itself as the drive to breathe. This need does not have to be consciously felt in order to be efficacious in driving respiration. It is clearly not consciously felt in a comatose patient who might be tested for a remaining rudimentary drive (e.g., with the "apnea" test). But even when the drive to breathe occurs in the absence of any self-awareness, its presence gives evidence of the organism's continued impulse to live. This drive is the organism's own impulse, exercised on its own behalf, and indispensable to its continued existence.[11]

As a vital sign, the *spontaneous action of breathing* can and must be distinguished from the technologically supported, *passive condition of being ventilated* (i.e., of having one's "breathing" replaced by a mechanical ventilator). The natural work of breathing, even apart from consciousness or self-awareness, is itself a sure sign that the organism as a whole is doing the work that constitutes—and preserves—it as a whole. In contrast, artificial, non-spontaneous breathing produced by a machine is not such a sign. It does not signify an activity of the organism as a whole. It is not driven by *felt need*, and the exchange of gases that it effects is neither an achievement of the organism nor a sign of its genuine vitality. For this reason, it makes sense to say that the operation of the ventilator can obscure our view of the arrival of human death—that is, the death of the human organism as a working whole. A ventilator causes the patient's chest to heave and the lungs to fill and thereby *mimics* the authentic work of the organism. In fact, it mimics the work so well that it enables some systems of the body to keep functioning—but it does no more than that. The simulated "breathing" that the ventilator makes possible is not, therefore, a *vital sign:* It is not a sign that the organism is accomplishing its vital work and thus remains a living whole.[12]

We have examined the phenomenon of breathing in order to understand and explain a living organism's "needful openness" to the world—a needful openness lacking in patients with total brain failure. Having done this, however, we must also emphasize that an animal cannot be considered dead simply because it has lost the ability to breathe spontaneously. Even if the animal has lost that capacity, other vital capacities might still be present. For example, patients with spinal cord injuries may be permanently apneic or unable to breathe without ventilatory support and yet retain full or partial possession of their conscious faculties. Just as much as striving to breathe, signs of consciousness are incontrovertible evidence that a living organism, a patient, is alive.

If there are no signs of consciousness *and* if spontaneous breathing is absent *and* if the best clinical judgment is that these neurophysiological facts cannot be reversed, Position Two would lead us to conclude that a once-living patient has now died. Thus, on this account, total brain failure can continue to serve as a criterion for declaring death—not because it necessarily indicates complete loss of integrated somatic functioning, but because it is a sign that this organism can no longer engage in the essential work that defines living things.

B. Comparison with the UK Standard

Although the terms may be different, the concepts presented here to defend the use of total brain failure as a reasonable standard for death are not wholly new. A similar approach to judging the vital status of a patient diagnosed as "brain dead," emphasizing the crucial importance of both spontaneous breathing and the capacity for consciousness, was advocated by the late British neurologist Christopher Pallis.[13] His conceptual justification for this argument was influential in gaining acceptance for a neurological standard in the United Kingdom.[14]

Like this report's Position Two, Pallis attempted to strike a balance between the need to be "functionalist" and the need to remain rooted in the biological facts of total brain failure. He stated in very direct terms that the relevant functions that were irreversibly absent from the patient with a destroyed brainstem were *the ability to breathe* and *the capacity for consciousness*. When challenged as to why these two functions should be singled out, Pallis pointed to what he called "the sociological context" for basic concepts of life and death. In the West, he maintained, this context is the Judeo-Christian tradition in which "breath" and "consciousness" are two definitive features of the human soul:

> The single matrix in which my definition is embedded is a sociological one, namely Judeo-Christian culture. . . . The "loss of the capacity for consciousness" is much the same as the "departure of the conscious soul from the body," just as "the loss of the capacity to breathe" is much the same as the "loss of the breath of life."[15]

Pallis also pointed to "the widespread identity, in various languages, of terms denoting *soul* and *breath*."[16] A challenge to this approach can be framed with two questions: First, are consciousness and breathing the *only* or the *most important* culturally significant features of the soul? And second, does this argument about traditional beliefs, bound to a particular culture, provide a sufficient rationale for a standard applicable to the transcultural, universal phenomenon of human death?

Position Two agrees with Pallis's emphasis on certain functions in preference to others, but it avoids the limitations of his approach, that is, its dependence on a particular culture. Position Two does this by taking the loss of the impulse to breathe and the total loss of engagement with the world as the cessation of the most essential functions of the organism as a whole. In this way, it builds upon an insight into biological reality, an insight latent in culture-bound notions of "breath of life" and "departure of the conscious soul from the body." It does so by articulating a philosophical conception of the biological realities of organismic life. To repeat, an organism is the unique sort of being that it is because it *can* and *must* constantly act upon and be open to its environment. From this philosophical-biological perspective, it becomes clear that a human being with a destroyed brainstem has lost the functional capacities that define organismic life.

On at least one important point, however, our Position Two and the UK neurological standard part company. The UK standard follows Pallis in accepting "death of the brainstem," rather than total brain failure, as a sufficient criterion for declaring a patient dead. Such a reduction, in addition to being conceptually suspect, is clinically dangerous because it suggests that the confirmatory tests that go beyond the bedside checks for apnea and brainstem reflexes are simply superfluous. As noted in Chapter Three [of *Controversies in the Determination of Death*] it is important to seek clarity on where a patient is on the path to the endpoint of total brain infarction. Only if the destructive cycle of infarction and swelling has reached this endpoint can the irreversibility of the patient's condition be known with confidence. Ultimately, the decision to perform these confirmatory tests (beyond those targeted at brainstem functions, for example, angiography or EEG) belongs to the attending clinician. The counsel offered here is one of caution in reaching a diagnosis with such important consequences. Only in the presence of a certain diagnosis of total brain failure do the arguments that seek to interpret this clinical finding hold weight.

NOTES

1. J. P. Lizza, "The Conceptual Basis for Brain Death Revisited: Loss of Organic Integration or Loss of Consciousness?" *Adv Exp Med Biol* 550 (2004): 52.

2. S. Laureys, A. M. Owen, and N. D. Schiff, "Brain Function in Coma, Vegetative State, and Related Disorders," *Lancet Neurol* 3, no. 9 (2004): 537–46.

3. H. Jonas, "Against the Stream," in *Philosophical Essays: From Ancient Creed to Technological Man* (Englewood Cliffs, NJ: Prentice-Hall, 1974), 138.

4. D. A. Shewmon, "Chronic 'Brain Death': Meta-Analysis and Conceptual Consequences," *Neurology* 51, no. 6 (1998): 1538–45.

5. This patient experienced a cardiac arrest in January 2004, more than twenty years after the diagnosis of "brain death." A report on the case, including the brain-only autopsy performed, appears in S. Repertinger, et al., "Long Survival Following Bacterial Meningitis-Associated Brain Destruction," *J Child Neurol* 21, no. 7 (2006): 591–5.

6. Wijdicks and Bernat, in a response to the Shewmon article, commented: "These cases are anecdotes yearning for a denominator." E. F. Wijdicks and J. L. Bernat, "Chronic 'Brain Death': Meta-Analysis and Conceptual Consequences," *Neurology* 53, no. 6 (1999): 1538–45.

7. Shewmon, "Brain and Somatic Integration," 467. Author's emphasis.

8. Jonas, "Against the Stream," 136.

9. Capron comments: "In part, any definition 'is admittedly arbitrary in the sense of representing a choice,' as the President's Commission stated in defending the view that the brain's function is more central to human life than are other necessary organs. . . . But the societally determined view of what constitutes death is not 'arbitrary in the sense of lacking reasons.' . . . The 'cultural context' of the standards for determining death includes the generally held view that human death, like the death of any animal, is a natural event. Even in establishing their 'definition,' members of our society act on the basis that death is an event whose existence rests on certain criteria recognized rather than solely invented by human beings." A. M. Capron, "The Report of the President's Commission on the Uniform Determination of Death Act," in *Death: Beyond Whole Brain Criteria*, ed. R. Zaner (The Netherlands: Kluwer Academic Publishers, 1988), 156–57. See also, A. M. Capron, "The Purpose of Death: A Reply to Professor Dworkin," *Indiana Law J* 48, no. 4 (1973): 640–6.

10. The account here focuses on the details of organismic life that are manifested in the "higher animals" or, perhaps more precisely, the *mammals*. How these arguments might be modified and extended to other sorts of organisms (e.g., bacteria or plants) is beyond the scope of this discussion.

11. The significance of this account of breathing may be more apparent if we contrast it with the more reductive account provided by Shewmon in his influential 2001 paper that criticized a "somatic integration rationale" for a whole brain standard for human death. Shewmon wrote:

> If "breathing" is interpreted in the "bellows" sense—moving air in and out of the lungs—then it is indeed a brain-mediated function, grossly substituted in [brain dead] patients by a mechanical ventilator. But this is a function not only of the brain but also of the phrenic nerves, diaphragm and intercostal muscles; moreover, it is not a somatically integrative function or even a vitally necessary one. . . . It is merely a condition for somatic integration itself. On the other hand, if "breathing" is understood in the sense of "respiration," which strictly speaking refers to the exchange of oxygen and carbon dioxide, then its locus is twofold: (1) across the alveolar lining of the lungs, and (2) at the biochemical level of the electron transport chain in the mitochondria of every cell in the body. (Shewmon, "Brain and Somatic Integration," 464)

In his eagerness to debunk what he considers the myth of lost somatic integration, Shewmon fails to convey the essential character of breathing. We might summarize his account of breathing as follows:

Breathing = Inflation and deflation of a bellows + Diffusion at the alveoli
    + Cellular respiration

But Shewmon misses the critical element: the *drive* exhibited by the whole organism to bring in air, a drive that is fundamental to the constant, vital working of the whole organism. By ignoring the essentially *appetitive* nature of animal breathing, Shewmon's account misses the relevance of breathing as incontrovertible evidence that "the organism as a whole" continues to be *open to* and *at work upon* the world, achieving its own preservation. The breathing that keeps an organism alive is not merely the operation of a "bellows" for which a mechanical ventilator might substitute. Bringing air into the body is an integral part of an organism's mode of being as a *needy* thing. More air will be brought in if metabolic need demands it and the body *feels* that need, as for example during exercise or in a state of panic or injury. The "respiration" taking place at the cellular level can be understood adequately only in the context of the work of the whole organism—the work of breathing.

12. If the view presented here is correct, that is, if the presence of spontaneous breathing truly reveals a persistent drive of the organism as a whole to live, we can better understand the force of a rhetorical question sometimes posed to those who view the loss of "higher" mental and psychological capacities as a sufficient criterion for declaring death. "Would you," they may be asked, "bury a patient who continues to breathe spontaneously?" Quite naturally, we recoil from such a thought, and we do so for reasons that the account given above makes clear. The striving of an animal to live, a striving that we can discern even in its least voluntary form (i.e., breathing), indicates that we still have among us a living being—and not a candidate for burial.

13. C. Pallis and D. H. Harley, *ABC of Brainstem Death,* 2nd ed. (London: BMJ Publishing Group, 1996); C. Pallis, "On the Brainstem Criterion of Death," in *The Definition of Death: Contemporary Controversies*, ed. S. J. Youngner, R. M. Arnold, and R. Schapiro (Baltimore: The Johns Hopkins University Press, 1999), 93–100.

14. Other countries have adopted this conceptual framework as well. The Canadian Forum that issued its recommendations in 2006 followed the UK approach in adopting "irreversible loss of the capacity for consciousness combined with the irreversible loss of all brain stem functions, including the capacity to breathe" as the definition of neurologically determined death. Shemie, S. D., C. Doig, B. Dickens, P. Byrne, B. Wheelock, G. Rocker, A. Baker, et al. "Severe Brain Injury to Neurological Determination of Death: Canadian Forum Recommendations." *Canadian Medical Association Journal* 174, no. 6 (2006): S1–13.

15. Pallis, "On the Brainstem Criterion of Death," 96.

16. Ibid.

Index